PRINCIPLES OF HEALTH
Allergies & Immune Disorders

PRINCIPLES OF HEALTH
Allergies & Immune Disorders

Editor
Michael A. Buratovich, PhD

SALEM PRESS
A Division of EBSCO Information Services, Inc.
Ipswich, Massachusetts

GREY HOUSE PUBLISHING

Cover photo: A health care worker administers a skin-prick allergy test. Image by Alex Raths. (Via iStock)

Copyright © 2021, by Salem Press, A Division of EBSCO Information Services, Inc., and Grey House Publishing, Inc.

Principles of Health: Allergies & Immune Disorders, published by Grey House Publishing, Inc., Amenia, NY, under exclusive license from EBSCO Information Services, Inc.

All rights reserved. No part of this work may be used or reproduced in any manner whatsoever or transmitted in any form or by any means, electronic or mechanical, including photocopy, recording, or any information storage and retrieval system, without written permission from the copyright owner. For permissions requests, contact proprietarypublishing@ebsco.com.

For information contact Grey House Publishing/Salem Press, 4919 Route 22, PO Box 56, Amenia, NY 12501.

∞ The paper used in these volumes conforms to the American National Standard for Permanence of Paper for Printed Library Materials, Z39.48 1992 (R2009).

Publisher's Cataloging-In-Publication Data
(Prepared by The Donohue Group, Inc.)
Names: Buratovich, Michael A., editor.
Title: Principles of health. Allergies & immune disorders / editor, Michael A. Buratovich, PhD.
Other Titles: Allergies & immune disorders | Allergies and immune disorders
Description: Ipswich, Massachusetts : Salem Press, a division of EBSCO Information Services, Inc. ; Amenia, NY : Grey House Publishing, [2021] | Includes bibliographical references and indexes.
Identifiers: ISBN 9781637000236
Subjects: LCSH: Immunologic diseases. | Allergy. | LCGFT: Reference works.
Classification: LCC RC582 .P75 2021 | DDC 616.079—dc23

FIRST PRINTING
PRINTED IN THE UNITED STATES OF AMERICA

Contents

Publisher's Note vii
Introduction ix
Contributors xi

Immune System 1
Antibodies 3
B-Lymphocytes 5
Endocrine disorders 10
Endocrinology 15
Endocrinology, pediatric 20
Home Health 22
Host-defense mechanisms 25
Hybridomas and monoclonal antibodies 31
Immune response 37
Immune response to bacterial infections 42
Immune response to fungal infections 45
Immune response to viral infections 47
Immunization and infectious disease 49
Immunology 56
Immunopathology 62
Inflammation 64
Metchnikoff advances the cellular theory
    of immunity 67
Neutrophil 70
Rheumatology 72
T Lymphocytes 78
Vaccine types 82

Immune System and Genetics 89
Agammaglobulinemia and genetics 91
Allergies and genetics 93
Antibodies and genetics 97
Genetic diseases 103
Immunogenetics 109

Allergies 115
Allergic bronchopulmonary aspergillosis 117
Allergies 118
Allergist and immunologist 127
Bites and stings 129
Coughing 132

Dermatitis 134
Ear infections and disorders 141
Eosinophilic esophagitis 148
Food allergies 151
Food allergy testing panels 155
Hay fever 159
Hives 162
Itching 163
Mold and mildew 165
Prevention of viral infections 167

Immune System Diseases 171

Immune Deficiencies
Acquired immunodeficiency syndrome (AIDS) . . 173
Human immunodeficiency virus (HIV) 179
HIV/AIDS-related cancers 183
Kaposi's sarcoma 187
Kawasaki disease 189
Leukemia 191
Leukopenia 200
Lymphocytosis 202
Ménière's disease 204
Metabolic disorders 205
Neutropenia 210
Purine nucleoside phosphorylase (PNP)
    deficiency 211
Severe combined immunodeficiency
    syndrome (SCID) 214
T-cell immunodeficiency syndrome 217

Autoimmune Diseases
Addison's disease 221
Autoimmune disorders 223
Autoimmune polyglandular syndrome 231
Congenital hypothyroidism 234
Crohn's disease 236
Cushing's syndrome 241
Diabetes mellitus 245
Eczema 254
Graft-versus-host disease (GVHD) 255
Guillain-Barré syndrome 259
Hashimoto's thyroiditis 264

Histiocytosis 266
Hyperthyroidism. 267
Idiopathic thrombocytopenic purpura 271
Juvenile idiopathic arthritis 273
Multiple sclerosis 276
Myasthenia gravis 282
Myositis. 285
Psoriasis and psoriatic arthritis. 287
Rheumatoid arthritis 296
Sjögren's syndrome. 300
Spondylitis 302
Systemic lupus erythematosus (SLE) 304
Thyroid disorders 310
Ulcerative colitis 313
Uveitis. 316
Vasculitis 318
Vitiligo. 321

Diseases 325
Anemia 327
Blood and blood disorders 332
Coronavirus infections 338
COVID-19 disease. 341
Cytomegalovirus (CMV) 345
Epstein-Barr virus 348
Goiter 352
Impetigo 354
Influenza 356
Insect-borne diseases 361
Measles 368
Nasopharyngeal disorders 371
Osteoarthritis 377
Rashes. 385

Rhinitis 388
Rhinoviruses 391
Roseola 393
Shingles. 396
Sinusitis. 399
Skin disorders 402

Medications 407
Prescription Medications
Anti-inflammatory drugs 409
Antihistamines 414
Antiviral drugs: Mechanisms of action 418
Antiviral drugs: Types. 422
Biological therapies 426
Corticosteroids 433
Decongestants. 438
Immunotherapy 440
Sublingual immunotherapy 447
Theophylline. 450

Natural Products, Herbal Supplements,
  and Other Alternatives
Idiopathic environmental intolerances. 455
Immune support. 458
Natural treatments for allergies 460
Natural treatments for asthma 464
Natural treatments for lupus 470
Natural treatments for rheumatoid arthritis . . . 472

Bibliography 477
Glossary. 505
Organizations 525
Subject Index 531

Publisher's Note

Allergies & Immune Disorders is the eighth volume in Salem's *Principles of Health* series, following *Depression, Prescription Drug Abuse, Nursing, Anxiety & Stress, Diabetes, Obesity,* and *Pain Management*.

This new resource introduces students and researchers to the fundamentals of allergies and immune disorders using easy-to-understand language for a solid background and a deeper understanding and appreciation of these important subjects.

This work begins with a comprehensive Editor's Introduction to the topic written by Michael A. Buratovich, PhD.

Following the Introduction, *Principles of Health: Allergies & Immune Disorders* includes 119 entries arranged in 6 broad categories:

Immune System describes major components and functionality of the immune system, which defends the body against infection. A complex network of cells and proteins, the immune system is designed to recognize foreign invaders and keep a record of every germ it defeats, allowing the body to destroy repeat infections quickly. Entries in this section include antibodies, endocrinology, immunology, and vaccine types.

Immune System and Genetics tells the story of B lymphocyte genetics to provide a better understanding of what happens in the immune system when problems occur. White blood cells, called lymphocytes, have the ability to actually alter their DNA in response to an immune system threat, making molecules that bind to the molecules of foreign substances. Among the topics discussed in this section are allergies and genetics, antibodies and genetics, genetic diseases, and immunogenetics.

Allergies are caused by an immune system's overreaction to normally harmless substances, and can range from mild symptoms like coughing and runny nose to life-threatening reactions. Millions of Americans experience allergies each year, and allergies are also a leading cause of chronic illness. Topics discussed in this section include bites and stings, dermatitis, food allergies and testing, hay fever, and hives.

Immune System Diseases looks at immunodeficiency (when the immune system does not adequately respond to infection) and autoimmune response (an overactive immune system that attacks healthy cells). Not all individuals with immunodeficiency develop autoimmunity, and not all individuals with autoimmunity are immunodeficient. However, certain immune system defects can lead to a high risk for developing autoimmunity. Immune deficiencies discussed in this section include AIDS/HIV, Kaposi's sarcoma, leukemia, and metabolic disorders. Autoimmune diseases that are covered include Addison's disease, Crohn's disease, Hashimoto's thyroiditis, juvenile idiopathic arthritis, and multiple sclerosis.

Diseases discuss the complex relationship between the immune system and common medical disorders and bacterial and viral infections. Certain disorders compromise the body's ability to fight off infection, and both bacteria and viruses can have a devastating effect on an individual with a compromised immune system. Articles in this section cover anemia, blood and blood disorders, COVID-19, influenza, insect-borne diseases, and osteoarthritis.

Medications offer information on prescription medications such as antihistamines, antiviral drugs, biological therapies, corticosteroids, and immunotherapy, as well as natural products and herbal supplements.

Essays begin with valuable top matter—Category, Definition, and Key Terms—and end with a helpful Further Information section.

This work also includes the following appendices:
- Bibliography;
- Glossary;
- Organizations;
- Subject Index

Salem Press extends appreciation to all involved in the development and production of this work. Names and affiliations of contributors to this work follow the Editor's Introduction.

Principles of Health: Allergies & Immune Disorders, as well as all Salem Press reference books, is available in print and as an e-book. Please visit www.salempress.com for more information.

Introduction

We are proud to present *Principles of Allergies & Immune Disorders*, which covers in detail the immune system, its function, and its dysfunction.

The immune system has intrigued humankind for centuries. The Greek historian Thucydides noted in his report of the plague that swept through Athens during 430 BCE that survivors of the disease were unlikely to die from a second exposure. Scholars called this phenomenon "immunity," derived from the Latin term "immunitas," which at the time referred to an exemption from paying taxes. Immunity came to mean that survival of an infection exempted an individual from further infection.

Humans have attempted to exploit immunity in many ways. The Chinese vaccinated themselves by inhaling powders made from dried smallpox lesion crusts as early as 1000 ACE. A different version of this procedure was "variolation," the insertion of smallpox crusts into the skin. By 1700, variolation had spread to Africa, India, and the Ottoman Empire. In 1717, Lady Mary Worthley Montagu, the wife of a British ambassador, learned about variolation in Constantinople and brought the practice to England. African slaves brought variolation to the Americas. One to two percent of those who underwent variolation died from it. Therefore, while safer than contracting smallpox (which had a 30 percent mortality rate), variolation was not risk-free.

The modern vaccination movement began with English doctor Edward Jenner, who discovered that milkmaids who had contracted cowpox from cows were immune to smallpox. Jenner used cowpox from sores on the hands of milkmaid Sarah Nelmes to inoculate an eight-year-old boy, James Phipps, in 1757. James developed a fever but little else, and the inoculation did not cause any disease. Thus, the smallpox vaccine was born.

Nearly a century later, in 1880, Louis Pasteur demonstrated that an attenuated cholera culture could induce immunity in chickens. Pasteur's experiment was the first demonstration of vaccination of a bacterial disease. In 1892, Waldemar Mordecai Haffkine developed a cholera vaccine for humans at the Pasteur Institute, which he successfully field-tested in India from 1893 to 1896.

In 1884, zoologist Élie Mechnikov studied single-cell organisms and phagocytes in starfish larvae. He pushed a rose thorn into the starfish's body and saw that the phagocytic cells moved to the thorn and clustered around it. From these observations, he proposed that cells are directly involved in defending the body against infection, a theory known as the cellular theory of immunology.

In 1890, Emil von Behring and Kitasato Shibasaburo reported that animals immunized with diphtheria and tetanus toxins produced something in their blood that neutralized or destroyed these toxins and induced resistance to infection. This resistance mechanism was transferable, and called "passive immunity." Passive immunity consisted of circulating antitoxins, later identified as antibodies, that mediated immunity; this contrasted with the cellular theory of immunity, in which phagocytic cells contend with foreign matter.

From 1901 to 1996, fifteen Nobel Prizes have been awarded for advances in immunology. Immunological advances are some of the most fascinating and heavily reported scientific discoveries.

Principles of Allergies & Immune Disorders has a rich introduction to the immune system and its essential parts, processes, and cell types. The human immune system is a complex, multipart system. Every component executes a particular function to form a working immune response. The opening section gives the reader an overview of the immune system, how it mounts an immune response, and the white blood cells that make it all happen.

The next section examines the genetics of the immune response. White blood cells called lymphocytes have the uncanny ability to rearrange their DNA to make molecules that specifically recognize and bind to molecules made by the microorganisms that invade our bodies. The Japanese scientist Susumu Tonegawa won the Nobel Prize for Physiology or Medicine in 1987 for his elucidation of the genetics of antibody diversity. This section tells the story of B lymphocyte genetics. It provides the reader with a foundation to help them better understand what happens when things go wrong.

The third section examines allergies, which are characterized by an overreaction of the immune response against pollens, animal hair, or other environmental components. This section examines the different types of allergies (seasonal, food-based, etc.) and their causes. While we might associate allergies with sneezing, runny noses, red itchy eyes, and wheezing, they are more far-reaching and no small matter. Allergies affect 10 to 30 percent of all children and adults in the United States and other industrialized countries. Allergies account for about 2.5 percent of all clinician visits, 2 million lost school days, 6 million lost workdays, and 28 million restricted workdays per year. Patients with allergies take twice the number of prescriptions as those without allergies, and prescription medications account for almost half the direct medical costs of allergies. Unfortunately, the economic burden of allergies in the United States is increasing. Medical expenditures for allergy treatments almost doubled from 2000 to 2005 ($6.1 billion to $11.2 billion). Understanding allergies and how to effectively treat them can improve someone's quality of life and economic well-being.

The fourth section examines the two main types of immune system diseases, immune deficiencies and autoimmune diseases. Immune deficiencies result from the absence of an integral component of the immune system or the dysfunction of a central immune system process. The subnormal immune response renders an individual susceptible to infections. Autoimmune diseases occur when the immune system fails to distinguish between an invading organism and the body's own cells and tissues. Different autoimmune diseases have distinct causes and manifestations. The entries in this section examine a host of these fascinating and potentially debilitating conditions. These entries also build upon our introduction to the immune system, explaining what happens during a breakdown or malfunction of one or more of its components.

The fifth section examines a host of different diseases and the immune responses that protect against them. These entries illustrate the immune system in action to rid our bodies of these diseases and prevent them from harming us.

The final section examines the medicines that help the immune system when infections occur or calm it down should the immune system become overactive and harmful. Anti-inflammatory medications, allergy medicines, and herbal and other natural treatments are discussed.

This volume is an excellent reference for anyone who seeks an introduction to understanding our immune system, the conditions that afflict it and cause it to afflict us, the challenges that infections present to the immune system, and the medicines that help it or calm it down.

—*Michael A. Buratovich, PhD*

Contributors

Richard Adler, PhD
University of Michigan, Dearborn

Rick Alan
Medical Writer and Editor

Samar Aslam, MD
South Nassau Communities Hospital

Steven Matthew Atchison
Auburn University

Michael Auerbach
Independent Scholar

Catherine Avelar, BS
Cornell University of Veterinary Medicine

Nancy Banasiak, MSN, APRN
Yale University School of Nursing

Barbara C. Beattie
Sarasota, Florida

Allison C. Bennett, PharmD
Duke University

Alvin K. Benson, PhD
Brigham Young University

Leonard Berkowitz, DO
South Nassau Communities Hospital

Milton Berman, PhD
University of Rochester

Matthew Berria, PhD
Independent Scholar

Thomas L. Brown, PhD
Wright State University School of Medicine

Michael A. Buratovich, PhD
Spring Arbor University

John T. Burns, PhD
Bethany College

Jeffrey R. Bytomski, DO
Duke University Medical Center

James J. Campanella, PhD
Montclair State University

Christine M. Carroll, RN, BSN, MBA
American Medical Writers Association

Rosalyn Carson-DeWitt
Everyday Health

Kerry L. Cheesman, PhD
Capital University

Nancy Handshaw Clark, PhD
American University of the Caribbean School of Medicine/ Kingston Hospital, Surrey, England

Amanda Dameron, MA
Blue Cross Blue Shield of Massachusetts

Tish Davidson, AM
Fremont, California

Patrick J. DeLuca, PhD
Mount St. Mary College

Lillian Dominguez, MD
Brown University

Patricia Stanfill Edens, RN, PhD, FACHE
Medical Writer

Ophelia Empleo-Frazier, MSN, GNP-BC, WCC, DCP
Yale University School of Nursing

C. Richard Falcon
Roberts and Raymond Associates, Philadelphia

L. Fleming Fallon Jr., MD, PhD, MPH
Bowling Green State University

Adi R. Ferrara, BS, ELS
Bellevue, Washington

MaryAnn Foote, MS, PhD
M. A. Foote Associates

Katherine B. Frederich, PhD
Eastern Nazarene College

Paul J. Frisch
Nanuet, New York

Soraya Ghayourmanesh, PhD
City University of New York

Sibdas Ghosh, PhD
University of Wisconsin, Whitewater

Jennifer L. Gibson, PharmD
Excalibur Scientific, LLC

H. Bradford Hawley, MD
Boonshoft School of Medicine, Wright State University

Robert M. Hawthorne Jr., PhD
Independent Scholar

Julie Henry, RN, MPA
Myrtle Beach, South Carolina

Carl W. Hoagstrom, PhD
Ohio Northern University

David Hornung, PhD
St. Lawrence University

Carina Endres Howell, PhD
Lock Haven University of Pennsylvania

Shih-Wen Huang, MD
University of Florida

Mary Hurd
East Tennessee State University

Karen E. Kalumuck, PhD
The Exploratorium, San Francisco

Roger H. Kennett, PhD
Wheaton College

Michael R. King, PhD
University of Rochester

Hillar Klandorf, PhD
West Virginia University

Jeffrey A. Knight, PhD
Mount Holyoke College

Ernest Kohlmetz, MA
Independent Scholar

Anita P. Kuan, PhD
Woonsocket, Rhode Island

Jeanne L. Kuhler, PhD
Auburn University, Montgomery

Nicholas Lanzieri
Pace University

Kathleen LaPoint, MS
Greensboro, North Carolina

Lorraine Lica, PhD
San Diego, California

Beatriz Manzor Mitrzyk, PharmD
Mitrzyk Medical Communications, LLC

Cherie Marcel, BS
Independent Scholar

Geraldine F. Marrocco, EdD, APRN, CNS, ANP-BC
Yale University School of Nursing

Grace D. Matzen
Molloy College

Ralph R. Meyer, PhD
University of Connecticut

Paul Moglia, PhD
Mount Sinai South Nassau Communities Hospital

Robin Kamienny Montvilo, RN, PhD
Rhode Island College

Anita Nagypál, PhD
Independent Scholar

Kimberly A. Napoli, MS
KanCom Biomedical Communications

Deanna M. Neff, MPH
Stow, Massachusetts

Bryan Ness, PhD
Pacific Union College

William D. Niemi, PhD
Russell Sage College

Jane C. Norman, PhD, RN, CNE
Tennessee State University

Colm A. Ó'Moráin, MA, MD, MSc, DSc
University of Dublin, Trinity College

RoseMarie Pasmantier, MD
State University of New York Health Science Center, Brooklyn

Ekta Patel, MD
Icahn School of Medicine at Mount Sinai

Laura J. Pinchot, BA
Clarion University of Pennsylvania

George R. Plitnik, PhD
Frostburg State University

Jevon Plunkett
Washington University

Victoria Price, PhD
Lamar University

Michael Raghunath, MD
Mount Sinai South Nassau

C. Mervyn Rasmussen, MD
Bremerton Naval Hospital, Washington

Andrew J. Reinhart, MS
Washington University School of Medicine

Alice C. Richer, RD, MBA, LD
Norwood, Massachusetts

Jeffrey B. Roberts, MD
Duke University Medical Center

Ana Maria Rodriguez-Rojas, MS
GXP Medical Writing, LLC

Eugene J. Rogers, MD
Chicago Medical School

Virginia L. Salmon
Northeast State Community College

Elizabeth D. Schafer, PhD
Loachapoka, Alabama

Miriam E. Schwartz, MD, MA, PhD
University of California, Los Angeles

Tom E. Scola
University of Wisconsin, Whitewater

Rebecca Lovell Scott, PhD, PA-C
College of Health Sciences

Gregory B. Seymann, MD
University of California, San Diego School of Medicine

Martha A. Sherwood, PhD
University of Oregon

Julie M. Slocum, RN, MS, CDE
Women and Infants' Hospital

Dwight G. Smith, PhD
Southern Connecticut State University

Sharon W. Stark, RN, APRN, DNSc
Monmouth University

Bethany Thivierge, MPH, ELS
Technicality Resources

Venkat Raghavan Tirumala, MD, MHA
Western Kentucky University

Maxine M. Urton, PhD
Xavier University

Charles L. Vigue, PhD
University of New Haven

Catherine J. Walsh, PhD
Mote Marine Laboratory

Barbara Woldin, BS
American Medical Writers Association

Geetha Yadav, PhD
Bio-Rad Laboratories Inc.

W. Michael Zawada, PhD
University of Colorado Health Sciences Center

Susan M. Zneimer, PhD, FACMG
US Labs

Immune System

The immune system is a vital part of the body that is constantly working to protect us from disease and illness. It is made up of various organs, cells, and proteins (antibodies) that work together to fight disease-causing germs like bacteria, viruses, parasites, or fungi. It also recognizes and neutralizes harmful substances and fights disease-causing changes (like cancer cells) in the body. The immune system is activated by substances, called antigens, that the body does not recognize. In some cases, the body mistakenly sees its own cells as foreign bodies and attacks them; this is called an autoimmune response. The two subsystems of the immune system—innate and adaptive—are closely linked. The innate, or nonspecific, immune system provides general defense against harmful pathogens, employing natural killer cells and phagocytes that "eat" harmful substances. The adaptive, or specific, immune system makes antibodies to fight particular germs that the body has previously come into contact with, and can adapt to fight bacteria or viruses as they change. This is also known as acquired immunity. Failures of the immune system can lead to devastating diseases, either because the immune system attacks itself or because it fails to defend against foreign antigens. The twenty-one essays in this section discuss the specifics of the immune system as well as how the immune system responds to bacterial, fungal, and viral infections. Topics also include infectious disease, vaccine types, and the cellular theory of immunity.

Antibodies	3
B-Lymphocytes	5
Endocrine disorders	10
Endocrinology	15
Endocrinology, pediatric	20
Home Health	22
Host-defense mechanisms	25
Hybridomas and monoclonal antibodies	31
Immune response	37
Immune response to bacterial infections	42
Immune response to fungal infections	45
Immune response to viral infections	47
Immunization and infectious disease	49
Immunology	56
Immunopathology	62
Inflammation	64
Metchnikoff advances the cellular theory of immunity	67
Neutrophil	70
Rheumatology	72
T Lymphocytes	78

Vaccine types 82

Antibodies

Category: Biology
Also known as: Gamma globulin proteins, immunoglobulin (Ig)
Anatomy or system affected: Blood, cells, circulatory system, immune system, lymphatic system
Specialties and related fields: Bacteriology, biochemistry, biotechnology, immunology, internal medicine, microbiology, oncology, pathology, pharmacology, preventive medicine, public health
Definition: An antibody is a protein produced by the body to recognize and eliminate specific foreign antigens, such as bacteria, viruses, or other microorganisms, by way of triggering the immune system. It is produced by white blood cells, also called "B lymphocytes."

KEY TERMS

constant region: The highly conserved C-terminal portion of the antibody
Fc-fusion proteins: specific proteins of interest fused to the Fc region of the antibody at its C-terminal end
heavy chain: the bigger subunits of an antibody
isotypes: the different classes of antibodies
light chain: the smaller subunits of an antibody
monoclonal antibodies: antibodies derived from a single parent clonal cell
variable region: the N-terminal portion of the antibody, which possesses antigen-binding sites and has variable amino acid sequences

STRUCTURE AND FUNCTIONS

An antibody is a Y-shaped protein unit, or tetramer, made of four individual subunits. Antibodies consist of two identical smaller subunits called "light chains" and two larger ones called "heavy chains." There are two families of light chains, called "kappa" and "lambda." Each immunoglobulin (Ig) class consists of either one of these two families of light chains and does not change through its life. There are approximately ten different types of heavy chains, and they contribute to the other classes of antibodies or immunoglobulins. The five major types of heavy chains are a, d, e, g, and m types. Each possesses a specific number of amino acids. Depending on the heavy chain present, the antibodies are classified into five major classes or isotypes: IgA, IgD, IgE, IgG, and IgM. Each isotype has a specific function, and more than one Ig isotype is required to eliminate a particular antigen. The presence of specialized proteins called "cytokines" can trigger the switching of one type of isotype to another.

Each light or heavy chain possesses a constant region conserved in its amino acid composition across different Ig types and a variable region that differs between B cells. The constant region is present in the C-terminal portion of the protein, and the variable region is present at the N-terminus. The variable region contains the antigen-binding sites and is thus responsible for binding to the specific antigen. The antibody displays maximum versatility in this region in possessing hundreds of binding sites and, as a result, can recognize and bind hundreds of different antigens. The tips of the variable region are

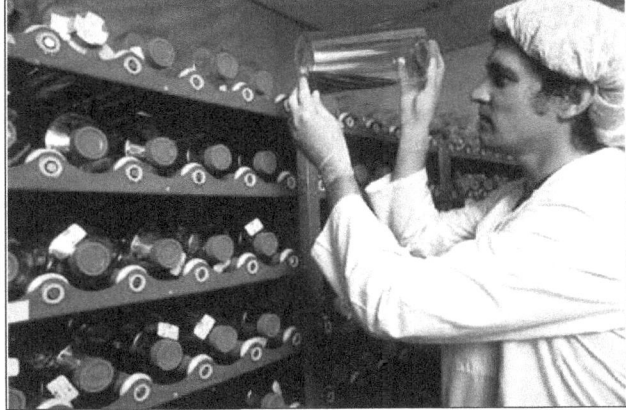

Unlimited quantities of monoclonal antibodies can be produced in a laboratory setting. Photo by Linda Bartlett. Image courtesy of the National Cancer Institute, via Wikimedia Commons. [Public domain.]

called "fragment antigen-binding" (Fab) regions. The constant region remains identical in all heavy or light chains of the antibodies. It is responsible for activating the complement system and can also initiate phagocytosis. The constant region is also identical between different isotypes. The base of this region consists of the fragment crystallizable (Fc) region. Once the antigen is bound to the antibody surface, the constant region of the antibody elicits an appropriate immune response.

When exposed to the antigen, the B cells transform into plasma cells and begin producing antibodies, utilizing the aid of helper T cells of the immune system. Antibodies, through their antigen-binding sites, bind with the antigen and form antigen-antibody complexes. Each antigen presents a surface that can be recognized and bound by the specific antibody. The antigen-antibody complex is a signal for destruction. The complex is engulfed by other specialized cells called "macrophages" or "lysed" by triggering a proteolytic pathway called a "complement pathway." This whole response is called the "humoral response" of the immune system.

DISORDERS AND DISEASES
An essential function of an antibody is to distinguish between "self" and "nonself" proteins. An antibody should bind only to nonself proteins. When this recognition capability is compromised, the result is the development of autoimmune diseases or disorders. An autoimmune disease can occur in specific organs, such as the thyroid gland, or the entire body, as with lupus or rheumatoid arthritis. Scleroderma, multiple sclerosis, vitiligo, psoriasis, and alopecia are other autoimmune diseases that can develop because of an attack on the body's proteins by antibodies.

PERSPECTIVE AND PROSPECTS
The study of antibodies began in the late nineteenth century when scientists discovered a "factor" or antitoxin that could react with antigens or toxins. Emil von Behring and Shibasaburo Kitasato introduced the term "antibody" in 1890. In the early twentieth century, the specificity of antibodies was demonstrated, and the methodology for studying antigen-antibody complexes was deduced. In 1959, Gerald Edelman and Rodney Porter independently published the three-dimensional structure of antibodies. Edelman and Porter received the Nobel Prize for this achievement in 1972. Since then, the field of antibody research has grown, and important discoveries have been made about the structure, functions, and utility of antibodies. Different types of antibodies have been discovered, and their genetic basis inferred.

In addition to affording immunity against pathogens, antibodies are integral agents in clinical diagnostics and treating various human diseases, including cancer and many infectious diseases. Antibody engineering involves the development of monoclonal antibodies directed against specific antigens involved in diseases. Some of these antibodies can be modified to carry drugs or radioactive substances to be delivered specifically to tumor cells in cancer. Several monoclonal antibodies such as *Herceptin* (trastuzumab), Rituxan (rituximab), and Remicade (infliximab) have been approved by the Food and Drug Administration (FDA) to treat various diseases. Fc-fusion proteins such as Enbrel (etanercept) have also been developed in the last decade to treat multiple diseases. Many monoclonal antibodies and Fc-fusion proteins are being tested in clinical trials. In addition, diagnostic tests may involve the detection of antibodies. Polyclonal antibodies were initially used to prevent viral illnesses and later in the treatment of antibody deficiencies.

Another primary application of antibodies is in scientific research. Some instrumental scientific techniques involve using antibodies, such as enzyme-linked immuno-sorbent assay (ELISA), Western blotting, flow cytometry, immunohistochemistry, immunohistochemistry, and immunocytochemistry.

These techniques are regularly employed in scientific experiments to understand the structure and function of proteins involved in various diseases.

—*Geetha Yadav, PhD and Samar Aslam, MD*

Further Information

An, Zhiqiang, editor. Therapeutic Monoclonal Antibodies: From Bench to Clinic. John Wiley & Sons, 2009.

Jefferis, Roy, Koicho Kato, and William R. Strohl, editors. Structure and Function of Antibodies. Mdpi AG, 2021.

Klein, Christian. Monoclonal Antibodies. Mdpi AG, 2018.

Lodish, Harvey, Arnold Berk, Chris A. Kaiser, Monty Krieger, and Anthony Bretscher. Molecular Cell Biology. 9th ed., W. H. Freeman & Co., 2021.

McCullough, Kenneth, and Raymond Spier. Monoclonal Antibodies in Biotechnology: Theoretical and Practical Aspects. Cambridge UP, 1990.

B-Lymphocytes

Category: Immunology
Also known as: B cells
Anatomy or system affected: Blood, bone marrow, immune system, lymphatic system
Specialties and related fields: Hematology, immunology, microbiology, oncology
Definition: A type of white blood cell that synthesizes and secretes antibodies.

KEY TERMS

antibodies: secreted glycoproteins that bind to foreign substances in our bodies and inactivate them, clump them, mark them for destruction, and facilitate their disposal; also known as immunoglobulins

antigens: foreign substances in the body that elicit an immune response

heavy chain: the larger polypeptide chain of an antibody

isotype switching: when activated B cells, by their interaction with T-helper cells change the type of antibody they are secreting to some other antibody subtype

light chain: the smaller polypeptide chain of an antibody

lymphopoiesis: the process of B-lymphocyte development

major histocompatibility complex (MHC) proteins: cell surface proteins that come in two types, class I and II that help antigen-presenting cells present antigen to lymphocytes (class II) and mark every nucleated cell in the body (class I); also called "human leukocyte antigens" (HLAs)

recombinase: the RAG-1 and RAG-2 protein complex that cuts and paste gene segments from the antibody gene cluster together to form unique antibodies that bind a wide range of antigens

INTRODUCTION

B lymphocytes are white blood cells that play integral roles in the adaptive immune system. B lymphocytes differentiate into plasma cells and memory B lymphocytes. Plasma cells secrete antibodies to fight infection and destroy abnormal cells such as cancer cells. Memory B lymphocytes are activated by contracting a disease or by vaccination. They confer long-lasting immunity to a specific disease. One subset of B lymphocytes can also infiltrate cancer tumors.

FUNCTION

The immune system is a complex of tissues, cells, and the chemicals these cells produce spread throughout the body. Its function is to rid the body of foreign microbes and damaged or abnormal body cells. The major organs of the immune system are the bone marrow, lymph nodes, thymus, and spleen. Immune system cells and a clear fluid called "lymph" move throughout the body in a series of channels called "lymphatic vessels" that are separate from the circulatory system.

The immune system has two divisions: the innate immune system and the adaptive immune system. The innate system consists of white blood cells (leukocytes) that respond rapidly to a wide range of microbes but cannot confer immunity against disease. The adaptive system has cells that respond more slowly to disease but can create long-lasting immunity. While cells in the innate system can attack many different microbes, each cell of the adaptive system recognizes and attacks only 1 type of microbe or damaged cell. B lymphocytes and T lymphocytes are the main cells of the adaptive immune system.

All cells have specific marker molecules on their surfaces that identify them as "self-cells" or "nonself-cells." Each B lymphocyte and T lymphocyte interacts with only one particular type of surface marker molecule that is displayed on the surfaces of microbes or abnormal cells and identifies them as nonself-cells. These marker molecules (often proteins) that elicit a reaction from B lymphocytes are called "antigens."

DEVELOPMENT

B lymphocytes develop in the bone marrow from hematopoietic stem cells. Hematopoietic stem cells can divide and differentiate into many different types of blood cells. As B lymphocytes mature, each cell develops a unique receptor on its surface that will bind only to a single, specific antigen on a foreign microbe or an abnormal body cell such as a cancer cell. Scientists believe the body can make over one billion unique B lymphocytes. Any B lymphocytes that develop receptors that will bind with marker molecules on healthy self-cells are elimi-

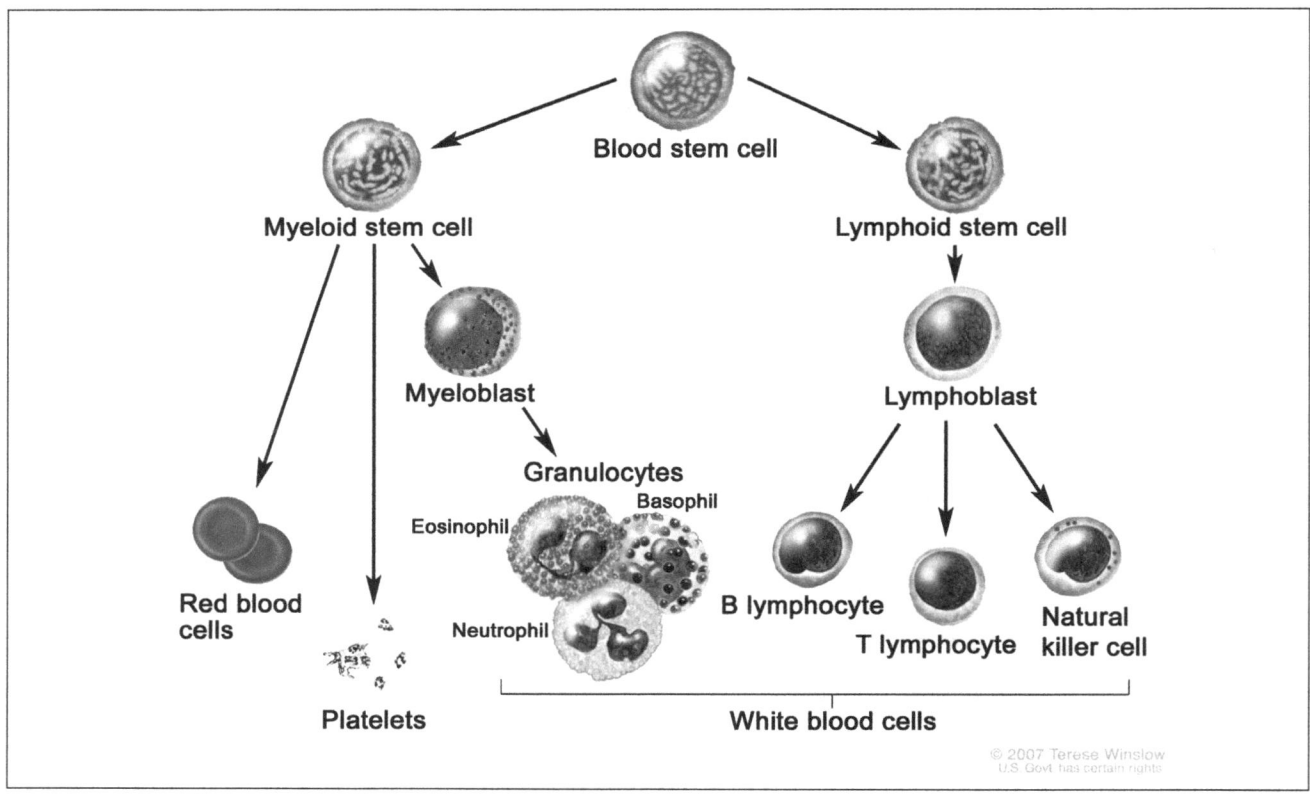

Blood cell development. A blood stem cell goes through several steps to become a red blood cell, platelet, or white blood cell. Image via the National Cancer Institute (cancer.gov).

nated while still in the bone marrow so as not to harm the body.

The B-cell receptor is a membrane-bound antibody. Antibodies consist of four polypeptides, two heavy chains, and two light chains. All antibodies have at their front end a variable region that differs from one antibody to another. Behind the variable region is the constant region that is the same for each specific antibody subtype.

The variable region of the heavy chain is encoded by a variable or V region, a diversity region or D region, and a J or joining region. The light chain variable region consists of a V region and a J region. The genes that encode the heavy chain are on chromosome 14, and the light chain has two different gene clusters, kappa, and lambda. The kappa gene cluster is on chromosome two, and the lambda gene cluster is on chromosome 22. The heavy chain gene cluster consists of 51 different *V* segments, six different *J* segments, 27 distinct *D* segments, and eight different constant regions. The kappa light chain gene cluster consists of 40 different V gene segments, five different J chain clusters, and a single constant region. The lambda gene cluster contains 30 V gene segments and four J gene segments, with four different constant regions.

During B-lymphocyte development or lymphopoiesis, the antibody gene clusters are rearranged to create proteins that bind an enormous variety of distinct antigens. The earliest stage of B-lymphocyte development is the early pro-B cell, which forms from the daughter cell after the hematopoietic stem cell divides. The early pro-B cell expresses proteins that rearrange the antibody gene cluster, RAG-1 & -2. The RAG proteins join a single D gene segment from one of the copies of the heavy chain gene cluster with a single J gene segment. Upon completion of the DJ joining, the early pro-B cell becomes a late pro-B cell. The RAG-1 & -2 recombinase further joins a single V segment with the DJ segment and joins the VDJ combination to the μ constant region gene. Successful cutting and pasting of the VDJ-μ gene segments mark the transition of the late pro-B cell to a large pre-B cell. If the cell fails to rearrange its heavy chain gene segments, the cell dies.

The large pre-B cell expresses the rearranged heavy chain and traffics it to the cell surface. Successful expression of the antibody heavy chain induces the cell to divide and become a small pre-B cell. Next, the small pre-B cell rearranges the light chain genes, beginning with the kappa genes first. If the cell fails to rearrange its kappa genes, then it moves to the lambda genes. VJ joining of the light chain gene segments makes a functional light chain, and expression of the light chain with the heavy chain places an antibody on the surface of the cell and designates the cell as an immature B cell. If the antibody strongly binds to any self-antigens in the bone marrow, it dies.

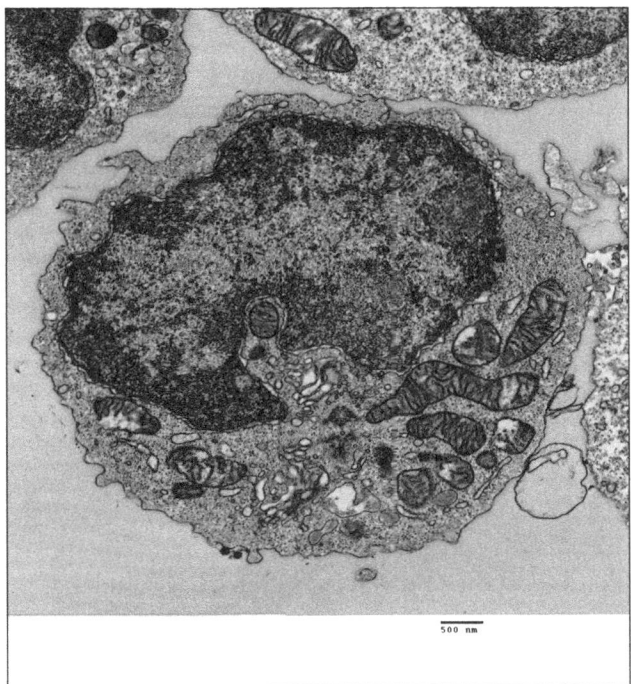

Transmission electron micrograph of a B cell from a human donor. Image by the National Institute of Allergies and Infectious Diseases (NIAID), via Wikimedia Commons.

The variability in antibody formation is remarkable. The heavy chain alone can encode at least 8262 (51 × 6 × 27) different heavy chain variable regions. If a heavy chain is coupled with a kappa light chain, then there are 200 (40 x 5) different light chains and 1.6 x 10^6 (8262 x 200) different possible antibodies that such rearrangements can form.

B-CELL ACTIVATION
Immature B lymphocytes can make either immunoglobulin D (IgD) or immunoglobulin M (IgM). The expression of IgD licenses the cell to leave the bone marrow and migrate to lymph nodes. The B cells that have IgM and IgD on their surfaces and have left the bone marrow are called "naïve B cells." Lymph nodes are enlargements of the lymphatic vessels, found in the neck, under the arms, and in the groin, where foreign and abnormal cells are filtered from lymph. When the naïve B lymphocyte enters the lymph node from the blood, they first enter the paracortical region. B cells migrate to the periphery of the lymph node, also known as the cortical region, where they form the primary lymphoid follicles. If a naïve B cell encounters an antigen that binds to its IgM receptor, the lymphocyte is activated and clones itself, producing massive numbers of identical cells. In the lymph node, the proliferating B cell forms a "germinal center," and a follicle with a germinal center is called a "secondary lymphoid follicle."

Most clone cells become plasma cells that secrete IgM antibodies (IgD antibodies are never secreted). Antibodies are large glycoproteins ten times smaller than a virus particle. They bind with any antigen identical to the one that activated the B lymphocyte. An activated B lymphocyte can produce 2000 antibodies per second for up to five days. These antibodies enter the lymphatic and circulatory systems where they attach to the surface of the abnormal cell or invading microbe. This either inactivates the target, causes it to clump with similar cells and be destroyed, or flags the target for destruction by another type of white blood cell. Producing enough antibodies to combat disease takes ten to seventeen days to reach maximal effectiveness, and during that time the individual will show symptoms of the illness.

Activated B lymphocytes also function as antigen-presenting cells that use major histocompatibility complex (MHC) class II proteins to present antigen to T-helper cells. The B lymphocyte presentation of antigen to T-helper cells activates the T cell if it receives two distinct signals. First, the antigen must bind to the T-cell receptor on the surface of the T-helper cells. Second, the T-helper cell has a cell surface protein called "CD40." CD40 must bind to CD40L on the surface of the B lymphocyte. This dual signal system guarantees that only the right cell presenting the right antigen in the proper context activates the T cell. The activated T cell then secretes cytokines that drive the B cell to switch the type of antibody it secretes. This phenomenon, called "isotype switching" requires a second rearrangement of the heavy chain antibody genes. An enzyme called "activation-induced deaminase," or AID, breaks the intervening deoxyribonucleic acid (DNA) removing all the constant regions between the VDJ and the decided upon antibody. The antibody the B cell eventually secretes depends upon the instructions it receives from the T-helper cell. For example, if the T-helper cell secretes IL-4 and IL-5, then the B cells will become an IgE secreting plasma cell. But if the T-helper cells secrete interferon-gamma, then the B lymphocyte will become an IgG secreting plasma cell.

Not all B lymphocytes become plasma cells. Most B lymphocytes are born and never experience antigen stimulation. A few B lymphocytes, under stimulation by cytokines secreted by helper T lymphocytes, become memory B lymphocytes, or memory B cells. These cells remain in the body for a long time (years to decades). If the same microbe is encountered again, memory B lymphocytes can ramp up antibody production in two to five days, destroying the invading microbe before it can make a person sick. This is the basis for long-term immunity to disease. Vaccines work by introducing a weakened or partial form of a microbe that does not make the individual sick but stimulates the production of plasma cells and memory B lymphocytes.

Another subset of B lymphocytes called "tumor-infiltrating B lymphocytes" (TIL-Bs) appears to migrate to solid cancer tumors and secrete tumor-specific antibodies. Tumor-infiltrating T lymphocytes (TIL-Ts) are also found in solid tumors, and more is known about how they work. TILs have been associated with substantial remission in metastatic melanoma. Experimentally, the presence of TILs also correlates with improved outcomes in ovarian, breast, colorectal, and non-small cell lung cancers.

Why, if the immune system is so effective in preventing illness, does it not wipe out cancer cells and keep the individual cancer-free? One reason is that cancer cells start as normal body cells. At some point, they are transformed because certain genes are inappropriately turned off or on, or are mutated. When this happens, the transformed cell still has many of the surface marker molecules that originally identified it as a self-cell. B lymphocytes that have receptors that would interact with healthy self-cell antigens are killed before they leave the bone marrow to prevent autoimmune diseases. In many cases, transformed cancer cells still look enough like self-cells that B lymphocytes do not recognize them as abnormal and do not mark them for destruction. If B lymphocytes respond to a transformed cell, the response may not be strong enough to be effective since the growth of cancer cells is not limited the way it is in healthy cells. In addition, some cancer cells make chemicals that inactivate or disrupt the functioning of immune system cells.

TREATMENT

The properties of the adaptive immune system can be manipulated in ways to prevent and treat cancer by using vaccines and monoclonal antibodies. Some cancers are primarily caused by viruses. By making a vaccine against the causative virus, it will be rapidly destroyed and cancer can be prevented. As of 2021, two cancer prevention vaccines have been approved.

Many strains of human papillomavirus (HPV) are known to cause cervical, vulvar, anal, penile, and mouth, and colon cancers. The virus is transmitted through sexual activity. Vaccination before puberty against the most common strains of HPV stimulates the adaptive immune system and creates memory B lymphocytes that provide long-term immunity. As of 2021, 3 HPV vaccines have been approved by the U.S. Food and Drug Administration (FDA). The FDA-approved HPV vaccines include a nonavalent HPV vaccine (Gardasil® 9, 9vHPV), a quadrivalent HPV vaccine (Gardasil®, 4vHPV), and a bivalent HPV vaccine (Cervarix®, 2vHPV). All three HPV vaccines protect against HPV types 16 and 18 that cause most HPV cancers. The distribution of these vaccines has substantially reduced the rate of HPV-caused cancers.

Hepatitis B is a viral infection that can cause liver cancer. Current recommendations in the United States call for children to receive a hepatitis B vaccine at birth. Research is underway to develop vaccines against other microbe-triggered cancers, including various lymphomas (Epstein Barr virus) and stomach cancer (*Helicobacter pylori* bacterium).

Research is also underway to design treatment vaccines to use in individuals with active cancers. As of 2015, only one treatment vaccine has been approved by the FDA. This vaccine, sipuleucel-T, can extend the life of men with metastatic prostate cancer but does not cure the disease. Other current cancer-treating vaccines include live Bacillus of Calmette et Guillen (BCG), which can treat early-stage bladder cancer, and talimogene laherparepvec, which can treat melanoma.

Another B-lymphocyte-related treatment is the use of targeted monoclonal antibodies (mAbs). Scientists first isolate B lymphocytes from laboratory mice that were vaccinated with a specific antigen and fuse them to cancer cells (myelomas). The resultant hybrid cells or "hybridomas" can successfully grow in culture, but also produce a specific type of antibody. After the hybridoma lines are screened to identify which cells produce the antibody of interest, which is a very labor-intensive process, those lines that make the desired antibody are grown in culture. Then the genes that encode the desired antibodies are transferred to a cell line that grows well in culture (e.g., Chinese Hamster Ovary cells) to make small antibody-producing factories. These antibodies are then purified and injected into the body where they attack or mark cancer cells. The effect is short-lived since no memory B cells are created.

The FDA has approved more than a dozen monoclonal antibody biologics for use with other cancer treatments. The mAb drugs can be recognized because their generic name ends in "mab" (e.g., alemtuzumab, trastuzumab). Some mAbs, called "conjugated mAbs," have a chemotherapy drug or radioactive isotope attached to the antibody to increase its effectiveness (e.g., brentuximab vedotin, ibritumomab tiuxetan). Although mAbs have side effects, these are less harsh than those of chemotherapy drugs.

—*Tish Davidson, AM and Michael A. Buratovich, PhD*

Further Information

Finn, O. J. "Immuno-Oncology: Understanding the Function and Dysfunction of the Immune System in Cancer." *Annals of Oncology*, vol. 23(Suppl 8), 2012, pp. iiv6-iiv9, annonc.oxfordjournals.org/content/23/suppl_8/viii6.full.

Melero, I., G. Gaudemack, W. Gerritsen, et al. "Therapeutic Vaccines for Cancer: An Overview of Clinical Trials." *Nature Reviews Clinical Oncology*, vol. 11, 2014, pp. 509-24.

Scott, Andrew M., Jedd D. Wolchok, and Lloyd J. Old. "Antibody Therapy of Cancer." *Nature Reviews Cancer*, vol. 12, 2012, pp. 278-87, www.nature.com/nrc/journal/v12/n4/full/nrc3236.html.

ENDOCRINE DISORDERS

Category: Diseases/Disorders
Anatomy or system affected: Endocrine system, glands
Specialties and related fields: Endocrinology
Definition: The endocrine system controls the metabolic processes of the body. Endocrine disorders occur when the normal function of the endocrine system is disrupted.

KEY TERMS

cyclic AMP: a chemical that acts as a second messenger to bring about a response by the cell to the presence of some hormones at their receptors

endocrine: the secretion of hormones directly into the bloodstream, rather than by way of a duct

feedback: the mechanism whereby a hormone inhibits its production; often involves the inhibition of the hypothalamus and tropic hormones

hypothalamohypophysial: relating to the hypothalamus and the hypophysis (pituitary gland)

target cell or organ: a cell or organ possessing the specific hormone receptors needed to respond to a given hormone

tropic: hormones that feed a particular physiological state

tropin: hormones that cause a "turning toward" a particular physiological state

PROCESS AND EFFECTS

Endocrine disorders include disturbances in the production of hormones that result from either insufficient or excessive activity and tissues unable to respond to hormones. First, we will review the location of the principal endocrine glands, the hormones secreted, and the normal functions of the hormones. The hormones are released into the bloodstream and are carried throughout the body, affecting target cells or organs that have receptors for the given hormone.

The pituitary gland, or hypophysis, is sometimes called the "master gland" because of its widespread influence on many other endocrine glands and the body. It is located in the midline on the lower part of the brain, just above the posterior part of the roof of the mouth. The pituitary has three lobes: the posterior lobe, the intermediate lobe, and the anterior lobe.

The posterior lobe does not synthesize hormones, but it does have nerve fibers coming into it from the brain's hypothalamus. The ends of these axons release two hormones that are synthesized in the hypothalamus, oxytocin and antidiuretic hormone (ADH). Oxytocin causes the contraction of the smooth muscles of the uterus during childbirth and the contraction of tissues in the mammary glands to release milk during nursing. ADH causes the kidneys to reabsorb water and thereby reduce urine volume to normal levels when necessary.

The intermediate lobe of the pituitary secretes melanocyte-stimulating hormone (MSH), a hormone with an uncertain role in humans but known to cause the darkening of melanocytes in animals. Sometimes, the intermediate lobe is considered to be a part of the anterior lobe.

The anterior lobe of the pituitary is controlled by releasing hormones produced by the hypothalamus and carried to the anterior lobe by unique blood vessels. In response to these releasing hormones, some stimulatory and some inhibitory, the anterior lobe produces thyroid-stimulating hormone (TSH), adrenocorticotropic hormone (ACTH), follicle-stimulating hormone (FSH), luteinizing hormone (LH),

> **INFORMATION ON ENDOCRINE DISORDERS**
>
> **Causes**: Malfunction of the endocrine system
>
> **Symptoms**: Wide-ranging and dependent on the region, including precocious puberty, dwarfism, thyroid problems, diseases such as diabetes
>
> **Duration**: Chronic
>
> **Treatments**: Hormonal therapy, medications

prolactin, and somatotropin or growth hormone (GH). TSH stimulates the thyroid to produce thyroxine, ACTH stimulates the adrenal cortex to produce some of its hormones, FSH stimulates the growth of the cells surrounding eggs in the ovary and causes the ovary to produce estrogen, LH induces ovulation (the release of an egg from the ovary) and stimulates the secretion of progesterone by the ovary, prolactin is essential for milk production and various metabolic functions, and GH is needed for normal growth.

The pineal gland, or epiphysis, is a neuroendocrine gland attached to the roof of the diencephalon in the brain. It produces melatonin, which is released into the bloodstream at night and has essential functions related to an individual's biological clock.

The thyroid gland is below the larynx in the front of the throat. It produces the hormones triiodothyronine (T3) and thyroxine (T4), which are essential for maintaining a normal level of metabolism and heat production and enabling normal development of the brain in young children. Scattered throughout the thyroid, parathyroid, and thymus glands are specialized cells called "C cells." These cells secrete the hormone calcitonin, which is involved in maintaining the correct blood levels of calcium. The thymus, located under the breast bone or sternum, produces the hormone thymosin that stimulates the immune system. Even the heart is an endocrine gland: It produces atrial natriuretic factor, which stimulates sodium excretion by the kidneys. The pancreas, located near the stomach and small intestine, produces digestive enzymes that pass to the duodenum, but also it produces insulin and glucagon in special cells called "pancreatic islets." Insulin causes the body's tissues to take up blood sugar (glucose), and glucagon causes stored glycogen to be broken down in the liver, increasing blood glucose levels.

The pair of adrenal glands, located on the kidneys, consists of two components: first, an outer cortex that produces glucocorticoids, mineralocorticoids, and sex steroids or androgens; and second, a medulla, or inner part, that secretes adrenaline and noradrenaline. The gonads, testes, or ovaries are located in the pelvic region and produce several hormones, including estrogen and progesterone, which are essential for reproduction in females, and testosterone essential for reproduction in males. The kidneys and digestive tract also produce hormones that regulate red blood cell formation and the functioning of the digestive tract, respectively.

COMPLICATIONS AND DISORDERS
A wide variety of endocrine disorders can be treated successfully. The ability to restore normal endocrine function with replacement therapy has long been one of the techniques for showing the existence of hypothesized hormones.

The posterior pituitary releases both oxytocin and ADH. Chemicals similar to oxytocin induce contractions in pregnant women so that birth will occur at a predetermined time. The other hormone released from the posterior pituitary, ADH, typically causes the reabsorption of water within the kidney's tubules. ADH deficiency causes diabetes insipidus, a condition in which the urinary system excretes many liters of water a day; the patient must drink vast quantities of water to stay alive. A synthetic form of ADH, desmopressin acetate, can be given in a nasal spray that diffuses into the bloodstream and thus restores the reabsorption of water by the kidneys.

The anterior lobe of the pituitary produces six known hormones. Special releasing hormones secreted by the hypothalamus and carried to the anterior lobe by the hypothalamohypophysial portal system of blood vessels stimulate the pituitary tropic hormones. Thus, the source of some anterior pituitary disorders can reside in the hypothalamus. Tumors of anterior pituitary cells can result in the overproduction of a hormone, or if the tumor is destructive, the underproduction of a hormone. Radiation or surgery destroys or extirpates tumors and thereby restores normal pituitary functioning.

Anterior pituitary hormones can be the basis of a variety of disorders. As with other hormones, there may be below-normal production of the hormone (hyposecretion) or overproduction of the hormone (hypersecretion). Because the pituitary hormones are often supportive of hormone secretion by the target organ or tissue, hyposecretion or hypersecretion of the tropic or supportive hormone leads to a similar change in the production of hormones by the target organ or tissue.

For example, hyperthyroidism, or Graves' disease, can be caused by excessive secretion of TSH by the pituitary, leading to hypersecretion of thyroxine or by nodules within the thyroid that produce excessive thyroxine. In the diagnosis process, blood levels of both TSH and thyroxine are usually measured to determine the specific cause of the disorder. Similarly, hypothyroidism can be induced by deficits at several levels. The lack of iodine in the diet can prevent the production of thyroxine, which requires iodide as part of its molecular composition. The production of thyroxine usually has a negative feedback effect on the hypothalamus and pituitary, reducing TSH production. The failure to produce thyroxine causes high TSH blood levels, and abnormal thyroid growth that results in a greatly enlarged thyroid called a "goiter." The addition of iodine to salt has eliminated the incidence of goiter in developed countries. However, hypothyroidism can still develop from other sources, even with an adequate supply of iodine in the diet. The usual treatment is to ingest a dose of thyroxine daily.

Other examples of anterior pituitary disorders include those involving changes in GH secretion. Undersecretion of GH can lead to short stature or even a type of dwarfism called "pituitary dwarfism," in which an individual has normal body proportions but is smaller than usual. Now it is possible to obtain human GH from bacteria genetically engineered to produce it. Replacement GH can be given during the standard growth years to enhance growth. A tumor sometimes develops in the pituitary cells that produce GH, and this can cause abnormally increased growth or gigantism. If the tumor develops during the adult years, only a few areas of abnormal growth can occur, such as in the facial bones and the bones of the hands and feet. This condition is called "acromegaly." Abraham Lincoln might have had abnormal levels of GH that caused gigantism in his youth and then acromegaly in his later years. Radiation or surgery of the anterior pituitary treats acromegaly. Alternatively, two drugs, octreotide, and lanreotide inhibit GH secretion by the anterior pituitary. Both medications also shrink pituitary adenomas in some patients.

Pineal gland tumors are associated with precocious puberty, in which children become sexually developed in early childhood. Melatonin normally inhibits sexual development during this period. Changes influence the pineal gland in the daily photoperiod. The highest melatonin levels appear in the blood during the night, especially during the long nights of winter. The pineal gland thus seems to be involved in the functioning of the body's biological clock. Seasonal affective disorder (SAD), a mental depression during late fall and winter, has been linked to seasonally high melatonin levels. Daily exposure to bright lights to mimic summer has been used to treat SAD. The pineal gland and melatonin are also being studied concerning jet lag and disorders associated with shift work.

The pancreatic islets also called the "islets of Langerhans," produce insulin and glucagon. Diabetes mellitus is caused by insufficient insulin production (type 1 or juvenile-onset diabetes) or the lack of functional insulin receptors on body cells (type 2 diabetes). Type 1 diabetes is treated with insulin injections, an implanted insulin pump, or even a transplant of fetal pancreatic tissue. Type 2 diabetes is treated with diet, weight loss, and specific medications. Weight loss induces an increase in insulin receptors. Long-term complications resulting from high blood sugar levels include damage to the kidneys, the blood vessels in the retina (diabetic retinopathy), the legs and feet, and the nerves (diabetic neuropathy).

Changes in the levels of steroid hormones (glucocorticoids, mineralocorticoids, or androgens) secreted by the adrenal cortex cause diseases. Hypersecretion of the glucocorticoid cortisol causes Cushing's syndrome, and hyposecretion of cortisol results in Addison's disease. Like the thyroid, the hormones produced by the adrenal cortex participate in a feedback loop mechanism with the pituitary and hypothalamus. Thus, when hormones released by the adrenal glands are low, the pituitary and hypothalamus try to compensate by secreting higher levels of their hormones. In Addison's disease, low levels of adrenal glucocorticoids cause increased ACTH release from the pituitary. Addison's disease is characterized by low blood pressure and a poor physiological response to stress: The administration of exogenous glucocorticoids treats Addison's disease. Extreme cases of adrenal insufficiency can bring about an "adrenal crisis." In this situation, an immediate injection of glucocorticoid hormone prevents death.

In addition to treating Addison disease, glucocorticoids, particularly cortisone, are used to treat inflammation; however, overuse can lead to adrenal cortex suppression by the negative feedback mechanism. When athletes abuse the androgen sex hormones to increase muscle mass, adrenal suppression can develop along with sterility and damage the heart. Masculinization occurs in women who have tumors of the androgen-producing cells of the adrenal glands. These women display several changes associated with increased male sex hormones, including beard growth and increased muscle development.

PERSPECTIVE AND PROSPECTS
The early history of endocrinology noted that boys who were castrated failed to undergo the changes associated with puberty. A. A. Berthold, in 1849 described the effects of castration in cockerels. The birds failed to develop large combs and wattles and failed to show male behavior. He could reverse these effects if testes were transplanted back into the cockerels. W. M. Bayliss and E. H. Starling, in 1902, first introduced the term "hormone" to refer to secretin. They found that the small intestine produces secretin in response to acid in the chyme and that secretin causes the pancreas to release digestive enzymes into the small intestine. Most important, F. G. Banting and G. H. Best, in 1922, reported their extraction of insulin from the pancreas of dogs and their success in alleviating diabetes in dogs through injections of insulin. Frederick Sanger in 1953 established the amino acid sequence for insulin and later won a Nobel Prize for this achievement.

Another Nobel Prize was awarded to Earl W. Sutherland, Jr., in 1971, for his demonstration in 1962 of the role of cyclic AMP as a second messenger in the sequence involved in the stimulation of cells by many hormones. Andrew V. Schally and Roger C. L. Guillemin, in 1977, received a Nobel Prize for their work in isolating and determining the structures of hypothalamic regulatory peptides.

More recent achievements in endocrinological research have centered on identifying receptors that bind with the hormone when the hormone stimulates a cell and on the genetic engineering of bacteria to produce hormones such as human growth hormone. The use of fetal tissues in endocrinological research and therapy—the host usually does not reject fetal implants—continues to be an area for future research.

—*John T. Burns, PhD and Sharon W. Stark, RN, APRN, DNSc*

Further Information
Griffin, James E., and Sergio R. Ojeda, editors. *Textbook of Endocrine Physiology*. 6th ed., Oxford UP, 2012.
Hadley, Mac E., and Jon E. Levine. *Endocrinology*. 6th ed., Pearson/Prentice Hall, 2007.
Henry, Helen L., and Anthony W. Norman, editors. *Encyclopedia of Hormones*. 3 vols., Academic Press, 2003.
Jameson, J. Larry, and Tinsley Randolph Harrison. *Harrison's Endocrinology*. McGraw-Hill, 2013.
Koch, Christian A., George P. Chrousos. *Endocrine Hypertension: Underlying Mechanisms and Therapy*. Humana Press, 2013.
Kronenberg, Henry M., et al., editors. *Williams Textbook of Endocrinology*. 12th ed., Saunders/Elsevier, 2011.
Laws, Edward R., et al. *Pituitary Disorders: Diagnosis and Management*. Wiley, 2013.
Martini, Frederic. *Fundamentals of Anatomy and Physiology*. 9th ed., Prentice-Hall, 2012.
Radovick, Sally, and Margaret H. MacGillivray. *Pediatric Endocrinology: A Practical Clinical Guide*. Humana Press, 2013.
Scanlon, Valerie, and Tina Sanders. *Essentials of Anatomy and Physiology*. 6th ed., F. A. Davis, 2011.
Shaw, Michael, editor. *Everything You Need to Know About Diseases*. Springhouse Press, 1996.
Wells, Ken R. "Endocrine System." *Gale Encyclopedia of Nursing and Allied Health*, edited by Kristine Krapp, Gale Group, 2002.

Endocrinology

Category: Specialty
Anatomy or system affected: Brain, endocrine system, glands, immune system, nervous system, pancreas, psychic-emotional system, reproductive system, uterus
Specialties and related fields: Biochemistry, genetics, gynecology, immunology
Definition: The science dealing with how the internal secretions from ductless glands in the body act both in normal physiology and in disease states.

KEY TERMS

adrenal gland: an endocrine gland situated immediately above the upper pole of each kidney; it consists of an inner part or medulla, which produces epinephrine and norepinephrine, and an outer part or cortex, which produces steroid hormones

endocrine pancreas: specialized secretory tissue dispersed within the pancreas called "islets of Langerhans," which are responsible for the secretion of glucagon and insulin

hypothalamus: the region of the brain called the "diencephalon," forming the floor of the third ventricle, including neighboring associated nuclei

metabolism: the process of tissue change, which may be synthetic (anabolic) or degradative (catabolic)

parathyroid gland: one of four small endocrine glands situated underneath the thyroid gland, whose main product is parathyroid hormone, which regulates serum calcium levels

pituitary gland: a small (0.5-gram), two-lobed endocrine gland that is attached by a stalk to the brain at the level of the hypothalamus

thyroid gland: a 20-gram endocrine gland that sits in front of the trachea and consists of two lateral lobes connected in the middle by an isthmus

SCIENCE AND PROFESSION

The rates of metabolic pathways in the body are controlled mainly by the endocrine system, in conjunction with the nervous system. These two systems are integrated into the neuroendocrine system, which controls the secretion of hormones by the endocrine glands. The study of endocrinology deals with the normal physiology and pathophysiology of endocrine glands. The endocrine glands that are the main focus of clinical endocrinologists are the hypothalamus, pituitary gland, thyroid, parathyroid, adrenal glands, endocrine pancreas, ovaries, and testes. The endocrine system regulates all body activities, including growth and development, homeostasis, energy production, and reproduction.

The hypothalamus is a highly specialized endocrine organ that sits at the brain's base and functions as the master gland of the endocrine system. It is the central integrator for the endocrine and nervous systems. The hypothalamus produces many chemical mediators that have direct control over the pituitary gland. These chemicals are made in the hypothalamus cells and reach the pituitary gland, which sits just below it, by a unique hypophyseal portal blood system. In adult humans, the pituitary is divided into the anterior lobe (adenohypophysis) and the posterior lobe (neural lobe).

Vasopressin and oxytocin are the two primary hormones made in the hypothalamus but stored in the posterior lobe of the pituitary for release when needed. Vasopressin (also known as antidiuretic hormone, or ADH) is a hormone that maintains a normal water concentration in the blood and is a regulator of circulating blood volume. Oxytocin is a hormone that is involved in lactation and obstetrical labor.

The hypothalamic-pituitary-thyroid axis is essential in the control of basal metabolic rate. Several releasing hormones secreted from the hypothalamus control the release of anterior pituitary hormones, which then cause the release of hormones at the end organ. Most of these hormones have the chemical structures of peptides. Thyrotropin-releasing hormone (TRH) was the first hypothalamic releasing hormone that was synthesized and used clinically. TRH, secreted in nanogram quantities, is a cyclic tripeptide that causes the release of a thyrotropin-stimulating hormone (TSH) from the thyrotropic cells of the anterior pituitary gland. The release of TSH is in microgram quantities and leads to an increase in thyroid hormone release by the thyroid gland. The amount of thyroid hormone synthesized is on the order of milligrams. Therefore, the secretion of minute amounts of TRH allows for the production of thyroid hormone that is a millionfold greater than the amount of TRH itself, an example of an amplifying cascade. The central nervous system can control all metabolic processes with minimal amounts of hypothalamic releasing hormones. This intricate system possesses controls to stop the production of too much hormone as well. Such negative feedback is an essential concept in endocrinology.

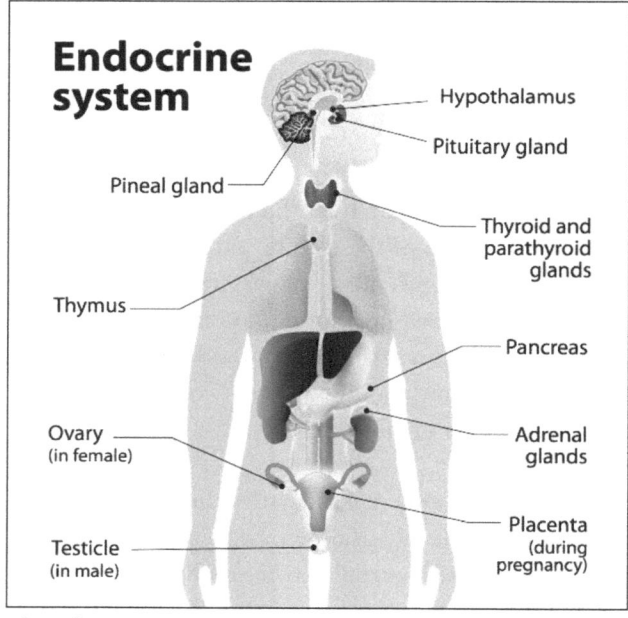

The endocrine system. Image via the U.S. Environmental Protection Agency (epa.gov).

Many hormones are subject to the laws of negative feedback control. In the case of the thyroid, an increased amount of thyroid hormone produced by the thyroid gland will cause the pituitary and hypothalamus to decrease the amounts that they make of TSH and TRH, respectively. TRH also causes a potent release of the anterior pituitary hormone called "prolactin." Thyroid hormone is essential in determining basal metabolism and is needed for proper development in the newborn child. The thyroid gland produces both thyroxine (T4), also called "tetraiodothyronine") and triiodothyronine (T3), both of which it synthesizes from iodine and the amino acid tyrosine.

The hypothalamic-pituitary-adrenal axis is critical in the reaction to stress, both physical and emotional. Corticotropin-releasing hormone (CRH) is a polypeptide, consisting of forty-one amino acids, that causes the production of the proopiomelanocortin molecule by the corticotropic cells of the anterior pituitary. The proopiomelanocortin molecule is cleaved by proteolytic enzymes to yield adrenocorticotropic hormone (ACTH, also called "corticotropin"), melanocyte-stimulating hormone, and lipotropin. It is ACTH made by the anterior pituitary, which then stimulates the adrenal cortex to produce steroid hormones. The primary stress hormone produced by the adrenal cortex in response to ACTH is the glucocorticoid cortisol. ACTH also has some control over the production of the mineralocorticoid aldosterone and the androgens dehydroepiandrosterone and testosterone. These steroids are synthesized from cholesterol. The production of cortisol (also known as "hydrocortisone") is subject to negative feedback by CRH and ACTH.

The hypothalamic-pituitary-gonadal axis is involved in the control of reproduction. Gonadotropin-releasing hormone (GnRH), also known as luteinizing hormone-releasing hormone (LHRH), is produced by the hypothalamus and stimulates the release of luteinizing hormone (LH) and follicle-stimulating hormone (FSH) from the gonadotrophic cells of the anterior pituitary. LH and FSH have different effects in men and women. In men, LH controls the production and secretion of testosterone by the Leydig cells of the testes. The release of LH is regulated by negative feedback from testosterone. FSH, along with testosterone, acts on the Sertoli cells of the seminiferous tubule of the testis at the time of puberty to start sperm production. In women, LH controls ovulation by the ovary and also the development of the corpus luteum, which produces progesterone. Progesterone is a steroid hormone that is critically important for the maintenance of pregnancy. FSH in women stimulates the development and maturation of a primary follicle and oocyte. The ovarian follicle in the nonpregnant woman is the leading site of production of estradiol. Estradiol is the principal estrogen made in the reproductive years by the ovary. It is responsible for the development of female secondary sexual characteristics.

Growth hormone-releasing hormone (GHRH) is a polypeptide with forty-four amino acids that stimulates the release of growth hormone (GH) from the somatotrophic cells of the anterior pituitary. The regulation of GH secretion is under dual control. While GHRH positively releases GH, somatostatin (a polypeptide with fourteen amino acids, also released from the hypothalamus) inhibits the release of GH. Somatostatin has a wide variety of functions, including suppressing insulin, glucagon, and gastrointestinal hormones. GH release from the pituitary circulates in the bloodstream and stimulates the production of somatomedins by the liver. Several somatomedins are produced, all of which profoundly affect growth, with the most important one in humans being somatomedin C, also called "insulin-like growth factor I (IGF I)." Molecular biological techniques have shown that many cells outside the liver also produce IGF I; in these cells, IGF I acts in autocrine or paracrine ways to cause the growth of the cells or to affect neighboring cells.

Prolactin is a peptide hormone that is secreted by the lactotrophs of the anterior pituitary. It is involved in the differentiation of the mammary gland cells. It initiates the production of milk proteins and other constituents. Prolactin may also have other functions, as a stress hormone or growth hormone. Prolactin is under negative tonic control. The inhibition of prolactin release is caused by dopamine, which is produced by the hypothalamus. Thus, while dopamine is usually considered a neurotransmitter, it acts as an inhibitory hormone in the case of prolactin release. Serotonin, also classically thought of as a neurotransmitter may cause the stimulation of prolactin release from the anterior pituitary.

DIAGNOSTIC AND TREATMENT TECHNIQUES
One of the most common medical problems seen by specialists in endocrinology is a patient with type 1 diabetes mellitus, sometimes also called "juvenile-onset" or "insulin-dependent" diabetes mellitus. "Insulin-dependent" is probably more appropriate, as not all patients with type 1 diabetes mellitus develop the disease in childhood. Type 1 diabetes is an autoimmune disease in which antibodies to different parts of the pancreatic beta-cell, the cell that usually produces insulin, are produced. Some of these antibodies are cytotoxic; that is, they destroy the pancreatic beta-cell. The most striking characteristic of patients with type 1 diabetes is that they produce very little insulin. The symptoms of type 1 diabetes include increased thirst, increased urination, blurring of vision, and weight loss. A doctor would confirm the diagnosis by running blood tests for glucose and insulin. The glucose level would be high, and the insulin level would be low. The treatment includes controlled diet, exercise, insulin therapy, and self-monitoring of blood glucose. With proper control of blood glucose, patients with type 1 diabetes can lead normal, productive lives.

Graves' disease is another autoimmune disease that endocrinologists commonly see. Graves' disease is caused by thyroid-stimulating immunoglobulin antibodies that bind to and activate TSH receptors. As a result, the thyroid gland produces too much thyroid hormone, enlarging in size. The antibodies also commonly affect the eyes, causing a characteristic bulging. The clinical symptoms of hyperthyroidism include increased heart rate, anxiety, heat sensitivity, sleeplessness, diarrhea, and abdominal pain. Patients often lose considerable weight, despite having a great appetite and eating large amounts of food. Sometimes, the diagnosis is missed, leading to an extensive evaluation for a variety of other diseases. Often, patients with Graves' disease have a family history of thyroid disease or other endocrine diseases.

The usual screening method for Graves' disease is a simple blood test for thyroid function, which includes testing for T4, T3, and TSH. In patients with Graves' disease, both T4 and T3 will be elevated, and TSH will be very low. If the blood test reveals this pattern, the next usual step is to proceed to a radioactive iodine uptake and scan test, which involves giving a small amount of radioactive iodine by mouth and having the patient return twenty-four hours later for a scan. The thyroid gland stores iodine and thus will accumulate radioactive iodine as well. The radioactive iodine emits gamma-ray energy that can be picked up by a solid-crystal scintillation counter placed over the thyroid gland. With this device, one can determine the percentage of iodine uptake and obtain a picture of the thyroid gland. The normal radioactive iodine uptake is about 10 to 30 percent of the dose, depending somewhat on the total body iodine derived from the diet. Patients with Graves' disease will have high radioactive iodine uptakes.

Those who suffer from Graves' disease can be treated by three different means depending on the circumstances. The first treatment that is often tried is antithyroid drugs, either propylthiouracil or methimazole. These drugs belong to the class of sulfonamides and inhibit the production of new thyroid hormones by blocking the attachment of iodine to the amino acid tyrosine. Another mode of therapy is the use of radioactive iodine. A dose of radioactive iodine (on the order of five to ten millicuries) is used to destroy part of the thyroid gland. The gamma-ray energy emitted from the iodine molecule that has traveled to the thyroid gland is enough to kill some thyroid cells. An alternative way to destroy the thyroid gland is to remove it surgically (thyroidectomy). Endocrinologists rarely send patients for surgery, as the other therapies are often effective. All treatments aim to bring the thyroid hormone level into the normal range and shrink the thyroid gland. After treatment, the patient's level of thyroid hormone sometimes falls to levels that are below normal. The symptoms of hypothyroidism are the opposite of hyperthyroidism and include fatigue, weight gain, cold sensitivity, constipation, and dry skin. If this happens, the patient is treated with thyroid hormone replacement. The dose is adjusted for each individual to produce normal levels of T4, T3, and TSH.

A less common but important endocrine disorder is a pituitary tumor that secretes prolactin, called a "prolactinoma." Prolactinomas are diagnosed earlier in women than in men. Women with the condition often complain of a lack of menstrual periods and spontaneous milk production from the breasts, known as galactorrhea. These tumors, which can be small, are called "microadenomas" because they are less than ten millimeters in size. They can affect men as well, causing decreased sex drive and impotence. Macroadenomas are tumors greater than ten millimeters in size. When the tumors increase in size, they can cause symptoms such as headache and decreased vision. It is important to note that most microadenomas never progress to macroadenomas. Vision loss and reduced eye movement can be seen with a macroadenoma and are the reason for immediate treatment.

Doctors screen patients for prolactinoma by running a blood test for prolactin. There are other reasons for mild elevations in prolactin levels, including certain psychiatric drugs such as phenothiazines or the antihypertensive drugs reserpine and methyldopa, primary hypothyroidism, cirrhosis, and chronic renal failure. If a pituitary tumor is suspected, then other biochemical tests of pituitary function are conducted to determine if the rest of the gland is functioning normally. At that time, imaging tests, such as computed tomography (CT) scanning or magnetic resonance imaging (MRI), can visualize the hypothalamic-pituitary area. Patients with macroadenomas will require treatment. In patients with little neurological involvement, medical therapy may be initiated. Bromocriptine, a semisynthetic ergot alkaloid that is an inhibitor of prolactin secretion, may be used. It has been shown that patients treated with this drug have a reduction in tumor size. Patients can be maintained on the medication indefinitely because prolactin levels return to pretreatment levels when the drug is stopped. If there is severe neurologic involvement with vision loss and other eye problems, immediate surgery may be indicated. There is a very high incidence of tumor recurrence after surgery, requiring medical or radiation therapy.

PERSPECTIVE AND PROSPECTS
The field of endocrinology is a continuously evolving one. Advances in biomedical technology, including molecular biology and cell biology, have made it a demanding job for the clinician to keep up with all the breakthroughs in the field. The challenge for endocrinology will be to apply many of these new technologies to novel treatments for patients with endocrine diseases.

An example of the progression of endocrinology can be seen in the history of pituitary diseases. The start of pituitary endocrinology is ascribed to Pierre Marie, the French neurologist who in 1886 first described pituitary enlargement in a patient with acromegaly (enlargement of the skull, jaw, hands, and feet) and linked the disease to a pituitary abnormality. During the first half of the twentieth century, many hypothalamic and pituitary hormones were isolated and characterized. The field of endocrinology was revolutionized by the development of radioimmunoassay, which allows sensitive and specific measurements of hormones Radioimmunoassay replaced bioassay techniques, which were laborious, time-consuming, and not always precise. This technique has allowed for rapid measurement of hormones and improved screening for endocrine diseases involving hormone deficiency or hormone excess.

The action of noninvasive imaging techniques has complemented the development of new hormone assays. Before the advent of CT scanning in the late 1970s, it was an ordeal to diagnose a pituitary tumor. Pneumoencephalography was often performed, which involved injecting air into the fluid-containing structures of the brain, with associated risk and discomfort to the patient. In the 1980s, with new generations of high-resolution CT scanners that were more sensitive than early scanners, smaller pituitary lesions could be detected and diagnosed. That decade also ushered in the use of MRI to diagnose disorders of the hypothalamic-pituitary unit. MRI has allowed doctors to evaluate the hypothalamus, pituitary, and nearby structures very precisely; it has become the method of choice for evaluating patients with pituitary disease. MRI can easily visualize the optic chiasm in the forebrain and the vascular structures surrounding the pituitary.

In patients who require surgery, advances have helped decrease mortality rates. Harvey Cushing pioneered the transsphenoidal technique in 1927 but abandoned it in favor of the transfrontal approach. The modern era of transsphenoidal pituitary surgery was developed by Gérard Guiot and Jules Hardy in the late 1960s. The transfrontal surgical procedure reaches the pituitary tumor by retracting the frontal lobes to visualize the pituitary gland sitting underneath. Transsphenoidal surgery done with an operating microscope to visualize the pituitary contents allows selective removal of the tumor, leaving the normal pituitary gland intact. The advantage of this approach from below, instead of from above, includes minimal brain movement and less blood loss. This technique requires a neurosurgeon with much skill and experience. There are also new drug treatments for patients with pituitary diseases, such as bromocriptine for use in patients with prolactinomas and octreotide (a somatostatin analog) to lower growth hormone levels in patients with acromegaly.

—*RoseMarie Pasmantier, MD*

Further Information

Bar, Robert S., editor. *Early Diagnosis and Treatment of Endocrine Disorders.* Humana Press, 2003.

Braverman, Lewis E., and David S. Cooper, editors. *Werner and Ingbar's The Thyroid: A Fundamental and Clinical Text.* 10th ed., Lippincott Williams & Wilkins, 2013.

"Diabetes." *MedlinePlus*, 2 Aug. 2021, medlineplus.gov/diabetes.html. Accessed 24 Aug. 2021.

"Endocrine Diseases." *MedlinePlus*, 17 Aug. 2021, medlineplus.gov/endocrinediseases.html. Accessed 24 Aug. 2021.

"Endocrine Glands." *MedlinePlus*, 5 Aug. 2021, medlineplus.gov/ency/article/002351.htm. Accessed 24 Aug. 2021.

Harmel, Anne Peters, and Ruchi Mathur. *Davidson's Diabetes Mellitus: Diagnosis and Treatment.* 5th ed., W. B. Saunders, 2004.

Imura, Hiroo, editor. *The Pituitary Gland.* 2nd ed., Raven Press, 1994.

Lebovitz, Harold E., editor. *Therapy for Diabetes Mellitus and Related Disorders.* 5th ed., American Diabetes Association, 2009.

Melmed, Shlomo, Ronald Koenig, Clifford Rosen, Richard Auchus, and Allison Goldfine. *Williams Textbook of Endocrinology.* 14th ed., Elsevier, 2019.

"Pituitary Tumors." *MedlinePlus*, 17 Aug. 2021, medlineplus.gov/thyroiddiseases.html. Accessed on 24 Aug. 2021.

Speroff, Leon, and Marc A. Fritz. *Clinical Gynecologic Endocrinology and Infertility.* 8th ed., Lippincott Williams & Wilkins, 2011.

"Thyroid Diseases." *MedlinePlus*, 17 Aug. 2021, medlineplus.gov/thyroiddiseases.html. Accessed 24 Aug. 2021.

ENDOCRINOLOGY, PEDIATRIC

Category: Specialty
Anatomy or system affected: Brain, endocrine system, glands, immune system, nervous system, pancreas, psychic-emotional system
Specialties and related fields: Biochemistry, genetics, immunology, neonatology, pediatrics
Definition: The study of the normal and abnormal function of the endocrine (ductless) glands in children and adolescents.

KEY TERMS

hormone: a chemical molecule produced in either the hypothalamus or one of the endocrine glands that is secreted and travels (usually via the bloodstream) to a target organ or specific receptor cells, causing a particular response

insulin: a hormone that is essential in regulating blood glucose, as well as in assimilating carbohydrates for growth and energy

pancreas: a large gland near the stomach that has both exocrine and endocrine functions and which produces insulin

pituitary gland: a tiny gland at the base of the brain that, with the hypothalamus, regulates most of the endocrine systems

thyroid: a gland in the anterior neck that regulates the level of the body's metabolism and which is instrumental in normal physical and mental growth

SCIENCE AND PROFESSION

Pediatric endocrinology is a major subspecialty, limited to children and adolescents, which involves the study of normal and abnormal functions of the endocrine system, which comprises the glands of internal or ductless secretions. These practitioners, referred to as endocrinologists or pediatric endocrinologists, are doctors of medicine or osteopathy who have completed three years of pediatric residency training and an additional two to three years of fellowship training in endocrinology.

Endocrinology is one of the most exciting and challenging fields in pediatrics because it requires a blend of basic science and technology in the clinical setting. Some of the diagnoses are very difficult, yet they are almost always wholly logical. Endocrinology is tightly related to other areas of pediatrics, such as adolescent medicine, genetics, growth, development, nutrition, and metabolism. These relationships make this field even more complex and intellectually stimulating.

Pediatric endocrinology and adult endocrinology are relatively young fields, probably beginning with the discovery in 1888 that "myxedema" (hypothyroidism) could be improved by feeding the patient thyroid extract. Both fields deal with the major endocrine glands and their disorders, such as diabetes mellitus or hypothyroidism. Still, there are several key differences, mostly related to growth (both physical and mental), potential, and genetics. Some significant areas of specific emphasis in pediatric endocrinology include diabetes mellitus (which presents very differently in children), growth disorders, sexual maturation and differentiation disorders, genetic disorders, and adolescent medicine.

DIAGNOSTIC AND TREATMENT TECHNIQUES

In pediatric endocrinology, as in all medical fields, history taking and physical examination are the starting points and usually the most valuable tools for diagnosis. Endocrinology is a specialty that is particularly aided by science. Blood and urine chemistries, hormone assays, chromosomal analyses, X-rays, computed tomography (CT) scans, magnetic resonance imaging (MRI), and a host of other sophisticated tests have advanced diagnoses and treatments. They have made this specialty one of the favorites for physicians who like science. Virtually all the known hormones can be assayed accurately and quickly.

Many of the treatments in endocrinology involve hormone therapy. Since insulin was first available for injection in 1922, there have been remarkable advances in treatment. In 1985, recombinant growth hormone was synthesized for the first time. This development has allowed endocrinologists to treat not only pituitary dwarfism but also other kinds of growth deficiencies, such as Turner syndrome.

Turner syndrome is a relatively common chromosomal abnormality affecting females and resulting in short stature and lack of sexual development. While these girls will never become fertile, the combination of growth hormone for height and other hormonal therapy to develop secondary sexual characteristics enables them to have a normal female body. Studies have shown that typical body image and the presence of menstruation are essential for these patients' self-esteem.

Diabetes mellitus is the most common significant endocrine disorder in both adults and children. What was commonly referred to as juvenile diabetes years ago is now called "diabetes mellitus, type 1." Unlike type 2, which usually presents insidiously in middle-aged and older adults, type 1 presents rapidly. The patient will need daily injectable insulin treatments. Diabetes in children is complex to manage because of the insulin treatment and the patients' growth, metabolism, fluctuating activity levels, and physiologic and psychological changes that occur, especially in adolescence.

Small portable and entirely accurate glucometers allow patients to measure blood glucose (sugar) at home, making diabetes management more straightforward. Tighter control of blood glucose will decrease or delay the onset of long-term complications of the disease, such as blindness, heart disease, and kidney disease. In the United States, newborn screening, which is now performed in all fifty states, has virtually eliminated cretinism—the tragic result of undiagnosed congenital hypothyroidism. These children were irreversibly developmentally disabled.

Enhanced techniques in pediatric surgery and neurosurgery, greatly aided by scans, play a role in treating some endocrine disorders. Small tumors and masses can be identified and often removed successfully. Often, endocrinologists and oncologists work together in concert with the surgeon.

Although this subspecialty is one of the most scientific and laboratory-based in pediatrics, it is also a field where emotional support, counseling, and mental health care are given. Children do not like being "different," and body image is critical in children, particularly teenagers. Even when a child appears normal, they resent the frustration of ongoing monitoring and treatment. It can result in rebellion, especially in children with diabetes. Often, a team approach is needed, which involves professionals, teachers, family, and peers.

PERSPECTIVE AND PROSPECTS
In the future, further research will almost certainly reveal even more dramatic advances for the diagnosis, treatment, and prevention of endocrine disorders. An implantable glucose pump, which can serve as a substitute pancreas, can dramatically change diabetic patients' lives. A method for rapidly analyzing blood glucose using the surface of the skin is Food and Drug Administration (FDA)-approved and readily available. These devices, constant glucose monitors (CGMs), drastically simplify measuring a patient's blood sugar. Furthermore, integration of the CGM software with cell phone apps, such as the DEXCOM system, provides continuous, visual readouts in real time. In addition, genetic engineering may revolutionize the approaches to treating many of these diseases.

—*C. Mervyn Rasmussen, MD*

Further Information

Bar, Robert S., editor. *Early Diagnosis and Treatment of Endocrine Disorders*. Humana Press, 2003.
Colaco, Prisca. *Atlas of Growth and Endocrine Disorders in Children*. ?Jaypee Brothers Medical Publishers Ltd., 2017.
"Diabetes in Children and Teens." *MedlinePlus*, 27 May 2021, medlineplus.gov/diabetesinchildrenandteens.html. Accessed 24 Aug. 2021.
"Growth Disorders." *MedlinePlus*, 17 Aug. 2021, medlineplus.gov/growthdisorders.html. Accessed 24 Aug. 2021.
Hanas, Ragnar. *Type 1 Diabetes in Children, Adolescents and Young Adults*. Class Health, 2019.
Handwerger, Stuart, editor. *Molecular and Cellular Pediatric Endocrinology*. Humana Press, 1999.
Harmel, Anne Peters, and Ruchi Mathur. *Davidson's Diabetes Mellitus: Diagnosis and Treatment*. 5th ed., W. B. Saunders, 2004.
Hirsch, Larissa. "Endocrine System." *KidsHealth*. Oct. 2018, kidshealth.org/en/parents/endocrine.html?ref=search. Accessed 25 Aug. 2021.
Little, Marjorie. *Diabetes*. Chelsea House, 1991.
Melmed, Shlomo, et al. *Williams Textbook of Endocrinology*. 12th ed., Saunders/Elsevier, 2011.
Sperling, Mark A., editor. *Pediatric Endocrinology*. 3rd ed., Saunders/Elsevier, 2008.
"Thyroid Diseases." *MedlinePlus*, 17 Aug. 2021, medlineplus.gov/thyroiddiseases.html. Accessed 24 Aug. 2021.
Wales, Jeremy K. H., and Jan Maarten Wit. *Pediatric Endocrinology and Growth*. 2nd ed., W. B. Saunders, 2004.

HOME HEALTH

Category: Issues/Overviews
Related terms: Home cleanliness, home hygiene, house cleaning, housekeeping, indoor air pollution

Definition: The recognition and removal of allergens, pathogens, and other pollutants found in the home or different living environments.

KEY TERMS

allergen: an ordinarily harmless substance—such as pet dander, pollen, or food proteins—that can cause an allergic reaction in some patients

dust: airborne pollutants that can include dead skin, hair, ash, pollen, fibers, and minerals from outdoor soils that can lead to allergies, respiratory diseases, and asthma

mold: a growth of fungus that occurs on food or in a home or other moist warm conditions

pathogen: a bacterium, virus, or other microorganism that can cause disease

pollen: a fine powdery substance, typically yellow, consisting of microscopic grains discharged from the male part of a flower that can trigger allergies or asthma

NATURAL POLLUTANTS

Every home contains natural pollutants that require regular removal to reduce health risks, prevent offensive odors, and eliminate stains and structural damage that devalue the structure. Most of these pollutants become airborne and are inhaled, creating subsequent health problems that range in severity from sneezing to difficulty breathing. Other pollutants may be unintentionally ingested, causing illness.

Airborne pollutants are collectively called "dust." The most common dust component in a home is dead skin particles shed by the home's residents. Dust also contains hair, ash, pollen, fibers, and minerals from outdoor soil. Overexposure to dust can lead to allergies, respiratory diseases, and asthma. Dust mites feed on the organic matter in dust. Mites most commonly live on mattresses, sheets, and pillows. Their excrement contains substances that can cause severe allergic reactions. Companies are now making tightly woven antiallergy encasings for mattresses and pillows. The use of air filters in the furnace, air conditioner, and vacuum cleaner reduces airborne contaminants.

The inhabitants of a house, such as humans, pets, and occasionally rodents, naturally shed hair, dander, saliva, urine, and feces. Such substances may trigger an allergic reaction in people or carry bacteria, viruses, or parasites that infect humans. Hair and dander may be removed by frequent vacuuming and dusting, and any bodily excretions should be cleaned with soap and water. Toilets should be disinfected regularly; closing the lid before flushing prevents the contents from being dispersed into the room as an aerosol.

Also living in homes may be insects such as flies, termites, ants, spiders, fleas, lice, cockroaches, and bedbugs. Many of these insects feed on garbage, food spills and crumbs that are not cleaned up, and food supplies that are not adequately packaged. Insects can transmit diseases to humans either directly by biting or indirectly by contaminating food with eggs or droppings. Natural or chemical pesticides, swatting, vacuuming, or flypaper eliminates insects from the home. Adequate containment of garbage, keeping kitchen floors swept and counters wiped clean, and storing food in airtight containers discourage their return.

Pollen from houseplants and cut flower arrangements diminish indoor air quality. Pollen may also drift inside through open windows and doors and be brought in on shoes and clothing, especially from plants next to the house. To reduce indoor pollen, keep houseplants and floral arrangements well hydrated. Trim outdoor plants near windows and doors so that their branches and leaves are away from openings. Although silk floral arrangements do not contain pollen, their complex surfaces trap dust. Clean silk floral arrangements regularly by spraying with compressed air.

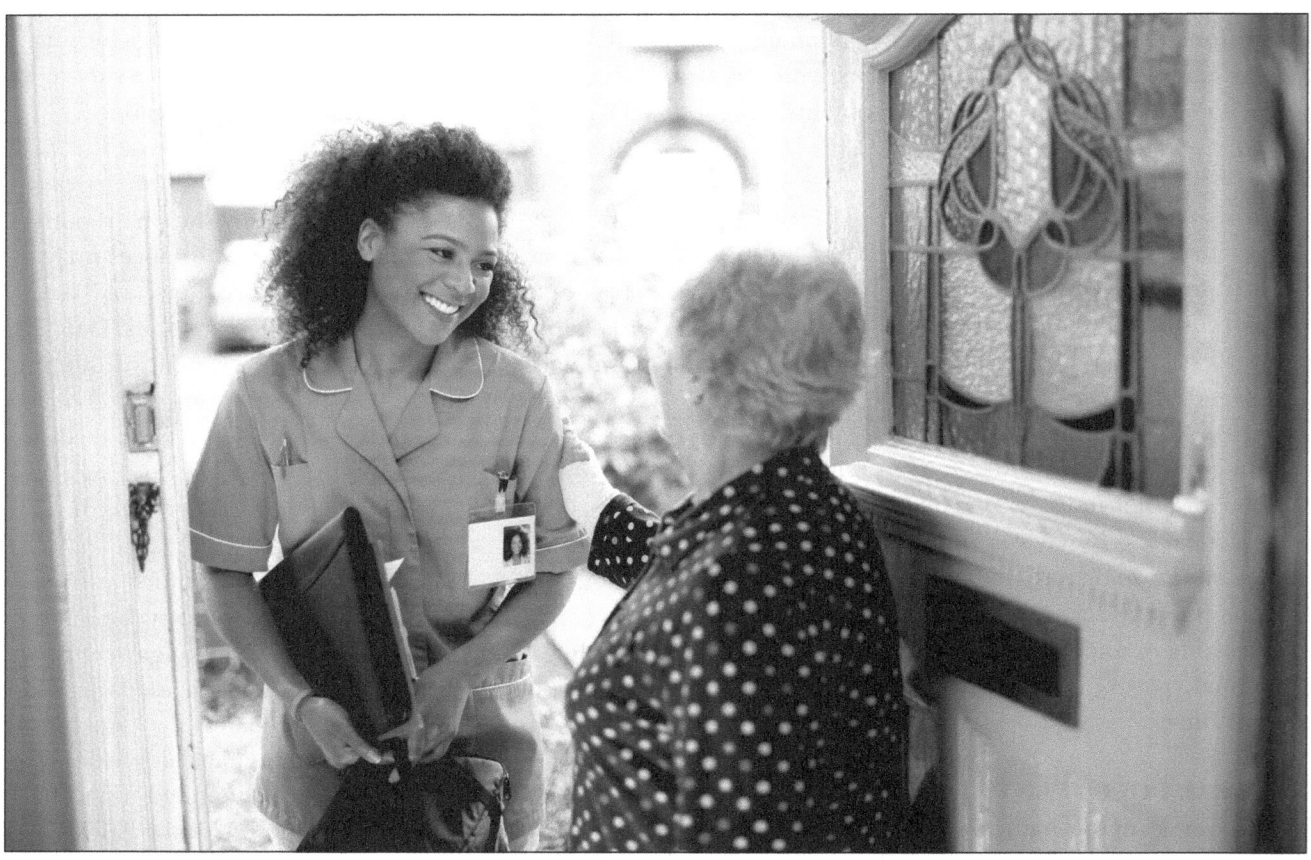
A clean home environment reduces common allergens. Photo via iStock.com/sturti. [Used under license.]

Mold, a type of fungus, grows in warm, damp areas such as inadequately ventilated bathrooms, kitchens, and basements. Mold releases spores into the air, which, when inhaled, may cause symptoms such as a dry cough, nasal congestion, eye irritation, and wheezing. Mold may be visible, but it is usually detected initially by its musty odor. It may be destroyed by scrubbing first with a detergent without ammonia in hot water and then with a 10 percent bleach solution. Discard porous materials such as carpeting and insulation that remain damp.

Bacteria and viruses may make a person ill when ingested or inhaled. They may be found on unwashed, uncooked fruits and vegetables and uncooked meats. Thoroughly wash all raw foods before eating them. Handling raw meat and neglecting to wash one's hands and the food preparation surface afterward may result in the contamination of other foods and subsequent pathogen ingestion. Surfaces that come in contact with raw meat juices should be thoroughly disinfected.

Bacteria and viruses may also be transmitted on surfaces commonly used by many people, such as doorknobs and telephones. Such surfaces should be regularly and frequently wiped with a disposable disinfectant cloth during cold and flu season.

CHEMICAL POLLUTANTS

Among other causes, the degassing of synthetic materials in newer homes, and poor ventilation that keeps the house airtight, may lead to sick building syndrome. Symptoms of sick building syndrome include eye irritation, scratchy or sore throat, nasal congestion, skin rash, and difficulty concentrating. The symptoms typically begin within one hour of entering a polluted structure and disappear within one hour of leaving it.

Another chemical pollutant is tobacco smoke. The ash becomes a component of dust; the odor lingers in soft surfaces such as curtains, upholstery, and clothing; and the second-hand smoke is inhaled by the other residents of the home, causing increased respiratory problems.

Carbon monoxide is an odorless, colorless gas that faulty furnaces or space heaters may give off. Exposure may cause flulike symptoms, severe headache, dizziness, trouble breathing, and even death. Carbon monoxide detectors in the home are recommended and may be found in combination with smoke detectors.

Radon is another invisible, odorless gas that is also radioactive. It results from the decay of uranium in the soil and seeps into a home through the foundation, where it can build up to dangerous levels. Radon increases the risk of lung cancer for those who breathe it. The U.S. Environmental Protection Agency (EPA) recommends that all homes be tested for radon below the third floor. Commercial radon reduction systems are available too.

Asbestos, used as pipe insulation, may be a pollutant in homes built between 1920 and 1978. Breathing high levels of exposed asbestos may result in an increased risk of cancer and lung disease. Homes built before 1978 may also contain lead paint. Flakes of this paint have a sweet taste, making the paint tempting to children. If they ingest the paint flakes, they can become ill with lead poisoning.

—*Bethany Thivierge, MPH*

Further Information

Allen, Joseph G., and John D. Macomber. *Healthy Buildings: How Indoor Spaces Drive Performance and Productivity*. Harvard UP, 2020.

"Do You Know the Hygiene Hot Spots in Your Home?" *BBC News*, 25 Jun. 2019, www.bbc.com/news/health-48746377.

"Hygiene Etiquette & Practice." *Centers for Disease Control and Prevention*, 27 Jul. 2016, www.cdc.gov/healthywater/hygiene/etiquette/index.html.

"What Is Home and Everyday Life Hygiene?" *International Scientific Forum on Home Hygiene*, www.ifh-homehygiene.org/what-home-hygiene.

"Why Home Hygiene Is Important." *Healthy House Institute*, 20 Jan. 2012, www.healthyhouseinstitute.com/blog-1156-Why-Home-Hygiene-is-Important.

Host-defense mechanisms

Category: Biology

Anatomy or system affected: Blood, cells, gastrointestinal system, immune system, skin, urinary system

Specialties and related fields: Hematology, immunology, preventive medicine, serology

Definition: Immunological methods the body uses to protect against external infectious agents and maintain internal homeostasis, such as those rooted in the skin, sweat, urine, tears, phagocytes, and "helpful" bacteria.

KEY TERMS

antibodies: proteins produced by immune cells called "lymphocytes"; antibodies bind to targets called "antigens" in a precise manner

antigen: any substance that causes the formation of a specific antibody; generally, a protein

complement: a series of serum proteins that, when activated, carry out a variety of immune functions; the most notable complement function is the lysis of a target

granulocyte: a white blood cell characterized by large numbers of cytoplasmic granules, including neutrophils, eosinophils, and basophils

innate immunity: nonspecific immunity in the sense that prior contact with an infectious agent is not required for proper innate immune response

interferons: a family of proteins; some of these proteins induce an antiviral state within a cell, while others serve to regulate aspects of the immune response

lymphocyte: either of two kinds of small white blood cells; B lymphocytes function to secrete antibodies, while T lymphocytes function to destroy virus-infected cells

macrophage: any of several forms of either circulating or fixed phagocytic cells of the immune system

neutrophil: a circulating white blood cell that serves as one of the principal phagocytes for the immune system

phagocyte: any cell capable of surrounding, ingesting, and digesting microbes or cell debris; in a certain sense, phagocytes function as scavengers

STRUCTURE AND FUNCTIONS

Humans exist in an environment that contains a wide variety of potentially infectious agents. These agents range from microscopic viruses—such as rhinoviruses that cause the common cold—to various bacteria and even macroscopic agents such as parasitic worms. In the absence of a functioning immune system, as is observed in persons with acquired immunodeficiency syndrome (AIDS) or congenital immune deficiencies, a person will eventually succumb to overwhelming infections.

Host-defense mechanisms consist of two major components: an innate system that is not dependent on prior exposure to an infectious agent and an acquired immunity that is stimulated by exposure to an agent. In general, the innate system functions in a nonspecific manner, while the acquired immune responses are highly specific.

The first major lines of host defense are the physical barriers to infection. These include the intact skin and the mechanical or physical barriers that serve to protect body openings. Few infectious agents are capable of penetrating intact skin. Numerous sweat glands and follicles are also associated with the skin. Their secretion of fatty acids or lactic acid serves to produce an acid environment that inhibits the growth of bacteria. In addition, the high salt content found on the body's surface also serves to inhibit growth. Bacteria that can resist the high levels of salt and acid, such as *Staphylococcus* or *Streptococcus*, tend to cause skin-related problems such as acne or boils.

Openings of the body, such as the mouth, anus, and vagina, exhibit both the physical barrier of the skin and a variety of other defense strategies. Secreted mucus serves to trap foreign particles, which can then be expelled, depending on the tissue, by the ciliary action of the cells, coughing or sneezing, or the washing action of saliva, urine, or tears. Many of these secretions also contain antibacterial or antiviral agents. Gastric juices contain hydrochloric acid, while the enzyme lysozyme, found in tears and saliva, serves to cause the breakdown of certain bacteria.

The normal flora of organisms found within the body also plays an essential role in defense. Bacteria in the mouth and gut serve to suppress any external agents that may find their way to those regions. Removal of the innate flora with antibiotics may result in yeast infections of the mouth or vaginal tract or ulceration by "opportunistic" gut organisms.

Penetration of the host by infectious agents initially brings into action other aspects of the innate immune system. Innate immunity takes the form of a series of "professional" phagocytes, cells that eat foreign particles such as bacteria; also included are chemical agents found in tissue and blood.

Two forms of phagocytes are in blood and tissues: neutrophils and monocytes/macrophages. Neutrophils represent the most numerous white cells in the blood, approximately 60 to 70 percent of the total. They can be recognized by their multilobed nuclei, which confer the ability to pass between the endothelial cells of capillaries into sites of tissue infections. When neutrophils locate a target, such as an infectious agent or a dead cell, they surround that target with membranous arms called "pseudopods" and ingest it. Once incorporated within this "phagosome," the particle is ready for killing and digestion.

The killing of ingested organisms such as bacteria involves a series of complicated reactions. The major products are highly reactive oxidizing agents such as peroxides or metabolic byproducts such as acid. At the same time, digestive organelles within the phagocyte, called "lysosomes," fuse with the phagosome. Lysosomes contain numerous digestive enzymes, and these function to digest the engulfed particle. In effect, the particle now ceases to exist.

Monocytes are most often observed in their differentiated macrophage stage. As professional phagocytes, macrophages function similarly to neutrophils. Unlike circulating cells such as neutrophils, however, macrophages constitute the mononuclear phagocytic system associated with many tissues in the body. Examples of tissue-associated macrophages are the Kupffer cells of the liver, the microglia of the brain, and certain alveolar cells of the lungs. In addition to serving a nonspecific phagocytic function, macrophages serve as antigen-presenting cells (APCs) for specific immune responses.

A variety of blood chemicals also can be associated with innate immunity. Complement represents a series of some twenty blood proteins, activated in a cascade fashion, which exhibit various pharmacologic activities. The complement pathway activates when exposed to certain bacteria. Components of the pathway can serve as chemoattractants for neutrophils. They can increase the efficiency of phagocytosis (opsonization). Most significantly, they form a membrane attack complex on the surface of a target, resulting in lysis.

Another type of blood cell may play a role in certain types of parasitic infections: the eosinophil. Granulocytes like the neutrophils, eosinophils contain within their granules digestive enzymes capable of being released against targets such as parasitic worms. The binding of these enzymes on the surface of a target damages the parasite's membrane, ultimately resulting in the parasite's death.

Acquired host defenses, while involving mechanisms similar to those of the innate systems, differ in one crucial way: they require prior exposure to the antigen. Acquired immunity consists of two major arms: humoral immunity, which represents substances soluble in the blood, and cellular immunity, which utilizes cells targeted against agents in a specific manner.

Humoral immunity centers primarily on proteins called "antibodies." Exposure to foreign antigens triggers a series of reactions among three distinct types of blood cells: antigen-presenting cells, T lymphocytes, and B lymphocytes. It is the B cell that secretes the antibodies.

The process starts when an APC encounters and phagocytizes an antigen. The APC digests the antigen and expresses the antigen's pieces, or determinants, on the cell's surface. The most common APC is the macrophage, but dendritic cells in the skin's dermis also present antigen. This portion of the process is analogous to the series of events associated with innate immunity. At this point, however, the determinant is "presented" to appropriate T and B lymphocytes. Only those lymphocytes that possess specific receptors for that antigenic determinant can interact with the APC; this aspect represents the specificity of the reaction. In association with a subclass of T lymphocytes called "T-helper cells" (also known as "CD4+ cells"), the B cell is stimulated to begin secreting large quantities of antibodies. The antibodies recognize and bind only those antigens against which they were produced.

The formation of antigen-antibody complexes is the key to the humoral response. The result of the reaction depends upon the form taken by the antigen. If the antigen is a toxin, antibody binding neutralizes it. When antibodies bind to a bacterium or virus, they "opsonize" it or significantly enhance the ability of phagocytes to engulf them. Antibody binding to a virus may also inhibit the agent's binding to a target cell, rendering the virus inactive.

The other arm of acquired immunity directly utilizes cellular defenses. The critical cell here is the T lymphocyte. T lymphocytes mature in an organ called the "thymus," near the thyroid in the neck, and provides the basis for the cells' name. One subset of T cells is the "killer" cells (or CD8+ cells) because of their function. They have receptors on their surfaces that bind to specific target cells that are usually virally infected. However, killer T cells are also associated with the rejection of foreign grafts. Once the T cell binds to the target, pharmacologically active granules are released that bind to and disrupt the target membrane. Thus, the humoral response is directed primarily against extracellular agents such as bacteria. In contrast, the cellular response is directed primarily against intracellular parasites.

DISORDERS AND DISEASES
In their most apparent form, the mechanisms of host defense protect against disease. Humans exist in an environment that is a sea of microorganisms. Most infections, while often uncomfortable, are not life-threatening. It is only when the immune system fails to function properly or is overwhelmed that illness results in the individual's death. Ironically, the study of these circumstances has provided much knowledge of the functioning of the immune system.

Throughout history, diseases have periodically plagued humanity. Epidemics of viral diseases such as polio and bacterial infections such as bubonic plague or cholera have killed untold millions of persons. Perhaps the most significant advances in medicine since the eighteenth century have been vaccination to prevent disease. Passive immunity temporarily augments host defenses. Active immunity mimics an actual infection, providing lifelong protection.

Passive immunity involves the acquisition of preformed antibodies by an individual. Antibodies from mother's milk are the most common form of passive immunization. The first milk made by a lactating mother, the colostrum, contains antibodies that protect her baby from childhood diseases. Preformed antibodies may also be given to a person exposed to potentially lethal toxins under circumstances where there may be insufficient time for a proper immune response. These can include persons exposed to snake venom or tetanus toxin. While temporarily providing protection, passively acquired antibodies survive in the individual only for a short period.

More commonly, vaccines provide active immunization by stimulating the acquired host defenses. These vaccines generally utilize inactivated or attenuated parasites that stimulate specific cellular or humoral responses. The prototypes of active immunization are the polio vaccines developed by Jonas Salk and Albert Sabin in the 1950s. Salk's vaccine utilizes a formalin-inactivated poliovirus, while Sabin's consists of an attenuated virus. While controversy exists regarding which is superior, both vaccines act in basically the same manner. Exposure to either vaccine results in the production of protective antibodies in the circulation of the individual. Should a vaccinated person become infected by poliovirus, their immune response would neutralize the virus before reaching its target in the central nervous system. There are analogous vaccines against previously common viral diseases such as smallpox, measles, and mumps and bacterial diseases such as pertussis (whooping cough) and diphtheria.

It is also important to remember that the humoral and cellular defense systems are not self-exclusive; each functions in conjunction with the other. Suppose the antigen in question is a bacterium. In that case, it is primarily the role of the humoral system to deal with the infection. Humoral immunity can take several forms. The antibody may bind to the cell's surface, inactivating the cell wall or membrane enzymes, resulting in the death of the cell. The antibody-antigen (bacterium) complex may also activate the complement pathway, resulting in either opsonization or a membrane attack complex by complement components. Indeed, antibody binding by itself may result in opsonization.

If the antigen is a virus-infected cell, the cellular portion of the response comes into play. Cytotoxic T cells can bind to the target through specific receptors, causing the death of the virus-infected cell. Suppose an antibody binds to viral receptors on the infected cell. In that case, cytotoxic cells with receptors for the antibody may show an increased affinity for the target in a process called "antibody-dependent cell-mediated cytotoxicity" (ADCC). The result is the death of the target. The antibody may also neutralize a cell-free virus before the particle can even infect the target cell. However, certain bacteria, such as the mycobacteria associated with tuberculosis and leprosy, are intracellular parasites. In such cases, it is the cellular immune system that plays a significant role in defense. In this manner, the humoral and cellular defense mechanisms complement each other.

Persons infected with the human immunodeficiency virus (HIV), the virus that causes AIDS, clearly illustrate the failure of the immune system to function. HIV infects the subclass of T lymphocytes known as T-helper cells. The eventual result is the death and depletion of this subclass of cells. As briefly described earlier, T-helper cells are central to the function of both the humoral and the cellular arms of acquired immunity. The interaction of these cells with B lymphocytes is necessary for both antibody production by these cells and their proliferation. The T-helper cell activates the CD8+ cytotoxic T cells, causing them to proliferate.

As AIDS progresses in the individual, the T-helper subclass becomes increasingly depleted. As a result, both the cellular and humoral immune systems become progressively less functional. The person becomes more susceptible to opportunistic organisms in the environment and eventually succumbs to a wide variety of diseases.

In rare congenital cases, only certain aspects of the immune system are nonfunctional. For example, children with B-cell deficiencies suffer from repeated bacterial infections. In contrast, yeast and viral infections rarely result in problems. However, children in whom the thymus fails to develop (DiGeorge or Nezelof syndromes) suffer from repeated viral infections but rarely from bacterial infections. These often tragic examples serve to illustrate the role of various cells within the host defense.

Severe combined immunodeficiency syndrome (SCID) affects approximately one of every 150,000 live births. This genetic disorder results from a lack of the enzyme adenosine deaminase (ADA), which ultimately causes a lack of functioning T cells. For years, patients with this disorder had been doomed to living in sterile bubble environments. They died at a young age because of their inability to fight even the mildest infection. Bone marrow transplants for patients with compatible donors can sometimes strengthen the immune system; however, this option is not available for everyone.

In 1990, two unrelated girls with SCID, four and nine years old, were test subjects for the first clinical gene therapy trial. T cells in their blood were isolated and cultured and given normal copies of the ADA gene. The genetically engineered T cells were then infused back into the patients for approximately two years. Both girls showed remarkable improvement, with near-normal levels of ADA and functioning immune systems, and were able to lead normal lives after that. These positive results remained several years after cessation of the actual gene therapy, indicating that this first clinical trial of gene therapy was a success. The door is now open for using gene therapy on other disorders, including the immune system.

Host defenses also help maintain the homeostatic process, defined as maintaining the status quo. An example of such a process is the immune system's role in protecting humans against various forms of cancer. Although immunosuppressed individuals appear to be at no greater risk for most cancers than normal persons, certain types of skin cancers and certain types of B-cell lymphomas arise more frequently in these persons. Thus, it is likely that the immune system plays at least some role in protecting the individual from certain forms of cancer. Artificial stimulation of the immune system can effectively treat sundry forms of advanced cancers. The process involves removing immune cells from the patient and incubating those cells with a form of interferon generally secreted by T-helper cells during their regulation of the immune response. The cells are infused back to the patient. The theory is that, by nonspecifically stimulating cytotoxic cells, some of those cells may serve to destroy the cancer. In some instances, patients have shown improvement.

Complex cellular interactions and regulatory circuitry drive the function of the immune system. The initial encounter with a foreign infectious agent utilizes an innate system that serves as the first line of defense. Then, through a learning process, a specific immune response is generated that provides a more rapid, more efficient means of generating protection.

PERSPECTIVE AND PROSPECTS

Humankind has tried to manipulate their immune system to protect against disease dates back more than a thousand years. To protect themselves against smallpox, the Chinese practiced variolation, in which people inhaled dried crusts obtained from the pocks of mild cases. The practice was copied by early Arabic physicians and eventually made its way to eighteenth-century Europe. In the late eighteenth century, an English country physician, Edward Jenner, observed that dairymaids who had recovered from a mild disease called "cowpox" rarely exhibited the scars associated with smallpox. Jenner reasoned that exposure to the cowpox agent would protect someone against smallpox. Jenner tested his theory and was proved correct. Smallpox became the first disease prevented by vaccination.

During the late nineteenth century, competition between French and German scientists resulted in much of the existing basic knowledge of host defenses. A Russian, Élie Metchnikoff, working with Louis Pasteur in Paris during the 1880s, developed the views of cellular immunity that are still current. In that same period, the work of Emil von Behring and Paul Ehrlich in Berlin established the role of humoral immunity in protecting against disease.

Active immunization remains the primary method by which an individual may be protected from disease. Still, the process lends itself to a variety of problems. Not all antigenic determinants of the bacterium or parasite in question are equally important. A response to some antigens may hinder the immune response to more essential determinants. Furthermore, some individuals react inappropriately to some vaccines, resulting in severe allergic reactions.

For these reasons, much research involves the attempt to isolate only the desired antigen for the vaccine. Vaccine research has taken several approaches. Purified components, rather than the entire organism, have been used in some vaccines. In some cases, the gene that encodes the desired antigen was isolated and spliced into the genetic material of a harmless organism. Such an approach produced a modified hepatitis B vaccine. The gene encoding the surface antigen of the virus was spliced into the genome of vaccinia, long used for vaccination against smallpox. When the individual is vaccinated, the hepatitis gene is expressed (though the vaccine does not make any live virus), and the person becomes immune to the disease. In theory, whole cocktails of vaccines can be prepared in a similar manner.

New illnesses and other environmental hazards that affect host defenses continue to arise. AIDS may be unusually lethal, but as a previously unknown disease, it is unique. Nevertheless, the ability of the host immune system to respond to new infectious agents remains a bulwark for maintaining the health of an individual.

—*Richard Adler, PhD and Karen E. Kalumuck, PhD*

Further Information

Adelman, Daniel C., et al., editors. *Manual of Allergy and Immunology*. 5th ed., Lippincott Williams & Wilkins, 2012.

Bibel, Debra Jan, editor. *Milestones in Immunology*. Springer, 1988.

Delves, Peter J., et al. *Roitt's Essential Immunology*. 13th ed., Wiley-Blackwell, 2017.

Frank, Steven A. *Immunology and Evolution of Infectious Disease*. Princeton UP, 2002.

Hall, Stephen S. *A Commotion in the Blood: Life, Death, and the Immune System*. Henry Holt, 1997.

Hawley, Louise, Richard J. Ziegler, and Benjamin L. Clarke. *Microbiology and Immunology*. Lippincott Williams & Wilkins, 2013.

Male, David K., et al., editors. *Immunology*. Elsevier/Saunders, 2013.

Murray, Patrick R., Ken S. Rosenthal, and Michael A. Pfaller. *Medical Microbiology*. 9th ed., Mosby/Elsevier, 2020.

Paul, William E., editor. *Immunology: Recognition and Response*. W. H. Freeman, 1991.

Playfair, J. H. L., and B. M. Chain. *Immunology at a Glance*. 10th ed., Wiley-Blackwell, 2013.

Punt, Jenni, et al. editors. *Kuby Immunology*. 8th ed., W. H. Freeman, 2018.

Hybridomas and Monoclonal Antibodies

Category: Immunogenetics
Anatomy or system affected: Blood, brain, eyes, gastrointestinal system, immune system, intestines, liver, lungs, lymphatic system, mouth, respiratory system, skin, throat
Specialties and related fields: Bacteriology, dermatology, epidemiology, gastroenterology, gynecology, hematology, immunology, internal medicine, microbiology, neurology, oncology, ophthalmology, osteopathic medicine, otorhinolaryngology, pathology, pharmacology, proctology, psychiatry, public health, pulmonary medicine, virology
Definition: Fusion of immortal mouse cancer cells with antibody-producing B cells to produce an immortal hybrid cell that secretes one type of antibody in perpetual culture.

KEY TERMS

antibody: a protein produced by plasma cells (matured B cells) that binds specifically to an antigen

antigen: a foreign molecule or microorganism that stimulates an immune response in an animal

antisera: a complex mixture of heterogeneous antibodies that react with various parts of an antigen; each type of antibody protein in the mixture is made by a different type (clone) of plasma cell

plasmacytoma: a plasma cell tumor that can be grown continuously in a culture

SIGNIFICANCE

In 1975, Georges Köhler and Cesar Milstein reported that fusion of spleen cells from an immunized mouse with a cultured plasmacytoma cell line resulted in the formation of hybrid cells called "hybridomas" that secreted the antibody molecules that the spleen cells had been stimulated to produce. Clones of hybrid cells producing antibodies with a desired specificity are called "monoclonal antibodies" and can be used as a reliable and continuous source of that antibody. These well-defined and specific antibody reagents have a wide range of biological uses, including basic research, industrial applications, and medical diagnostics and therapeutics.

A NEW WAY TO MAKE ANTIBODIES
Because of their specificity, antisera have long been used as biological reagents to detect or isolate molecules of interest. They have been useful for biological research, industrial separation applications, clinical assays, and immunotherapy. One disadvantage of conventional antisera is that they are heterogeneous collections of antibodies against a variety of antigenic determinants present on the antigen that has elicited the antibody response. In an animal from which antisera is collected, the mixture of antibodies changes with time, so that the types and relative amounts of specific antibodies are different in samples taken at different times. This variation makes standardization of reagents difficult and means that the amount of characterized and standardized antisera is limited to that available from a particular sample.

The publication of a report by Georges Köhler and Cesar Milstein in the journal *Nature* in 1975 describing production of the first monoclonal antibodies provided a method to produce continuous supplies of antibodies against specific antigenic determinants. Milstein's laboratory had been conducting basic research on the synthesis of immunoglobulin chains in plasma cells, mature B cells that produce large amounts of a single type of immunoglobulin. As a model system, they were using rat and mouse plasma cell tumors (plasmacytomas). Prior to 1975, Köhler and Milstein had completed a series of experiments in which they had fused rat and mouse plasmacytomas and determined that the light and heavy chains from the two species associate randomly to form the various possible combinations. In these experiments they used mutant plasmacytoma lines that would not grow in selective culture media, while the hybrid cells complemented each other's deficiencies and multiplied in culture.

After immunizing mice with sheep red blood cells (SRBC), Köhler and Milstein removed the spleen cells from the immunized mice and fused them with a mouse plasmacytoma cell line. Again, the selective media did not allow unfused plasmacytomas to grow, and unfused spleen cells lasted for only a short time in culture so that only hybrids between plasmacytoma cells and spleen cells grew as hybrids. These hybrid plasmacytomas have come to be termed hybridomas.

Shortly after the two types of cells are fused by incubation with a fusing agent such as polyethylene glycol, they are plated out into a series of hundreds of small wells so that only a limited number of hybrids grow out together in the same well. Depending on the frequency of hybrids and the number of wells used, it is possible to distribute the cells so that each hybrid cell grows up in a separate cell culture well.

On the basis of the number of spleen cells that would normally be making antibodies against SRBC after mice have been immunized with them, the investigators expected that one well in about 100,000 or more might have a clone of hybrid cells making antibody that reacted against this antigen. The

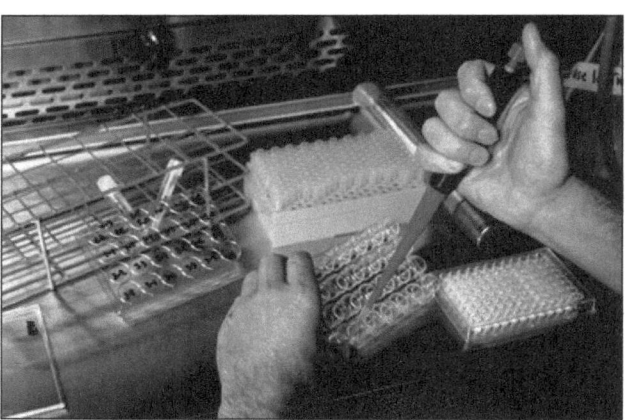
Monoclonal antibodies. Photo by Linda Bartlett, via Wikimedia Commons.

supernatants (liquid overlying settled material) from hundreds of wells were tested, and the large majority were found to react with the immunizing antigen. Further work with other antigens confirmed that a significant fraction of hybrid cells formed with spleen cells of immunized mice produce antibodies reacting with the antigen recently injected into the mouse. The production of homogeneous antibodies from clones of hybrid cells thus became a practical way to obtain reliable supplies of well-defined immunological reagents.

The antibodies can be collected from the media in which the cells are grown, or the hybridomas can be injected into mice so that larger concentrations of monoclonal antibodies can be collected from fluid that collects in the abdominal cavity of the animals.

SPECIFIC ANTIBODIES AGAINST ANTIGEN MIXTURES
One advantage of separating an animal's antibody response into individual antibody components by hybridization and separation of cells derived from each fusion event is that antibodies that react with individual antigenic components can be isolated even when the mouse is immunized with a complex mixture of antigens. For example, human tumor cells injected into a mouse stimulate the production of many different types of antibodies. A few of these antibodies may react specifically with tumor cells or specific types of human cells, but, in a conventional antisera, these antibodies would be mixed with other antibodies that react with any human cell and would not be easily separated from them. If the tumor cells are injected and hybridomas are made and screened to detect antibodies that react with tumor cells and not with most normal cells, it is possible to isolate antibodies that are useful for detection and characterization of specific types of tumor cells. Similar procedures can also be used to make antibodies against a single protein after the mouse has been immunized with this protein included in a complex mixture of other biological molecules such as a cell extract.

Following the first report of monoclonal antibodies, biologists began to realize the implications of being able to produce a continuous supply of antibodies with selected and well-defined reactivity patterns. There was discussion of "magic bullets" that would react specifically with and carry specific cytotoxic agents to tumor cells without adverse effects on normal cells. Biologists working in various experimental systems realized how specific and reliable sources of antibody reagent might contribute to their investigations, and entrepreneurs started several biotechnology companies to develop and apply monoclonal antibody methods. This initial enthusiasm was quickly moderated as some of the technical difficulties involved in production and use of these antibodies became apparent; with time, however, many of the projected advantages of these reagents have become a reality.

MONOCLONAL REAGENTS
A survey of catalogs of companies selling products used in biological research confirms that many of the conventional antisera commonly used as research reagents have been replaced with monoclonal antibodies. These products are advantageous to the suppliers, being produced in constant supply with standardized protocols from hybrid cells, and the users, who receive well-characterized reagents with known specificities free of other antibodies that could produce extraneous and unexpected reactions when used in some assay conditions. Antibodies are available against a wide range of biomolecules reflecting current trends in research; examples include antibodies against cytoskeletal proteins, protein kinases, and oncogene proteins, gene products involved in the transition of normal cells to cancer cells such as those involved in apoptosis.

Immunologists were among the first to take advantage of monoclonal antibody technology. They were able to use them to "trap" the spleen cells making antibodies against small, well-defined molecules called "haptens" and to then characterize the antibodies produced by the hybridomas. This enabled them to define classes of antibodies made against specific antigenic determinants and to derive information about the structure of the antibody-binding sites and how they are related to the determinants they bind. Other investigators produced antibodies that reacted specifically against subsets of lymphocytes playing specific roles in the immune responses of animals and humans. These reagents were then used to study the roles that these subsets of immune cells play in responses to various types of antigens.

Antibodies that react with specific types of immune cells have also been used to modulate the immune response. For example, antibodies that react with lymphocytes that would normally react with a transplanted tissue or organ can be used to deplete these cells from the circulation and thus reduce their response against the transplanted tissue.

MONOCLONAL ANTIBODIES AS DIAGNOSTIC REAGENTS

Monoclonal antibodies have been used as both in vitro and in vivo diagnostic reagents. By the 1980s, many clinical diagnostic tests such as assays for hormone or drug levels relied upon antisera as detecting reagents. Antibodies reacting with specific types of bacteria and viruses have also been used to classify infections so that the most effective treatment can be determined. In the case of production of antibodies for typing microorganisms, it has frequently been easier to make type-specific monoclonal antibodies than it had been to produce antisera that could be used to identify the same microorganisms.

Companies supplying these diagnostic reagents have gradually switched over to the use of monoclonal antibody products, thus facilitating the standardization of the reactions and the protocols used for the clinical tests. The reproducibility of the assays and the reagents has made it possible to introduce some of these tests that depend upon measurement of concentrations of substances in urine as kits that can be used by consumers in their own homes. Kits have been made available for testing glucose levels of diabetics, for pregnancy, and for the presence of certain drugs.

Although the much-hoped-for "magic bullet" that would eradicate cancer has not been found, there are several antibodies in use for tumor detection and for experimental forms of cancer therapy. Monoclonal antibodies that react selectively with cancer cells but not normal cells can be used to deliver cytotoxic molecules to the cancer cells. Monoclonal reagents are also used to deliver isotopes that can be used to detect the presence of small concentrations of cancer cells that would not normally be found until the tumors grew to a larger size.

Since 1986, when the Food and Drug Administration (FDA) approved the first therapeutic monoclonal antibody for allograft rejection in renal transplants, more than thirty other monoclonal antibodies have been approved, and hundreds more are undergoing clinical trials. Most of these are used in the treatment of cancers or autoimmune diseases such as Crohn's disease or rheumatoid arthritis. During this time, monoclonals have been particularly effective in the treatment of Hodgkin's lymphoma and other lymphoid malignancies.

HUMAN MONOCLONAL ANTIBODIES

Initially, the majority of monoclonal antibodies made against human antigens were mouse antibodies derived from the spleens of immunized mice. When administered to humans in clinical settings, the disadvantage of the animal origin of the antibodies soon became apparent. The human immune system recognized the mouse antibodies as foreign proteins and produced an immune response against them, limiting their usefulness. In addition, the mouse antibodies were unable to carry out certain immune functions such as effectively binding to human Fc receptors. Even when the initial response to an antibody's administration was positive, the immune reaction against the foreign protein quickly limited its effectiveness. To avoid this problem, human monoclonal antibodies have been developed using several methods. The first is the hybridization of human lymphocytes stimulated to produce antibodies against the antigen of interest with mouse plasmacytomas or later with human plasmacytoma cell lines. This method has been used successfully, although it is limited by the ability to obtain human B cells or plasma cells stimulated against specific antigens, because it is not possible to give an individual a series of immunizations and then remove stimulated cells from the spleen. Limited success has resulted from the fusion of circulating lymphocytes from immunized individuals or fusion of lymphocytes that have been stimulated by the antigen in cell cultures. Investigators have reported some success in making antitumor monoclonal antibodies by fusing lymph node cells from cancer patients with plasmacytoma cell lines and screening for antibodies that react with the tumor cells.

There has also been some success at "humanizing" mouse antibodies using molecular genetic techniques. In this process, the portion of the genes that make the variable regions of the mouse antibody protein that reacts with a particular antigen is spliced in to replace the variable region of a human antibody molecule being produced by a cultured human cell or human hybridoma. What is produced is a human antibody protein that has the binding specificity of the original mouse monoclonal antibody. When such antibodies are used for human therapy, the reaction against the injected protein is reduced compared to the administration of the whole mouse antibody molecules. A variation on this method is the production of chimeric antibodies by exchanging the variable domain from a mouse antibody with

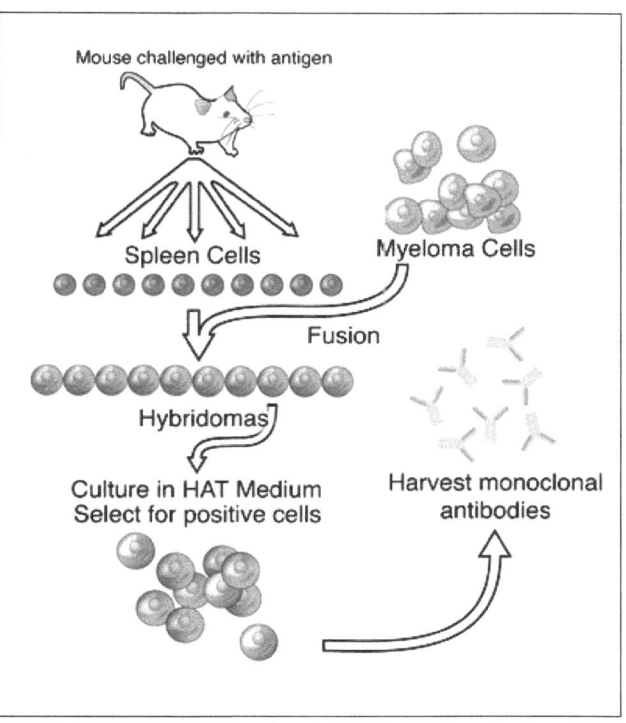

Overview of hybridoma technology and monoclonal antibody creation. By Adenosine (Own work), via Wikimedia Commons.

the desired specificity with the human variable domain from a human antibody of the desired Ig class.

Another application of antibody engineering is the production of bispecific antibodies. This has been accomplished by fusing two hybridomas making antibodies against two different antigens. The result is an antibody that contains two types of binding sites and thus binds and cross-links two antigens, bringing them into close proximity to each other.

RECOMBINANT ANTIBODIES

Advances in molecular genetic techniques and in the characterization of the genes for the variable and constant regions of antibody molecules have made it possible to produce new forms of monoclonal antibodies. The generation of these recombinant antibodies is not dependent upon the immunizing of animals but on the utilization of combinations of antibody genes generated using the in vitro techniques of genetic engineering. Geneticists discovered that genes inserted into the genes for fibers expressed on the surface of bacterial viruses called "bacteriophages" are expressed and detectable as new protein sequences on the surface of the bacteriophage. Investigators working with antibody genes found that they could produce populations of bacteriophage expressing combinations of antibody-variable genes. Molecular genetic methods have made it possible to generate populations of bacteriophage expressing different combinations of antibody-variable genes with frequencies approaching the number present in an individual mouse or human immune system. The population of bacteriophage can be screened for binding to an antigen of interest, and the bacteriophage expressing combinations of variable regions binding to the antigen can be multiplied and then used to generate recombinant antibody molecules in culture.

As phage display technology was further developed and useful antibodies derived, it was found that random mutagenesis of the isolated antibody gene could also be used to derive a panel of mutant binding sites with higher affinity binding than the antibody detected in the original screening.

Recombinant deoxyribonucleic acid (DNA) technology has also made it possible to modify the procedures for immunization and production of human monoclonal bodies. A process referred to as DNA immunization involves introducing the gene for the target antigen in a form that results in the expression of the protein and an immune response against it. Also mice that have had their own immunoglobulin genes replaced by the corresponding human genes can be immunized to produce human monoclonal antibodies.

Researchers have also experimented with introducing antibody genes into plants, resulting in plants that produce quantities of the specific antibodies. Hybridomas or bacteriophages expressing specific antibodies of interest may be a potential source of the antibody gene sequences introduced into these plant antibody factories.

MONOCLONAL ANTIBODIES IN PROTEOMICS

Coincident with the development of genomic methods for determination of gene expression at the RNA level has been an interest in detection of relative levels of protein expression. Incorporation of monoclonal antibodies into microarrays that allow the comparison of the expression of proteins from different cells or tissues has since been developed and will likely continue to be important in both basic research and clinical assays.

—*Roger H. Kennett, PhD*

Further Information

Chames, Patrick, et al. "Therapeutic Antibodies: Successes, Limitations, and Hopes for the Future." *British Journal of Pharmacology,* vol. 157, no. 2, 2009, pp. 220-33.

Gibbs, W. W. "Plantibodies: Human Antibodies Produced by Field Crops Enter Clinical Trials." *Scientific American*, vol. 277, no. 5, 1997, p. 44.

Hoogenboom, H. R. "Designing and Optimizing Library Selection Strategies for Generating High-Affinity Antibodies." *Trends in Biotechnology,* vol. 15, no. 2, 1997, pp. 62-70.

Kontermann, Roland, and Stefan Dübel, editors. *Antibody Engineering*. 2nd ed., Springer, 2013.

Nevoltris, Damien, and Patrick Chames, editors. *Antibody Engineering: Methods and Protocols*. 3rd ed., Humana Press, 2018.

Ossipow, Vincent, and Nicolas Fischer. *Monoclonal Antibodies: Methods and Protocols*. 2nd ed., Humana, 2014.

Rüker, Florian, and Gordana Wozniak-Knopp, editors. *Introduction to Antibody Engineering*. Springer, 2020.

Springer, Timothy. *Hybridoma Technology in the Biosciences and Medicine*. Springer, 2013.

Steinitz, Michael, editor. *Human Monoclonal Antibodies: Methods and Protocols*. 2nd ed., Humana Press, 2019.

Stigbrand, T., et al. "Twenty Years with Monoclonal Antibodies: State of the Art." *Acta Oncologica*, vol. 35, no. 3, 1996, pp. 259-65.

Van de Winkel, J. G., et al. "Immunotherapeutic Potential of Bispecific Antibodies." *Immunology Today*, vol. 18, 1997, pp. 562-74.

Immune response

Category: Biology
Anatomy or system affected: Blood, cells, circulatory system, glands, liver, lymphatic system, spleen
Specialties and related fields: Cytology, hematology, immunology, microbiology, preventive medicine, serology
Definition: A system that includes the spleen, thymus, lymphatic system, and specialized cells and protects the body from foreign substances.

KEY TERMS

antibody: any of the proteins produced in the body during an immune response; recognizes and attacks foreign antigen substances

antigen: a substance within the human body recognized as foreign either by antibodies or by special immune cells; the cause behind the stimulation of the immune response

autoimmunity: an abnormal immune reaction against antigens

immunosuppression: a decrease in the effectiveness of the immune system

pathogen: any disease-causing organism, including a virus, bacterium, protozoan, mold or yeast, or other parasites

STRUCTURE AND FUNCTIONS

The immune system is capable of recognizing and identifying many different substances foreign to the human body. For the immune system to function properly, it must receive, interpret, and transmit large amounts of information about invaders outside or within the body. These constant and everchanging threats to the body must be met and destroyed by one complex system—namely, the human immune system. Many organs and parts of the body play a significant role in maintaining resistance; some have more important roles than others, but all parts must work in unison. The circulatory and lymphatic systems, along with specific organs, are of primary importance in the overall workings of the immune system.

Blood. Besides the outer protective layer of the skin and mucous membranes, the first line of defense in the immune system includes the blood in the circulatory system. About 50 percent of human blood is plasma. Plasma contains mainly water, but also proteins, carbohydrates, vitamins, hormones, and cellular waste. The other half of blood is composed of white cells, red cells, and platelets. The red blood cells, called "erythrocytes," are responsible for moving oxygen from the lungs to the other parts of the body. Special cells called "platelets" or "thrombocytes" enable the blood to form clots, thus preventing severe bleeding. An unborn child produces red and white blood cells in the spleen and liver, while a newborn makes blood cells in the center of bones, called the "marrow." After maturity, the bone marrow produces all red and most white blood cells. Although the red cells and platelets are vital, the white cells play a major role in the immune system.

In a broad sense, white blood cells surround and engulf foreign matter and adjacent dying cells in a process called "phagocytosis." The function is possible since the white blood cells can move, unlike red corpuscles, by pushing their bodies out and pulling forward. Red corpuscles flow with the blood within the circulatory system. White blood cells flow within the bloodstream but move in the lymph vessels, where they work to defend the body against diseases. White blood cells can destroy some of the bacteria and foreign matter they engulf. However, sometimes the corpuscle dies from the toxins produced by the bacteria. The resulting formation of pus is an accumulation of dead white blood cells.

Three major types of white blood cells, known collectively as leukocytes, are involved in immune responses. All three types of leukocytes, granulocytes, monocytes, and lymphocytes, arise from areas in either bone marrow, the spleen, or the liver.

The granulocytes are about twice the size of a red blood cell, originate from red bone marrow, and live only about twelve hours. Under the classification of granulocytes, distinct cells have different structures, sizes, and shapes. These specialized granulocytes include neutrophils, eosinophils, and basophils. None of these cells has a specific memory for future immune responses. Neutrophils eat and digest small foreign matter with the help of special enzymes. Between 40 and 75 percent of the white blood cells in the human body are neutrophils. When these highly mobile neutrophil cells arrive at an injury site, they release their enzymes and degrade the surrounding tissues. Eosinophils are similar to neutrophils but seem specialized in fighting infection caused by parasites because of the array of toxic proteins they secrete. They are also effective against fungal, bacterial, viral, or protozoan infections. Basophils are smaller cells that account for less than 1 percent of the white blood cells found in the blood. After being born in the bone marrow, they travel throughout the body playing roles in fighting fungal and worm infections and allergies. They also regulating immune responses and prevent coagulation by releasing heparin. Basophils cannot engulf and destroy foreign matter.

The second group of leukocytes includes the monocytes, the largest cells found in the blood.

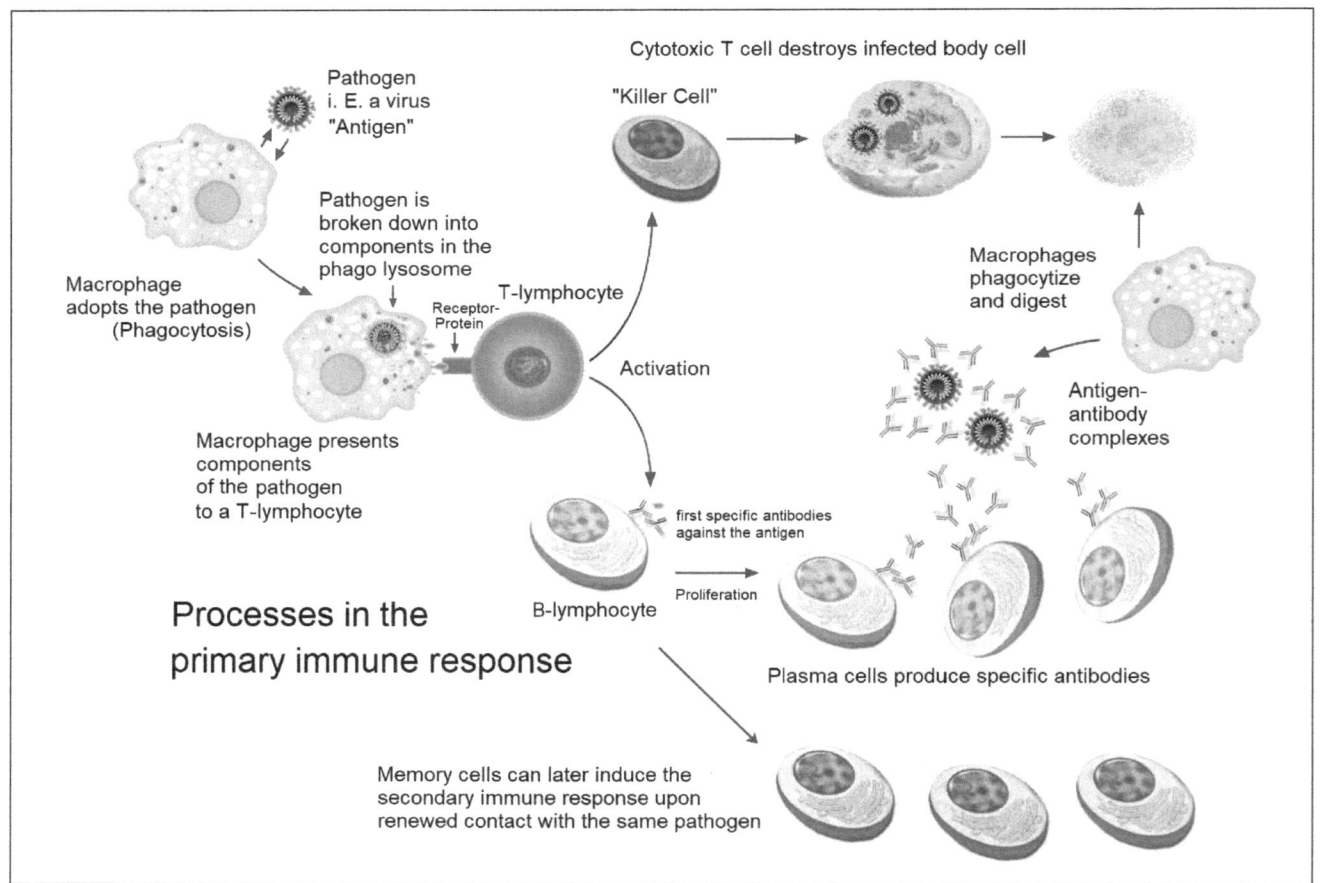

Overview of the processes involved in the primary immune response. Image by Sciencia58, via Wikimedia Commons. [CC 4.0].

Monocytes are two to three times as large as red cells, yet they are not very numerous, making up 3 to 9 percent of all the leukocytes in the blood. After only a few days in the blood, they move to areas between tissues. Over months or years, the monocytes enlarge ten times in size to specialize in phagocytosis. After this growth, they are called "macrophages." They are also called "terminal cells" since they cannot divide and thus do not reproduce.

The third type of leukocyte, and the most complex white blood cells, are called "lymphocytes" because they come from the lymph system and bone marrow. The T lymphocytes can differentiate into helper, killer, and suppressor cells. Besides recognizing foreign matter precisely, they can live freely in the blood, grow larger and divide, and then change back to their original form after working against the invader. Lymphocytes circulate throughout the body, moving from the bloodstream through the lymph fluid and into the blood. The two major types of lymphocytes are T lymphocytes (also called "T cells") and B lymphocytes (also called "B cells"). Both T and B cells can recognize foreign matter and hook onto it. Some of these special "memory" cells remain in the body for life, preventing a specific invader from causing illness when reencountered in the future. These specialized cells must have a way to travel through the body; one of these transport systems is the lymphatic system.

The lymphatic system. This system is a closed network of vessels that help circulate fluids from the body and return them to the bloodstream. The lymphatic system also defends against disease-causing foreign materials, known as "antigens." The smallest components of the lymph system are the lymphatic capillaries that run parallel to the blood capillaries. The fluid, or lymph, within lymphatic capillaries comes from the liquid that moved across the cell membranes from tissues throughout the body. These capillaries merge into larger lymphatic vessels that fuse into a collecting area called a "lymph node." The lymph fluid is drained into trunks that join one of two collecting ducts. The larger left thoracic duct collects lymph from the lower part of the abdomen, the legs, and the left side of the upper body before emptying into a vein near the neck and shoulder. The right lymphatic duct does the same for the right side of the upper body. After leaving the collecting ducts, the lymph fluid becomes part of the blood plasma in the veins and returns to the right atrium of the heart. Lymph does not flow like blood in veins and arteries; instead, it is controlled by muscular activity.

The spleen. This lymphatic organ is in the upper left abdominal cavity, behind the stomach, and under the diaphragm. The hollow spaces within the spleen are filled with blood, making it soft and elastic. The white blood cells in the lining of these open cavities engulf and destroy foreign materials, as well as damaged red blood cells that pass through the spleen.

The thymus. This gland lies between the lungs and above the heart, just behind the upper part of the breast bone. It contains many white cells; some are inactive, but others develop and leave the thymus to become functional in the immune system.

The liver. Well protected by the ribs, the liver sits in the upper right of the abdominal cavity below the diaphragm. Since it is the largest gland in the body, it plays a significant role in metabolism while also aiding the body's ability to clot blood. In addition, various liver cells, called "macrophages," help in destroying damaged red blood cells. The liver's connection to the immune system is its ability to destroy foreign substances through phagocytosis.

Bone marrow. Marrow is in the center of bones. There are two types of marrow, red or yellow marrow. Red marrow that aids in the formation of white and red blood cells. The yellow marrow stores fat and does not produce blood cells. Most white blood cells originate from bone marrow hematopoietic stem cells. After their birth in the bone marrow, a subset of lymphocytes travel through the bloodstream to the thymus gland. There, they undergo special processing that changes them into mature T lymphocytes (the letter *T* indicates that they came from the thymus gland). The other lymphocytes that do not reach the thymus after leaving the bone marrow are named B lymphocytes (*B* because they came from bone marrow). These B lymphocytes are abundant in lymph nodes, the spleen, bone marrow, secretory glands, intestinal lining, and reticuloendothelial tissue.

THE RESPONSES OF THE IMMUNE SYSTEM
Failures of the immune system can lead to devastating diseases, either because the immune system attacks itself or because it fails to defend against outside foreign antigen matter. An antigen can be any substance that stimulates the body to fight, ranging from a bacterial infection to the virus that causes acquired immunodeficiency syndrome (AIDS).

When the body fights against an antigen, the immune system can produce two types of response, either a cellular immune response or a humoral immune response. The cellular response involves specific cells that recognize, attack, and destroy the invading pathogen or antigen. It is the primary response against most viruses, fungi, parasitic organisms, and bacteria (for example, mycobacteria) and transplanted tissues. The humoral immune response, which consists of complement and antibodies, is the body's primary defense against most other bacteria. The two systems work together, however, communicating by complex chemical mediators.

Another way of looking at how the body fights to keep itself healthy is to separate the immune responses into either primary or secondary responses. The second time a given antigen enters the body, the immune system attacks it with the secondary immune response stored in special immune memory cells. The secondary immune response is faster and more extensive than the primary response. This immune memory is specifically designed for each antigen. It provides immunity to the wide variety of diseases and conditions to which one is exposed daily.

The body begins to build this memory before birth by inventorying all the molecules within the body. Foreign substances not in this memory are considered to be antigens, which will activate an immune response. When the immune system first encounters an antigen, it mounts a primary response that produces lymphocytes sensitized to the invader. Many B lymphocytes can respond to create the appropriate antibody molecules, which are then released into the lymph and transported to the blood. This process may last several weeks. During this primary immune response, the B cells and T cells serve as memory cells. Because immunological memory for the antigen is stored, if the immune system encounters this antigen in the future, the memory cells can react more quickly and effectively. In this secondary immune response, the antibodies are ready to respond by attaching to the surfaces of the antigens. There must be a specific type of antibody produced for every type of antigen. These new antibodies may survive only a few months, but the memory cells live much longer.

There are four main ways that antibodies help neutralize antigens. The antibody can pull together clusters of invading organisms to prevent them from spreading (agglutination). Second, when some antibodies bind to antigens, they activate blood proteins called the "complement system" to punch holes in the invader and destroy it. The antibody can also combine with the antigen, which makes it easier for leukocytes to destroy it. By covering the outside of viruses or toxins, antibodies can neutralize their harmful activity. Given the multifaceted utility of antibodies, it is essential to establish antibody memory. It is this particular memory that leads to future immunity.

These memory cells are responsible for the four different types of immunity, two are acquired actively, and two are acquired passively. The first type is naturally acquired active immunity, which results after exposure to a live pathogen that causes a disease. The second type, artificially acquired active immunity, is gained after a vaccination. The immune response is triggered after an injection of weakened or dead pathogens is received. However, the body does not suffer the severe symptoms of the disease. An example would be a smallpox vaccination. The third type of immunity is artificially acquired passive immunity, gained through an injection of prepared antibodies. This method is passive since another person made the antibodies (gamma-globulin). This type of immunity usually does not last more than a few weeks, and the person will be susceptible to that pathogen in the future. Naturally acquired passive immunity occurs when the antibodies pass to the fetus from the mother. This type of immunity only includes those antibodies available in the blood of the mother. This process gives an infant certain short-term immunities for the first year of life.

These types of immunity are usually desirable, but there are occasions when an immune response is unwanted, such as after an organ transplant. Tissue or organ transplantation from one person to another may cause the body to reject the foreign tissue, triggering an immune response and possibly destroying the new organ. Consequently, matching the tissue between the recipient and the donor may delay or even prevent the immunological rejection of the transplant. The transplant recipient also receives immunosuppressive drugs, including steroids, calcineurin inhibitors, and antiproliferative agents that interfere with their ability to form antibodies. Other medications, including daclizumab, basiliximab, rituximab, and antithymocyte globulin, can destroy the lymphocytes that help produce antibodies. Unfortunately, the recipient is often left unprotected against infections since the immune system is not functioning normally.

PERSPECTIVE AND PROSPECTS

In the same way that the discovery of penicillin shocked the world, immunology has created endless possibilities in medicine. When surgeons found that they could transplant an organ from one person to another, the interest in immunology exploded.

This field of medicine has discovered that several factors can diminish the power of the immune system. Improper diet, stress, disease, and excessive physical activity levels can depress the immune system. Other factors that can modify immunity include age, genetics, and metabolic and environmental factors. The susceptibility of the young and the very old to infections illustrate these anatomical, physiological, and microbial factors. For the young, the system is immature, while the aged have suffered a lifetime of assaults from pathogens. The impact of psychological stress is challenging to measure, yet it can negatively affect the immune system.

Unanswered questions remain about how the immune system relates to other body systems. The relationships among the brain and nervous system, hormones, and the respiratory system leave many areas ripe for further study.

Recent research has identified the significant importance of Class I major histocompatibility proteins (IMHCPs) in the cellular immune system. When disease-associated proteins occur in a cell, they are broken into pieces by its proteolytic machinery. I-MHCPs attach to antigen fragments and transport them to the cell surface. The I-MHCP/antigen complex is "presented" to the body's immune cells at the cell surface. The I-MHCPs holding an antigen fragment can attach to specific immature T cells. Once such a T cell and IMHCP-antigen complex hook up, the T cell divides vigorously. This critical link between the cellular immune system and I-MHCPs is illustrated by diseases like AIDS, which kills T cells.

Class II MHCPs (II-MHCPs) interact similarly in antibody production by the humoral immune system. Understanding the genes used in the production of the I-MHCPs and the IIMHCPs has led to methods to control their production, possibilities for the eventual cure of AIDS, emerging cancer treatments, and a better understanding of the production of antibodies.

Additional information is needed on defects in the system, as are explanations for its dysfunctions. With a more profound knowledge of immunology, it may be possible to conquer AIDS, allergies, and asthma and develop birth control methods based on the immune response. Doctors may cure cancer, diabetes, herpes, infertility, multiple sclerosis, and rheumatoid arthritis. The possibilities are endless and could also include perfecting transplants of organs and skin grafts and preventing congenital disabilities and even obesity. Those at risk for genetic disorders could be diagnosed through molecular diagnostic tests. Human gene therapy might even cure those with existing genetic conditions. Genetically engineered drugs and gene replacement therapy could relieve the stress on the human immune system. Until these methods become feasible, however, individuals must protect the natural immunity supplied by their bodies.

—Maxine M. Urton, PhD

Further Information

Adelman, Daniel C., et al., editors. *Manual of Allergy and Immunology*. 5th ed., Lippincott Williams & Wilkins, 2012.

Goering, Richard, et al. *Mims' Medical Microbiology and Immunology*. 6th ed., Elsevier, 2018.

Immune Web, www.*immuneweb*.org.

Janeway, Charles A., Jr., et al. *Immunobiology: The Immune System in Health and Disease*. 7th ed., Garland Science, 2007.

Male, David K., et al., editors. *Immunology*. 8th ed., Elsevier/Saunders, 2018.

Marieb, Elaine N., and Suzanne Keller. *Essentials of Human Anatomy and Physiology*. 12th ed., Pearson/Benjamin Cummings, 2017.

Martin, Seamus J., et al. *Roitt's Essential Immunology*. 13th ed., Blackwell, 2017.

Punt, Jenni, et al., editors. *Kuby Immunology*. 8th ed., W. H. Freeman, 2018.

Tortora, Gerard J., and Bryan Derrickson. *Principles of Anatomy and Physiology*. 16th ed., John Wiley & Sons, 2020.

Immune response to bacterial infections

Category: Immune response

Definition: The immune response is how the body recognizes and defends itself against infections, including bacterial infections. The more effective the body's immune response, the more successfully it combats the development and severity of infection. A breakdown of the immune response can have dire consequences.

KEY TERMS

adaptive immunity: acquired immunity to a previous infection or vaccination; involves specialized immune cells and antibodies that destroy foreign cells and remember what those substances look like to prevent future infection

antigen: a toxin or other foreign substance that induces an immune response in the body, especially the production of antibodies

antigen-presenting cells: type of immune cell that boosts immune responses by showing antigens on its surface to other cells of the immune system; a type of phagocyte

B lymphocyte: a type of white blood cell that makes antibodies; develops from stem cells in the bone marrow

helper T cells: a type of immune cell that stimulates killer T cells, macrophages, and B cells to make immune responses

killer T cells: a type of immune cell that can kill certain cells, including foreign cells, cancer cells, and cells infected with a virus; can be separated from other blood cells, grown in a laboratory, and given to patients

lymphocyte: a form of small leukocyte (white blood cell) occurring especially in the lymphatic system; includes natural killer cells, T cells, and B cells

macrophage: a type of white blood cell that surrounds and kills microorganisms, removes dead cells, and regulates the action of other immune cells

mucous membrane: the moist, inner lining of some organs and body cavities, such as the nose, mouth, lungs, and the stomach

neutrophil: the most abundant type of white blood cell; forms an essential part of the innate immune system

phagocyte: a type of immune cell that can surround and kill microorganisms, ingest foreign material, remove dead cells, and boost immune response; monocytes, macrophages, and neutrophils are all phagocytes

suppressor T cells: a lymphocyte that can suppress antibody production by other lymphoid cells; blocks the actions of other lymphocytes to keep the immune response from becoming overactive

T lymphocyte: a type of white blood cell important to adaptive immunity; searches out and destroys invading organisms

The immune system defends itself against infectious organisms (pathogens) such as bacteria by utilizing physical barriers that prevent bacteria from entering the body and detecting and eliminating bacteria after they enter the body. Cells, proteins, tissues, and organs work together in a coordinated response, the immune response, to defend against microorganisms.

When a bacterial infection develops, the immune system responds through a series of steps by activating specific cells and producing substances that recognize and react to invading microorganisms or antigens. Bacterial antigens are generally proteins present on the surface of a bacterium.

TYPES OF IMMUNITY

Physical barriers are the immune system's first line of defense. They comprise the skin, mucous membranes, mucus, and tears. Unless damaged through injury or other means, the skin generally protects against invasion by microorganisms. Mucous membranes (the linings of the mouth, nose, and eyelids) are effective barriers. They are generally coated with secretions, such as lysozyme, that fight microorganisms. Organisms that penetrate physical barriers are identified and eliminated by white blood cells and antibodies. Adaptive immunity, comprised of cell-mediated and antibody-mediated immunity, is an essential defense component against bacterial infection. In antibody-mediated or humoral immunity, the immune response is mediated by antibodies (immunoglobulins), specific proteins produced in response to antigens. Cell-mediated immunity is mediated by effector T cells (T lymphocytes).

CELLS INVOLVED IN AN IMMUNE RESPONSE

The immune system consists of a coordinated network of cells, tissues, and organs. White blood cells, or leukocytes, circulate and detect and destroy microbes. Two basic types of leukocytes are phagocytes and lymphocytes. Phagocytes ingest invading organisms, and lymphocytes help recognize invaders and eliminate them. The neutrophil is the most common type of phagocyte and primarily fights bacteria; infection generally triggers an increase in neutrophil numbers. Leukocytes circulate in the bloodstream to provide a coordinated effort for the immune system to monitor and protect against bacterial infection.

B and T lymphocytes (B and T cells) have separate functions: B cells seek targets and send defenses, and T cells, in various forms, destroy the invading organism. With stimulation by antigens, T cells comprise several forms, or classes, of effector T cells: killer (cytotoxic), helper, and suppressor.

Killer T cells destroy specific target cells. Helper T cells help other cells, such as B cells, produce antibodies; they also help activated killer T cells destroy foreign cells (macrophages), enabling the killer T cells to ingest foreign cells efficiently. T cells also produce cytokines that activate other cells. B cells have receptors on their surface, where antigens attach stimulate cells to become antibody-secreting cells.

PRIMARY AND SECONDARY IMMUNE RESPONSE

A primary immune response occurs the immune system encounters antigens. At subsequent encounters with the same antigens, a secondary immune response occurs. Before an infection, precursor T or B cells are present as resting cells. Still, the immune system activates T cells or triggers B lymphocytes to produce antibodies during an adaptive immune response. After initially encountering an antigen, sufficient amounts of antibody take several days to produce, with only small amounts formed during the first few days; circulating antibodies are undetectable until about one week after the initial encounter. The primary immune response is relatively slow, with antigens first needing to be recognized, processed, and presented by antigen-presenting cells. Antibody levels need to reach sufficient levels for the host to develop resistance (which may take several days or weeks).

A second encounter with microbial antigens leads to an accelerated immune response, called the "secondary or memory response." During the secondary response, memory B cells "remember" and rapidly recognize antigens. Memory B cells then multiply and change into plasma cells and secrete large amounts of antibodies in only one to two days. Similarly, memory T cells rapidly develop into effector cells. The secondary immune response is swift, efficient, and effective. This specific immune response prevents people from contracting certain diseases more than once.

ANTIGEN-PRESENTING CELLS

The primary immune response is initiated when an antigen penetrates epithelial surfaces and comes into contact with macrophages or other antigen-presenting cells. An antigen-presenting cell is usually either a macrophage or a dendritic cell. In combination with either a B or T cell, it is required for an immune response. Antigens, such as bacterial cells, are ingested and processed by antigen-presenting cells and then presented to lymphocytes to initiate the immune response.

Processing by macrophages results in the attachment of antigen fragments to cell surface molecules known as major histocompatibility complex (MHC). The macrophage presents the antigen-MHC complex to helper T cells, recognizing processed antigen and developing into effector T cells. When a macrophage presents antigen to a B cell, the B cell generates antibodies specific for that antigen.

CELL SIGNALING

Helper T cells provide signals, such as interleukins or cytokines that stimulate cells to proliferate and function more efficiently. The interaction between an antigen-presenting macrophage and a helper T cell results in secretion of interleukin-1 from macrophages that, in turn, stimulate helper T cells to mature and produce other cytokines, including interleukin-2 and -4. Interleukin-2 stimulates the proliferation of other T cells, and interleukin-4 causes B cells to develop into antibody-secreting plasma cells. Interleukin-2 also activates killer T cells to destroy cells with antigens on their surfaces. When interleukin-4 stimulates a B cell, the B cell grows and divides to form an army of identical B cells, each capable of producing large amounts of identical antibody molecules.

IMPACT

The immune system prevents and defends against bacterial infections. Antibody-mediated and cell-mediated immune responses are generated during almost all infections. Still, the magnitude and importance of each response vary, depending on the host and the infectious agent. As people age, they usually become immune to more microorganisms. The immune system comes into contact with increasing numbers of antigens throughout a person's life. In general, adults and teenagers tend to get fewer bacterial infections than younger children because their bodies have learned to recognize and immediately attack antigens to which they are exposed.

—*Catherine J. Walsh, PhD*

Further Information

Coico, Richard, and Geoffrey Sunshine. *Immunology: A Short Course*. 6th ed., Wiley-Blackwell, 2009. A clear and comprehensive introduction to essential topics in modern immunology.

DeFranco, Anthony L., Richard M. Locksley, and Miranda Robertson. *Immunity: The Immune Response in Infectious and Inflammatory Disease*. Oxford UP, 2007. An introduction for undergraduates and medical students to the immune response to infection. Includes chapters on the immune response to specific microorganisms.

Mak, Tak W., and Mary E. Saunders. *Primer to the Immune Response*. Academic Press/Elsevier, 2008. Provides an understandable introduction to immunology. A resource for college students, students studying medicine, and those in health professions.

IMMUNE RESPONSE TO FUNGAL INFECTIONS

Category: Immune response
Also known as: Mycoses

Anatomy or system affected: Blood, brain, eyes, gastrointestinal system, immune system, intestines, liver, lungs, lymphatic system, mouth, reproductive system, respiratory system, skin, throat

Specialties and related fields: Dermatology, gastroenterology, gynecology, hematology, immunology, internal medicine, microbiology, neurology, oncology, ophthalmology, otorhinolaryngology, pathology, pulmonary medicine

Definition: The immune response is how the body recognizes and defends itself against invading microbes, including fungi. The more effective the body's immune response, the more successfully it combats the development and severity of infection. A breakdown of the immune response can have dire consequences.

KEY TERMS

complement: a complex of more than thirty proteins in the blood that coordinate to attack invading cells and destroy them

fungal spores: a microscopic body, usually the product of sexual or asexual reproduction, that is specially adapted for dispersal, survival, extended periods of dormancy

neutropenia: an abnormally low number of neutrophils in the blood

neutrophils: the most abundant white blood cell in the bloodstream, filled with microscopic granules, that gobble up and digest invading microorganisms and debris

BASIC IMMUNE SYSTEM COMPONENTS

Skin and mucous membranes are the first line of defense against microbes. If these are penetrated, the body's immune response becomes active. Lymphocytes, specialized white blood cells, react to the presence of antigens on the surface of invading fungal spores or molds. The two major types of lymphocytes are T cells (T lymphocytes) and B cells (B lymphocytes). T cells attack antigens directly. B cells produce antibodies, circulating proteins that bind to specific antigens and make it easier for immune cells to destroy the antigens.

Other contributors to the immune response to fungal infections include macrophages and other phagocytes, which are blood cells that surround and digest foreign bodies; complement, which are specialized proteins in the blood that act in sequence to mediate inflammation and the immune response; and neutrophils, which are circulating white blood cells that play a significant role in destroying fungal pathogens.

Lymphocytes may develop a "memory" of invading antigens they encounter. This allows the immune system to respond faster and more efficiently to future exposure to the same antigens. For superficial, noninvasive infections, this memory is not long-lasting. Hence, a recurrence of infection often occurs after treatment has been discontinued.

IMMUNE RESPONSE TO FUNGI IN HEALTHY PERSONS

Humans inhale or ingest thousands of fungal spores every day. Of the more than 200,000 species of fungi, fewer than 100 are associated with human infection. In healthy persons, most potentially pathogenic fungi produce mild, even subclinical, transitory infection, if any infection. In these situations, the body's immune system has responded quickly and effectively to the pathogens.

Some fungal pathogens, however, challenge the body's immune response, even in healthy persons. *Histoplasma capsulatum*, in its yeast form, can be resistant to killing by macrophages. *H. capsulatum* can multiply within macrophages. Progressive pulmonary infection or disseminated disease may result. *Candida albicans* may bind to complement, and by so doing, can short-circuit the immune response. *Coccidioides immitis* contains a substance in its wall that resists its destruction, a critical step in the immune response. *Cryptococcus neoformans*, unlike other pathogenic fungi, is an encapsulated yeast. The capsule helps to impair the destruction of the fungus by phagocytes. Despite setbacks by such challenges, in most healthy persons, the immune response recoups, with T-cell-mediated responses and the proliferation of neutrophils playing a significant role.

With most fungal pathogens, antibodies do not contribute significantly to the immune response. *C. neoformans* is an exception, so much so that rising titers of antibodies against *C. neoformans* are evidence of recovery from illness. In contrast, high titers of *C. immitis*-specific antibodies are associated with the dissemination and a worsening clinical course.

IMMUNE RESPONSE TO FUNGI IN IMMUNOCOMPROMISED PERSONS

Invasive fungal infections are a significant threat to immunocompromised persons. Both underlying disease and therapy can compromise the immune response and cause it to malfunction, resulting in an increased risk for severe and systemic fungal infections. Leukemia, diabetes ketoacidosis, sarcoidosis, chronic granulomatous disease, and acquired immunodeficiency syndrome (AIDS) are diseases that directly impact the functioning of the immune response. Leukemia can severely deplete neutrophils, resulting in neutropenia, a low level of circulating neutrophils. Diabetes ketoacidosis impairs lymphocytes by increasing serum acidity. The lesions caused by sarcoidosis and chronic granulomatous disease interfere with the functioning of macrophages. The human immunodeficiency virus (HIV) causes AIDS by attacking and destroying helper T cells. Consequently, T-cell-mediated immunity is compromised.

Agents used to treat cancer and AIDS or suppress rejection of solid or stem-cell transplants and high-dose, long-term therapy with corticosteroids increases the risk for severe and systemic fungal infections by suppressing the immune response. In particular, they cause neutropenia and depression of the T-cell-mediated immune response. Neutropenia is a significant contributor to the emergence of disseminated candidiasis and severe aspergillosis, zygomycosis, and hyalohyphomycosis (caused by *Fusarium* species). High-dose, long-term use of corticosteroids impairs both macrophage and neutrophil function. This contributes to the development of severe aspergillosis, cryptococcosis, and zygomycosis (also called "mucormycosis").

IMPACT

With the increase in immunocompromised persons from disease (such as AIDS) and treatment (such as immunosuppressive chemotherapy), fungal infections have become a major cause of morbidity and mortality. These infections include particularly virulent strains and fungi rarely observed as pathogenic in the past. A greater understanding of the factors contributing to the breakdown of the immune response in these situations has become critical to controlling these opportunistic infections.

—*Ernest Kohlmetz, MA*

Further Information

Kavanaugh, Kevin, editor. *New Insights in Medical Mycology*. Springer, 2007.

Ryan, Kenneth J., and George Ray. *Sherris Medical Microbiology: An Introduction to Infectious Diseases*. 5th ed., McGraw-Hill Medical, 2010.

Shoman, Shmuel, and Stuart M. Levitz. "The Immune Response to Fungal Infections." *British Journal of Haematology*, vol. 129, 2005, pp. 569-82.

Immune response to viral infections

Category: Immune response
Definition: The immune response is how the body recognizes and defends itself against infections, including viral infections. The more effective the body's immune response, the more successfully it combats the development and severity of infection. A breakdown of the immune response can have dire consequences.

KEY TERMS

apoptosis: the death of cells which occurs as a normal and controlled part of organism growth or development

cellular response: does not involve antibodies; utilizes the activation of phagocytes, antigen-sensitized cytotoxic T cells and the release of cytokines in response to an antigen

humoral response: targets pathogens circulating in bodily fluids, or "humors"; involves the transformation of B lymphocytes into plasma cells that produce and secrete antibodies to a specific antigen

interferon: proteins made by lymphocytes released in response to a viral infection; part of a group of cytokines that "interfere" with viral replication

cytotoxic T-cells: a type of lymphocyte that kills foreign cells, cancer cells, and virally-infected cells

natural killer cells: a type of white blood cell with enzymes that can kill tumor cells or cells infected with a virus

Viral infections are caused by viral particles that replicate in the host cell. These viral particles then produce more genetic material for new particles and incorporate their genetic material into the host cell's genome. As part of its immune response, the human immune system attacks these viral particles to undermine their effect on the body.

Viruses are fought with specific and nonspecific mechanisms, involving either a humoral or cellular response. These two immune responses involve the formation of specific antibodies generated to kill viral antigens, the production of interferon by host cells to inhibit viral function, and the production of natural killer cells that recognize and kill the virus.

SPECIFIC TYPES

Humoral immune response. A humoral (body fluid) response to viral infection blocks or neutralizes the viral particles' ability to infect a host cell. The immunoglobulin genes in the human immune system are integrally involved in this process. When viruses infect a human host cell, they are considered foreign antigens. The human host cell will then generate antibodies that recognize the specific antigen. Once an antibody is formed, it will continue to replicate and attack the antigen, thereby neutralizing the viral impact on the host cell.

Cellular immune response. Cellular response to viral infection kills the virus by attacking proteins that reside on viral cell surfaces, such as glycoproteins, or by attacking core proteins of the virus. This attack is made by T-cell lymphocytes that will recognize the cell surface proteins of a virus. The killer T cells will destroy the cell and the virus in the cell. Another cellular response is the production of interferons, which are hormones produced by the body when viruses are present.

SPECIFIC METHODS

Interferons. Interferons (IFNs) are proteins made by lymphocytes produced in the human immune system released in response to a viral infection. IFNs are part of a group of cytokines that "interfere" with viral replication within the human host cell. They also activate other immune cells, such as natural killer cells and macrophages, and increase the recognition of viral infections for other immune cells to respond. Before a virus kills a human cell, it first produces and releases IFNs. These IFNs will then communicate with neighboring host cells to set off a chain reaction to produce and release protein factors called "interferon-stimulated genes," which will fight the virus.

Cytotoxic T-cell lymphocytes. Cytotoxic T-cell lymphocytes (CTLs) are virus-specific cells that recognize specific viral antigens that have been synthesized or produced within a human cell. These cells are located on the cell surface on virtually all somatic cells in the human body, so they can respond to practically all the viral antigens it recognizes. CTLs can destroy these viral particles. However, CTLs, in the process of destroying viral particles, also destroy the involved human cell, which could lead to more damage and injury to the human body. Liver damage, for example, is caused by the virus-specific CTL rather than by the virus itself in the case of hepatitis B infection.

Natural killer cells. Antidependent cell-mediated cytotoxicity (ADCC) is a mechanism in the human immune system and part of cell-mediated immunity that involves effector cells to lyse or kill a pathogen (such as a virus) that antibodies have bound. Thus, as part of the humoral immune response, antibodies are released to bind to a viral particle, thereby allowing other cells in the immune system to attach to the antibody-antigen complex and destroy it directly.

One ADCC method includes activating natural killer (NK) cells that recognize part of the antibody attached to the virus. NK cells are large granular lymphocytes produced by the immune system that make up approximately 2 to 5 percent of peripheral blood lymphocytes. Once attached to the viral-antibody complex, these NK cells release cytokines, such as interferons and cytotoxic granules, that enter the target cell and promote cell death by triggering the apoptosis (regulated cell death) process. This process is similar but independent of responses by CTLs.

IMPACT

All living organisms, including humans, have to develop protective mechanisms against infectious organisms, including viruses if they are to survive. The complexity of the many infectious particles found on Earth has forced the human body to develop numerous complicated methods to fight these foreign substances. These methods, which include producing and releasing vast amounts of specific and nonspecific proteins to fight infection, define the immune response.

—*Susan M. Zneimer, PhD, FACMG*

Further Information

Coffin, J. M., S. H. Hughes, and H. E. Varmus, editors. *Retroviruses*. Cold Spring Harbor Laboratory Press, 2002. Also available at www.ncbi.nlm.nih.gov/books/nbk19403. This volume is a significant source of information on retroviruses, their classification, production, and replication; it also examines how retroviruses infect host cells.

Koyoma, Shohei, et al. "Innate Immune Response to Viral Infection." *Cytokine*, vol. 43, no. 3, 2008, pp. 336-41. A review of the different types of immune response to virus infections, including the involvement of immune receptors, the recognition of viruses, signaling pathways and communication for immune response, and the factors inhibiting host immune response.

Lane, Thomas, editor. *Chemokines and Viral infection*. Springer, 2006. This book examines the functional roles of chemokines and their receptors in the immune response against well-known viral pathogens.

Murphy, Kenneth, Paul Travers, and Mark Walport. *Janeway's Immunobiology*. 7th ed., Garland Science, 2008. The standard textbook in graduate and medical-school immunology courses because of its clear writing style, organization, and scientific accuracy. Includes color illustrations.

Nathanson, Neal, et al. *Viral Pathogenesis and Immunity*. 2nd ed., Academic Press/Elsevier, 2007. A compilation of articles on all significant viral infections that includes discussions of pathogenesis, host response, virus-host interactions, and the control of viruses.

Stetson D. B., and R. Medzhitov. "Type I Interferons in Host Defense." *Immunity*, vol. 25, 2006, pp. 373-81. Summarizes the various roles that interferons play in the immune response to pathogens. Discusses the classification of interferons and their role in the viral response.

IMMUNIZATION AND INFECTIOUS DISEASE

Category: Prevention
Also known as: Vaccination
Anatomy or system affected: Blood, immune system, lymphatic system
Specialties and related fields: Allergist, epidemiology, hematology, immunology, microbiology, pharmacology, public health, virology
Definition: The injection, ingestion, or inhalation of suspension of immunogens (molecules that produce an immune response), or a vehicle that causes the synthesis of immunogens, that elicit a protective immune response against a specific infection.

KEY TERMS

adjuvant: a substance given with a vaccine that enhances the immune response elicited by it

antigen: a foreign substance that elicits an immune response when inoculated into a living organism

attenuated: weakened or partial organisms

conjugate: the attachment of molecules that tend to elicit weak immune responses, such as carbohydrates, to large molecules that enhance the immunogenicity of the attached molecules.

excipient: an inactive substance that serves as the vehicle or medium for a drug, vaccine, or other material

immunity: the ability of an immune system to recognize, neutralize, and destroy an infecting organism, protecting the individual from infection

inoculation: the introduction of a substance or group of substances into a living organism

lipid nanoparticles: a shell of cholesterol and other fat-soluble molecules that house an internal mRNA core, and fuse with host cells to deliver the messenger ribonucleic acid (mRNA) payload

INTRODUCTION

Immunization, also known as "vaccination," is the administration of a substance (a vaccine) through inoculation, ingestion, or nasal inhalation to stimulate a person's immune system and aid it in fighting a particular disease. Persons who receive a vaccine are considered immunized against a particular pathogen.

The period from 1870 to the start of World War I is considered the golden age of immunology. During this time, Louis Pasteur discovered proof of the germ theory of disease, Élie Metchnikoff proposed the cellular theory of immunity, and several critical new vaccines became available, many developed by Pasteur himself.

Vaccination remains the most critical protection against viral infections, primarily because of the lack of effective treatment options once a viral infection is established. Similarly, there is renewed interest in vaccine development internationally due to the decreasing effectiveness of antibiotics in treating bacterial infections.

No proper vaccines exist against protozoan diseases such as malaria, fungal diseases such as candidiasis, chlamydia, helminthiasis (parasitic worm infection), or human immunodeficiency virus (HIV), although research in all of these areas is ongoing. The development of a malaria vaccine and an HIV vaccine have seen some promising early results.

Infectious diseases are not the only possible targets of vaccines. Some researchers are investigating vaccines' potential for contraception and treating and preventing diseases such as cocaine addiction, Alzheimer's, and cancer. Others are looking to improve the effectiveness of antigens in stimulating immunity with the use of additives called "adjuvants." In addition, a great deal of research focuses on combining existing vaccines into a reduced total number of injections in the vaccine schedule (the recommended timeline for a given vaccine or vaccines).

Before the invention of vaccines, scientists and other naturalists noticed that people who recovered from certain diseases, such as smallpox were immune to the disease. Reportedly, Chinese physicians were the first to exploit this phenomenon to prevent disease by drying and grinding up smallpox scabs that children then inhaled. In England, contaminating a fresh skin cut, called "variolation," with scabs from smallpox wounds became common in the eighteenth century. Most often, localized skin reactions occurred; severe smallpox cases were less common. Although only 1 percent of people became seriously sick after variolation, the mortality rate was as high as 50 percent.

English physician Edward Jenner occasionally encountered patients who did not respond with the usual reactions to variolation. According to one story, a milkmaid had told Jenner that she would not get smallpox because she had already had cowpox. This mild disease causes lesions on the udders of cows and would sometimes infect the hands of milkmaids. Jenner then began to deliberately inoculate people with cowpox in superficial wounds in an attempt to prevent smallpox. The term "vaccination," from the Latin *vacca*, or "cow," was coined to recognize Jenner's work.

Because viral diseases cannot be effectively treated once established, vaccination is usually the only practical method of controlling them. Controlling viral disease requires that an entire population be immune to it. A phenomenon called "herd immunity" is established if most of the population is immune. With herd immunity, disease outbreak is limited to sporadic cases, avoiding the epidemic spread of disease. Two centuries after Jenner, smallpox was eliminated worldwide by vaccination. The bifurcated needle, developed in the 1960s and used to scratch the skin and deliver a drop of vaccine, is considered the single most successful medical device ever developed because it helped eliminate the scourge of smallpox.

PRINCIPLES AND RESULTS OF VACCINATION

A vaccine is a suspension of organisms, or pieces of organisms, delivered to the immune system in various ways. Vaccines offer the immune system a biochemical example of the disease microbe used by the body to induce immunity. Both antibody-based or humoral immunity and cell-based immunity depend on the formation of immunologic memory. Once vaccinated, immunologic memory is responsible for the rapid neutralizing responses that prevent disease after exposure.

Jenner's inoculations worked because the cowpox virus, which is not a severe pathogen, is closely related to the smallpox virus. The injection by skin scratches provoked a primary immune response against the proteins of the cowpox virus in the recipients, leading to the formation of antibodies and long-term memory cells. Exposure to the smallpox virus and its proteins would then lead to the rapid neutralizing response characteristic of immune people. A vaccinia virus vaccine eventually replaced the cowpox vaccine.

TYPES OF VACCINES AND THEIR CHARACTERISTICS

There are now several basic vaccine types: attenuated microbe vaccines, inactivated whole-agent vaccines, toxoids, subunit vaccines, conjugated vaccines, and nucleic acid vaccines.

Attenuated microbe vaccines. Attenuated microbe vaccines use living but weakened (attenuated) viruses that cannot cause disease in healthy persons. Live attenuated viruses infect and multiply in the cells of the recipient. Attenuated microbes are usually viral strains derived after mutations accumulated during long-term artificial culture or through genetic manipulation. These microbes no longer cause disease, yet they still can cause a low-level infection that generates immunity. Live vaccines more closely mimic an actual infection.

Lifelong immunity is often achieved without booster immunizations, and an effectiveness rate of 95 percent is not unusual. This long-term effectiveness of live viral vaccines probably occurs because the attenuated viruses replicate in the body, increasing the initial dose and acting as a series of secondary, or booster, immunizations. Examples of live vaccines include those that protect against smallpox, measles, mumps, rubella, and the oral polio vaccine, no longer available in the United States. Some newer live-virus vaccines against rotavirus, dengue fever, and other diseases are artificial virus combinations. In development, scientists start with a particular virus's genetic backbone. Genes from a pathogenic virus are added, and those proteins are produced in infected cells of the vaccine recipient.

The best-known example of a live attenuated bacterial vaccine is the bacillus Calmette-Guérin (BCG) vaccine, which has been used for some time, though with limited efficacy, to combat tuberculosis. More recently, it has shown some success as a treatment for superficial or early-stage bladder cancers. Albert Calmette and Camille Guérin made BCG by modifying tuberculosis bacteria from cows in culture to provide immunity without causing the disease. The delivery of the microbes' proteins is internal and, therefore, distinct from both oral and injectable vaccines. Newer, genetically modified, live-attenuated vaccines against tuberculosis and typhoid fever are in development.

Attenuated vaccines are not recommended for people whose immune systems are compromised. Because of advances in chemotherapy treatments for cancer, increases in the number of organ transplant recipients taking immunosuppressive drugs, and an increase in the number of people immunocompromised by diseases like HIV and acquired immunodeficiency syndrome (AIDS), the use of attenuated microbe vaccines should be carefully considered. If available, inactivated vaccines are substituted. A separate danger of such vaccines is the theoretical possibility that the live microbes can mutate back to a virulent form.

Inactivated whole-agent vaccines. Inactivated whole-agent vaccines use microbes that have been killed, usually by formalin or phenol chemical treatment. Inactivated virus vaccines used in humans include those for rabies, influenza, and polio, the latter of which was adopted for use in the United States after 2003. Inactivated bacterial vaccines include those for pneumococcal pneumonia and cholera. Several long-used inactivated vaccines have been replaced by newer, more effective subunit vaccines, including those for pertussis, whooping cough, and typhoid fever.

Toxoids. Toxoid vaccines are composed of toxins that have been inactivated through chemical or genetic means. As vaccines, they are directed at the toxins produced by a pathogen. Tetanus and diphtheria toxoids have long been part of the standard childhood immunization series. They require a series of injections for complete immunity, followed by boosters every ten years. Many older adults have not received boosters, so they are likely to have low levels of protection.

Subunit vaccines. Subunit vaccines use only those molecules or fragments from a microorganism that best stimulates an immune response or have the highest "antigenicity." Genetic modification techniques produce subunit vaccines. For example, the vaccine against the hepatitis B virus consists of a portion of the viral protein coat produced by genetically modified yeast. In contrast, "recombinant vaccines" are produced by genetically modified organisms that synthesize the desired antigenic fraction. The recombinant flu vaccine provides an example of a recombinant vaccine. Recombinant flu vaccines express the influenza genes for the surface hemagglutinin (HA) protein in a virus (baculovirus) that infects insect cells. The insect cells synthesize a plethora of HA protein, which is purified and packaged into a flu vaccine.

Subunit vaccines are inherently safer because they cannot reproduce in the recipient. They also contain little or no extraneous material and, therefore, tend to produce fewer adverse effects. Similarly, it is possible to separate the fractions of a disrupted bacterial cell, retaining the desired antigenic fractions. The newer acellular vaccines for whooping cough contained in the DTaP (diphtheria, tetanus, and pertussis) vaccine use this approach.

Conjugated vaccines. Conjugated vaccines, also referred to as glycoconjugates, have been developed because of the poor immune response of children to vaccines based on the capsular polysaccharides surrounding the cell wall of certain bacteria. Polysaccharides are T-independent antigens. Therefore, the child's immune system only responds to the vaccine through their B cells (lymphocytes). Immunologic memory depends on the contributions of T cells. Therefore, polysaccharides do not stimulate immunity until the age of fifteen to twenty-four months.

In glycoconjugate technology, the polysaccharides are chemically bonded to proteins such as diphtheria or tetanus toxoid. The protein recruits T cells to the vicinity where the polysaccharides and B cells interact. The B cells receive the chemical signal necessary to form immunologic memory from the T cells. This approach has led to the very successful vaccines for *Haemophilus influenzae* type B, *Streptococcus pneumoniae*, and *Neisseria meningitidis* that give significant protection, even at two months of age.

Deoxyribonucleic acid (DNA) vaccines. Experimental DNA vaccines contain the genes that code for antigens. The development of DNA vaccines requires that the genes from the pathogen be isolated and analyzed. DNA vaccines would stimulate an immune response to the free-floating antigen secreted by cells and against the antigens displayed on cell surfaces. DNA vaccines would contain copies of a few of the pathogen's genes, so the vaccine would not cause disease.

DNA vaccines are relatively easy and inexpensive to design and produce. Naked DNA vaccines, which consist of DNA administered directly into the body, could be mixed with molecules that facilitate its uptake by the body's cells. Naked DNA vaccines for influenza and herpes viruses are under investigation.

Messenger ribonucleic acid (mRNA) vaccines. In 1990, Agnes Jani and Phillip Felgner and their colleagues injected mRNA into the muscles of laboratory animals and observed protein synthesis. In 1992, Bloom and colleagues from the Scripps Research Institute in La Jolla, California, reversed diabetes insipidus in Brattleboro rats by injecting vasopressin mRNA into their hypothalamus. These two studies demonstrated the ability of injected RNA to induce the expression of specific proteins. However, these studies also showed the caveats of mRNA injection, including its short half-life and the tendency for the immune system to recognize mRNA and destroy it.

Further research revealed that efficient delivery of mRNAs by encasing them in lipid nanoparticles increased mRNA uptake by cells and prevented recognition of the RNA by the immune system. Using modified bases during the synthesis of mRNAs not only increases their half-lives but significantly decreases their immunogenicity. The production of mRNA vaccines is rapid, inexpensive, and highly scalable.

mRNA vaccines made by Pfizer-BioNTech (BNT162b2) and Moderna (mRNA-1273) were granted Emergency Use Authorization (EUA) by the U.S. Food and Drug Administration (FDA) on December 11, 2020 and December 18, 2020, respectively, for the COVID-19 pandemic. Both vaccines encode the severe acute respiratory syndrome (SARS)-CoV-2 spike protein and induce excellent immune responses against SARS-CoV-2. Other mRNA vaccines for Zika virus, influenza, respiratory syncytial virus, human immunodeficiency virus, and several types of cancer are in development.

Recombinant vector vaccines. Recombinant vector vaccines, also experimental, use an attenuated pathogen to introduce DNA to cells. A vector is a harmless virus or bacterium used as a carrier. Certain harmless or attenuated viruses are used to carry portions of the genetic material from other microbes. The carrier viruses then ferry the microbial DNA to cells and display the pathogen's antigens on the cell's surface. The harmless organism mimics a pathogen and provokes an immune response. Recombinant vector vaccines closely mimic a natural infection, effectively stimulating the immune system. Recombinant vector vaccines for HIV, rabies, and measles are under investigation.

Adenovirus-based vaccines for COVID-19 include the Oxford-AstraZeneca (ChAdOx1), Johnson & Johnson (JNJ-78436735), and Sputnik V (Gam-*COVID*-Vac) vaccines. The FDA awarded the Johnson & Johnson vaccine EUA on February 27, 2021. The Oxford-AstraZeneca vaccine has been approved for use in the European Union, Vietnam, Argentina, Bangladesh, Brazil, the Dominican Republic, El Salvador, India, Malaysia, Mexico, Nepal, Pakistan, the Philippines, Sri Lanka, South Korea, and Taiwan. Adenovirus-based vaccines are also available for Ebola.

VACCINE SAFETY

Variolation, the first attempt to provide immunity to smallpox, sometimes caused the disease it was intended to prevent. At that time, however, the risk was considered worthwhile. The orally delivered live attenuated polio vaccine was effective at reducing polio in the face of an epidemic. On rare occasions, it caused a mild form of the disease. Therefore, the lower-risk inactivated poliovirus vaccine was adopted in the developed world when epidemics were rarer.

In 1999, a rotavirus vaccine for children was withdrawn from the market because several recipients developed a life-threatening intestinal obstruction called "intussusception." Eventually, further re-

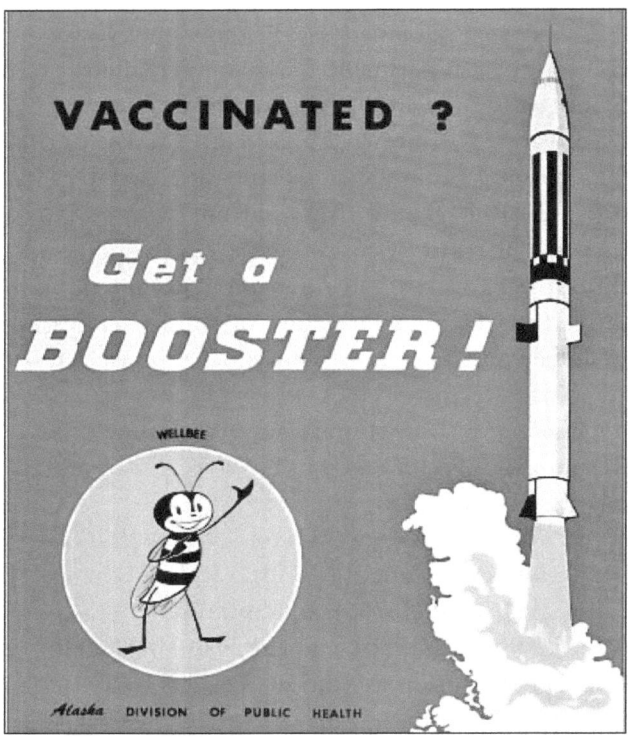

Widespread campaigns such as the CDC's run of the "Wellbee" mascot promoted immunization and vaccination, which have reduced risks for certain diseases in many parts of the world. Image courtesy of

search that the vaccine was not the cause, and some experts suggested that it be reintroduced in developing countries where the incidence of rotavirus is high. New, safer versions of the vaccine were introduced in 2006 and 2008.

Public reaction to such risks has changed. Most parents have never seen a case of polio or measles and, therefore, tend to view the risk of these diseases as remote. Rumored reports of harmful effects often lead people to avoid certain vaccines. A contrived connection between the MMR (measles, mumps, rubella) vaccine and autism has received widespread publicity. Autism is a poorly understood developmental condition that causes a child, in part, to withdraw to varying degrees from everyday reality, namely other persons. Because autism is usually diagnosed at the age of eighteen to thirty months, the age range in which vaccination is common in the United States

and Europe, some persons claimed a cause-and-effect connection between the vaccines and autism. Medically, however, experts overwhelmingly agree that autism is a condition with a significant genetic component that begins before birth. Moreover, the first study to propose a causal link between the MMR vaccine and autism, published in 1998 by former surgeon Andrew Wakefield, was shown to be fraudulent and officially retracted. The significant increase in autism diagnoses is caused primarily by the vastly expanded definition of autism spectrum disorders and not by adopting certain vaccines. All testimony to the contrary has been discredited.

Thimerosal is a mercury-containing organic compound. Since the 1930s, it has been widely used as a preservative in vaccines to help prevent bacterial contamination. Still, many parents refuse to immunize their children for fear of a link between autism, for example, and the use of vaccines containing thimerosal, an ethyl mercury-based preservative. Scientific evidence does not support this link. In 2004, the Institute of Medicine conducted a scientific review of thimerosal. It concluded that "the evidence favors rejection of a causal relationship between thimerosal-containing vaccines and autism." Since then, nine additional studies have found no link between thimerosal-containing vaccines and autism spectrum disorder. Nevertheless, thimerosal is no longer used in the production of most single-shot vaccines in the United States.

CHALLENGES OF VACCINATION

The economics of vaccination. Although interest in vaccine development declined with the introduction of antibiotics, it has intensified in recent years. Fear of litigation had contributed to decreased development of new vaccines in the United States and Europe. However, the passage of the National Childhood Vaccine Injury Act in 1986, which limited vaccine manufacturers' liability in the United States, helped reverse this trend. Even so, to the pharmaceutical industry, vaccines are inherently less attractive economically than drug treatments that last for extended periods.

Cultivation of vaccine microbes and antigens. To develop a vaccine, the laboratory must grow the pathogen in large quantities. The early successful viral vaccines were developed by animal cultivation. The vaccinia virus for smallpox was grown on the shaved bellies of calves, for example. However, some viruses, such as polio, measles, and mumps, will not grow in anything except living human cells. The introduction of vaccines against these and other such viral diseases awaited the development of cell culture techniques. Cell cultures from human sources enabled the growth of these viruses on a large scale.

A valuable biological resource for the cultivation of viruses is the chick embryo. Viruses for several vaccines, including influenza, are grown in the various anatomic compartments of the egg. However, recombinant vaccines and DNA vaccines do not need a cell or animal host to grow the vaccine's microbe. Recombinant vaccines avoid a major problem with certain viruses that have not been grown in cell culture, such as hepatitis B. (The first hepatitis B vaccine used viral antigens extracted from the blood of chronically infected humans because no other source was available.)

Distribution and delivery of vaccines. Diarrheal diseases are a major cause of infant mortality in developing countries, where costs and distribution of vaccines also pose unique problems. For example, a vaccine that must be refrigerated would be nearly useless in countries that lack reliable electrical service. As an alternative, edible, plant-derived vaccines of several types are undergoing clinical trials.

IMPACT

Infectious disease places a heavy burden on public health in many parts of the world. The cost in terms of human suffering, social hardship, and economic cost is enormous. Consequently, preventing and combating these diseases are keys to the economic development of many underdeveloped regions.

Many diseases are vaccine-preventable. The introduction of immunization has been one of the most extraordinary and most cost-effective interventions in human health. The health impact of vaccination programs is tremendous, perhaps surpassed in significance only by measures to prevent poverty and introduce clean water sanitation systems.

—Kimberly A. Napoli, MS

Further Information

Allen, Arthur. *Vaccine: The Controversial Story of Medicine's Greatest Lifesaver*. Norton, 2007.

Centers for Disease Control and Prevention. "Autism and Vaccines." www.cdc.gov/vaccinesafety/concerns/autism.html.

Deer, Brian. *The Doctor Who Fooled the World*. Johns Hopkins UP, 2020.

Delves, Peter J., et al. *Roitt's Essential Immunology*. 13th ed., Wiley, 2017.

DeStefano, Frank, Cristofer S. Price, and Eric S. Weintraub. "Increasing Exposure to Antibody-Stimulating Proteins and Polysaccharides in Vaccines Is Not Associated with Risk of Autism." *Journal of Pediatrics*, vol. 163, no. 2, pp. 561-67.

Hackett, Charles J., and Donald A. Harn Jr., editors. *Vaccine Adjuvants: Immunological and Clinical Principles*. Humana, 2006.

Hamborsky, Jennifer, Andrew Kroger, and Charles Wolfe, editors. *Epidemiology and Prevention of Vaccine-Preventable Diseases*. 13th ed., Public Health Foundation, 2015. Centers for Disease Control and Prevention. Accessed 31 Dec. 2015.

Merino, Noël. *Vaccines*. Greenhaven, 2015.

Pardi, Norbert, Michael J. Hogan, Frederick W. Porter, and Drew Weissman. "mRNA Vaccines—A New Era in Vaccinology." *Nature Reviews Drug Discovery*, vol. 17, 2018, pp. 261-79.

Plotkin, Stanley A., Walter A. Orenstein, and Paul A. Offit, editors. *Vaccines*. 6th ed., Saunders, 2013.

Immunology

Category: Specialty
Anatomy or system affected: Blood, cells, immune system
Specialties and related fields: Cytology, hematology, microbiology, preventive medicine, serology
Definition: The study of the immune system, its protection of the body from foreign agents, and its malfunction in autoimmune diseases, in which the body's defenses react against the body's cells or tissues.

KEY TERMS

antibody: a protein produced by lymphocytes in response to an antigen; binds only to a specific antigen

antigen: any substance perceived by immunological defenses to be foreign and against which antibody is produced; generally, a protein

autoantibody: an antibody produced against tissue antigens within a host—that is, self-antigens

complement: a series of about twenty serum proteins that, when sequentially activated by immune complexes, may trigger cell damage

determinant: a region on the surface of an antigen capable of creating an immune response or of combining with an antibody produced by an immune response

Hashimoto's disease: thyroiditis; among the earliest characterized autoimmune diseases

lymphocyte: a small white blood cell constituting about 25 percent of all blood cells; two basic types are B cells (antibody production) and T cells (cellular immunity)

systemic lupus erythematosus (SLE): commonly called "lupus"; a chronic inflammatory disease characterized by an arthritic condition and a rash

tolerance: the state in which an organism does not normally react against its tissue

SCIENCE AND PROFESSION

The field of immunology deals with the ability of the immune system to react against an enormous repertoire of stimulation by antigens. In most instances, these antigens are foreign infectious agents such as viruses or bacteria. Inherent in this process is the ability to react against nearly any known determinant, whether natural or artificially produced. The most reactive antigenic determinants are proteins, though, to a lesser degree, other substances such as carbohydrates (sugars), lipids (fats), and nucleic acids may also stimulate a response.

In general, the body exhibits tolerance during constant exposure to its tissue. The precise reasons behind tolerance are vague, but the basis for the lack of response lies in two central mechanisms: the elimination during the development of immunological cells capable of responding to the body's tissue and the active prevention of existing reactive cells from responding to self-antigens. When this regulation fails, autoimmune disease may result.

There are two major types of immunological defense: humoral immunity and cell-mediated immunity. Humoral immunity refers to the soluble substances in blood serum, primarily antibodies, and complement. In contrast, cellular immunity refers to the portion of the immune response directly mediated by cells. Though these processes are sometimes categorized separately, they do interact with and regulate each other.

Antibodies are produced by cells called "B lymphocytes" in response to foreign antigens. These proteins bind to the antigen in a specific manner, resulting in a complex that can be removed readily by phagocytic white blood cells. More important, in the context of autoimmunity, antibody-antigen complexes also activate the complement pathway, a series of some twenty enzymes and serum proteins. The result of activation is the lysis of the antigenic targets. In general, the targets are bacteria; in autoimmune diseases, the target may be any cell in the body.

The cellular response utilizes any of several types of cytotoxic cells. These can include a specialized lymphocyte called the "T cell" (because of its development in the thymus) or another unusual large granular lymphocyte called the "natural killer" (NK) cell. NK and cytotoxic T cells function similarly—by binding to the target and releasing toxic granules in apposition to its cell membrane.

Though autoimmune diseases differ in scope, they do tend to exhibit certain common factors. The pathologies associated with most of these illnesses result in part from producing autoantibodies, antibodies produced against the body's cells or tissues. If the antibody binds to tissue in a particular organ, complement is activated in the tissue, destroying those organs. For example, Goodpasture's syndrome is characterized by the deposition of autoantibodies directed against the glomerulus membrane in the kidneys. Complement activation can result in severe organ pathology and subsequent kidney failure.

Suppose the autoantibody binds to soluble material in blood serum. In that case, the resultant antibody-antigen complexes are carried along in the circulation. There is the possibility that they will lodge in various areas of the body. For example, systemic lupus erythematosus (SLE) produces autoantibodies against soluble nucleoprotein released from cells as they undergo normal death and lysis. The immune complexes frequently lodge in the kidney, where they can cause renal failure.

However, all autoimmune diseases do not result solely from autoantibody production. Though a precise role for either cytotoxic T cells or NK cells in human autoimmune disease has not been fully confirmed, several observations make such an association likely. First, large T cells are found in certain organ-specific diseases, including thyroiditis and pernicious anemia. Second, animal models of similar diseases show a specific role for such cells in the pathology of these diseases. Thus, it is likely that these cells do participate in organ destruction.

Autoimmune disorders are categorized in the form of a disease spectrum. At one end of the spectrum, one can place organ-specific diseases. For example, Hashimoto's disease is an autoimmune thyroid disorder characterized by autoantibodies against thyroid antigens. The extensive infiltration and proliferation of lymphocytes are observed (although, as described above, their roles are unproved), along with the subsequent destruction of follicular tissue.

Likewise, diabetes mellitus, type 1 (formerly called "juvenile-onset diabetes"), is an organ-specific autoimmune disease. In this case, however, autoantibodies are directed against the beta cells of the pancreas, which produce insulin. In pernicious (or megaloblastic) anemia, antibodies are produced against intrinsic factor, a molecule necessary for uptake of vitamin B_{12}. People with pernicious (or megaloblastic) anemia suffer from a lack of absorption of the vitamin. Addison's disease, from which U.S. president John F. Kennedy suffered, is a potentially life-threatening condition resulting from antibody production against the adrenal cortex. Myasthenia gravis (MG) is characterized by severe heart or skeletal muscle weakness caused by antibodies directed against neurotransmitter receptors on the muscle. Cells from any organ may be potential targets for the production of an autoantibody.

Certain organ-specific autoimmune diseases in the spectrum are characterized not by antibodies directed against any specific organ but by cellular infiltration triggered in some manner by less specific autoantibodies. For example, biliary cirrhosis, an inflammatory condition of the liver, is characterized by the obstruction of bile flow through the liver ductules. Though extensive cellular infiltration is observed, serum antibodies are directed against mitochondrial antigens found within all cells. Certain types of chronic hepatitis also exhibit an analogous situation.

In some cases, antibodies may be directed against circulatory cells. Antibodies directed against red blood cells may cause subsequent lysis of the cells, leading to hemolytic anemia. Antibodies directed against blood platelets can cause a reduction in the number of those cells, resulting in thrombocytopenia purpura. Often, these are temporary conditions that have resulted from the binding of a pharmacologic chemical such as an antibiotic to the cell's surface, which triggers an immune response. A more severe condition is hemolytic disease of the newborn (HDN), one example being hemolytic disease of the newborn (formerly erythroblastosis fetalis) or Rh disease. In this case, a mother lacking the Rh protein on her blood cells may produce an immune response against that protein, which is present in the blood of the fetus she is carrying during pregnancy. Before 1967, when an effective preventive measure became available, HDN was a severe problem for many pregnancies. An analogous situation occurs with other cell types.

At the other end of the autoimmune spectrum are those diseases that are not cell- or organ-specific but result in widespread lesions in various body parts. Lupus received its name from the butterfly rash often seen on patients' faces, which resembles a wolf bite (*lupus* is Latin for "wolf"). However, pathologic changes can be found at various sites in the body, including the kidneys, joints, and blood vessels. Likewise, rheumatoid arthritis is characterized by the production of rheumatoid factor, an antibody molecule directed against other antibodies in blood serum. The resultant immune complexes lodge in joints, causing joint pain and destruction associated with severe arthritis.

In most cases, the specific reason for the production of autoantibodies is unknown. Genetic factors are certainly involved since some autoimmune diseases run in families. Bacterial or viral infections may trigger some. Viral antigens may be expressed on the surfaces of specific cells, or the virus itself may be attached to the cell. Heart muscle appears to express antigenic determinants in common with certain streptococcal bacteria. A mild "strep throat" may be followed several weeks later by severe rheumatic fever.

The binding of drugs to cell surfaces may trigger an immune response. For example, penicillin may bind to the surfaces of red blood cells, triggering hemolytic anemia. Likewise, the hypnotic/sedative apronal (*Sedormid*) may bind to the membrane of platelets.

Most cases of autoimmune disease, however, are triggered by no apparent cause. They may "simply" involve a breakdown of the normal regulatory mechanisms associated with the immune response.

DIAGNOSTIC AND TREATMENT TECHNIQUES
The regulation of self-reactive lymphocytes is necessary for maintaining tolerance by the immune system. When regulation breaks down or is otherwise defective, either humoral or cellular immunity is generated against the cells or tissues. The resultant pathology may be simply a painful nuisance or may have potentially fatal consequences. The difference relates to the extent of damage to particular organs, in the case of organ-specific autoimmune reactions, or to the level of tissue damage in systemic disease.

Despite differences in pathology, the mechanisms of tissue damage are similar in most autoimmune diseases. Most involve the formation of immune complexes. Either antibodies bind to cell surfaces, or immune complexes form in the circulation. In either case, the result is complement activation. Components of the complement pathway, in turn, can either directly damage cell membranes or trigger the infiltration of a variety of cytotoxic cells.

Because the damage associated with most autoimmune diseases results from parallel processes, treatment methods vary little in theory from one illness to another. Most involve the treatment of resultant symptoms; for example, the use of aspirin to reduce minor inflammation and, when necessary, the use of steroids to reduce the level of the immune response. Recently, the focus has shifted from treating symptoms only to attacking the underlying disease mechanism with disease-modifying drugs. Some of these drugs include methotrexate, azathioprine, cyclosporine, and hydroxychloroquine. Newer immune modulators (such as infliximab and etanercept) and monoclonal antibodies (such as rituximab) are used in some autoimmune conditions that are refractory to other measures.

The treatment of autoimmune diseases does not eliminate the problem. The disease remains, but under ideal conditions, it is held under control. At the same time, there exists the danger of side effects of treatment. For example, most methods that reduce the level of the immune response are nonspecific; reducing the severity of the autoimmune disease may cause the patient to become more susceptible to infections by bacteria or viruses.

Specific approaches have been successful in the palliative treatment of some forms of autoimmune disease. For example, patients with MG exhibit significant muscle weakness. An MG patient may have difficulty breathing and may experience extreme fatigue, in severe cases being unable to open their mouth or eyelids. Associated with the disease are autoantibodies produced against the receptor for the neurotransmitter acetylcholine (ACh), the chemical utilized by nerves in regulating movement by the muscle. By blocking the ACh receptor, these antibodies inhibit the ability of nerves to control muscle movement. In effect, the patient loses control of the muscles.

Patients with MG often exhibit abnormalities of the thymus, the gland associated with T-cell production. In addition, there is evidence that the thymus contains ACh receptors that are particularly antigenic (perhaps exacerbating the illness). Removal of the thymus, even in adults, often aids in reducing the symptoms of the disease. Though not superfluous in adults, the thymus carries out its primary functions during the early years of life through adolescence. Thus, its removal generally has few significant implications.

Often, MG will respond to more conventional forms of treatment. Steroid treatment will often reduce symptoms. Metabolic controls may also aid in reducing symptoms. For example, during normal neural function that involves ACh, the enzyme cholinesterase degrades ACh, thereby regulating muscle movement. Anticholinesterase drugs that prolong the presence of ACh at the site of the receptor on the muscle have also been of benefit to some patients.

SLE is among the most common systemic autoimmune diseases. The disease usually strikes women in the prime of life, between the ages of twenty and forty. It is characterized by a butterfly rash over the facial region and weakness, fatigue, and fever. In many respects, the symptoms are those of severe arthritis. As the disease progresses, tissue or organ degradation may occur in the kidney or heart.

The specific cause of the symptomology is the formation of immune complexes, which consist of antibodies against cell components such as deoxyribonucleic acid (DNA) or nucleoprotein. Complexes in the kidney have been large enough to observe with the electron microscope, mainly when the complexes contain cell nuclei. Regions of the skin characterized by inflammation and a rash have similar complexes. The immune complexes are sometimes ingested (phagocytized) by scavenger neutrophils, which make up the most significant proportion (65 percent) of white blood cells. The presence of these so-called lupus erythematosus (LE) cells, white cells with ingested antibody-bound nuclei, was at one time used for the diagnosis of lupus.

As is true for many autoimmune diseases, the control of lupus involves the use of steroids and other immunosuppressive drugs. These have included drugs such as cyclosporin, which blocks T-cell function, and antimitotic drugs such as azathioprine or methotrexate, which block the proliferation of immune cells, as well as immune modulators such as rituximab. Generalized immunosuppression as a side effect is a concern. Often, using combinations of steroids and immunosuppressives makes it possible to use lower concentrations of each, increasing the drugs' effectiveness and reducing the danger of toxicity.

Other palliative treatments of symptomology can increase patient comfort. For example, aspirin may be used to reduce inflammation or joint pain. Topical steroids can reduce the rash. Since lupus may significantly increase the photosensitivity of the skin, staying out of direct sunlight, or at least covering the surface of the skin, may reduce skin lesions. It should be emphasized again that these treatments deal only with symptoms; none will cure the disease.

Since some systemic diseases result from immune complex disorders, a reduction of such complexes benefits some patients. Treatment involves a process called "plasmapheresis." Plasma, the liquid portion of the blood, is removed from the patient (a small proportion at a time). The immune complexes are separated from the plasma. Though a temporary measure, since other complexes continue to form, the process does prove useful.

Rheumatoid arthritis is another common autoimmune disorder. As is true of most autoimmune diseases, rheumatoid arthritis is primarily a disease of women. Symptomatology results from the lodging of immune complexes in joints, resulting in the inflammation of those joints. Many cases result from the formation of antibodies directed against other antibody molecules—a case of the immune system turning against itself. Pathology results from complement activation and the infiltration of various cells into the joint; the result is damage to both cartilage and bone.

Medical treatment usually begins with aspirin or other nonsteroidal anti-inflammatory agents. Other common treatments increase patient comfort: rest, proper exercise, and weight loss, if necessary. In severe cases, steroids, immune modulators, or monoclonal therapy may be necessary.

In general, autoimmune diseases are characterized by alternating periods of symptomatology and remission. Since the precise origin of most of these disorders is unknown, prevention remains difficult. Treatments are generally similar in reducing inflammation as the first line of intervention, with immunosuppression as a last resort.

PERSPECTIVE AND PROSPECTS
During the 1950s, F. Macfarlane Burnet published his theory of clonal selection. Burnet believed that antibody specificity was predetermined in the B cell as it underwent development and maturation. Selection of the cell by the appropriate antigen resulted in the proliferation of that specific cell, a process of clonal selection.

However, Burnet also had to account for tolerance—the inability of immune cells to respond against their antigens. Burnet theorized that exposure to self-antigens, or determinants, resulted in the ablation of any self-reactive cells during prenatal development. Only those self-reactive immune cells directed against sequestered antigens survived.

Though Burnet's theories have reached the level of dogma in the field of immunology, they fail to account for certain autoimmune disorders. Although not appreciated during Burnet's time, W. W. Gull and others recognized autoimmune disorders as early as 1866. In that year, W. W. Gull demonstrated the link between chilling, and a syndrome called "paroxysmal hemoglobinuria." When external tissue such as skin is exposed to cold, large amounts of hemoglobin are discharged into the urine. In the "correct" circumstances, the body does react against itself. In 1904, Karl Landsteiner established the autoimmune basis for the disease by demonstrating the role of complement in the lysis of red blood cells, causing the release of hemoglobin and the symptomatology of the disorder. Furthermore, he demonstrated that one could cause the lysis of normal cells by mixing them with sera from patients who had hemoglobin in their urine.

Hashimoto's disease was among the first organ-specific autoimmune diseases to be described. The disease was first described in 1912 by Hakaru Hashimoto, a Japanese surgeon. The immune basis for the disease was established independently by Ernest Witebsky and Noel Rose in the United States, and by Deborah Doniach and Ivan Roitt in Great Britain, in 1957.

Since the 1950s, dozens of autoimmune disorders have been described. Treatment of these disorders remains, for the most part, nonspecific. Research in the area has examined the precise triggers for autoimmune diseases and developed ways to suppress specifically those immune reactions responsible for the symptomatology. Successes have been associated with vaccines directed against components involved with the reactions under investigation. For example, since the production of autoantibodies is the basis for some forms of the disease, the generation of additional antibody molecules directed against determinants on the autoantibodies at fault could neutralize those components' effects. This procedure could be likened to a police department that arrests its dishonest officers. There is a precedent for such an operation. Newborn children of mothers suffering from MG synthesize just such antibodies against the inappropriate MG antibodies that have crossed the placenta. Synthesis does seem to alleviate the symptoms of the disease.

There is no question that autoimmune disorders represent an aberrant form of the immune response. Nevertheless, understanding the underlying mechanism will shed light on exactly how the immune system is regulated. For example, it remains unclear how antibody production is controlled following a normal immune response. In the presence of an antigen, antibody levels increase for days to weeks, reach a plateau, and then slowly decrease as additional production comes to a halt. How the shutdown takes place remains nebulous.

Tolerance does not result solely from an absence of T or B cells that respond to antigens; it involves an active suppression of the process. A more detailed understanding of the process will generally lead to a more thorough understanding of the immune system.

—*Richard Adler, PhD*

Further Information

Delves, Peter J., et al. *Roitt's Essential Immunology*. 13th ed., Blackwell, 2017. Several chapters deal specifically with immune disorders. Concise, with a large number of illustrations, but does require a basic knowledge of biology.

Fettner, Ann Giudici. *Viruses: Agents of Change*. McGraw-Hill, 1990. Though argumentative in her approach, Fettner provides a simple discussion of the role of viruses in disease. Included are sections on autoimmunity and the possible roles played by viruses.

Frank, Steven A. *Immunology and Evolution of Infectious Disease*. Princeton UP, 2002. Blends research from molecular biology, immunology, pathogen biology, and population dynamics to discuss how and why parasites vary to escape recognition by the immune system, vaccine design, and the control of epidemics.

Janeway, Charles A., Jr., et al. *Immunobiology: The Immune System in Health and Disease*. 6th ed., Garland Science, 2005. An excellent text that provides a lucid and comprehensive examination of the immune system, covering such topics as immunobiology and innate immunity, the recognition of antigen, the development of mature lymphocyte receptor repertoires, the adaptive immune response, and the evolution of the immune system.

Parham, Peter. *The Immune System*. 3rd ed., Garland Science, 2009. An introductory immunology text details how cells and molecules work together to defend the body against invading microorganisms describes situations in which the immune system cannot control disease, and examines what happens when the immune system overreacts.

Punt, Jenni, et al. *Kuby Immunology*. 8th ed., W. H. Freeman, 2018. An excellent text that gives an overview of the immune system and its role with cells and organs and discusses such topics as the generation of B-cell and T-cell responses, immune effector mechanisms, and the immune system in health and disease.

Rose, Noel R., and Ian. R. Mackay, editors. *The Autoimmune Diseases*. 6th ed., Academic Press/Elsevier, 2019. A well-written textbook containing thorough discussions of autoimmune disorders. Primarily for those with a background in immunology, but it does provide much basic information.

IMMUNOPATHOLOGY

Category: Specialty
Anatomy or system affected: All
Specialties and related fields: Dermatology, genetics, hematology, immunology, pathology, serology
Definition: The study of disease processes with an immunological basis or pathogenesis involving either B cells (antibodies) and complement or T cells, including damage to tissues and cells caused by hypersensitivity reactions.

KEY TERMS

antibody: a molecule of the immune system, produced by B cells and targeted toward eliminating a specific antigen

B cells: also known as B lymphocytes; the antibody-producing cells of the immune system

congenital: something that is present at birth

hypersensitivity: reactions in which the immune system response is exaggerated

immunodeficiency: a state in which the immune system components that are meant to protect an individual are in a weakened state or absent altogether

T cells: also known as T lymphocytes; the immune system cells involved in cellular immunity and regulation of the immune response

SCIENCE AND PROFESSION

Immunopathology is the subdiscipline of immunology that deals with the four basic types of pathologies caused by the immune system: autoimmune disorders, congenital immunodeficiencies, acquired immunodeficiencies, and hypersensitivity reactions. Physicians who deal with such disorders are trained in immunology and/or pathology.

Autoimmune disorders are those in which the body fails to distinguish between self and nonself, leading to an attack by the immune system on the tissues or organs of the body. There are many autoimmune disorders, and the symptoms are highly varied, depending on the site and extent of the attack. Some disorders are tissue-specific, while others affect tissues and organs throughout the body. Examples of autoimmune disorders are multiple sclerosis (MS), systemic lupus erythematosus (SLE), and myasthenia gravis.

Congenital (primary) immunodeficiencies are those conditions in which there is an absence or a failure of the immune system at birth. Often, they result from a failure of one or more components of the immune system to develop during the fetal stages. Most congenital deficiencies have a genetic basis. An example of a primary immunodeficiency disorder is DiGeorge syndrome, in which T cells are deficient due to a developmental problem of the thymus. The most severe of these disorders is severe combined immunodeficiency disorder (SCID). In this disorder, neither B nor T cells develop or function properly. Complement deficiencies fall into this category as well. Complement is a series of proteins that combine to attack invading cells, such as bacteria.

Acquired (secondary) immunodeficiencies are those that arise later in life, following a change in some environmental condition or exposure, such as accidents or surgery that damages or removes the spleen or lymph nodes, radiation exposure that damages the bone marrow, and cancers that attack or destroy parts of the immune system. Lymphocytic leukemias (malignancies of bone marrow precursors of B and T cells) are an example of acquired immune system diseases. Malnutrition or the use of certain drugs (especially opiates) may also negatively affect the immune response. Finally, viruses, such as the human immunodeficiency virus (HIV), can attack and suppress the human immune system components, leading to a deficient ability to defend the body from daily attacks by microorganisms. Some acquired immunodeficiencies occur without an identified cause.

In contrast to the immunodeficiency syndromes, hypersensitivity reactions are those in which the immune system overreacts in its attempt to keep the body healthy, and by doing so, causes localized or systemic reactions that can range from annoying to life-threatening. Hypersensitivity reactions are classified according to their molecular mechanism of action. They may overlap with other categories, such as autoimmune disorders. Type I reactions are those which most people would recognize as allergies. Here, a series of chemicals, including immunoglobulin E (IgE), are released into the bloodstream, triggering the effects commonly associated with allergies: runny nose, itchy eyes, and difficulty breathing. The most severe case is anaphylaxis, sometimes seen in individuals with allergies to bee or wasp venom or certain food substances. Type II reactions are those in which existing antibodies in the bloodstream bind to antigens that are seen as foreign and begin the process of tissue destruction. Examples include transfusion reactions, in which the wrong blood type is given to an individual, and erythroblastosis fetalis (hemolytic disease of the newborn), in which maternal antibodies attack a developing fetus with a different set of antigens. Type III disorders consist of the formation of large immune complexes that deposit in the blood vessel walls or kidneys, leading to vasculitis and glomerulonephritis. Type IV reactions involve T-cell-mediated attacks; they include contact dermatitis (such as poison ivy reactions) and transplant rejection.

DIAGNOSTIC AND TREATMENT TECHNIQUES
Specialists who deal with immunopathologies may provide treatments that vary widely, as do the disorders themselves. The goal of all therapy is to restore the immune system to its normal balance to continue to protect the body from the constant barrage of invading microorganisms. Individuals with immune system deficiencies must avoid contact with other individuals as much as possible since most viruses and bacteria spread through personal contact. Prophylactic regimens of antibiotics, antivirals, and antifungals are helpful in most of those with immunodeficiencies. Still, in those with more severe forms, bone marrow transplants are the treatment of choice. The use of passive immunization-transferring antibodies from healthy individuals into those with immunodeficiencies is helpful in some cases. In acquired immunodeficiency syndrome (AIDS), drug combinations, or "cocktails," aim to suppress the replication of HIV, which attacks the T cells and keeps them from functioning.

Because most hypersensitivity reactions are temporary immunopathologies, their treatment involves short-term therapies to restore balance to the system. Antihistamines, for instance, help many allergy sufferers, as do air purifiers and lifestyle changes. Careful tissue and blood typing can eliminate or lower the instances of the other types of hypersensitivities.

Treatment for autoimmune disorders is also quite variable because of the wide variety of manifestations and underlying causes. Treatments commonly include immunosuppressive drugs and the replacement of hormones or other chemicals that the body is lacking.

PERSPECTIVE AND PROSPECTS

Since immunology itself is a field that is still in its infancy, recognition of immune disorders and their treatments is relatively new. Paul Ehrlich first described autoimmunity at the turn of the twentieth century. He called the phenomenon "horror autotoxicus," a name that struck fear in patients and providers alike. Hypersensitivity reactions, especially allergies, were recognized hundreds of years ago. Various chemical prescriptions were used to control the symptoms. Still, it was not until the mid-twentieth century that the molecular basis of allergies began to be understood. Immunodeficiencies are still being described, and the understanding of their basis is quite incomplete.

Some immunodeficiencies, if detected early enough, may be candidates for future gene therapy. In those cases where a single gene defect can be identified, introducing the functional gene into the developing tissue may reverse the course of the disease, partially or entirely. Other options include transplantation of the thymus or bone marrow to allow normal functioning of the immune system components.

One of the most exciting potential treatments for secondary immunodeficiencies is vaccination. The ability to block AIDS through early immunization looks promising, although still many years away from use.

—*Kerry L. Cheesman, PhD*

Further Information

Abbas, Abul K., Andrew H. Lichtman, and Shiv Pillai. *Basic Immunology: Functions and Disorders of the Immune System.* 6th ed., Saunders/Elsevier, 2019.

Clark, William R. *In Defense of Self: How the Immune System Really Works.* Oxford UP, 2007.

"Disorders of the Immune System." *American Academy of Allergy, Asthma, and Immunology,* 17 Jan. 2014, www.niaid.nih.gov/research/immune-system-disorders. Accessed 29 Aug. 2021.

Fischer, A. M., et al. "Naturally Occurring Primary Deficiencies of the Immune System." *Annual Review of Immunology,* vol. 15, 1997, pp. 93-124.

"Immune System and Disorders." *MedlinePlus,* 18 Aug. 2021, medlineplus.gov/immunesystemanddisorders.html. Accessed 29 Aug. 2021.

Janeway, Charles A. *Immunobiology: The Immune System in Health and Disease.* 7th ed., Garland Science, 2007.

Majno, Guido, and Isabelle Joris. "Part III: Immunopathology." *Cells, Tissues, and Disease: Principles of General Pathology.* 2nd ed., Oxford UP, 2004, pp. 523-610.

"Overview of the Immune System." *American Academy of Allergy, Asthma, and Immunology,* 30 Dec. 2013, www.niaid.nih.gov/research/immune-system-overview. Accessed 29 Aug. 2021.

Inflammation

Category: Diseases/Disorders
Anatomy or system affected: All
Specialties and related fields: Family medicine, internal medicine, pathology, rheumatology
Definition: The reaction of blood-filled living tissue to injury.

KEY TERMS

chemotaxis: movement of white blood cells toward a gradient of increasing or decreasing concentration of a particular substance

histamine: a small molecule released by cells in response to injury and allergic and inflammatory reactions, causing contraction of smooth muscle and dilation of capillaries

interleukins: members of a class of glycoproteins produced by leukocytes that regulate immune responses

leukocytes: colorless, nucleated, amoeboid cells that circulate throughout the blood and body fluids and destroy or isolate foreign substances and infectious agents, including lymphocytes, granulocytes, monocytes, and macrophages

CAUSES AND SYMPTOMS

In inflammation, the following changes are seen locally: redness, swelling, heat, pain, and loss of function. These changes are chemically mediated. Inflammation may be caused by microbial infection; physical agents such as trauma, radiation, and burns; chemical toxins; caustic substances such as strong acids or bases; decomposing or necrotic tissue; and immune system reactions. Acute inflammation is of relatively short duration (from a few minutes to a day), while chronic inflammation lasts longer. The local changes associated with inflammation include the outflow of fluid into the spaces between cells and the inflow or migration of white blood cells (leukocytes) to the area of injury. Chronic inflammation is characterized by the presence of leukocytes and macrophages and the proliferation of new blood vessels and connective tissue.

Inflammation is a protective mechanism for the body. Redness is attributable to increased blood flow to the injured area. Swelling is caused by the flow of fluid into the spaces between cells. Heat is produced by a combination of increased blood flow and chemical reactions in the local area. Pain results from the presence of two main chemicals found in the bloodstream: prostaglandins and bradykinin. Loss of function results from pain (the body limits movement to reduce discomfort) and swelling (interstitial fluid limits movement).

Acute inflammation. Many chemicals are involved in acute inflammation. Mediators of inflammation originate from blood plasma and both damaged and normal cells. Vasoactive amines are a class of chemicals that increase the permeability of blood vessels and cell walls. The most well studied of these are histamine and serotonin. Histamine is stored in granules in mast cells found in both tissue and basophils, the latter being a type of cell found in the blood. Serotonin is found in mast cells and platelets; it is another type of cell found in the bloodstream. These substances cause vasodilation (expansion of the walls of blood vessels) and increased vascular permeability (leakage through the walls of small vessels, especially veins). Histamine and serotonin can be released by trauma or exposure to cold. Other chemicals that circulate in the blood can release histamine. Two of these are part of the complement system; another is called "interleukin-1." The effects of histamine diminish after approximately one hour.

INFORMATION ON INFLAMMATION

Plasma proteases comprise three interrelated systems that explain much about inflammation: the complement, kinin, and clotting systems. The complement system comprises twenty different proteins involved in reactions against microbial agents that invade the body. The various chemicals act in a cascade, like falling dominoes: Each sets off another in sequence. The result of these chemical actions is to increase vascular permeability, promote chemotaxis (the attraction of living cells to specific chemicals), engulf invading microorganisms, and destroy pathogens through a process called "lysis."

The kinin system releases bradykinin, a chemical substance that causes contraction of smooth muscle tissue, dilation of blood vessels, and pain. The duration of action for bradykinin is brief because the enzyme kininase inactivates it. Bradykinin does not promote chemotaxis.

The clotting system is made up of a series of chemicals that form a solid mass. The most encountered example is the scab that forms at a cut in the skin. Like the complement system, the clotting system is a cascade of thirteen different chemicals. In addition to producing a solid mass, the clotting system also increases vascular permeability and promotes chemotaxis for white blood cells.

Other substances are involved in acute inflammation. Among the most important of these is a class called "prostaglandins." Several different prostaglandin molecules have been isolated; they are derived from the membranes of most cells. Prostaglandins cause pain, vasodilation, and fever. Aspirin counteracts the effects of prostaglandins, which explains the antipyretic (fever-reducing) and analgesic (pain-reducing) properties of the drug.

Another group of substances involved in acute inflammation is leukotrienes. The primary sources for these molecules are leukocytes, and some leukotrienes are found in mast cells. This group promotes vascular leakage but not chemotaxis. They also cause vasoconstriction (a decrease in the diameter of blood vessels) and bronchoconstriction (a decrease in the diameter of air passageways in the lungs). The effect of these leukotrienes is to slow blood flow and restrict air intake and outflow. A different type of leukotriene is found only in leukocytes. This type enhances chemotaxis but does not contribute to vascular leakage. In addition, leukotrienes cause white blood cells to stick to damaged tissues, speeding the removal of bacteria and promoting healing.

Other chemical substances are known to be involved with inflammation: platelet-activating factor, tumor necrosis factor, interleukin-1, cationic (positively charged) proteins, neutral proteases (enzymes that break down proteins), and oxygen metabolites (molecules resulting from reactions with oxygen). The sources of these are generally leukocytes, although some are derived from macrophages. They reinforce the effects of prostaglandins and leukotrienes.

There are four different outcomes for acute inflammation. There may be a complete resolution in which the injured site is restored to normal; this outcome usually follows a mild injury or limited trauma where there has been only minor tissue destruction. Healing with scarring may occur, in which injured tissue is replaced with scar tissue rich in collagen, giving it strength but at the cost of normal function; this outcome follows more severe injury or extensive destruction of tissue. There may be the formation of an abscess, which is characterized by pus, and which follows injuries that become infected with pyogenic (pus-forming) organisms. The fourth outcome is chronic inflammation.

Chronic inflammation. Acute inflammation may be followed by chronic inflammation. This reaction occurs when the organism, factor, or agent responsible for the acute inflammation is not removed or when the normal healing processes fail to occur. Repeated episodes of acute inflammation may also lead to chronic inflammation. The stages of acute inflammation seem to remain for long periods. In addition, chronic inflammation may begin insidiously, such as with a low-grade infection or other processes that do not display the usual signs of acute inflammation; tuberculosis, rheumatoid arthritis, and chronic lung disease are examples of this third alternative.

Chronic inflammation typically occurs in one of the following conditions: prolonged exposure to potentially toxic substances such as asbestos, coal dust, and silica that are nondegradable; immune reactions against one's tissue (autoimmune diseases such as lupus and rheumatoid arthritis); and persistent infection by an organism that is either resistant to drug therapy or insufficiently toxic to cause an immune reaction (such as viruses, tuberculosis, and leprosy). The characteristics of chronic inflammation are similar to those of acute inflammation but are less dramatic and more protracted.

—*L. Fleming Fallon Jr., MD, PhD, MPH*

Further Information

Challem, Jack. *The Inflammation Syndrome: Your Nutritional Plan for Great Health, Weight Loss, and Pain-Free Living.* Rev. ed., Wiley-Blackwell, 2010.

Dartt, Darlene A. *Immunology, Inflammation and Diseases of the Eye.* Academic Press, 2011.

Gallin, John I., and Ralph Snyderman, editors. *Inflammation: Basic Principles and Clinical Correlates.* 3rd ed., Raven Press, 1999.

Górski, Andrzej, Hubert Krotkiewski, and Michal Zimecki, editors. *Inflammation*. Kluwer, 2001.

Guha, Sushovan, Sunil Krishnan, and Bharat B. Aggarwal. *Inflammation, Lifestyle, and Chronic Disease: The Silent Link*. CRC Press, 2012.

Kumar, Vinay, Abul K. Abbas, and Nelson Fausto, editors. *Robbins and Cotran: Pathologic Basis of Disease*. 8th ed., Saunders/Elsevier, 2010.

McPherson, R. "Inflammation and Coronary Artery Disease: Insights from Genetic Studies." *The Canadian Journal of Cardiology*, vol. 28, no. 6, 2012, pp. 662-66.

Meggs, William Joel, and Carol Svec. *The Inflammation Cure*. Contemporary Books, 2004.

Preddy, Victor R., and Ronald R. Watson. *Bioactive Food as Interventions and Related Inflammatory Diseases*. Elsevier/Academic Press, 2013.

Yian, Gu, and Nikolas Scarmeas. "Dietary Inflammation Factor Rating System and Risk of Alzheimer Disease in Elder." *Alzheimer Disease and Associated Disorders*, vol. 25, no. 2, 2011, pp. 149-54.

Metchnikoff advances the cellular theory of immunity

Categories: Biology; Health and medicine
Anatomy or system affected: Blood, immune system, lymphatic system
Specialties and related fields: Bacteriology, immunology, internal medicine, microbiology, virology
Definition: Demonstrated that amoeboid white blood cells combat disease by engulfing and killing bacteria. He was the first modern pathologist to view inflammation as part of the healing. process.

KEY TERMS
amoeboid movement: a type of cellular movement that features crawling-like movement caused by extensions of the cytoplasmic projections called "pseudopodia"
orthobiosis: sound and correct living that leads to longevity and well-being
phagocytosis: a process by which cells engulf and ingest particles

SUMMARY OF EVENT

The genius of science frequently manifests itself under unexpected circumstances. A line of research that, to the layperson, would probably be seen as obscure and peripheral to bettering the human condition can produce a result that, when viewed in a particular light, proves to hold the key to some fundamental physical or biological process. Such is the phenomenon of cellular immunity, whose significance the Russian zoologist Élie Metchnikoff stumbled upon in 1882 while studying the development of invertebrate embryos.

Thanks to the work of Louis Pasteur, Robert Koch, and others, the pathology of infectious disease and the microbial nature of many of the agents was already well known. However, the crucial role of white blood cells in fighting infection was not. Immunity to diseases following infection was thought to arise primarily out of a host's production of specific antitoxins. Pasteur favored the depletion theory for recovery from primary infection. postulating that bacteria used up some vital growth factor and could no longer reproduce, thus limiting disease.

As a professor of zoology at the university in Odessa, Russia, Metchnikoff labored far from the European biomedical research centers. A passionate Darwinist professed atheist and political radical, he followed his fellow Russian Alexander Kovalevsky in choosing comparative embryology as the discipline most likely to elucidate evolutionary relationships in the animal kingdom.

Believing that "ontogeny recapitulates phylogeny," Metchnikoff reasoned that studying developmental stages of the simplest multicellular invertebrates would yield fundamental insights into the evolutionary process. At the same time, following the lead of Rudolf Virchow, who maintained that pathology ultimately derived from disturbances of cells

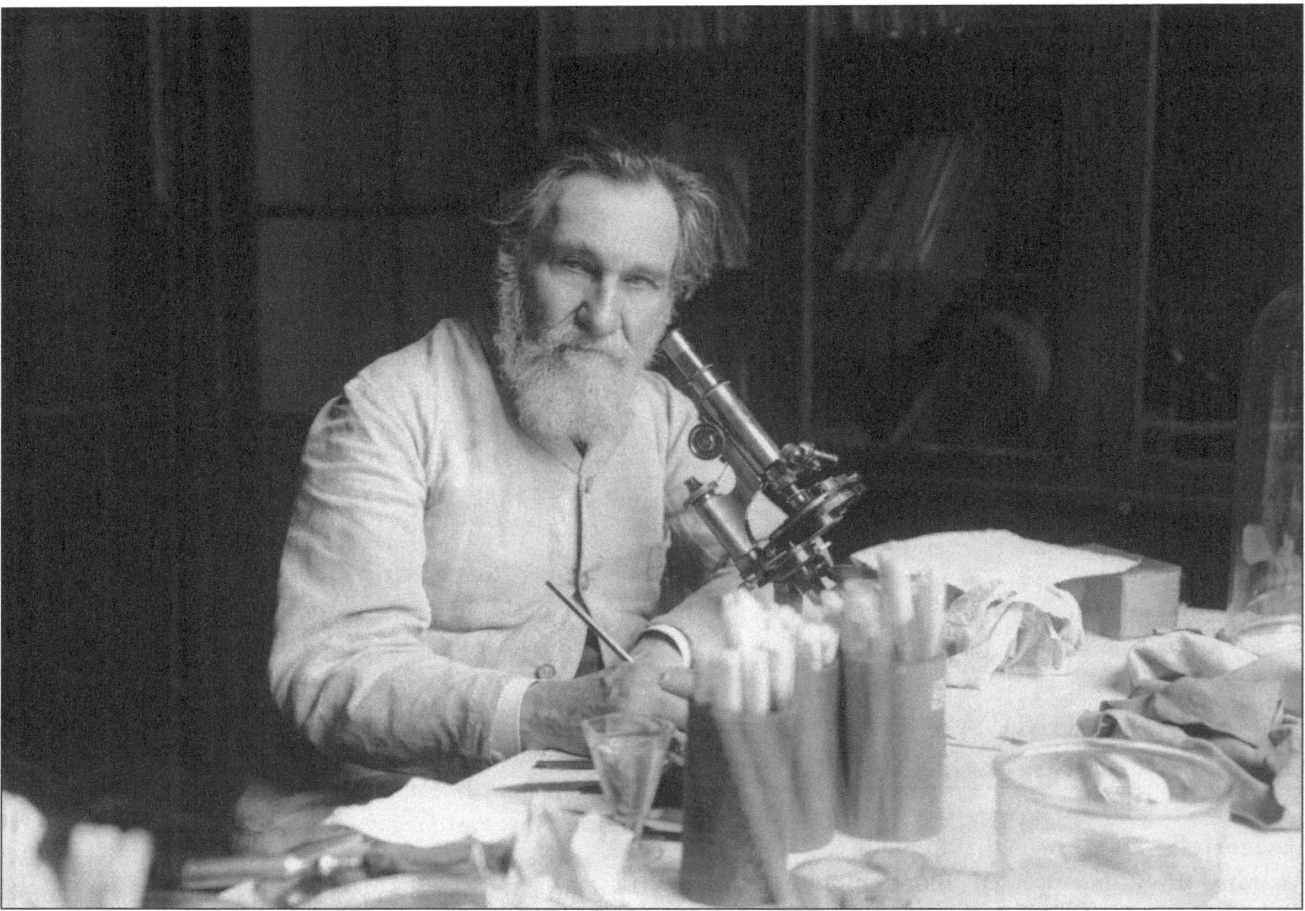
Metchnikoff. Photo via Wikimedia Commons. [Public domain.]

and could be understood only at the cellular level, Metchnikoff directed his microscope at inflammation. At a congress of naturalists and physicians in Odessa in 1882, he first set forth his hypothesis that phagocytosis was the basis of the healing process. Following the assassination of Czar Alexander II, academic freedom at Russian universities took a sharp downturn. Metchnikoff emigrated, settling first in Messina, Italy, where he had done his doctoral research. His wife's inheritance freed him from the necessity of paid employment, both in Italy and later at the Pasteur Institute in Paris.

While observing the development of starfish embryos, Metchnikoff noticed that amoeboid cells that migrated to form the digestive surface bore a solid resemblance to vertebrate leukocytes and wondered if the amoeboid cells would behave similarly. He verified that pricking the embryos with a fine thorn caused the cells to migrate to the injury site. The cells enveloped dye particles, thus providing further evidence that the ability of such cells to engulf foreign particles, including bacteria, played a role in protection against disease.

Metchnikoff next turned to *Daphnia* (water fleas), small, nearly transparent arthropods with a defined gut and body cavity. He noted that amoeboid cells in the cavity fluid engulfed and destroyed spores of a parasitic fungus to which the organism had some immunity. His first paper reporting these discoveries on the intracellular digestion of invertebrates (1883) attracted little attention from the medical community. Still, Metchnikoff persisted, extrapolating his findings to inflammation following trauma and maintaining that the migration of white blood cells to infection sites, pus formation, and changes in other cells associated with inflammation were part of an active process by which the body combated disease organisms. This ran contrary to prevailing medical opinion and plunged Metchnikoff into the thick of a raging conflict between rival schools of pathology.

Metchnikoff's work attracted the attention of Louis Pasteur, who, in 1888, offered him a position with the newly opened Pasteur Institute. Metchnikoff became the institute's director following Pasteur's death in 1895, continuing an active research program until the outbreak of World War I all but closed the institute. While at the institute, he delivered a series of lectures and then published two major books summarizing his findings: *Leçons sur la pathologie comparée de l'inflammation* (1892; *Lectures on the Comparative Pathology of Inflammation*, 1893) and *L'immunité dans les maladies infectieuse* (1901; *Immunity in Infective Diseases*, 1905). In these books, he maintained that the phagocyte was the chief means of defense against disease and that circulating antibodies, the so-called humoral factors, were secondary in importance.

SIGNIFICANCE
By 1901, the two schools of immunology—cellular and humoral—had become sharply drawn along national lines, with the French, led by the Russian expatriate Metchnikoff, championing the role of the cell. The Germans, headed by Koch's successor Paul Ehrlich, maintaining that circulating chemicals, rather than cells, constituted the key to defense against disease.

The development of specific therapies supported the German school. Ehrlich had demonstrated that guinea pigs fed increasing doses of lethal vegetable toxins developed immunity to them and that the immunity derived from a chemical present in blood serum. Working with diphtheria and cholera, diseases whose causative agents produce potent toxins, Ehrlich's laboratory in Berlin produced animal sera effective against these scourges. Cellular immunity, in contrast, appeared to be relatively nonspecific.

By the time the Nobel Prize committee decided to award the Nobel Prize in Physiology or Medicine jointly to Metchnikoff and Ehrlich in 1908, the humoral theory of immunity appeared to have triumphed over cellular theory. Metchnikoff had become convinced that a well-balanced intestinal flora held the key to prolonging human life. He devoted much of his energies in the last decade of his life to promoting yogurt consumption to achieve a condition he called "orthobiosis."

In choosing to make a joint award to two rivals whose theories, in 1908, appeared to some extent to be in opposition, the Nobel committee anticipated the eventual integration of the two theories into a comprehensive model of immune system function. In his *History of Immunology* (1989), Arthur Silverstein noted that the controversy between humoral and cellular theories of immunity provided a striking example of how nonscientific events (notably the Franco-Prussian War) shape research. He considers it a case in which the triumph of one concept (the humoral theory) stifled developments dependent on the other, to the detriment of science. Metchnikoff's death in 1916 left no distinguished proponent of his theory to take up the mantle, and cellular immunology remained on the back burner for decades.

The discovery of antibiotics revived interest. Antibiotics function by depressing growth rates rather than killing bacteria outright, giving white blood cells an advantage. Serum factors have little effect on antibiotic effectiveness, but a robust cellular immune system is essential.

—Martha A. Sherwood, PhD

Further Information

Lagerkvist, Ulf. *Pioneers of Microbiology and the Nobel Prize.* World Scientific, 2003. Describes Metchnikoff's research and provides an insider's view of the workings of the Nobel committee that awarded him the prize in 1908.

Metchnikoff, Elie. *Lectures on the Comparative Pathology of Inflammation.* Translated by F. A. Starling and E. H. Starling. Dover, 1968. Metchnikoff's book about inflammation, with a new introduction by scholar Arthur M. Silverstein.

Silverstein, Arthur M. *A History of Immunology.* Academic Press, 1989. The long chapter on cellular versus humoral immunity integrates many threads, including philosophy and nationalism.

Silverstein, Arthur M. *Paul Ehrlich's Receptor Immunology: The Magnificent Obsession.* Academic Press, 2002. Emphasis is on Ehrlich and the Berlin school but contains considerable information on Metchnikoff, especially his conflicts with Ehrlich.

Tauber, Alfred I. *Metchnikoff and the Origins of Immunology: From Metaphor to Theory.* Oxford UP, 1991. A thorough account of the scientific aspects of Metchnikoff's work.

Neutrophil

Category: Biology
Anatomy or system affected: Immune system, circulatory system
Specialties and related fields: Immunology, hematology, cytology
Definition: A neutrophil is a white blood cell that fights infection and is the most abundant white blood cell type.

KEY TERMS

white blood cells: white blood cells function in the immune system and are made in the bone marrow.

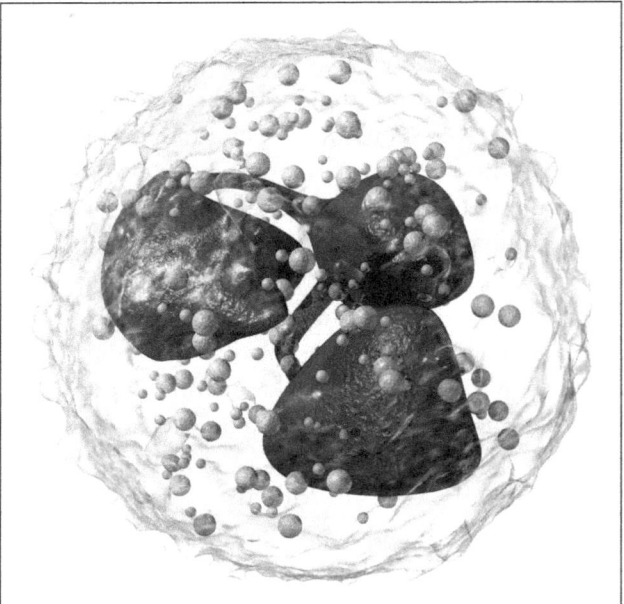

3D rendering of a neutrophil. Image by Blausen Medical, via Wikimedia Commons. [CC 4.0.]

There are many types of white blood cells, including granulocytes, monocytes, and lymphocytes

polymorphonuclear leukocytes: polymorphonuclear leukocyte, or PMN, is another term for neutrophil, based on the irregular shaped multilobed nuclei characteristic of this cell type

granulocytes: granulocytes are a type of white blood cell with granules that contain enzymes released during infection or other immune responses such as allergy; the different types of granulocytes include neutrophils, eosinophils, and basophils

phagocytosis: a phagocyte is a cell that eats, *phago* derived from the Greek word "for eat"

STRUCTURE AND FUNCTIONS

Neutrophils play essential roles in the immune system. They are the most abundant white blood cell type and the first cells to arrive at the site of infection or injury. Neutrophils comprise about 55 to 75 percent of a normal white blood cell count, with normal cell counts ranging from 2 to 7 billion cells per liter of blood. Along with eosinophils and basophils, neutrophils comprise a type of white blood cell known as "granulocytes," so named because they contain small "granules" or grain-like shapes within their cytoplasm. These granules store microbe-fighting enzymes. Neutrophils specialize in the capture, engulfment, and killing of microorganisms.

Neutrophils are produced in the bone marrow and are short-lived, with life spans measured in hours. It takes about one week for a neutrophil to develop from a progenitor cell into a mature neutrophil in the bone marrow. The bone marrow produces about 100 billion neutrophils every day. Once produced, neutrophils live only about four to ten hours in the bloodstream or one to two days if they migrate into tissue. The bone marrow stores many granulocytes that can be mobilized quickly in response to infection. This granulocyte depot prevents the rapid depletion of neutrophils during an infection. Newly formed cells have a round nucleus, but as cells mature, the nucleus becomes more irregular and lobular, giving multiple nuclei. Because of their multilobed nuclei, these cells are often referred to as polymorphonuclear leukocytes. Neutrophils are characterized histologically by cytoplasmic granules, nuclear features, and staining characteristics and functionally by their role in immune responses against infectious microorganisms.

When the body detects an invasion of foreign organisms, the body's cells send out chemical signals that recruit cells to the site of invasion. An essential feature of the role of neutrophils in immune defense is their mobility; unlike some of the other white blood cells, neutrophils aren't limited to a specific area of circulation. They can move freely through the walls of veins and into tissues of the body to immediately attack antigen. The neutrophils are the first cells to respond and travel through the bloodstream to the site of infection. Once at the site of infection, neutrophils attach themselves to walls of blood vessels and enter surrounding tissue to attack invaders and prevent more organisms from entering the blood.

A primary function of neutrophils is phagocytosis and the killing of microorganisms. Although neutrophils utilize an arsenal of antimicrobial weapons to destroy their target, phagocytosis, or "cell-devouring" is one of their primary strategies. Neutrophils surround and engulf bacteria and other microorganisms. The granules of the neutrophil, filled with enzymes that can digest many types of cellular material, are released to destroy the organisms. At the same time, neutrophils can also release potent forms of reactive oxygen-based molecules—such as superoxide or hydrogen peroxide—that can destroy bacteria in a process known as "oxidative burst." Even in dying, neutrophils have developed a method to kill their targets. Under certain conditions, a neutrophil can undergo a process called "NETosis," a form of cell death that releases a mesh-like network of fibers containing antimicrobial enzymes and chemicals. Scientists have termed these neutrophil extracellular traps (NET).

DISORDERS AND DISEASES

Usually, the body regulates the production of neutrophils and other white blood cells to respond to infection or injury. Abnormal neutrophil counts may result from infections or another condition. Too many or too few neutrophils in the bloodstream can indicate blood disorders with the potential to be severe conditions. Neutrophilia, a high number of neutrophils in the blood, can result from infection or reaction to a medication. Neutrophilia is generally associated with acute inflammation, although it may result from certain diseases such as chronic myelogenous leukemia, a type of cancer of blood-forming tissues. More common is a disorder called "neutropenia," an abnormally low number of neutrophils in the blood. Neutropenia most often occurs in cancer patients undergoing chemotherapy. However, it can also result from inherited disorders that affect the immune system and some acquired diseases. Neutropenia significantly increases the risk of life-threatening bacterial infection.

PERSPECTIVE AND PROSPECTS

Neutrophils are critical in immune response and are first responders to infection. In addition to direct uptake and destruction of invading pathogens, neutrophils also secrete chemicals that recruit reinforcements, including other specialized cell types, to the site of infection to assist with immune defense. Although neutrophils are the most abundant circulating leukocyte, their full spectrum of biological functions in the immune system is still emerging. An enhanced understanding of the full capabilities of neutrophils can hopefully lead to improved treatment options for diseases involving neutrophils.

—*Catherine J. Walsh, PhD*

Further Information

Bain, Barbara J. *Blood Cells: A Practical Guide*. 5th ed., Wiley Blackwell, 2015. A guide for identifying different blood cells and includes information on blood collection and clinical laboratory tests.

Gabrilovich, Dmitry, editor. *The Neutrophils: New Outlook for Old Cells*. 3rd ed., Imperial College P, 2013. Provides an overview of the biology of neutrophils, including the role of neutrophils in cancer and ways to use neutrophils in treatment.

Territo, Mary. "Neutrophilic Leukocytosis." *Merck Manual*, www.merckmanuals.com/home/blood-disorders/white-blood-cell-disorders/neutrophilic-leukocytosis. Accessed 19 Jan. 2017. The information provided on this website focuses on neutrophilic leukocytosis, or a high number of leukocytes, including possible diseases associated with the condition.

"Types of White Blood Cells." *New Health Advisor*, www.newhealthadvisor.com/Types-of-White-Blood-Cells.html. Accessed 21 Sept. 2017. An informative website with general information about the types of white blood cells important in human health, including a short video explanation on white blood cell types.

"White Blood Cell Disorders." *Dana-Farber/Boston Children's Cancer and Blood Disorders Center*, www.danafarberbostonchildrens.org/conditions/blood-disorders/white-blood-cell-disorders.aspx. Accessed 19 Jan. 2017. A website that includes a brief description of some white blood cell disorders in children and possible treatments.

Rheumatology

Category: Specialty
Anatomy or system affected: Bones, hands, hips, immune system, joints, knees, legs, musculoskeletal system
Specialties and related fields: Geriatrics and gerontology, immunology, orthopedics, pharmacology
Definition: The field of medicine is concerned with the diagnosis and treatment of joint inflammation and bone or joint destruction and the surgical repair of damaged joints.

KEY TERMS

acute: referring to a disease process of sudden onset
arthritis: joint inflammation
capillary exudate: a group of substances secreted by the capillaries as part of the inflammatory process
chronic: referring to a lingering disease process
joint: the conjunction of two or more bones

SCIENCE AND PROFESSION

Rheumatology is concerned with the major diseases of bones and joints: arthritis, osteoarthritis, other arthritic disorders such as gouty arthritis, and ankylosing spondylitis, among a host of others.

The onset of rheumatoid arthritis is usually in middle age. It strikes three times as many women as men. Understanding rheumatoid arthritis requires an understanding of the body's skeletal system—the bones and bone structures, as well as the tissues between and around bones and joints.

There are 206 bones in the human body. Some are support mechanisms that hold the body erect and support its weight, including the spine, hips, and legs. Some bones form defensive "cages" that protect body organs, such as the skull and the ribs. Some bones are involved in movement, specifically the spine, shoulders, arms, hands, hips, legs, and feet.

Bones are composed of three main sections. The tough membranous tissue covering the bone, the periosteum, contains the blood vessels that nourish bone cells and the nerve fibers that sense pain and pressure. The outer layer of the bone itself is compact bone; it forms the hard exterior. Inside is a spongy inner structure called "cancellous" (chambered) bone. Cancellous bone contains the marrow that manufactures blood cells, and it also stores fat cells.

When bones meet, the structure formed is called a "joint" or "articulation." Some joints are fixed, such as the ribs and the bones of the skull; these are fibrous joints covered with a tough, fibrous adhesive material that connects them, prohibiting movement and maintaining the integrity of the protective cage.

Some joints are capable of motion. Moving joints are of two types: synovial joints and cartilaginous joints. An example of the latter is the spine, where each vertebra is connected to its neighbor by a spinal disk made of cartilage. Cartilaginous joints are capable of movement, but they have nowhere near the mobility of the synovial joints, so-called because they are filled with synovial fluid, a liquid resembling the white of an egg.

There are six synovial joints: ball-and-socket, ellipsoidal, hinge, pivot, saddle, and gliding joints. Ball-and-socket joints are in the shoulders (humerus) and hips (femur). Such joints include a long bone that ends with a ball-shaped structure that fits neatly into a round, concave socket. Ball-and-socket joints are capable of the widest range of movement. Ellipsoidal joints are modifications of the ball-and-socket structures, where the bones are not round but oval. They are found in the wrists and ankles. The elbows and knees are hinge joints, which permit only bending and extending motions, up and down or side to side, as with a standard door hinge. In pivot joints, one bone contains a small cup or arch that accepts a point of another bone, permitting it to rotate on its axis. The two bones at the top of the spine, which govern the range of motion of the head, are examples. A saddle joint consists of two bones shaped somewhat like saddles; they fit snugly into each other and allow a wide range of movement. The joint connecting the thumb to the rest of the hand is the only saddle joint in the human body. The bones of gliding joints are almost flat; their surfaces slide over one another, permitting limited motion forward and back or from side to side. Some of the wrist bones are gliding joints.

The synovial joints are the most intricate and mobile of all the joints, and they are also the most prone to disease. The synovial joint capsule is a complex structure that encloses the moving bones and other tissues. It consists of the capsular ligament, which forms the joint capsule; the joint cavity, an open space between bones that allows free mobility; and the synovial membrane, a thin, smooth tissue that secretes synovial fluid. The synovial fluid fills the joint cavity and lubricates bone surfaces. Bones do not rub against each other; they are too rough and would become abraded. They are separated by a covering of smooth, white tissue called "articular cartilage" that permits smooth movement and absorbs impact. Just outside the joint capsule are bursae, small pouches that store synovial fluid.

In rheumatoid arthritis, the first signs of disease are pain and inflammation in the synovial joint capsule. This initial manifestation may be attributable to several factors, such as bacterial infection or injury. The reasons that an acute episode of pain and inflammation in the synovial joints progresses to chronic rheumatoid arthritis are unknown. It is suspected that genetic factors may be involved; the disease often runs in families. Blood components called "rheumatoid factors" are present in the majority of rheumatoid arthritis patients. However, the role of these factors in the development of disease is unclear because rheumatoid factors also occur in people who do not develop rheumatoid arthritis.

In some patients, rheumatoid arthritis is relatively benign, with pain and inflammation controlled by medication and other support techniques. The disease progresses to devastating bone deformities and complete loss of mobility in the affected joints in other patients. How this degeneration occurs is related to a disruption in the body's normal reaction to infection or injury. Pain and inflammation are protective mechanisms with which the body attempts to compensate for a disease or disorder. The following sequence of events occurs typically when a synovial joint sustains damage from infection, physical injury, or a toxic substance.

Tissue injury, whether resulting from trauma or infection, causes the release of chemical mediators from surrounding cells. These chemicals include prostaglandins, leukotrienes, histamine, serotonin, and bradykinin. Collectively, they cause the local blood vessels to enlarge (vasodilate), increasing blood flow to the affected area and causing redness and heat.

Ordinarily, the capillaries, the tiny blood vessels that supply nutrients to the cells, have openings in their walls so small that only tiny bits of matter can get through. During inflammation, they become more permeable; the openings in the capillary walls enlarge so that the capillaries can deliver larger substances to the affected area. This group of substances forms the capillary exudate, and it flows copiously into the affected area, causing swelling. The exudate consists of lymphocytes, which produce antibodies to fight infection; neutrophils; and macrophages, specialized white blood cells that facilitate the removal of tissue debris, dead cells, and other material. These white blood cells can also release other substances, such as superoxide, an agent used by white blood cells to kill bacteria, which can also damage healthy tissue. Another is interleukin-1, an agent that promotes healing and stimulates lymphocytes to produce antibodies. A third agent released by the white blood cells, fibrinogen, effectively closes off the area of inflammation, preventing the spread of inflammation.

In typical situations, after neutralizing the agent causing the inflammation, the capillaries return to their normal size, specific white blood cells remove the protective shield, and the healing process begins. In rheumatoid arthritis, the orderly process that begins with pain and inflammation and ends with healing is disrupted by various events. Instead of neutralizing the trauma, the anti-inflammatory phase can set off a chain of events that progressively worsens the condition.

Why this disruption occurs is not yet known, but there are four major theories. The first is the genetic predisposition to the disease, a factor that may or may not relate to the other three. The second theory is that rheumatoid arthritis is an immune-complex disease. Ordinarily, when the body fights an infectious microorganism that has invaded the body, lymphocytes produce antibodies that combine with the antigens characteristic of the microorganism. This antigen/antibody combination is the immune complex, and white blood cells remove it. In this theory, the process is altered. Instead of being removed by white blood cells, the immune complex lodges in the synovial membrane and causes continuing inflammation. Capillaries continue to release exudate, whose constituents cause cell proliferation, thickening of the synovial membrane, and destruction of articular cartilage and bone tissue.

The autoimmune theory is similar, but in this case, the causative agent is not a foreign substance but something natural within the body. For example, if a specific protein released by a gland finds its way into a joint, it may be regarded as a foreign, infective agent. Thus, it will set off an immune response and cause inflammation, initiating the same process described above.

The fourth theory links rheumatoid arthritis to viral or bacterial infection. It has been noted that fever, malaise, and enlarged lymph nodes—common symptoms of infection—are often seen in patients with rheumatoid arthritis. Furthermore, rheumatoid arthritis sometimes coincides with bacterial pneumonia, tuberculosis, hepatitis, sexually transmitted diseases, and diseases caused by viruses, such as mumps and measles.

The progress of rheumatoid arthritis is variable. In some patients, it is characterized by occasional flare-ups (episodes of acute pain and inflammation) and periods of remission (times when the patient is relatively comfortable). In others, the disease causes progressive, insidious destruction of the joint and may involve other organs of the body. Articular cartilage may be destroyed, and the joint may become immobilized, an excruciating condition. The bones in the joint may fuse, becoming one solid mass. The bones may also become dislocated. In about 30 to 35 percent of patients, rheumatoid nodules develop. These hard, solid lumps usually occur at the elbows but may also be found at the knees, ankles, and feet. In advanced cases, nodules may be discovered in the heart muscle, the lungs, and other organs where they could impair organ function.

The American Rheumatism Foundation has codified the diagnosis of rheumatoid arthritis. This organization lists seven symptoms and suggests that the presence of any four should confirm the diagnosis of rheumatoid arthritis (although patients with two or more of the symptoms should not be excluded). The seven symptoms are morning stiffness lasting an hour or more; arthritis in three or more joints; arthritis in hands, fingers, or wrists; arthritis occurring symmetrically (e.g., in both hands, elbows, or knees); rheumatoid nodules; the presence of rheumatoid factor; and X-ray evidence of bone deterioration.

DIAGNOSTIC AND TREATMENT TECHNIQUES

Once a patient is suspected of having rheumatoid arthritis, the physician may wish to conduct further laboratory tests to assess the severity of the disease and, from that analysis, develop a treatment regimen. In addition to testing for rheumatoid factor, the physician will check the patient's erythrocyte (red blood cell) sedimentation rate (ESR). This test helps to determine the presence of inflammatory activity. Another blood test looks for C-reactive protein (CRP). CRP also indicates inflammatory activity; levels rise during an acute attack and fall during a period of remission. Synovial fluid is analyzed to discover changes that occur during inflammation. For example, during inflammatory episodes, the color of the fluid becomes significantly darker, turning yellow or green. Ordinarily quite transparent and viscous, the synovial fluid becomes cloudy and has a thinner consistency. Many more tests are available to the physician to help them evaluate the severity of the disease, including an analysis of the various substances involved in the immune process.

There is no cure for rheumatoid arthritis, but most patients improve with the therapies available. Despite treatment, however, 5 to 10 percent will eventually be disabled by bone deterioration and destruction.

Treatment depends on the severity of the condition. The regimen can involve rest and immobilization of the affected joint, or it may include a wide range of medications, from aspirin to potent, often toxic compounds. In advanced cases, the joint deformity may be so severe as to require surgery or prosthetic implants.

The therapy goals are to relieve pain, reduce inflammation, and maintain the function of the joint. Ideally, the physician would also like to halt the progress of the disease. Some medications in use today promise to slow or stop the progress of the disease, but nothing is available to cure it.

For the relief of pain, the physician has many medications available, many of which will also reduce inflammation. These include a group of drugs called "nonsteroidal anti-inflammatory drugs" (NSAIDs). NSAIDs as a class include the salicylates, such as aspirin, ibuprofen, acetaminophen, and at least twenty other drugs currently in use in the United States.

Far and away, the most significant number of patients with rheumatoid arthritis are treated with NSAIDs. Many of the NSAIDs are perfectly safe when used in lower doses. The high doses usually required to control the pain of rheumatoid arthritis, however, can cause significant adverse reactions. A significant percentage of patients given some NSAIDs develop side effects severe enough to warrant stopping the drug. Many develop gastrointestinal (GI) problems ranging from stomachaches to bleeding ulcers, which can be fatal.

NSAIDs reduce the production of prostaglandins, substances released in the capillary exudate that are partially responsible for the inflammatory process. At the inflamed synovial joint, this attribute of NSAIDs is a desirable one. In the stomach, however, NSAIDs can cause problems. One of the prostaglandins helps protect the stomach lining from damage by the organ's highly acid contents. NSAIDs can remove this protection, allowing stomach acids to attack the lining, causing irritation and inflammation. Therefore, some physicians prescribe an NSAID with a prostaglandin analog, such as misoprostol, in the hope of avoiding or reducing GI distress. Misoprostol has problems of its own, however, such as causing severe diarrhea in some patients.

The patient with severe rheumatoid arthritis has a painful, debilitating illness that does not respond to NSAIDs and progresses to deformity. The available medications are both more potent and more toxic. A group of agents called "disease-modifying drugs" promise to reduce the degenerative processes in rheumatoid arthritis. These drugs include gold compounds, D-penicillamine, drugs used to treat malaria, and sulfasalazine. These drugs alter the course of rheumatoid arthritis, but they do not relieve pain or inflammation. Therefore, they must be given with NSAIDs. They all have a high potential for toxicity and must be used carefully, with constant monitoring, to avoid serious side effects.

In some cases, physicians find it necessary to prescribe corticosteroids to patients with rheumatoid arthritis. These drugs present a problem because rheumatoid arthritis is a lifelong condition, and toxicity and physical changes often occur with long-term steroid therapy. Sometimes corticosteroids are given as short-term therapy to achieve a rapid reduction of inflammation. In this case, there is a danger of a severe rebound reaction upon cessation of the drug. A corticosteroid may be injected into the joint, an effective short-term procedure to bring fast relief of pain and inflammation in an acute situation. However, high-dose corticosteroid injections into joints diminish the activity of cartilage-making cells and accelerate cartilage destruction. Therefore, interarticular injections should utilize low-dose corticosteroids.

Immunosuppressive therapy is sometimes prescribed for patients with rheumatoid arthritis. Immunosuppressive agents are, to some extent, highly toxic, and they are reserved for patients who have not responded to other treatments.

Exercise and physical therapy are helpful to the patient with rheumatoid arthritis. During acute inflammation, passive exercise within pain limits, with the limb manipulated by another person or the patient, will help keep the joints mobile and prevent muscle tightening. After the inflammation has subsided, active exercise is recommended to maintain muscle mass and mobility, but the activity should never be strenuous or fatiguing.

Flexion contracture, a condition in which the muscles that move the joint become stiff and shortened, may respond to exercise. However, if the contracture has become established, more intensive exercise, splinting, or orthopedic treatment may be necessary.

Orthopedic surgery can correct fused or dislocated joints in the body, and in some cases, an implant of metal or plastic (arthroplasty) replaces a fused or badly deteriorated joint. The two most successful implant procedures are total replacement of the hip or knee. During a hip replacement, the surgeon reveals the joint where the ball of the femur nests in the socket of the acetabulum, a cavity in the hipbone. The surgeon replaces the femur ball with a metal or plastic ball attached to a shaft that is anchored inside the femur. The socket is replaced as well, usually with a plastic cup that is secured into the hipbone. The implant can give the patient instant relief from pain and restore mobility. The length of time that the hip replacement will last vary, but many patients receive years of relief from a single operation. A similar procedure replaces the hinge joint of the knee, and although knee replacement is not as successful as hip replacement, it has helped many patients.

PERSPECTIVE AND PROSPECTS

Rheumatoid arthritis afflicts about 1 percent of all populations. While the disease is not life-threatening, it is one of the most significant crippling disorders globally. Most patients can be treated successfully by medication, exercise, and other support measures. The disease is progressive in most patients. After ten years, 80 percent of patients will have some degree of deformity, ranging from minor destruction of bone and cartilage to complete joint fusion.

Physicians see most patients with moderate-to-severe rheumatoid arthritis. Other patients medicate themselves with over-the-counter painkillers and rarely if ever, see a physician. In these patients, the disease is mild, with acute episodes occurring only sporadically.

Currently, there is no perfect therapy for rheumatoid arthritis, in the sense that there is no one agent or family of agents that promise to be safe and effective in all patients. The danger of significant adverse reactions exists with the most effective drugs, particularly in those patients who require high doses to control the pain and inflammation of the most severe forms of the disease.

Pharmaceutical science continues to search for new medications that will relieve pain and inflammation without damaging side effects. This inveterate search is for new drugs that stop the progress of the disease safely and effectively. There is also the hope that rheumatoid arthritis will be curable or preventable one day.

Orthopedic surgeons continue to improve the techniques for alleviating the effects of bone and joint destruction in some patients. New prosthetic appliances are designed and produced constantly to widen the range of joint replacement procedures.

—*C. Richard Falcon*

Further Information

American College of Rheumatology. *American College of Rheumatology*, 2013.
Isenberg, David A., et al., editors. *Oxford Textbook of Rheumatology*. 3rd ed., New York: Oxford UP, 2004.
Lahita, Robert G. *Rheumatoid Arthritis: Everything You Need to Know*. Rev. ed., Avery, 2004.
Litin, Scott C., editor. *Mayo Clinic Family Health Book*. 4th ed., HarperResource, 2009.
Mayo Clinic. *Mayo Clinic on Arthritis*. HarperCollins, 2005.
MedlinePlus. "Rheumatoid Arthritis." *MedlinePlus*, 26 Aug. 2013.
Parker, James N., and Philip M. Parker, editors. *The 2002 Official Patient's Sourcebook on Rheumatoid Arthritis*. Icon Health, 2002.
Shlotzhauer, Tammi L., and James L. McGuire. *Living with Rheumatoid Arthritis*. 2nd ed., Johns Hopkins UP, 2003.
Sutton, Amy L., editor. *Arthritis Sourcebook: Basic Consumer Health Information About Osteoarthritis, Rheumatoid*

Arthritis, Other Rheumatic Disorders, Infectious Forms of Arthritis, and Diseases with Symptoms Linked to Arthritis. 3rd ed., Omnigraphics, 2012.

Yung, Raymond L. "What Is a Rheumatologist?" *American College of Rheumatology*, Aug. 2012.

T Lymphocytes

Category: Immune response
Anatomy or system affected: Blood, bone marrow, immune system, lymphatic system, thymus
Specialties and related fields: Bacteriology, hematology, immunology, oncology, virology
Definition: Specialized white blood cells that are essential components of the immune system.

KEY TERMS

antigen: a toxin or other foreign substance that induces an immune response

antigen presentation: the process by which antigen-presenting cells introduce protein antigens to lymphocytes in the form of short peptide fragments

antigen-presenting cell: a varied collection of immune cells including dendritic cells, macrophages, and B lymphocytes that process and present antigens for recognition by T lymphocytes.

histocompatibility leukocyte antigens: cell surface molecules expressed by antigen-presenting cells that present antigenic peptides to T lymphocytes; also known as major histocompatibility complex (MHC) proteins

lymphocyte: a type of white blood cell that has a single round nucleus, and resides, mostly, in the lymphatic system.

T-cell receptor: a T-lymphocyte-specific cell surface protein that recognizes and binds specific antigens

T-cytotoxic cell: a subtype of T lymphocyte that has the CD8 cell surface glycoprotein, and attacks and destroys tumor cells and viral-infected cells

T-helper cell: a subtype of T lymphocyte that secretes signaling molecules called "lymphokines" that induce the maturation and activation of B lymphocytes, macrophages, and T-cytotoxic cells

thymus: a lymphoid organ that lies just over the upper part of the heart and produces mature T cells for the immune system

DEFINITION

T lymphocytes are white blood cells of the adaptive immune system that help fight disease. There are several subgroups of T lymphocytes with different immune system functions: cytotoxic T lymphocytes (CTLs), helper T lymphocytes, memory T lymphocytes, regulatory T lymphocytes, and tumor-infiltrating T lymphocytes (TILs). Laboratory manipulation of TILs makes them useful for cancer treatments.

FUNCTION

Some background on the immune system is helpful in understanding how T lymphocytes function and the role they play in fighting infections. The immune system is a complex of tissues, cells, and chemicals produced by these cells that spread throughout the body. Its function is to rid the body of foreign microbes and damaged or abnormal body cells (such as cancer cells). The major organs of the immune system are the bone marrow, lymph nodes, thymus, and spleen. Immune system cells and a clear fluid called "lymph" move throughout the body in a series of channels called "lymphatic vessels" that are separate from the blood-based circulatory system.

The immune system has two divisions, the innate immune system, and the adaptive immune system. The innate system consists of white blood cells (leukocytes) that respond rapidly to a wide range of microbes but that cannot confer immunity against disease. While a cell in the innate system can attack many different kinds of microbes, each cell of the adaptive system recognizes and attacks only one type of microbe or damaged cell. T lymphocytes and B lymphocytes are the major cells of the adaptive immune system. Adaptive system cells respond more slowly when first encountering a microbe but can "remember" exposure to that microbe in a way that creates long-lasting immunity to a particular disease.

All cells have marker molecules on their surface that act as a "uniform" that identifies them as "self cells" or "nonself cells." Self markers do not cause an immune response in a healthy person. Nonself marker molecules, also called "antigens," stimulate an immune system reaction. As a distinctive feature of the adaptive immune system, every T lymphocyte or B lymphocyte develops a unique receptor on its surface that will interact only with one highly specific nonself antigen.

DEVELOPMENT
T lymphocytes originate in bone marrow from hematopoietic stem cells, which are cells that have the potential to differentiate into many kinds of blood cells. Immature T lymphocytes leave the bone marrow and travel to the thymus, an organ behind the breastbone. Here they undergo a complicated maturation process that results in 2 major types of T lymphocytes. One type has the CD8 protein on its surface and is called a "CD8+ cell." The other carries the CD4 protein and is called a "CD4+ cell." In addition to these proteins, every one of these cells has a different T-cell-specific antigen receptor on its surface.

While in the thymus, the pre-T lymphocytes rearrange their gene segments for the T-cell receptor. The T-cell receptor consists of two polypeptides, an alpha, and a beta chain. The genes that encode the alpha protein are on chromosome 14 and those that encode the beta chain are on chromosome seven. Early in its sojourn in the thymus, the pre-T lymphocyte rearranges its genes for the beta protein.

The beta chain gene cluster consists of approximately 52 variable or V gene segments, two D or diversity gene segments, and about 13 J or joining gene segments. In response to interleukin-2 (IL-2) and interleukin-7 (IL-7), secreted by the thymic epithelium, the pre-T lymphocyte synthesizes two proteins, RAG-1 & -2, that cut and paste a specific D segment with a single J segment. Then the pre-T lymphocyte makes another enzyme called the "V(D)J recombinase" that attaches a single V gene segment to the joined DJ segments. The joining of the VDJ segment to the constant region (μ segment) produces a mature beta-chain gene.

Once a mature beta chain of the T-cell receptor appears on the cell surface, the pre-T lymphocyte expresses the CD4 and CD8 proteins on its surface. It is called a "double positive" or DP cell at this point in its development. DP cells begin to rearrange the genes for the alpha subunit of the T-cell receptor. The alpha gene cluster contains between 70 to 80 copies of the V segment, no D segments, and about 61 copies of the J segment. The joining of a single V segment with a single J segment and a constant region produces a mature alpha chain of the T-cell receptor. The pairing of the mature alpha and beta chains of the T-cell receptor constitutes a functional T-cell receptor. The joining of multiple V with multiple J regions allows for extensive mixing and matching of distinct gene segments. Such wide variability allows T cells to deploy a cadre of receptor proteins that can recognize a kaleidoscope of different antigens.

Any pre-T lymphocytes whose T-cell receptors to molecules on healthy tissue cells die before they leave the thymus so as not to harm the body—a process called "negative selection." Likewise, any pre-T lymphocytes that fail to rearrange their T-cell receptor genes and produce a functional T-cell receptor also undergo programmed cell death. However, all T-cell receptors must interact with human leukocyte antigens (HLAs) on the surfaces of dendritic cells in the thymus. If they fail to bind to HLAs, the pre-T lymphocytes also die, an example of positive selection. The pre-T lymphocyte then stops expressing either CD8 or CD4 and becomes a CD4-positive T-helper cell or a CD8-expression T-cytotoxic cell. Mature T lymphocytes exit the thymus and move to the peripheral circulation or lymphatic system.

ACTIVATION
To activate T lymphocytes, dendritic cells, a type of antigen-presenting cell that constantly circulates through the body, present antigen to the T lymphocyte. The dendritic cell finds a foreign microbe or an abnormal cell, engulfs or "eats" the cell, and takes some of the engulfed cell's proteins, and traffics them to their surfaces, bound to an MHC protein. This process is called "antigen presentation." The first step of activation occurs if the T-cell receptor on the T lymphocyte surface fits the antigen presented on the surface of the antigen-presenting cell. However, T lymphocyte activation requires a second signal. T lymphocytes also have on their surfaces a protein called "CD28." CD28 must bind to the B7 protein complex on the surface of the antigen-presenting cell. This dual signal tells the T lymphocyte that the right cell has presented the antigen and has approved T lymphocyte activation. In the absence of either signal, the T lymphocyte remains inactivated.

The activated T lymphocyte produces IL-2 and a fully functional IL-2 receptor. IL-2 is a potent T-lymphocyte growth factor, and the T lymphocyte divides vigorously, a phenomenon called "clonal expansion." IL-2 expression also activates nearby CD8+ CTLs that recognize the same antigen. Dendritic cells can, likewise, present antigens to CD8+ cells and activate them. The CD8+ cell undergoes clonal expansion, dividing rapidly to produce a large number of identical cells.

After leaving the thymus, CTLs move through the body, looking for microbes or abnormal cells that match their T-cell receptors. When a CTL finds a match, it attaches to the cell and releases chemicals that kill this rogue cell. CTLs play an integral role in fighting viral infections.

A few CD8+ cells become memory T lymphocytes instead of CTLs. Memory cells remain in the body for many years and are the basis for long-term immunity. If the same microbe invades the body again, memory T lymphocytes and memory B lymphocytes respond quickly to control the invader before the individual becomes sick.

When a dendritic cell presents an antigen to a CD4+ T lymphocyte whose receptor matches its foreign surface protein, the CD4+ cell is activated and becomes either a helper T lymphocyte or a regulatory T lymphocyte. There are at least three subgroups of helper T lymphocytes: Th1, Th2, and Th17. Helper cells cannot kill other cells directly. Instead, they secrete chemicals that coordinate the immune system response. One subset of helper cells, Th2, secretes cytokines that stimulate B lymphocytes to produce antibodies against foreign or abnormal cells. Another, Th1, helps CTLs become more effective killers. In addition, some T-helper cells, so-called T follicular helper or Tfh cells, establish memory B cells. Other T-helper cells become memory T lymphocytes.

Some CD4+cells are exposed to a cytokine called "transforming growth factor-beta" (TGF-ß) and become regulatory T lymphocytes. Regulatory T lymphocytes monitor the activity of other T lymphocytes, help prevent immune response against normal body cells, and wind down the immune response once a microbe has been eliminated.

Both CD4+ and CD8+ cells can become tumor-infiltrating T lymphocytes (TILs). Researchers are still learning about TILs and how they can be used to fight cancer.

TREATMENT
The body is exposed to thousands of different microbes each day, and a healthy immune system effec-

tively eliminates most of them before an individual becomes sick. The immune system, however, has challenges in eliminating cancer cells. Cancer cells start as normal body cells with all the surface proteins that identify them as self cells. At some point, these normal cells transform into cancer cells, but they often continue to have enough of the surface proteins that originally marked them as self cells to escape detection by dendritic cells and T lymphocytes. If the immune system does respond to transformed cells, the response may not be effective since the growth of cancer cells is not limited the way it is in healthy cells. In addition, some cancer cells make chemicals that turn off or disrupt the functioning of immune system cells.

As of 2015, the U.S. Food and Drug Administration (FDA) has approved only 1 T-lymphocyte cancer treatment vaccine. Unlike preventative vaccines, patients receive treatment vaccines after they already have cancer. The drug, called "Sipuleucel-T," is used to treat advanced prostate cancer. Scientists take cells from the patient's immune system and expose them in the laboratory to chemicals that turn them into dendritic cells with a special molecule artificially attached to stimulate a strong immune response against prostate cancer cells. The drug does not cure the cancer but can prolong life.

Another approach to treating cancer uses TILs and manipulates them in the laboratory to fight certain cancers. The process is called "adoptive cell therapy" (ACT), and it was first used to successfully treat metastatic melanoma. A surgeon excises a portion of the patient's melanoma tumor that contains TILs. In the laboratory, the tumor is minced and grown in culture with interleukin 2 (IL-2), a cytokine that stimulates T-cell growth. In a few weeks, the T lymphocytes destroy the tumor leaving a culture of billions of TIL cells—many more than the body could make—that is reintroduced into the patient. Since these cells are clones of self TILs, the immune system does not reject them, and they can infiltrate and successfully attack metastatic melanoma tumors.

Originally, ACT worked only with melanoma tumors, but researchers are working on perfecting ways to use a harmless virus to genetically engineer the patient's own TIL cells to make them more effective against difficult to treat cancers such as acute lymphoblastic leukemia. The cells are taken from the patient, manipulated and cloned in the laboratory, and then re-introduced into the patient. This process is called "chimeric antigen receptor" (CAR) T-cell therapy. The results are promising. The FDA has approved several CAR T-cell treatments, including Abecma (idecabtagene vicleucel), Breyanzi (lisocabtagene maraleucel), Kymriah (tisagenlecleucel), Tecartus (brexucabtagene autoleucel), and Yescarta (axicabtagene ciloleucel). Kymriah is approved for the treatment of acute lymphoblastic leukemia. Yescarta, Kymriah, and Breyanzi are approved for the treatment of B-cell lymphoma. Yescarta is also approved for the treatment of follicular lymphoma. Tecartus is approved for mantle cell lymphoma, and Abecma is approved for the treatment of multiple myeloma. CAR T-cell treatments are not without their caveats. Patients can suffer from high fevers and dangerously low blood pressure, brain swelling, confusion, seizures, and severe headaches. CAR T-cell therapy is being tested in clinical trials against many kinds of cancer. A searchable list of current clinical trials can be found at www.clinicaltrials.gov.

—*Tish Davidson, AM and Michael A. Buratovich, PhD*

Further Information

Abbas, Abul K., Andrew H. Lichtman, and Shiv Pillai. *Cellular and Molecular Immunology.* 10th ed., Elsevier, 2021.

Burton, Thomas. "Immunotherapy Treatments for Cancer Gain Momentum." *Wall Street Journal*, 12 Oct. 2017, www.wsj.com/articles/immunotherapy-treatments-for-cancer-gain-momentum-1507825152?mod=searchresults_pos17&page=1.

Kershaw, Michael H., J. A. Westwood, C. Y. Slaney, and P. K. Darcy. "Clinical Application of Genetically Modified T Cells in Cancer Therapy." *Clinical and Translational Immunology*, vol. 3, 2014, p. e16., www.nature.com/cti/journal/v3/n5/full/cti20147a.html

Man, Yang-gao, et al. "Tumor-Infiltrating Immune Cells Promoting Tumor Invasion and Metastasis: Existing Theories." *Journal of Cancer*, vol. 4, no. 1, 2013, pp. 84-95.

Martin, Seamus, Dennis R. Burton, Ivan M. Roitt, and Peter J. Delves. *Roitt's Essential Immunology*. 13th ed., Wiley-Blackwell, 2017.

Pardoll, Drew. "T Cells Take Aim at Cancer." *Proceedings of the National Academy of Sciences*, vol. 99, no. 25, 2012, pp. 15840-42, www.pnas.org/content/99/25/15840.full.

VACCINE TYPES

Category: Prevention
Also known as: Immunization
Anatomy or system affected: Blood, immune system, lymphatic system
Specialties and related fields: Allergist, epidemiology, hematology, immunology, microbiology, pharmacology, public health, virology
Definition: The injection, ingestion, or inhalation of suspension of immunogens (molecules that produce an immune response), or a vehicle that causes the synthesis of immunogens, that elicit a protective immune response against a specific infection.

KEY TERMS

adjuvant: a substance given with a vaccine that enhances the immune response elicited by it

antigen: a foreign substance that elicits an immune response when inoculated into a living organism

attenuated: weakened or partial organisms

conjugate: the attachment of molecules that tend to elicit weak immune responses, such as carbohydrates, to large molecules that enhance the immunogenicity of the attached molecules.

excipient: an inactive substance that serves as the vehicle or medium for a drug, vaccine, or other material

immunity: the ability of an immune system to recognize, neutralize, and destroy an infecting organism, protecting the individual from infection

inoculation: the introduction of a substance or group of substances into a living organism

lipid nanoparticles: a shell of cholesterol and other fat-soluble molecules that house an internal mRNA core, and fuse with host cells to deliver the messenger ribonucleic acid (mRNA) payload

VACCINES

A vaccine is a suspension of immunogens (molecules that produce an immune response or stimulate the production of antibodies) such as weakened or dead pathogenic (disease-causing) cells or cellular components. The act of administering a vaccine, or immunization, is called "vaccination." Persons who receive a vaccine are considered immunized against a particular pathogen. Vaccines may contain a pathogen, suspending fluid, adjuvants, excipients, and preservatives.

Several types of vaccines are given to humans. These types include live attenuated, inactivated, component or subunit, toxoid, conjugate, deoxyribonucleic acid (DNA), and recombinant vector vaccines. Live attenuated vaccines contain living but altered bacteria or viruses that do not cause disease. Inactivated or killed vaccines contain killed bacteria or inactivated viruses that do not cause disease. Component or subunit vaccines contain parts of the whole bacteria or viruses. Toxoid vaccines contain toxins (or poisons) produced by the pathogen that have been made harmless. Conjugate vaccines allow the immune system to recognize certain bacteria disguised by a polysaccharide outer coating and therefore respond. DNA and recombinant vector vaccines are in the experimental stage and both use genetic material to stimulate an antibody response.

Some vaccines are combinations of pathogens for different diseases, such as measles, mumps, and rubella (or MMR vaccine). Most vaccines are administered by injection into the muscle (intramuscular); however, some may be given into the skin (subcutaneous), by mouth, or into the nose (intranasal).

Active immunity is classified as natural (after pathogen exposure and infection) or acquired (after vaccination). Passive immunity is also classified as natural (across the placenta during pregnancy) or acquired (injection of antibodies or immunoglobulins pooled from several donors). Immunoglobulins are prepared antibodies that are given to a person who has already been infected or who is at risk of acquiring an infection, thereby providing passive immunization. In this case, the immune system does not need to produce antibodies protecting the body.

Herd immunity occurs when most of, but not all, the people in a given population are immune to a pathogen. If there is an outbreak or exposure to a pathogen, those who are immune will sometimes naturally protect those who are not immune from getting the disease; however, those who are not immune are still more likely to get the disease and spread it to others.

MECHANISMS OF ACTION

A vaccine is given to intentionally expose the immune system to a pathogen in a safe, controlled manner so that the immune system can react and develop antibodies to that pathogen or antigen. Antibodies are large proteins that help fight infection and control disease. Many antibodies disappear after destroying the invading antigens, but the cells involved in antibody production remain and become memory cells. Memory cells "remember" the original antigen and then defend against it if the antigen attempts to reinfect a person. This protection is called "immunity." Therefore, after sufficient antibodies have been developed, the immune system that is reexposed to that pathogen will react within minutes to hours; the pathogen will be destroyed before a full-fledged infection and organ damage can occur. B cells are a type of lymphocyte (white blood cell) that makes antibodies. B cells use antibodies to identify, inactivate, and help destroy these pathogens.

Vaccines, which protect from the disease without the serious symptoms, have a high effectiveness rate (usually 95 to 99 percent). Vaccine failure, meaning that the vaccine administration did not result in antibody production, is uncommon. Several factors can lead to vaccine failure, including having an already compromised immune system and the inadequate storage or administration of the vaccine. The immune response to a pathogen may decrease over time, so vaccines known as boosters restore antibodies. Protective immunity lasts longer with boosters.

A suspending fluid (such as sterile water or saline) is needed to allow the vaccine to be administered. Preservatives and stabilizers, such as albumin, phenols, and glycine, keep the vaccine from being changed. Adjuvants, or enhancers, help the vaccine work. Adjuvants help promote an earlier, more potent response and a more persistent immune response to the vaccine. Antibiotics prevent the growth of bacteria during the production and storage of the vaccine. Eggs are used to grow the pathogen, and egg protein is found in influenza and yellow fever vaccines. Formaldehyde is used to inactivate bacterial products for toxoid vaccines and to kill unwanted viruses and bacteria that might contaminate the vaccine during production. Monosodium glutamate and 2-phenoxy-ethanol are preservatives that help the vaccine remain unchanged during the vaccine's exposure to heat, light, acidity, or humidity. Thimerosal is a mercury-containing preservative that helps prevent contamination and the growth of bacteria.

Most vaccines are given to prevent disease and are effective only if administered to the person before he or she is exposed to the pathogen or disease; most vaccines must be given by a certain age to ensure effectiveness. Also, most vaccine-preventable diseases can cause serious or life-threatening infections in infants and young children. For example, exposure and infection with polio can occur at a very young age and can cause paralysis, so the vaccine should be given to infants as soon as possible. Immunity to some pathogens can be transferred from a pregnant woman to her fetus, but this immunity wanes once the newborn is older than six months of age. Breastfeeding can also help extend immunity to some diseases, but even this is limited.

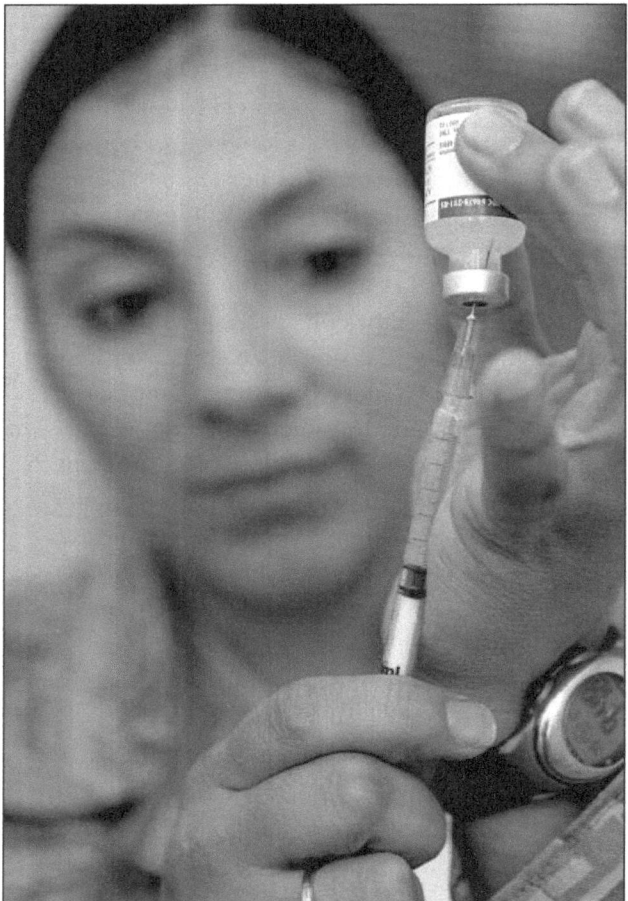

Senior Airman Sonia Vega of the 32nd Expeditionary Aerospace Medical Squadron prepares a vaccine at Balad Air Base. Photo by Staff Sgt. Joshua Garciavia, via Wikimedia Commons.

Certain vaccines (such as pneumococcal or hepatitis B vaccines) are given once in a lifetime unless a booster is needed. The seasonal influenza vaccine, however, is given annually because hundreds of influenza-like viruses exist; also, the seasonal variations or types of viruses that are prevalent change every year. Vaccination schedules have been developed for children, adolescents, and adults that indicate when these persons should receive doses of required vaccinations or boosters.

TYPES OF VACCINES

The selection of the type of vaccine depends on fundamental information or factors about the pathogen. These factors include how the pathogen infects cells and how the immune system responds to it. Practical considerations include the regions of the world where the vaccine would be used. Pros and cons are associated with each type of vaccine.

Live attenuated vaccines. Live attenuated vaccines are usually created from the naturally occurring pathogen. The pathogen's ability to cause serious infection is attenuated, or weakened, by manipulating the virus or bacteria in a laboratory environment, but these vaccines can still induce antibody production or protective immune responses. Attenuation of the pathogen usually is done by "passing" or growing the virus or bacteria from culture to culture before it is formulated into a vaccine. Live attenuated vaccines elicit strong cellular and antibody responses and often confer lifelong immunity with only one or two doses. Not everyone can safely receive live attenuated vaccines, however. People with weakened immune systems cannot be given live vaccines because of the risk they will develop disease symptoms.

These types of vaccines usually need to be refrigerated to stay potent. Proper storage then becomes critical in maintaining vaccine efficacy. Examples of live attenuated vaccines include measles, mumps, and rubella (MMR vaccine), oral polio vaccine

(OPV), the nasal form of influenza (flu) vaccine, and the varicella vaccine (chickenpox vaccine).

Inactivated vaccines. Inactivated vaccines contain a killed pathogen that cannot cause the disease but can stimulate antibody production. Pathogens can be inactivated with chemicals such as formaldehyde. Inactivated vaccines are more stable and safer than live vaccines. These vaccines usually do not require refrigeration and are easily stored and transported in freeze-dried form, making them useful in situations requiring long transportation or with less-developed medical infrastructure. Most inactivated vaccines, however, produce a weaker immune response than do live vaccines. Several additional doses or booster shots, therefore, are needed to maintain immunity. Examples of inactivated vaccines include inactivated polio vaccine (IPV) and inactivated (injectable form) influenza vaccine.

Component or subunit vaccines. Component or subunit vaccines are made by using only parts of the pathogen. These vaccines cannot cause disease, but they can stimulate the body to produce an immune response against the disease. Component vaccines contain only the essential antigens, but not all the other molecules, of the pathogen, so the chance of an adverse reaction to the vaccine is lessened.

These vaccines can contain anywhere from one to twenty or more antigens. Identifying what antigens best stimulate the immune system can be a tricky, time-consuming process. A recombinant component vaccine has been created for the hepatitis B virus. Hepatitis B genes that code for important antigens were inserted into common baker's yeast. The yeast then produced the antigens, which were collected and purified for use in the vaccine.

A conjugate vaccine is another type of component vaccine that has been developed for bacteria that possesses an outer coating of sugar molecules called "polysaccharides." The polysaccharide coating disguises the internal antigens of the bacterium so that the immune system does not recognize or respond to it. Vaccines help the immune system link the polysaccharide coating to the bacterium and, therefore, allow antibodies to produce immunity to that pathogen. Examples of component vaccines include *Haemophilus influenzae* type B (Hib) vaccine, hepatitis B (Hep B) vaccine, hepatitis A (Hep A) vaccine, and pneumococcal conjugate vaccine.

Toxoid vaccines. Toxoid vaccines are made by treating the toxin produced by the pathogen with heat or chemicals, such as formalin (a solution of formaldehyde and sterilized water). For pathogens that secrete toxins or harmful chemicals, a toxoid vaccine may be used when the toxoid is the main cause of illness. Toxins are inactivated and do not produce disease. Detoxified toxins are called "toxoids." After vaccination with a toxoid vaccine, the immune system produces antibodies that block the toxin. Examples of toxoid vaccines include those against diphtheria and tetanus.

DNA vaccines. Experimental DNA vaccines contain the genes that code for antigens. The development of DNA vaccines requires that the genes from the pathogen be isolated and analyzed. DNA vaccines would stimulate an immune response to the free-floating antigen secreted by cells and against the antigens displayed on cell surfaces. DNA vaccines would contain copies of a few of the pathogen's genes, so the vaccine would not cause disease.

DNA vaccines are relatively easy and inexpensive to design and produce. Naked DNA vaccines, which consist of DNA administered directly into the body, could be mixed with molecules that facilitate its uptake by the body's cells. Naked DNA vaccines for influenza and herpes viruses are under investigation.

mRNA vaccines. In 1990, Agnes Jani and Phillip Felgner, and their colleagues injected messenger ribonucleic acid (mRNA) into the muscles of laboratory animals and observed protein synthesis. In 1992, Bloom and colleagues from the Scripps Research Institute in La Jolla, California reversed diabetes insipidus in Brattleboro rats by injecting vasopressin mRNA into their hypothalamus. These two studies demonstrated the ability of injected RNA to induce the expression of specific proteins. However, these studies also showed the caveats of mRNA injection, including its short half-life and the tendency for the immune system to recognize mRNA and destroy it.

Further research revealed that efficient delivery of mRNAs by encasing them in lipid nanoparticles not only increased mRNA uptake by cells but also prevented recognition of the RNA by the immune system. Using modified bases during the synthesis of mRNAs not only increases their half-lives, but significantly decreases their immunogenicity. The production of mRNA vaccines is rapid, inexpensive, and highly scalable.

mRNA vaccines made by Pfizer-BioNTech (BNT162b2) and Moderna (mRNA-1273) were granted Emergency Use Authorization (EUA) by the FDA on December 11, 2020, and December 18, 2020, respectively, for the COVID-19 pandemic. Both vaccines encode the SARS-CoV-2 spike protein and induce excellent immune responses against SARS-CoV-2. Other mRNA vaccines for Zika virus, influenza, respiratory syncytial virus, human immunodeficiency virus, and several types of cancer are in development.

Recombinant vector vaccines. Recombinant vector vaccines, also experimental, use an attenuated pathogen to introduce DNA to cells. A vector in this case is a harmless virus or bacterium used as a carrier. Certain harmless or attenuated viruses are used to carry portions of the genetic material from other microbes. The carrier viruses then ferry the microbial DNA to cells and display the antigens of the pathogen on the cell's surface. The harmless organism mimics a pathogen and provokes an immune response. Recombinant vector vaccines closely mimic a natural infection, effectively stimulating the immune system. Recombinant vector vaccines for human immunodeficiency virus (HIV), rabies, and measles are under investigation.

Adenovirus-based vaccines for COVID-19 include the Oxford-AstraZeneca (ChAdOx1), Johnson & Johnson (JNJ-78436735), and Sputnik V (Gam-COVID-Vac) vaccines. The FDA awarded the Johnson & Johnson vaccine EUA on February 27, 2021. The Oxford-AstraZeneca vaccine has been approved for use in the European Union, Vietnam, Argentina, Bangladesh, Brazil, the Dominican Republic, El Salvador, India, Malaysia, Mexico, Nepal, Pakistan, the Philippines, Sri Lanka, South Korea, and Taiwan. Adenovirus-based vaccines are also available for Ebola.

CONTROVERSY
State laws in the United States mandate that children in daycare and students be immunized against certain diseases. Some exceptions are allowed. Still, many parents refuse to immunize their children for fear of a link between autism, for example, and the use of vaccines containing thimerosal, an ethylmercury-based preservative. Scientific evidence does not support this link. In 2004, the Institute of Medicine conducted a scientific review of thimerosal and concluded that "the evidence favors rejection of a causal relationship between thimerosal-containing vaccines and autism." Since then, nine additional studies have found no link between thimerosal-containing vaccines and autism spectrum disorder. Nevertheless, thimerosal is no longer used in the production of most single-shot vaccines in the United States.

The link between vaccines and autism comes from a fraudulent paper published in 1997 in the prestigious medical journal *The Lancet* by a British physician named Andrew Wakefield. Not only has no one been able to replicate Wakefield's results, but intensive investigation by the British journalist Brian Deer established that Wakefield's research project contained serious procedural errors, undisclosed financial conflicts of interest, and ethical violations. The paper was retracted, and Wakefield lost his medical license for endangering children and failing to disclose significant financial interests connected to the project. A follow-up study led by Brent Taylor at the Royal Free Hospital Medical School, London, published in 2002, examined 498 autistic children and failed to establish any link between vaccination and either inflammatory bowel disease or autism. Further work has corroborated Taylor's findings. A 2011 Institute of Medicine examined side effect data of eight vaccines given to children and adults and found no link with autism spectrum disorder. A 2013 CDC study of the antigens in vaccines established that increased exposure to these antigens is not the cause of autism spectrum disorder.

To alert persons to adverse effects associated with vaccine administration, and to educate parents and others about what to expect after receiving a vaccine, an information sheet must be given to each person before he or she can be vaccinated.

IMPACT
Disease prevention is the key to public health, and it is always better to prevent a disease than to have to treat it. Vaccination is considered one of the most important medical discoveries in all of human history. Diseases can cause suffering, permanent disability, and death. Vaccines prevent disease in those who get vaccinated and protect those who come into contact with unvaccinated persons. Vaccination has controlled many infectious diseases that were once common, including polio, measles, diphtheria, pertussis (whooping cough), rubella (German measles), mumps, tetanus, and influenza. It even led to the complete eradication of smallpox from the human population.

Not all countries have the same level of vaccination requirements as the United States. Given the current global nature of travel and business, exposure to many diseases is likely. Vaccination minimizes the risk of developing a disease and its associated complications. When persons travel outside the United States, additional vaccinations may be needed. One should consult a physician within a minimum of four weeks of traveling to determine what vaccines, if any, are needed.

—*Beatriz Manzor Mitrzyk, PharmD*

Further Information
Centers for Disease Control and Prevention. "Vaccines and Immunizations." www.cdc.gov/vaccines/.
Centers for Disease Control and Prevention. "Immunization Schedules: Resources for Parents." www.cdc.gov/vaccines/schedules/parents-adults/resources-parents.html.
Centers for Disease Control and Prevention. "Autism and Vaccines." www.cdc.gov/vaccinesafety/concerns/autism.html.
Deer, Brian. *The Doctor Who Fooled the World*. Johns Hopkins UP, 2020.
DeStefano, Frank, Cristofer S. Price, and Eric S. Weintraub. "Increasing Exposure to Antibody-Stimulating Proteins and Polysaccharides in Vaccines Is Not Associated with Risk of Autism." *Journal of Pediatrics*, vol. 163, no. 2, pp. 561-67.
Merino, Noël. *Vaccines*. Greenhaven, 2015.
Pardi, Norbert, Michael J. Hogan, Frederick W. Porter, and Drew Weissman. "mRNA Vaccines—A New Era in Vaccinology." *Nature Reviews Drug Discovery*, vol. 17, 2018, pp. 261-79.
Plotkin, Stanley A., Walter A. Orenstein, and Paul A. Offit. *Vaccines*. 7th ed., Saunders/Elsevier, 2017.
Shoenfeld, Yehuda, and Nancy Agmon-Levin. *Vaccines and Autoimmunity*. Wiley, 2015.
"Vaccines." *National Institute of Allergy and Infectious Disease*. National Institutes of Health, 13 Aug. 2020, www.niaid.nih.gov/research/vaccines.

IMMUNE SYSTEM AND GENETICS

This section discusses the role genes play in immune response. White blood cells (called lymphocytes) have the unique ability to rearrange their DNA to make molecules to specifically recognize and bind to molecules that invade the body. An explanation of B lymphocyte genetics will provide a better understanding of what happens in the immune system when things go wrong. Topics discussed in this section include genetic diseases, the Genome Project, immunogenetics—which investigates the embryonic development and activation of immune cells to better understand organ transplant rejection, autoimmunity, allergies, and immunodeficiencies—and the study of antibodies to improve antibody production methods.

  Agammaglobulinemia and genetics 91
  Allergies and genetics 93
  Antibodies and genetics 97
  Genetic diseases 103
  Immunogenetics 109

Agammaglobulinemia and Genetics

Category: Diseases/Syndromes
Also known as: Bruton's agammaglobulinemia; X-linked agammaglobulinemia (XLA); hypogammaglobulinemia
Anatomy or system affected: Blood, immune system, lymphatic system
Specialties and related fields: Hematology, immunology, pathology
Definition: A disorder of the immune system resulting from a failure of white blood cells, called "B lymphocytes," to develop. These cells are the source of the antibodies or immunoglobulins, which defend the body against infections.

KEY TERMS

autosomal recessive inheritance: a genetic trait or condition that occurs when someone inherits one copy of a mutated, or changed, gene from each parent
common variable immunodeficiency: an immune system disorder caused by abnormally low blood levels of antibodies
gene deletions: the loss of all or part of a gene, possibly resulting in a change in RNA and protein made from that gene; found in cancer and in other genetic diseases and abnormalities.
hematopoietic cells: immature cells that can develop into all types of blood cells, including white blood cells, red blood cells, and platelets
hyper-IgM syndrome: a group of rare primary immunodeficiency disorders characterized by an inability of B lymphocytes to mature and make secondary, high-affinity antibodies
immunoglobulin replacement: intravenous or subcutaneous treatment to increase antibodies with immunoglobulins, a blood product derived from blood donors

RISK FACTORS

The disease is inherited as X-linked recessive. The defective gene is on the X chromosome, one of two sex chromosomes (the Y chromosome is the other one). In males, who have only one X chromosome, a defective gene causes agammaglobulinemia. In females with two X chromosomes, a defective gene on one chromosome is insufficient to cause disease. Still, it makes the woman a carrier capable of passing the abnormal gene to her children. Males cannot pass the disease to their sons, but they can pass the defective gene to their daughters, who will then be carriers. Rarely, spontaneous gene mutations cause the condition to appear without the mother carrying the mutation. These random mutations occur more often in the male gamete. While the mother of a boy with X-linked agammaglobulinemia (XLA) has an 80 percent chance of being a carrier, the maternal grandmother is a carrier in only 25 percent of cases. XLA affects about three to six in one million males.

ETIOLOGY AND GENETICS

Mutations in the Bruton's tyrosine kinase (*BTK*) gene cause XLA. The *BTK* gene was named in honor of the physician who first described the illness in 1952. The *BTK* gene is quite large, with nineteen exons encoding the 659 amino acids of the Btk enzyme and spanning 37.5 kilobase pairs (kb) on the long arm of the X chromosome (Xq21.33-q22). The *BTK* molecular location is from base pair 100,491,097 to base-pair 100,527,837 on the X chromosome. More than eight hundred different mutations have been described on the international mutation database. The Btk enzyme belongs to the Tec family of cytoplasmic tyrosine kinases. It is expressed in hematopoietic cells, predominantly B cells. Btk is necessary for the development, differentiation, and functioning (signaling) of B cells. Btk deficiency prevents B cell development from the pro-B cell to pre-B cell transition. The failure of pro-B cells to transition to pre-B cells leads to a severe reduction in circulating B lymphocytes. An absence of mature B cells causes a failure of the humoral immune response and a distinct inability to produce immunoglobulins. The specific *BTK* gene mutation may influence the severity of the illness. However, environmental factors and functional aspects of other components of the immune system are also important influences.

Gross gene deletions of varying lengths may produce contiguous deletion syndrome affecting the X22q region. The defects in nearby genes (*TIMM8A*, *TAF7L*, and *DRP2*) can complicate the problems of XLA by adding neurological impairment, sensorineural deafness, and dystonia. There are numerous other genetic causes for hypogammaglobulinemia or agammaglobulinemia, such as autosomal recessive agammaglobulinemia, hyper-IgM syndromes, and common variable immunodeficiency.

SYMPTOMS

Patients with XLA are healthy at birth but start to have infections after a few months when the antibodies passed from the mother begin to dwindle. Patients have problems with common viral infections, particularly with encapsulated bacteria (*Streptococcus pneumoniae* and *Haemophilus influenzae*) and a parasite (*Giardia lamblia*). Children usually receive their diagnosis during a hospitalization for a severe infection between two and five years of age.

SCREENING AND DIAGNOSIS

When measured during routine blood tests, the serum IgG level is typically lower than 200 milligrams per deciliter (mg/dL) in affected individuals. IgM and IgA are often low as well. Complete blood counts (CBCs) show a marked reduction in B lymphocytes (CD19+ cells) in the peripheral blood. Typically, B lymphocytes constitute 10 to 15 percent of total lymphocytes, but The B lymphocytes of XLA patients only compose 1 to 2 percent of their total lymphocytes. Finally, molecular genetic testing for *BTK* mutations can definitively diagnose patients, detect female carriers, and diagnose prenatal cases.

TREATMENT AND THERAPY

Since its initial clinical description in 1952, the primary treatment has been immunoglobulin replacement. Patients receive intravenously administered immunoglobulins once a month or subcutaneous immunoglobulins each week. The dosages are adjusted to maintain a trough serum IgG level of 500 to 800 mg/dL to provide a satisfactory clinical response. Antibodies and other measures are em-

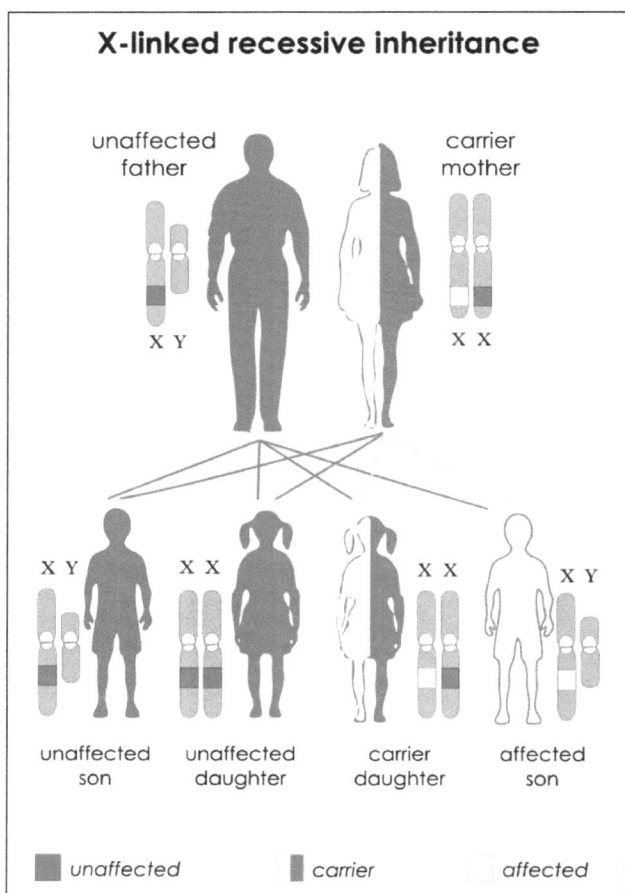

X-linked Recessive inheritance. Image via Wikimedia Commons. [Public domain.]

ployed when needed to manage infections. Live virus vaccines, such as the oral polio vaccine, should be avoided. Bone marrow or umbilical cord stem cell transplants from compatible donors effectively cure XLA. However, stem cell transplantation usually is not considered appropriate because of its risk and the need for aggressive immunosuppression of the patient's bone marrow before the procedure.

PREVENTION AND OUTCOMES
Parents of children who suffer from XLA should receive genetic counseling. Fortunately, early diagnosis and aggressive treatment now enable most patients to lead moderately healthy and productive lives.

—*H. Bradford Hawley, MD*

Further Information
Broides, Amon, Wenjian Yang, and Mary Ellen Conley. "Genotype/Phenotype Correlations in X-Linked Agammaglobulinemia." *Clinical Immunology*, vol. 118, 2006, pp. 195-200.

"BTK." *Genetics Home Reference*. U.S. National Library of Medicine, Feb. 2012. Accessed 14 Jul. 2014.

Conley, Mary Ellen, et al. "Primary B Cell Immunodeficiencies: Comparisons and Contrasts." *Annual Review of Immunology*, vol. 27, 2009, pp. 199-227.

Conley, Mary Ellen, and Vanessa C. Howard. "X-Linked Agammaglobulinemia." *Gene Reviews*. U of Washington, Seattle, 17 Nov. 2011. Accessed 14 Jul. 2014.

Howard, Vanessa, et al. "The Health Status and Quality of Life of Adults with X-Linked Agammaglobulinemia." *Clinical Immunology*, vol. 118, 2006, pp. 201-8.

Ikegame, Kazuhiro, et al. "Allogeneic Stem Cell Transplantation for X-linked Agammaglobulinemia Using Reduced Intensity Conditioning as a Model of the Reconstitution of Humoral Immunity." *Journal of Hematology & Oncology*, vol. 9, no. 9. 13 Feb. 2016, doi:10.1186/s13045-016-0240-y.

Mohamed, Abdalla J., et al. "Bruton's Tyrosine Kinase (Btk): Function, Regulation, and Transformation with Special Emphasis on the pH Domain." *Immunological Reviews*, vol. 228, 2009, pp. 58-73.

Taneja, A., E. Muco, and A. Chhabra. *Bruton Agammaglobulinemia*. StatPearls Publishing, Jan. 2021 [Updated 29 Jul. 2021], www.ncbi.nlm.nih.gov/books/NBK448170/.

ALLERGIES AND GENETICS

Category: Diseases/Disorders
Also known as: Atopy; allergic rhinitis; hay fever; atopic dermatitis; anaphylaxis
Anatomy or system affected: Blood, brain, eyes, gastrointestinal system, immune system, intestines, liver, lungs, lymphatic system, mouth, psychic-emotional system, reproductive system, respiratory system, skin, throat
Specialties and related fields: Dermatology, gastroenterology, hematology, immunology, ophthalmology, otorhinolaryngology, pharmacology, pulmonary medicine
Definition: A damaging immune response by the body to substances like pollen, fur, foods, or dust, to which it has become hypersensitive.

KEY TERMS
allergen: an ordinarily harmless substance—such as pet dander, pollen, or food proteins—that can cause an allergic reaction in some patients
atopy: a condition that underlies allergic diseases, characterized by high levels of immunoglobulin E (IgE), that is highly influenced by genetics
immunotherapy: treatment for allergies, also known as allergy shots, in which a small amount of allergen is injected into a patient to develop immunity
major histocompatibility complex class II (MHCII): genomic region that encodes human leukocyte antigen proteins that influence allergies
patch test: skin test used to diagnose allergies in which a substance is placed in a small metal disk and applied to the skin for a few days

INTRODUCTION

Allergies are a disorder of the immune system. Allergic reactions occur when the immune system responds strongly to ordinarily harmless substances, such as pet dander, pollen, or proteins in food, which are referred to as "allergens." Individuals can develop an allergy because of a genetic susceptibility inherited from their parents and subsequent exposure to that allergen; however, they also can develop allergies without any genetic risk factors.

RISK FACTORS

Individuals have a higher risk of developing allergies if they have family members with allergies or asthma. They also have a higher risk of developing an allergy if they already have asthma or one or more allergies, suggesting a shared genetic origin. Children are more likely to develop allergies than adults, and allergies are more common in firstborn children and children in smaller families. Those most at-risk in the United States are Puerto Ricans and African Americans, followed by Caucasians. Allergies are also more common in urban than rural environments and more common in developed than in developing countries. Other environmental factors (such as exposure to cigarette smoke and pollution) and medical factors (such as infections, autoimmune disease, diet, and stress) can also affect allergy risk. Understanding the factors that contribute to allergy development is critical, as the number of people with allergies has increased worldwide.

ETIOLOGY AND GENETICS

Multiple factors modulate risk for allergic diseases without a single causal agent; however, genetic predisposition is the most critical factor influencing whether a person will develop allergies. Atopy, characterized by high levels of immunoglobulin E (IgE), is a condition that underlies allergic diseases and is highly influenced by genetics. According to the American Academy of Allergy, Asthma, and Immunology, people who do not have a genetic predisposition toward developing allergic conditions have about a 15 percent risk of developing allergies. Suppose one or more of a person's parents or siblings have allergies. In that case, the risk for developing allergies is 30 to 60 percent or 25 to 35 percent, respectively. Monozygotic twins, who share 100 per-

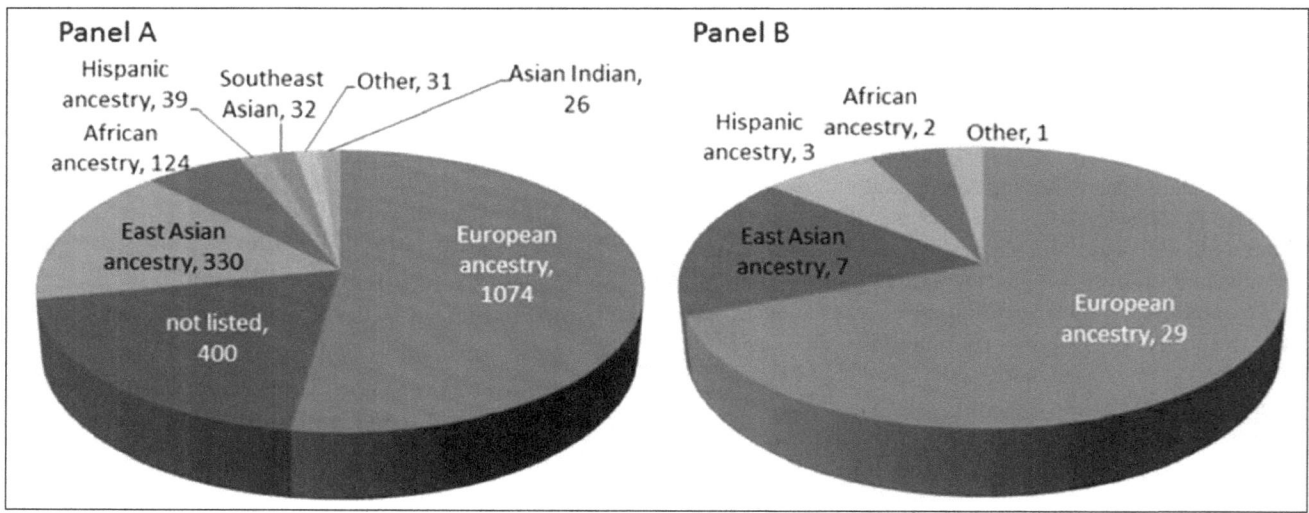

Published genome-wide association studies (GWAS) to date according to ethnicity and race for all catalogued GWAS (Panel A) and asthma GWAS (Panel B). Data generated from the National Human Genome Research Institute's GWAS catalog website. Image via National Center for Biotechnology Information (NCBI).

cent of their deoxyribonucleic acid (DNA), are more likely to have the same type of allergy than are dizygotic twins, who share 50 percent of their DNA, suggesting that genetic factors are essential in allergy risk. Even in monozygotic twins, only about 50 to 60 percent of twins share the same allergic condition, demonstrating that nongenetic factors also influence allergies. As a result, allergy is considered a complex genetic disease because it does not follow the laws of Mendelian inheritance.

Because multiple allergic conditions exist and allergies are also influenced by exposure to allergens, determining specific genetic risk factors for allergies is challenging. Researchers have conducted large-scale genome-wide association studies to uncover mutations that might play a role in allergy development. Several candidate susceptibility genes for allergic diseases have been identified: human leukocyte antigen DRB1 (HLA-DRB1), high-affinity IgE receptor (MS4A2), interleukins 4, 13, and 33 (IL4, IL13, and IL33), filaggrin FLG, DENND1B, and the alpha chain of the IL-4 receptor (IL4R), among others. DNA methylation—the epigenetic addition of methyl groups to DNA—may also affect gene expression and contribute to allergy development or its absence.

Several linkage studies suggest that the major histocompatibility complex class II region (MHC II) Major histocompatibility complex (MHC) influences allergy. This genomic region contains human leukocyte antigen (HLA) genes, which encode antigen-presenting proteins on the cell surface. Genetic variation in HLA genes determines the specificities of HLA proteins and whether the immune system will respond to a particular allergen. Several HLA haplotypes have been associated with specific allergies, such as the reported association between the HLA-DRB1*15:01 allele and ragweed pollen allergies. Other HLA haplotypes are associated more generally with allergies, such as the association between particular HLADQB1*03 alleles and higher levels of IgE.

Other candidate genes for allergies include those related to immunoglobulins. Polymorphisms in the MS4A2 gene FCER1B gene that encodes for the beta chain of the high-affinity receptor for IgE affect the extent to which the immune system responds against allergens and have been associated with allergy. Additionally, polymorphisms in genes encoding the IL13 and IL4 receptor alpha chain are associated with increased serum IgE levels and allergy risk. Another group of immunoglobulin-related genes, the T-cell immunoglobulin and mucin domain (TIM) family genes have been associated with protection from developing allergies. The PHF11 gene, which could be involved in immunoglobulin synthesis, is another immunoglobulin-related gene consistently linked to allergy risk.

Other genes associated with allergy in multiple studies include various components of the immune response. The CD14 gene encodes a cell-surface receptor intended to detect bacterial proteins. Still, variation in this gene is also associated with allergic responses to harmless allergens. Additionally, genes encoding transcription factors involved in developing T-regulatory cells, such as GATA3, which regulates Th2 cytokine responses, and TBX21, which regulates Th2 cytokine responses, have also been associated with allergy.

Because both genes and environmental factors in combination influence allergy risk, some researchers have investigated gene-gene and gene-environment interactions. For example, individuals who had specific polymorphisms in CD14 had a high or low allergy risk depending on whether they had pets, were exposed to tobacco smoke, or lived on a farm in childhood. Additionally, interactions between polymorphisms in different genes, such as GATA3 and IL13, can affect allergy risk. Moreover, ethnic background affects allergy susceptibility versus protection. The DENND1B variant is associated with asthma development in European-descended children and protection in African Americans.

SYMPTOMS

Allergy symptoms vary widely. Sneezing, runny nose, and sore throat are common with seasonal allergies, sometimes called "hay fever" or "allergic rhinitis." Allergic reactions can also affect the eyes, leading to redness, watery or itchy eyes, and swelling. Some allergies affect the skin, leading to rashes or hives. Others cause gastrointestinal symptoms such as vomiting or diarrhea. More severe allergic reactions can lead to anaphylaxis, which may include the symptoms listed above in addition to low blood pressure, difficulty breathing, or shock.

SCREENING AND DIAGNOSIS

A doctor may perform a skin test or blood test to test for allergies. In one type of skin test, a small drop of the possible allergen is either placed onto skin followed by scratching with a needle over the drop or injected into the skin. In another type of skin test, known as a "patch test," the potential allergen is placed in a small metal disk applied to the skin and kept there for a few days. If the individual is allergic to a substance, the test site will become red, swollen, and itchy with skin tests. Another way to test for allergies involves taking a blood sample. The medical laboratory adds the allergen to the blood and then measures the immune response to the allergen. If the body produces many antibodies to attack the allergen, the individual is allergic to the tested substance.

TREATMENT AND THERAPY

Several medications are available to relieve allergies. Oral and nasal antihistamines, such as diphenhydramine (Benadryl) and loratadine (Claritin), help with allergic rhinitis by blocking the action of histamine, a substance the body releases during an allergic reaction. Nasal sprays containing corticosteroids, such as mometasone (Nasonex) and fluticasone (Flonase), or nonsteroidal anti-inflammatory drugs (NSAIDs), such as cromolyn sodium (NasalCrom), are sprayed into the nose to reduce inflammation. Topical corticosteroids are also often used to treat skin allergies. Decongestants can also be used to alleviate allergy symptoms, sometimes in combination with antihistamines, as in fexofenadine (Allegra-D). Leukotriene receptor antagonists, such as Singulair, are another treatment that may be used to reduce inflammation-related allergy symptoms.

Immunotherapy, or allergy shots, is another treatment for allergies. People who receive immunotherapy have small amounts of allergens injected into their bodies. The doses of these allergens are increased over at least three to five years to develop the body's immunity to them. When the patient experiences minimal symptoms for two seasons or more, the treatment ceases.

PREVENTION AND OUTCOMES

Some allergies, such as those to dairy and eggs, can be outgrown, while others, such as peanut allergies, tend to be lifelong. The simplest way to prevent allergic conditions or reduce symptoms is to minimize exposure to the problematic allergen. For example, breastfeeding infants for four to six months, introducing low-risk solid foods, and then gradually exposing infants to highly allergenic foods such as cow's milk and peanuts may help prevent allergy development; long delays have been found to increase that risk, however. Another promising prevention strategy may be to reduce early skin exposure to soaps and food residues. Eating a healthy diet and managing stress can also effectively help alleviate allergy symptoms.

—*Jevon Plunkett and Jeffrey A. Knight*

Further Information

"Allergic Reactions." *American Academy of Allergy, Asthma, and Immunology*, 20 Sept. 2020, www.aaaai.org/tools-for-the-public/conditions-library/allergies/allergic-reactions. Accessed 2 Sept. 2021.

"Allergic Reactions: Tips to Remember." AAAAI.org. American Academy of Allergy, Asthma & Immunology, 2013. Accessed 28 Jul. 2014.

Ambardekar, Nayana. "Who Gets Allergies." *WebMD*, 27 Aug. 2021, www.webmd.com/allergies/who-gets-allergies. Accessed 2 Sept. 2021.

Contie, Vicki, Lesley Earl, Belle Waring, and Harrison Wein. "Red, Itchy Skin? Get the Skinny on Dermatitis." *NIH News in Health*. NIH Office of Communications and Public Liaison, Apr. 2012. Accessed 18 Jul. 2014.

Contopoulos-Ioannidis, D. G., I. N. Kouri, and J. P. Ioannidis. "Genetic Predisposition to Asthma and Atopy." *Respiration*, vol. 74, no. 1, 2007, pp. 8-12.

Grammatikos, A. P. "The Genetic and Environmental Basis of Atopic Diseases." *Annals of Medicine*, vol. 40, no. 7, 2008, pp. 482-95.

Ober, Carole, and Tsung-Chieh Yao. "The Genetics of Asthma and Allergic Disease: A 21st Century Perspective." *Immunological Reviews*, vol. 242, no. 1, 2011, pp. 10-30.

Paul, Marla. "Food Allergy Is Linked to Skin Exposure and Genetics." *Northwestern Now*, 6 Apr. 2018, news.northwestern.edu/stories/2018/april/food-allergy-is-linked-to-skin-exposure-and-genetics. Accessed 31 Jan. 2019.

"Prevention of Allergies and Asthma in Children." *The American Academy of Allergy, Asthma, Immunology*, www.aaaai.org/conditions-and-treatments/library/allergy-library/prevention-of-allergies-and-asthma-in-children. Accessed 31 Jan. 2019.

"Stinging Insect Allergy." *American Academy of Allergy, Asthma, and Immunology*, 28 Sept. 2020, www.aaaai.org/tools-for-the-public/conditions-library/allergies/stinging-insect-allergy. Accessed 2 Sept. 2021.

Thomsen, S. F., K. O. Kyvik, and V. Backer. "Etiological Relationships in Atopy: A Review of Twin Studies." *Twin Research and Human Genetics*, vol. 11, no. 2, 2008, pp. 112-20.

Torres-Borrego, J., A. B. Molina-Terán, and C. Montes-Mendoza. "Prevalence and Associated Factors of Allergic Rhinitis and Atopic Dermatitis in Children." *Allergologia et Immunopathologia*, vol. 36, no. 2, 2008, pp. 90-100.

Westly, Erica. "Seeking a Gene Genie." *Nature*, vol. 479, no. 7374, 2011, pp. S10-S11.

Xiumei Hong, et al. "Genome-Wide Association Study Identifies Peanut Allergy-Specific Loci and Evidence of Epigenetic Mediation in US Children." *Nature Communications*, vol 6, no. 1, 2015, doi:10.1038/ncomms7304.

ANTIBODIES AND GENETICS

Category: Immunogenetics
Anatomy or system affected: Blood, immune system, lymphatic system
Specialties and related fields: Hematology, immunology
Definition: Antibodies provide the mainline defense (immunity) in all vertebrates against infections caused by bacteria, fungi, viruses, or other foreign agents. Antibodies are used as therapeutic agents to prevent specific diseases and identify antigens in a wide range of diagnostic procedures. Large quantities of antibodies have also been produced in plants for use in human and plant immunotherapy. Because of their importance to human and animal health, antibodies are widely studied by geneticists seeking improved antibody production methods.

KEY TERMS

B cells: a class of white blood cells (lymphocytes) derived from bone marrow responsible for antibody-directed immunity

B-memory cells: descendants of activated B cells that are long-lived and that synthesize large amounts of antibodies in response to subsequent exposure to the antigen, thus playing an important role in secondary immunity

helper T cells: a class of white blood cells (lymphocytes) derived from bone marrow that prompts the production of antibodies by B cells in the presence of an antigen

lymphocytes: types of white blood cells (including B cells and T cells) that provide immunity

plasma cells: descendants of activated B cells that synthesize and secrete a single antibody type in large quantities and play an important role in primary immunity

ANTIBODY STRUCTURE

Antibodies, also known as immunoglobulins (Igs), are produced by plasma cells responding to a specific foreign molecule known as an antigen. Most antigens are proteins or proteins conjugated to sugars. Antibodies recognize, bind to, and inactivate antigens that have been introduced into an organism by various pathogens such as bacteria, fungi, and viruses.

The simplest form of the antibody molecule is a Y-shaped structure with two identical "heavy chains" and two identical "light chains." These chains are held together by chemical bonds. The lower portion of each chain has a constant region of similar amino acids in all antibody molecules, even among different species. The remaining upper part of each chain, known as the "variable region," differs in its amino acid sequence from other antibodies. The three-dimensional shape of the tips of the variable region (antigen-binding site) allows for the recognition and binding of target molecules (antigens). The high-affinity binding between antibody and antigen results from a combination of hydrophobic, ionic, and van der Waals forces. Antigen-binding sites have specific attachment points on the antigen called "epitopes" or "antigenic determinants."

ANTIBODY DIVERSITY

There are five classes of antibodies (IgG, IgM, IgD, IgA, and IgE), each with a distinct structure, size, and function. IgG is the principal immunoglobulin and constitutes about 80 percent of all antibodies in the serum.

ANTIBODY GENE REARRANGEMENT AND B-CELL DEVELOPMENT

The variable region of the heavy chain is encoded by a variable or V region, a diversity region or D region, and a J or joining region. The light chain variable region consists of a V region and a J region. The genes that encode the heavy chain are on chromosome 14, and the light chain has two different gene clusters, kappa and lambda. The kappa gene cluster is on chromosome two, and the lambda gene cluster is on chromosome 22. The heavy chain gene cluster consists of 51 different *V* segments, six different *J* segments, 27 distinct *D* segments, and eight

CLASSES, LOCATIONS, AND FUNCTIONS OF ANTIBODIES

Class	Location	Function
IgG	Blood plasma, tissue Fluid, fetuses	Produces primary and secondary immune responses; protects against bacteria, viruses, and toxins; passes through the placenta and enters fetal bloodstream, thus protecting fetuses.
IgM	Blood plasma	Acts as a B-cell surface receptor for antigens; fights bacteria in primary immune response; powerful agglutinating agent.
IgD	Surface of B cells	Prompts B cells to make antibodies (especially in infants).
IgA	Saliva, milk, urine, tears, respiratory and digestive systems	Protects surface linings of epithelial cells, digestive, respiratory, and urinary systems.
IgE	In secretion with IgA, skin, tonsils, respiratory and digestive systems	Acts as a receptor for antigens causing mast cells (often found in connective tissues surrounding blood vessels) to secrete allergy mediators; excessive production causes allergic reactions (including hay fever and asthma).

constant regions. The kappa light chain gene cluster consists of 40 different V gene segments, five different J chain clusters, and a single constant region. The lambda gene cluster contains 30 V gene segments and four J gene segments, with four constant regions.

During B-lymphocyte development or lymphopoiesis, the antibody gene clusters are rearranged to create proteins that bind an enormous variety of distinct antigens. The earliest stage of B-lymphocyte development is the early pro-B cell, which forms from the daughter cell after the hematopoietic stem cell divides. The early pro-B cell expresses proteins that rearrange the antibody gene cluster, RAG-1 & -2. The RAG proteins join a single D gene segment from one of the copies of the heavy chain gene cluster with a single J gene segment. Upon completion of the DJ joining, the early pro-B cell becomes a late pro-B cell. The RAG-1 & -2 recombinase joins a single V segment with the DJ segment and the VDJ combination to the μ constant region gene. Successful cutting and pasting of the VDJ-μ gene segments mark the transition of the late pro-B cell to a large pre-B cell. If the cell fails to rearrange its heavy chain gene segments, the cell dies.

The large pre-B cell expresses the rearranged heavy chain to test it out. The cell traffics the heavy chain to the cell surface. Antibody heavy chain proteins couple with light chain proteins, but the large pre-B cell has yet to rearrange the antibody light chain gene clusters. Therefore, the large pre-B cell couples the heavy chain a "surrogate light chain" to ensure that it properly traffics to the cell surface. The surrogate light chain is made of two proteins, VpreB and lambda 5. The surrogate light chain is a practice light chain for the heavy chain to ensure that it functions properly. Think of the surrogate light chain as a pair of training wheels for the antibody bicycle.

Successful expression of the antibody heavy chain induces the cell to divide and become a small pre-B cell. Next, the small pre-B cell rearranges the light chain genes, beginning with the kappa genes first. If the cell fails to rearrange its kappa genes, then it moves to the lambda genes. VJ joining of the light chain gene segments makes a functional light chain, and expression of the light chain with the heavy chain places an antibody on the cell's surface, designating it as an immature B cell. If the antibody strongly binds to any self-antigens in the bone marrow, it dies.

The variability in antibody formation is remarkable. The heavy chain alone can encode at least 8262 ($51 \times 6 \times 27$) different heavy chain variable regions. Suppose a heavy chain is coupled with a kappa light chain. In that case, there are 200 (40×5) different light chains and 1.6×10^6 (8262×200) different possible antibodies that such rearrangements can form.

PRODUCTION OF ANTIBODIES: IMMUNE RESPONSE

Immunity is a state of bodily resistance brought about by the production of antibodies against an invasion by an antigen.

The immune response is mediated by white blood cells known as lymphocytes that are made in the bone marrow. There are two types of lymphocytes: T cells, which are formed when lymphocytes migrate to the thymus gland, circulate in the blood, and become associated with lymph nodes and the spleen; and B cells, which are formed in the bone marrow and move directly to the circulatory and the lymph systems. B cells are genetically programmed to produce antibodies. Each B cell synthesizes and secretes only one type of antibody, which can recognize a discrete region (epitope or antigenic determinant) of an antigen with high affinity. Generally, an antigen has several different epitopes. Each B cell produces different antibodies that bind to one of the many epitopes on the same antigen. All of the antibodies

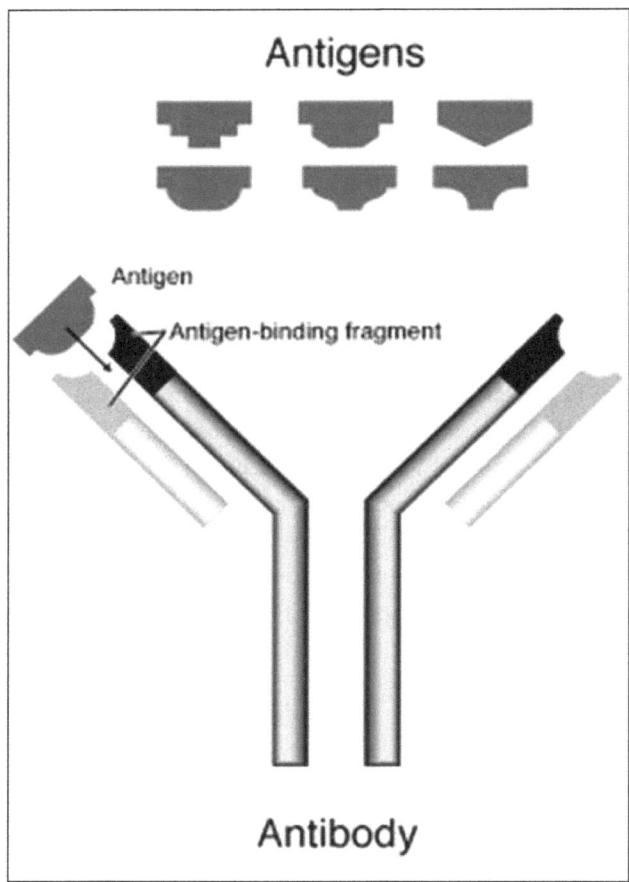

Antibody. Courtesy: National Human Genome Research Institute, via Wikimedia Commons. [Public domain.]

in this set referred to as "polyclonal" antibodies, react with the same antigen.

The adaptive immune response controls infections more effectively than the nonspecific innate response (bodily defenses against infection—such as skin, fever, inflammation, phagocytes, natural killer cells, and some other antimicrobial substances—that are not part of the immune system proper). The immune system has three characteristic responses to antigens: diverse, which effectively neutralizes or destroys various foreign invaders, whether they are microbes, chemicals, dust, or pollen; specific, which effectively differentiates between harmful and harmless antigens; and anamnestic, which has a memory component that remembers and responds faster to a subsequent encounter with an antigen. The primary immune response involves the first combat with antigens. In contrast, the secondary immune response includes the memory component of a first assault. As a result, humans typically get some diseases (such as chickenpox) only once; other infections (such as cold and influenza) often recur because the causative viruses mutate, thus presenting a different antigenic face to the immune system each season.

An antibody-mediated immune response involves several stages: detection of antigens, activation of helper T cells, and antibody production by B cells. White blood cells known as macrophages continuously wander through the circulatory system and the interstitial spaces between cells, searching for antigen molecules. Once an antigen is encountered, the invading molecule is engulfed and ingested by a macrophage. Helper T cells become activated by coming in contact with the antigen on the macrophage. In turn, an activated helper T cell identifies and activates a B cell. The activated T cells release cytokines (a class of biochemical signal molecules) that prompt the activated B cell to divide. Immediately, the activated B cell generates two types of daughter cells: antibody-producing cells (each of which synthesizes and releases millions of antibody molecules into the bloodstream in a single day) and B memory cells (which have a life span of a few months to a year, depending on the immunoglobulin cell from which they derive). The B memory cells are the component of the immune memory system that, in response to a second exposure to the same type of antigen, produces antibodies in larger quantities and at faster rates over a longer time frame than the primary immune response. A similar cascade of events occurs when a macrophage presents an antigen directly to a B cell.

POLYCLONAL AND MONOCLONAL ANTIBODIES

Plasma cells originate from different B cells and manufacture distinct antibody molecules since each B cell was presented with a specific portion of the same antigen by a helper T cell or macrophage. Thus a set of polyclonal antibodies is released in response to an invasion by a foreign agent. Each group of polyclonal antibodies will launch the assault against the foreign agent by recognizing different epitopes of the same antigen. The polyclonal nature of antibodies has been well recognized in the medical field.

In the case of multiple myeloma (a type of cancer), one B cell out of billions in the body proliferates uncontrollably. Eventually, this event compromises the total population of B cells of the body. The immune system will produce huge amounts of IgG originating from the same B cell, which recognizes only one specific epitope of an antigen; therefore, this person's immune system produces a set of antibodies referred to as "monoclonal" antibodies. Monoclonal antibodies form a population of identical antibodies that all specifically recognize one epitope. Thus, someone with this condition may suffer frequent bacterial infections because of a lack of antibody diversity. Indeed, a bacterium whose antigens do not match the antibodies manufactured by the overabundant monoclonal B cells has a selective advantage.

The high-affinity binding capacity of antibodies with antigens has been employed in both therapeutic and diagnostic procedures. However, a manufacturing challenge remains: the effectiveness of commercial preparations of polyclonal antibodies can vary widely from batch to batch. In some instances of immunization, certain epitopes of a particular antigen are strong stimulators of antibody-producing cells. At other times, the immune system responds more vigorously to different epitopes of the same antigen. Thus, one batch of polyclonal antibodies may have a low level of antibody molecules directed against a major epitope and not be as effective as the previous batch. Researchers such as S. K. Rasmussen and others have been developing methods in which multiple stable cell lines produce desired monoclonal antibodies to address such inconsistency between batches. Afterward, these multiple batches are combined in a single-batch preparation.

Instead, it may be desirable to produce a cell line that will produce monoclonal antibodies with a high affinity for a specific epitope on the antigen for commercial use. Such a cell line would provide a consistent and continual supply of identical (monoclonal)

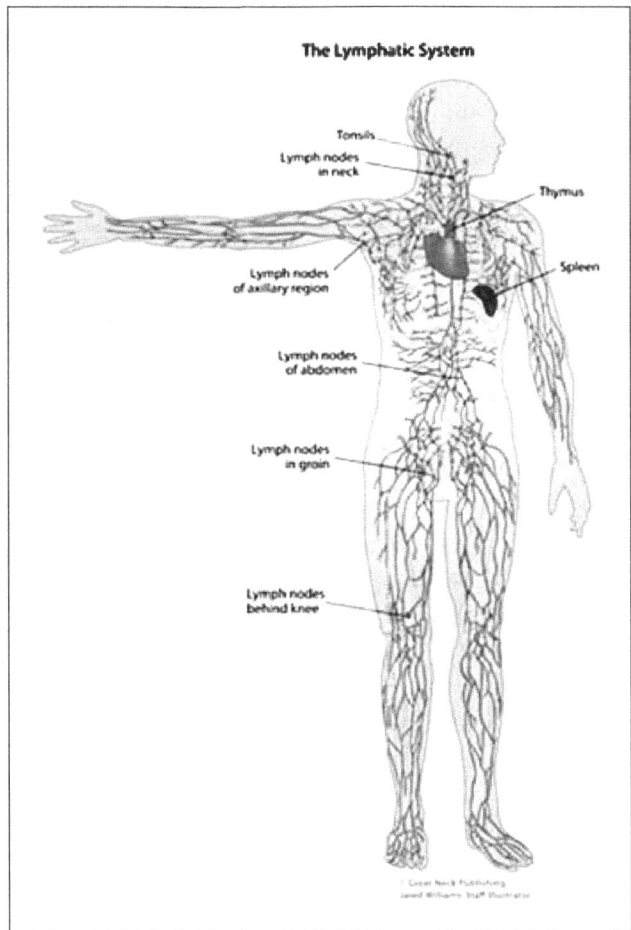

Lymphatic System: The lymphatic system works with the circulatory system to circulate fluids and antibodies to fight illness and disease. [© EBSCO.]

antibodies. Monoclonal antibodies can be produced by hybridoma cells, which are generated by the fusion of cancerous B cells and normal spleen cells obtained from mice immunized with a specific antigen. After the initial selection of hybridomas, monoclonal antibody production is maintained in culture. In addition, the hybridoma cells can be injected into mice to induce tumors that, in turn, will release large quantities of fluid containing the antibody. This fluid containing monoclonal antibodies can be collected periodically and used immediately or stored for future use. Various systems used to produce monoclonal antibodies include cultured lymphoid cell lines, yeast cells, *Trichoderma reesei* (ascomycetes), insect cells, *Escherichia coli*, *Escherichia coli* monoclonal antibodies, and monkey and Chinese hamster ovary cells. Transgenic organisms and plant cell cultures are potential systems for antibody expression.

IMPACT AND APPLICATIONS

The high-affinity binding capacity of antibodies can potentially inactivate antigens in vivo (within a living organism). Likewise, antibodies may also be employed in many therapeutic and diagnostic applications. In addition, it is a very effective tool in both immunological isolation and detection methods.

Monoclonal antibodies may outnumber all other products being explored by various biotechnology-oriented companies to treat and prevent disease. For example, many strategies for treating cancerous tumors and the inhibition of human immunodeficiency virus (HIV) replication employ monoclonal antibodies. HIV is a retrovirus whose genetic material is ribonucleic acid, or RNA, but makes a deoxyribonucleic acid (DNA) copy from an RNA template. HIV causes acquired immunodeficiency syndrome (AIDS). Advances in plant biotechnology have made it possible to use transgenic plants to produce monoclonal antibodies on a large scale for therapeutic or diagnostic use. Indeed, one of the most promising applications of plant-produced antibodies in immunotherapy is passive immunization (for example, against *Streptococcus mutans*, the most common cause of tooth decay). Large doses of the antibody are required in multiple applications for passive immunotherapy to be effective. Transgenic antibody-producing plants may be one source that can supply huge quantities of antibodies safely and cost-effectively. Hybrid IgA-IgG molecules produced by transgenic plants prevent the colonization of *S. mutans* in culture.

Antibodies expressed in soybeans at a level of 1 percent of total protein may cost approximately one hundred dollars per kilogram of antibody. $100/kg of antibody is relatively inexpensive in comparison with the cost of traditional antibiotics. Transgenic plants can act as bioreactors for the large-scale production of antibodies with no extensive purification schemes. Antibodies have been expressed in transgenic tobacco roots and then accumulated in tobacco seeds. Suppose this technology could obtain a stable accumulation of antibodies in more edible plant organs such as potato tubers. In that case, it could potentially allow for long-term storage and safe and easy delivery of specific antibodies for immunotherapeutic applications. Plant-produced antibodies ("plantibodies") may be more desirable for human use than microbial-produced antibodies; plant-produced antibodies undergo eukaryotic rather than prokaryotic (bacterial) posttranslational modifications. Human glycosylation (a biochemical process whereby sugars are attached to the protein) is more closely related to plants than bacteria.

The potential use of antibody expression in plants for altering existing biochemical pathways has also been demonstrated. For example, germination mediated by a phytochrome (a biochemical produced by plants) has been changed by utilizing plant-produced antibodies. In addition, antibodies expressed in plants have been successfully used to immunize host plants against pathogenic infection; for example, tobacco plants have already been immunized with antibodies against viral attacks. This approach has great potential to replace the traditional methods (use of chemicals) in controlling pathogens.

—*Sibdas Ghosh, PhD and Tom E. Scola*

Further Information

"Antibodies." *Genetics & Inherited Conditions.* Salem Press, 2010.

Coico, Richard, and Geoffrey Sunshine. "Antibody Structure and Function." *Immunology: A Short Course.* 6th ed., Wiley-Blackwell, 2009, pp. 41-60.

Diamos Andrew G., et al. "High Level Production of Monoclonal Antibodies Using an Optimized Plant Expression System." *Frontiers in Bioengineering and Biotechnology*, vol. 7, 2020, p. 472, www.frontiersin.org/article/10.3389/fbioe.2019.00472.

Dübel, Stefan, and Janice M. Reichert, editors. *Handbook of Therapeutic Antibodies.* 3 vols. Wiley-VCH, 2014.

Glick, Bernard R., and Jack J. Pasternak, editors. *Molecular Biotechnology: Principles and Applications of Recombinant DNA.* 4th ed., ASM, 2010.

Harlow, Ed, and David Lane, editors. *Using Antibodies: A Laboratory Manual.* Rev. ed., Cold Spring Harbor Laboratory Press, 1999.

Kontermann, Roland, and Stefan Dübel, editors. *Antibody Engineering.* 2nd ed., Springer, 2010.

Mayforth, Ruth D. *Designing Antibodies.* Academic, 1993.

Rasmussen, S. K., et al. "Recombinant Antibody Mixtures: Optimization of Cell Line Generation and Single-Batch Manufacturing Processes." *BMC Proceedings*, vol. 5 (Suppl. 8), 2011, p. 02.

Raz, E. *Immunostimulatory DNA Sequences.* Springer, 2001.

Smith, Mathew D. "Antibody Production in Plants." *Biotechnology Advances*, vol. 14, no. 3, 1996, pp. 267-81.

Story, Lachel. "Body Defenses." *Pathophysiology: A Practical Approach.* 2nd ed., Jones, 2015, pp. 31-50.

Wang, Henry Y., and Tadayuki Imanaka, editors. *Antibody Expression and Engineering.* American Chemical Society, 1995.

Genetic diseases

Category: Diseases/Disorders
Anatomy or system affected: All
Specialties and related fields: Embryology, genetics, internal medicine, neonatology, obstetrics, pediatrics
Definition: A variety of disorders transmitted from parent to child through chromosomal material; most people experience disease related to genetics in some form, and research into this area is yielding a greater understanding of the relationship between disease and hereditary proclivities toward illness, as well as new strategies for early detection and prevention or therapy.

KEY TERMS

autosomal recessive disease: a disease that is expressed when two copies of a defective gene are inherited, one from each parent; present on non-sex-determining chromosomes

chromosomes: rod-shaped structures in each cell that contain genes, the chemical elements that determine traits

deoxyribonucleic acid (DNA): the chemical molecule that transmits hereditary information from generation to generation

dominant gene: a gene that can express its effect when an individual has only one copy of it

gene: the hereditary unit, composed of DNA, that resides on chromosomes

inheritance: the passing down of traits from generation to generation

X-linked: a term used to describe genes or traits that are located on the X chromosome; a male needs only one copy of an X-linked gene for it to be expressed

CAUSES AND SYMPTOMS

Hereditary units called "genes" determine the majority of the physical and biochemical characteristics of an organism. Genes are composed of a chemical compound called "deoxyribonucleic acid" (DNA). They are organized into rod-shaped structures called "chromosomes" that reside in each cell of the body. Each human cell carries forty-six chromosomes arranged as twenty-three pairs, each composed of several thousand genes. Twenty-two of the chromosome pairs are homologous pairs; similar genes are located at similar sites on each chromosome. The remaining chromosomes are the sex chromosomes. Human females bear two X chromosomes, and human males possess one X and one Y chromosome.

HUMAN CHROMOSOMES
Genetic diseases are caused by defects in the number of chromosomes, their structure, or the genes on the chromosome (mutation). Shown here is the human complement of chromosomes (twenty-three pairs) and three errors of chromosome number (trisomies, or three instances of a particular chromosome instead of just two) that lead to the genetic disorders Patau syndrome (trisomy no. 13), Edwards syndrome (trisomy no. 18), and the more common Down syndrome (trisomy no. 21).

During the formation of the reproductive cells, the chromosome pairs separate, and one copy of each pair is randomly included in the egg or sperm. Each egg will contain twenty-two autosomes (non-sex chromosomes) and one X chromosome. Each sperm will have twenty-two autosomes and either one X or one Y chromosome. The egg and sperm fuse at fertilization, which restores the proper number of chromosomes. The genes inherited from the baby's parents will determine its sex and much of its physical appearance and future health and well-being.

Genetic diseases are inherited due to the presence of abnormal genes in the reproductive cells of one or both parents of an affected individual. There are two broad classifications of genetic disease: those caused by defects in chromosome number or structure and those resulting from a much more minor flaw within a gene. Within the latter category, there are four predominant mechanisms by which the disorders can be transmitted from generation to generation: autosomal dominant inheritance, in which the defective gene is inherited from one parent; autosomal recessive inheritance, in which defective genes are inherited from both parents, who themselves may show no signs of the disorder; X-linked chromosomal inheritance (often called "sex-linked"), in which the flawed gene has been determined to reside on the X chromosome; and multifactorial inheritance, in which genes interact with each other and environmental factors.

Errors in chromosome numbers include extra and missing chromosomes. The most common chromosomal defect observed in humans is Down syndrome, caused by three copies of chromosome 21 instead of the usual two. Down syndrome occurs at a frequency of about one in eight hundred live births, this frequency increasing with increasing maternal age. The symptoms of this disorder include intellectual disability, short stature, and numerous other medical problems. The most common form of Down syndrome results from the failure of the two copies of chromosome 21 to separate during reproductive cell formation. Upon fusion with a normal reproductive cell at fertilization produces an embryo containing three copies of chromosome 21.

Gross defects in chromosome structure include duplicated and deleted portions of chromosomes and broken and rearranged chromosome fragments. For example, Prader-Willi syndrome results from the deletion of a small piece of chromosome 15. Children affected with this disorder are prone to intellectual disability, obesity, and diabetes. *Cri du chat* (literally, "cat cry") syndrome is associated with a large deletion in chromosome 5. Affected infants exhibit facial abnormalities, are severely intellectually disabled, and produce a high-pitched, catlike wail.

Genetic diseases caused by defects in individual genes result when defective genes are propagated through many generations, or a new genetic flaw develops in a reproductive cell. New genetic defects arise from various causes, including environmental assaults such as radiation, toxins, or drugs. More than four thousand such gene disorders have been identified.

Manifestation of an autosomal dominant disorder requires the inheritance of only one defective gene from one parent afflicted with the disease. Inheritance of two dominant faulty genes, one from each parent, is possible but generally creates such severe consequences that the child dies while still in the womb or shortly after birth. Someone bearing one copy of the gene has a 50 percent chance of transmitting that gene and the disease to their offspring.

Among the most common autosomal dominant diseases are hyperlipidemia and hypercholesterolemia. These disorders result in elevated lipids and cholesterol levels in the blood, which contribute to artery and heart disease. The symptoms usually occur during adulthood, frequently after the affected individual has had children, and potentially transmitted the faulty gene.

Huntington's chorea causes untreatable neurological deterioration and death, and symptoms do not appear until affected individuals are at least in their forties. Children of parents who have Huntington's chorea may have already made reproductive decisions without knowing that they might carry the defective gene. They risk a 50 percent chance of transmitting the disease to their offspring.

Autosomal recessive genetic diseases require that an affected individual bear two defective gene copies, inheriting one from each parent. Usually, the parents are simply carriers of the defective gene; their one normal copy masks the effect of the one flawed copy. If two carriers have offspring, those children have a 25 percent chance of receiving two copies of the defective gene and inheriting the disease and a 50 percent chance of being asymptomatic carriers.

Cystic fibrosis is an autosomal recessive disease that occurs at a rate of about one in two thousand live births among Caucasians. The defective gene product causes improper chloride transport in cells, resulting in thick mucous secretions in the lungs and other organs. Sickle cell disease, another autosomal recessive disorder, is the most common genetic disease among African Americans in the United States. Abnormality in the protein hemoglobin, the component of red blood cells that carries oxygen to all the body's tissues, leads to deformed blood cells that are fragile and easily destroyed.

X-linked genetic diseases are transmitted by faulty genes located on the X chromosome. In X-linked recessive disorders, which are more common, females need two copies of the defective gene to acquire such a disease. Women carry only one flawed copy, making them asymptomatic carriers of the disorder. With only a single X chromosome, males need only one copy of the defective gene to express an X-linked disease. Males with X-linked disorders inherit the defective gene from their mothers since fathers must contribute a Y chromosome to male offspring. All male offspring of a carrier female will have a 50 percent chance of inheriting the defective gene and developing the disease. In the rare case of a female with two bad X-linked genes, 100 percent of her male offspring will inherit the disease gene. Assuming that the father does not carry the defec-

---

INFORMATION ON GENETIC DISEASES

Causes: Abnormal genes in the reproductive cells of one or both parents, environmental factors causing mutations

Symptoms: Varies widely; can include mental retardation, respiratory dysfunction, neurological deterioration, progressive muscle deterioration, cleft palate, spina bifida, anencephaly, heart abnormalities

Duration: Typically lifelong

Treatments: Typically alleviation of symptoms through surgery, drug therapy, hormone therapy, dietary regulation

tive gene, her female offspring will be carriers. There are more than 250 X-linked disorders, some of the more common being Duchenne muscular dystrophy (DMD). DMD causes progressive muscle deterioration and early death; hemophilia; and red-green color blindness, which affects about 8 percent of Caucasian males.

Multifactorial inheritance, which accounts for many genetic diseases, is caused by the complex interaction of one or more genes with each other and with environmental factors. This group of diseases includes many disorders that, anecdotally, "run in families." Representative conditions include cleft palate, spina bifida, anencephaly, and some inherited heart abnormalities. Other diseases appear to have a genetic component predisposing an individual to be susceptible to environmental stimuli that trigger the disease. These include cancer, hypertension, diabetes, schizophrenia, alcoholism, depression, and obesity.

DIAGNOSIS AND DETECTION
Most, but not all, genetic diseases manifest their symptoms immediately or soon after the birth of an affected child. Rapid recognition of such a medical condition and its accurate diagnosis is essential for parents and medical personnel's proper treatment and management of the disease. Medical technology has developed swift and precise diagnostic methods, in many cases allowing testing of the fetus before birth. In addition, tests are available that determine an individual's carrier status for many autosomal recessive and X-linked diseases. Combining these test results with genetic counseling of individuals and couples at risk of transmitting a genetic disease to their offspring helps them make informed decisions about their reproductive futures.

Errors in chromosome number and structure are detected in an individual by analyzing their chromosomes. A skin biopsy or blood sample is taken, the cells in the sample are cultured, and the chromosomes within each cell are stained with special dyes for observation through a microscope. A picture of the chromosomes, called a "karyotype," is taken. The patient's chromosome array is compared with that of a normal individual. Extra or missing chromosomes or alterations in chromosome structure indicate the presence of a genetic disease. The analysis of karyotypes is the method used to detect Down, Prader-Willi, and cri du chat syndromes, among others.

Specific laboratory tests can effectively detect defects in chromosome number and structure in the fetus before birth. Samples may be collected from the fetus by amniocentesis or by chorionic villus sampling. In amniocentesis, a needle is inserted through the pregnant woman's abdomen and uterus into the fluid-filled sac surrounding the fetus. A sample of this fluid, the amniotic fluid, is withdrawn. The amniotic fluid contains fetal cells sloughed off by the fetus. The cells are grown for several weeks until there are enough to perform chromosome analysis. This procedure is performed only after sixteen weeks' gestation to ensure adequate amniotic fluid for sampling.

Chorionic villus sampling relies on a biopsy of the fetal chorion, a membrane surrounding the fetus composed of cells that have the same genetic constitution as the fetus. A catheter is inserted through the pregnant woman's vagina and into the uterus until it is in contact with the chorion. The small sample of this tissue that is removed contains enough cells to perform karyotyping immediately, permitting diagnosis by the next day. Chorionic villus sampling can be performed as early as the eighth or ninth week of pregnancy. This earlier testing gives the procedure an advantage over amniocentesis. Earlier determination of whether a fetus carries a genetic disease allows safer pregnancy termination if the parents choose this course.

Karyotype analysis is limited to the diagnosis of genetic diseases caused by extensive chromosome abnormalities. The majority of hereditary disorders are caused by gene flaws that are too small to see microscopically. For many of these diseases, diagnosis is possible through either biochemical testing or DNA analysis.

Many genetic disorders cause a lack of a specific biochemical necessary for normal metabolism. These types of diseases are frequently referred to as "inborn errors of metabolism." Many of these errors can be detected by the chemical analysis of fetal tissue. For example, galactosemia is a disease that results from the lack of galactose-1-phosphate uridylyltransferase (GALT). Infants with this disorder cannot break down galactose, one of the major sugars in milk. If left untreated, galactosemia can lead to developmental disabilities, cataracts, kidney and liver failure, and death. Tests for galactosemia include detection of excessively high blood levels of galactose. If galactose levels are high, then a test called the "Beutler assay" measures GALT enzyme activity. Beutler assays on fetal cells obtained from amniocentesis or chorionic villus sampling determine GALT activity and effectively diagnoses galactosemia in unborn babies. If necessary, the infant can be placed on a galactose-free diet immediately after birth.

DNA analysis can be used to determine whether a genetic disease has been inherited when either the chromosomal location of the gene, the chemical sequence of the DNA, or particular DNA sequences commonly associated with the gene in question (called "markers") are known.

Genes are composed of sequences of four chemical elements of DNA: adenine (A), guanine (G), thymine (T), and cytosine (C). Sometimes the proper DNA sequence of a gene and the changes in the sequence that cause disease are known. Direct analysis of the DNA of an individual suspected of carrying a particular genetic disorder is possible in these cases. For example, in sickle cell disease, a single nucleotide base change leads to the disorder. Genetic tests for conditions like sickle cell disease require a tissue sample from the fetus. The fetal DNA is isolated from the cells and analyzed with highly specific probes that can detect the presence of the defective gene that will lead to sickle cell disease. With genetic data in hand, parents can make informed decisions about the fetus's future or the care of an affected child.

Occasionally a disease gene itself has not been precisely isolated or had its DNA sequence determined. Still, sequences very near the gene of interest have been analyzed. Suppose specific variations within these neighboring sequences are always present when the gene of interest is flawed. In that case, these nearby sequences can then be used as markers for the presence of the defective gene. When the variant sequences are present, so is the disease gene. Prenatal testing for cystic fibrosis has been done by looking for such variant sequences.

Individuals who come from families in which genetic diseases tend to occur can be tested as carriers, so they will know the risk of passing a particular disease to their offspring. For example, individuals whose families have a history of cystic fibrosis but who themselves are not affected may be asymptomatic carriers. Suppose they have children with individuals who are also cystic fibrosis carriers. In that case, they have a 25 percent chance of passing two copies of the defective gene to their offspring. DNA samples from the potential parents can be analyzed for the presence of a defective gene. The decision of partners to have children changes if both know they are carriers of a genetic disease. However, suppose only one or neither of them is a carrier. In that case, their offspring will not be at risk of inheriting cystic fibrosis, as it is an autosomal recessive disease. Carrier testing is possible for many genetic diseases and disorders that appear late in life, such as Huntington's chorea.

Many of the gene flaws of multifactorial diseases, which interact with environmental factors to produce disease, have been identified. Individuals who know they have a gene that puts them at risk for certain disorders can incorporate preventive measures into their lifestyle, thus minimizing their chances of developing the disease. For example, certain cancers, such as colon and breast cancer, have a genetic component. Individuals who test positive for the genes that predispose them to develop cancer can modify their diets to include cancer-fighting foods and receive frequent medical checkups to detect cancer development at its earliest, most treatable stage. Those with genes that contribute to arteriosclerosis and heart disease can modify their diets and increase exercise. Likewise, those with a genetic predisposition for alcoholism can avoid alcohol consumption.

PERSPECTIVE AND PROSPECTS

The scientific study of human genetics and genetic disease is relatively new, beginning in the early twentieth century. However, there are many early historical records that recognize that certain traits are hereditarily transmitted. Ancient Greek literature is peppered with references to heredity, and the Jewish book of religious and civil laws, the Talmud, describes in detail the inheritance pattern of hemophilia and its ramifications for circumcision.

The Augustinian monk Gregor Mendel worked out many of the principles of heredity by manipulating the pollen and eggs of pea plants over many generations. His work was conducted from the 1860s to the 1870s but was unrecognized by the scientific community until 1900.

At about this time, many disorders were being recognized as genetic diseases. Pedigree analysis, a way to trace inheritance patterns through a family tree, has been used since the mid-nineteenth century to track the incidence of hemophilia in European royal families. This analysis indicates that the disease was transmitted through females (indeed, hemophilia is an X-linked disorder). In the early twentieth century, Archibald Garrod, a British physician, recognized certain biochemical disorders as genetic diseases and proposed precise mechanisms for their transmission.

In 1953, Francis Crick and James D. Watson discovered the structure of DNA; thus began studies on the molecular biology of genes. This research resulted in the monumental discovery in 1973 that pieces of DNA from animals and bacteria could be cut and spliced together into a functional molecule. This recombinant DNA technology fostered a revolution in genetic analysis, in which pieces of human DNA can be removed and put into bacteria. The bacteria then replicate millions of copies of the human DNA, permitting detailed analysis. These recombinant molecules also produce human gene products, such as RNA and protein, thereby facilitating the study of normal and aberrant genes.

The recombinant DNA revolution spawned the development of DNA tests for genetic diseases and carrier status. Knowledge of what a normal gene product is and does is constructive in treating genetic conditions. For example, Duchenne muscular dystrophy is caused by the lack of a protein called "dystrophin." Providing function dystrophin into the skeletal muscles of the individual is one possible treatment of this disease.

Ultimately, medical science seeks to treat genetic diseases by providing a functional copy of the flawed gene to the affected individual. The introduction of normal copies of the defective gene would cure the genetic disorder. However, gene therapy that does not change the genetic of reproductive cells does not change the inheritance of future generations.

—*Karen E. Kalumuck, PhD*

Further Information

Cooper, Necia Grant, editor. *The Human Genome Project: Deciphering the Blueprint of Heredity.* Rev. ed., University Science Books, 1994.

"GeneTests." www.ncbi.nlm.nih.gov/sites/GeneTests.

Genetic Alliance, www.geneticalliance.org.

Gormley, Myra Vanderpool. *Family Diseases: Are You at Risk?* Genealogical Publishing, 2007.

Hereditary Disease Foundation, www.hdfoundation.org.

Jorde, Lynn B., John C. Carey, and Michael J. Bamshad. *Medical Genetics*. 4th ed., Mosby/Elsevier, 2010.

Judd, Sandra J., editor. *Genetic Disorders Sourcebook: Basic Consumer Information About Hereditary Diseases and Disorders*. 4th ed., Omnigraphics, 2010.

King, Richard A., Jerome I. Rotter, and Arno G. Motulsky, editors. *The Genetic Basis of Common Diseases*. 2nd ed., Oxford UP, 2002.

Lewis, Ricki. *Human Genetics: Concepts and Applications*. 10th ed., McGraw-Hill, 2012.

McCance, Kathryn L., and Sue E. Huether, editors. *Pathophysiology: The Biologic Basis for Disease in Adults and Children*. 6th ed., Mosby/Elsevier, 2010.

Marshall, Elizabeth L. *The Human Genome Project: Cracking the Code Within Us*. Franklin Watts, 1997.

Milunsky, Aubrey, and Jeff M. Milunsky, editors. *Genetic Disorders of the Fetus: Diagnosis, Prevention, and Treatment*. 6th ed., Wiley-Blackwell, 2010.

Nyhan, William L., and Georg F. Hoffmann. *Atlas of Inherited Metabolic Diseases*. 4th ed., CRC Press, 2020.

Petris, Gianluca, editor. *Curing Genetic Diseases through Genome Reprogramming*. Academic Press, 2021.

Springhouse Corporation. *Everything You Need to Know About Diseases*. Author, 1996.

Trivedi, Bijal P. *Breath from Salt: A Deadly Genetic Disease, a New Era in Science, and the Patients and Families Who Changed Medicine*. ?BenBella Books, 2020.

Wingerson, Lois. *Mapping Our Genes: The Genome Project and the Future of Medicine*. Plume, 1991.

Immunogenetics

Category: Immunogenetics

Definition: Immunogenetics studies the major histocompatibility (MHC) genes that identify self-tissues, the genes in B lymphocytes that direct antibody synthesis, and the genes that direct the synthesis of T lymphocyte receptors. This same genetic control that directs immune cell embryonic development and activation from an antigenic challenge also explains the basis of organ transplant rejection, autoimmunity, allergies, immunodeficiency, and potential therapies.

KEY TERMS

apoptosis: cell death that is programmed as a natural consequence of growth and development through normal cellular pathways or signals from neighboring cells

cytokines: soluble intercellular molecules produced by cells such as lymphocytes that can influence the immune response

downstream: describes the left-to-right direction of deoxyribonucleic acid (DNA) whose nucleotides are arranged in sequence with the 5' carbon on the left and the 3' on the right; the direction of ribonucleic acid (RNA) transcription of a genetic message with the beginning of a gene on the left and the end on the right

haplotype: a sequential set of genes on a single chromosome inherited together from one parent; the other parent provides a matching chromosome with a different set of genes

monoclonal antibodies: antibodies with one particular target that have been generated in large quantities from a single hybrid parent cell formed in a laboratory

transposon: a sequence of nucleotides flanked by inverted repeats capable of being removed or inserted within a genome

GENES, B CELLS, AND ANTIBODIES

The fundamental question that led to the development of immunogenetics is how scientists can make the thousands of specific antibodies that protect people from the thousands of organisms they encounter. Frank Macfarlane Burnet proposed the clonal selection theory, which states that an antigen (i.e., anything not-self, such as an invading microorganism) selects, from the thousands of different B cells, the receptor on a particular B cell that fits it like a key fitting a lock. That cell is activated to make a clone of plasma cells, producing millions of soluble antibodies with attachment sites identical to the receptor on that B-cell surface. The problem facing scientists interested in a genetic explanation for this capability was the need for more genes than the number found in the entire human genome.

Susumu Tonegawa first recognized that many antibodies produced in the lifetime of a human did not have to have the equivalent number of physical genes on their chromosomes. From his work, Tonegawa determined that the genes responsible for antibody synthesis are arranged in tandem segments on specific chromosomes relating to specific parts of antibody structure. The amino acids that form the two light polypeptide chains and the two heavy polypeptide chains making up the IgG class of antibodies are programmed by nucleotide sequences of deoxyribonucleic acid (DNA) that exist on three different chromosomes. Light chain genes are found on chromosomes 2 and 22. The specific nucleotide sequences code for light polypeptide chains. Half the chain has a constant amino acid sequence, and the other half has a variable sequence. The amino acid sequences of the heavy polypeptide chains are constant over three-quarters of their length, with five primary sequences identifying five classes of human immunoglobulins: IgG, IgM, IgD, IgA, and IgE. The other quarter length has a variable sequence that, together with the variable sequence of the light chain, forms the antigen-binding site. The nucleotide sequence coding for the heavy chain is part of chromosome 14.

The actual light chain locus is organized into sequences of nucleotides designated variable (V), joining (J), and constant (C) segments. The multiple options for the different V and J segments and mixing the different V and J segments cause many different DNA light chain nucleotide sequences and the synthesis of different antibodies. The same rearrangement occurs between various nucleotide sequences related to the V, diversity (D), and J segments of the heavy chain locus. The recombination of segments appears to be genetically regulated by recombination signal sequences downstream from the variable segments and recombination activating genes that function during B-cell development. Genetic recombination is complete with the immature B cell committed to producing one kind of antibody. The diversity of antibody molecules is explained by the messenger ribonucleic acid (mRNA) transcript coding for either the light polypeptide chain or the heavy polypeptide chain is formed containing exons transcribed from recombined gene segments during B-cell differentiation. The unique antigen receptor-binding site is formed when the variable regions of one heavy and one light chain come together during the formation of the completed antibody in the endoplasmic reticulum of the mature B cell. The B-cell antigen receptor is an attached surface antibody of the IgM class. The binding of the antigen to the specific B cell activates its cell division and the formation of a clone of plasma cells that produce a unique antibody. If this circulating B cell does not contact its specific antigen within a few weeks, it will die by apoptosis. During plasma cell formation, the class of antibody protein produced switches typically from IgM to IgG by forming an mRNA transcript containing the exon nucleotide sequence made from the IgG heavy chair C segment rather than the heavy chain C segment for IgM. The intervening nucleotide sequence of the IgM constant segment is deleted from the chromosome as an excised circle reminiscent of the transposon or plasmid excision process. This switch forms an IgG antibody having the same antigen specificity as the IgM antibody because the variable regions of the light and heavy polypeptide chains remain the same. Although the activation and development of B cells by some antigens may not need T-cell involvement, it is believed that T-cell cytokines influence class switching and most B-cell activity.

MAJOR HISTOCOMPATIBILITY GENES

In humans, the major histocompatibility (MHC) genes encoding "self-antigens" are also called the "HLA complex" and are located on chromosome 6. The nucleotides that compose this DNA complex encode for two sets of cell surface molecules designated MHC Class I and MHC Class II antigens. The Class I region contains loci *A*, *B*, and *C*, which encode for MHC Class I A, B, and C glycoproteins on every nucleated cell in the body. Because the *A*, *B*, and *C* loci comprise highly variable nucleotide sequences, numerous kinds of A, B, and C glycoproteins characterize humans. All people inherit MHC Class I *A*, *B*, and *C* genes as a haplotype from their parents. Children will have tissues with half of their Class I A, B, and C antigens like their mother and half like their father's. Siblings could have tissue antigens that are identical or dissimilar based on their MHC I glycoproteins. Body surveillance by T lymphocytes involves T cells recognizing self-glycoproteins. Cellular invasion by a virus or any other parasite results in processing an antigen and its display in the MHC Class I glycoprotein cleft. T-cytotoxic lymphocytes with T-cell receptors specific to the antigen-MHC I complex will attach to the antigen and activate the clonal selection. Infected host cells are killed when activated cytotoxic T cells bind to the surface and release perforins, causing apoptosis.

MHC Class II genes are designated *HLA-DPA1* and *HLA-DPB1*, *HLA-DQA1* and *HLA-DQB1*, and *HLA-DRA* and *HLA-DRB1*. These genes encode glycoprotein molecules that attach to the cell surface in a and ß pairs. A child will inherit the six genes as a group or haplotype, three a and ß glycoprotein gene pairs from each parent. During glycoprotein synthesis, the child will also have glycoprotein molecules made from the maternal and paternal a and ß pairings.

The Class II MHC molecules are on the membranes of macrophages, B cells, and dendritic cells.

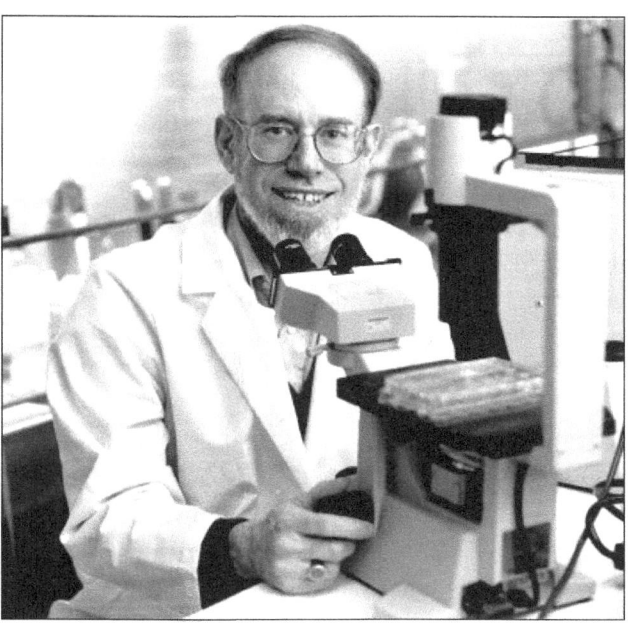

Jay Berzofsky, Head, Molecular Immunogenetics and Vaccine Research Section, Vaccine Branch, National Cancer Institute. Photy by Bill Branson, via Wikimedia Commons

These specialized cells capture antigens and attach antigen peptides to the three-dimensional grooves formed by combined a and ß glycoprotein pairs. The antigen attached to the Class II groove is presented to the T-helper cell, with the receptor recognizing the specific antigen while bound to the Class II self-antigen. The specific T-helper cell forms a specific clone of effector cells and memory cells.

GENES, T-HELPER CELLS, AND T-CYTOTOXIC CELLS

The thousands of specific T-cell receptors (TCR) available to any specific antigen one might encounter in a lifetime are formed from progenitor T cells in the human embryonic thymus. The TCR comprises two dissimilar polypeptide chains designated a and ß or ? and d. They are similar in structure to immunoglobulins and MHC molecules. They have regions of variable amino acid sequences and constant amino acid sequences arranged in loops called "domains." This basic structural configuration places all three molecules in a chemically similar grouping designated the immunoglobulin superfamily. The genes of these molecules are derived from a primordial supergene that encoded the basic domain structure.

The exons encoding the a and ? polypeptides are designated V, J, and C gene segments in sequence and associate with recombination signal sequences similar to the immunoglobulin light chain gene. The ß and d polypeptide genes are designated VDJ and C exon segments in sequence associating with recombination signal sequences similar to the immunoglobulin heavy chain genes. Just as there are multiple forms for each immunoglobulin variable gene segment, there are multiple forms for the variable TCR gene segments. Thymocytes, T-cell precursors in the thymus, undergo chance recombinations of gene segments. These genetic recombinations, as well as the chance combination of a completed a polypeptide with a completed ß polypeptide, provide thousands of completed specific TCRs ready to be chosen by an invading antigen and to form a clone of either T-helper cells or T-cytotoxic cells.

IMMUNOGENETIC DISEASE
The HLA genes of the major histocompatibility complex identify every human being as distinct from all other things, including other human beings, because of the MHC Class I and Class II antigens. Surveillance of self involves B- and T-cell antigen recognition because of MHC self-recognition. How well individual human beings recognize self and their response to antigen in an adaptive immune response are determined by MHC haplotypes and the genes that make immunoglobulins and T-cell receptors. These same genes can explain various disease states, such as autoimmunity, allergy, and immunodeficiency.

Because immunoglobulin structure and T-cell receptor formation are based on a chance mechanism, problems involving self-recognition may occur.

Thymocytes with completed T-cell receptors are protected from apoptosis when they demonstrate self-MHC molecule recognition. Alternatively, the thymic epithelial cells present thymocytes with self-antigens processed by specialized macrophages bearing MHC Class I and Class II molecules. Thymocytes reacting with high-affinity receptors to processed self-antigens undergo apoptosis. There is also a negative selection process within the bone marrow that actively eliminates immature B cells with membrane-bound autoantibodies that react with self-antigens. Despite these selective activities, autoreactive T cells and B cells can be part of circulating surveillance, causing autoimmune disease of either single organs or multiple tissues.

Autoimmune diseases occur in families, and there is growing evidence that an individual with a particular HLA haplotype has a greater risk for developing a particular disease. For example, ankylosing spondylitis develops more often in individuals with *HLA-B27* than those with another *HLA-B* allele, and rheumatoid arthritis is associated with several common *HLA-DRB1* alleles. Myasthenia gravis and multiple sclerosis are two neurological diseases caused by autoantibodies. There is evidence that they are related to the restricted expression of T-cell variable genes. Genomic studies provide evidence for the possibility that autoimmune induction occurs because of molecular mimicry between human host proteins and microbial antigens. Among the cross-reacting antigens that have been implicated are papillomavirus E2 and the insulin receptor, and poliovirus VP2 and the acetylcholine receptor.

The genetics of immunity also involves the study of defective genes that cause primary immunodeficiency infectious disease. The deficiency can decrease an adaptive immune response involving B cells, T cells, or both, as is the case with severe combined immunodeficiency disorder (SCID). There is evidence that SCID can demonstrate either autosomal recessive or X-linked inheritance. One such defect is on the short arm of chromosome 11. It involves a mutation of recombination-activating genes that are necessary for the rearrangement of immunoglobulin gene segments and the T-cell receptor gene segments. The inability to recombine the VD and J variable segments prevents the development of active B cells and T cells with various antigen receptors. SCID is essentially incompatible with life and characterized by severe opportunistic infections caused by even usually benign organisms.

Tissue rejection after transplantation remains an integral cause of transplant failure that markedly affects morbidity. Cytokines play a significant role in transplant rejection. Dutch researchers discovered that specific alleles of the genes that encode IL-6 and the IL-6 receptor in the recipient donor but not in the transplant recipient could predict the recipient's susceptibility to transplant rejection.

Allergies have a genetic component, and atopy, an abnormal IgE response, is common to certain families. There is evidence that children have a 30 percent chance of developing an allergic disease if one parent is allergic. In comparison, those children with two allergic parents have a 50 percent chance. The genetic control of IgE production can be related to TH2 lymphocyte cytokine stimulation of class switching from the constant segment of IgG to the constant segment of IgE on chromosome 14 in an antigen-selected cell undergoing clonal selection.

IMPACT
Understanding the genetic basis for immune reactions results in novel approaches to protection against disease and improvements in health. Researchers are pursuing therapeutics to control B-cell responses in autoimmune diseases and IgE responses in allergic reactions. Clinical laboratories provide detailed histocompatibility and immunogenetics testing for solid organ and stem cell transplantation and blood and platelet transfusions to reduce graft-versus-host the incidence and severity of graft-versus-host disease.

Immunotherapy capitalizes on a person's immune system to fight cancers or infectious diseases, either by actively stimulating the production of natural antibodies or by passively introducing antibodies engineered in a laboratory. With active stimulation, specific immunity may be induced with vaccines, or nonspecific immunity may be induced with interferons or interleukins. Monoclonal antibodies that target specific cell-surface antigens achieve passive immunity. Several therapeutic monoclonal antibodies have been approved for use in humans by the U.S. Food and Drug Administration (FDA), particularly in treating colorectal cancer, non-Hodgkin lymphoma, and some types of leukemia. Conversely, other therapeutic monoclonal antibodies have been produced and marketed to suppress immune responses in rheumatoid arthritis and allergic asthma. Researchers who employ related technologies are trying to develop biomarkers that will track the progression of immune disorders and measure their response to various treatment modalities.

Immunogenetics has led to new fields of study in public health, such as medical anthropology, which includes determining how people of certain races or ethnicities are genetically predisposed to certain diseases. Another new field of study is the immunology of aging, which includes attempting to determine the effect of genetic variation on the natural aging process. One crucial issue in this field is how to boost the immune response in the elderly to vaccines, especially those for influenza and pneumonia.

—*Patrick J. DeLuca, PhD and Bethany Thivierge, MPH*

Further Information
Abbas, Abul K., Andrew H. Lichtman, and Shiv Pillai. *Basic Immunology: Functions and Disorders of the Immune System.* 6th ed., Elsevier, 2019.
Flajnik, Martin F., Nevil J. Singh, and Steven M. Holland. *Paul's Fundamental Immunology.* Lippincott Williams & Wilkins, 2022.

Genetics Home Reference. "HLA-DRB1." *Genetics Home Reference*. U.S. NLM, 28 Jul. 2014. Accessed. 4 Aug. 2014.

Male, David. *Immunology: An Illustrated Outline*. 6th ed., CRC Press, 2021

McKusick, Victor A., and Paul J. Converse. "*142857 Major Histocompatibility Complex, Class II, DR Beta-1; HLA-DRB1." *OMIM.org*. Johns Hopkins U, 25 Jun. 2014. Accessed 4 Aug. 2014.

Oksenberg, Jorge R., and David Brassat, editors. *Immunogenetics of Autoimmune Disease*. Springer, 2006.

Owen, Judith A., Janis Kuby, Jenni Punt, and Sharon A. Stranford. *Immunology*. 7th ed., Macmillan, 2013.

Pines, Maya, editor. *Arousing the Fury of the Immune System*. Howard Hughes Medical Institute, 1998.

Poppelaars, Felix, Mariana Gaya da Costa, Siawosh K. Eskandari, Jeffery Damman, Marc Seelen. "Donor Genetic Variants in Interleukin-6 and Interleukin-6 Receptor Associate with Biopsy-Proven Rejection Following Kidney Transplantation." *Scientific Reports*, vol. 11, 2021, p. 16483, doi.org/10.1038/s41598-021-95714-z.

ALLERGIES

This section delves into common allergies caused by an immune system's overreaction to substances the body normally considers harmless. Causes, symptoms, and potential therapies are discussed for such familiar conditions as insect bites and stings, allergies to foods, hay fever, dermatitis, and hives. The fifteen articles in this segment give detailed accounts of immune system hypersensitivity as well as possible preventative measures, like diet alterations and other treatments. Also covered are the many products available for allergy testing, many of which have no medical validation. Allergic reactions range from mild to life-threatening, so it is important to properly diagnose disorders and come up with a plan for treatment.

    Allergic bronchopulmonary aspergillosis 117
    Allergies 118
    Allergist and immunologist 127
    Bites and stings 129
    Coughing 132
    Dermatitis 134
    Ear infections and disorders 141
    Eosinophilic esophagitis 148
    Food allergies 151
    Food allergy testing panels 155
    Hay fever 159
    Hives 162
    Itching 163
    Mold and mildew 165
    Prevention of viral infections 167

Allergic bronchopulmonary aspergillosis

Category: Diseases/Conditions
Anatomy or system affected: Lungs, respiratory system
Definition: Allergic bronchopulmonary aspergillosis (ABPA) is an allergic lung disorder. It is related to the fungus *Aspergillus fumigatus* (AF). ABPA also occurs as a lung infection that spreads to other parts of the body (more common in persons with suppressed immune systems) and as a fungal growth (aspergilloma) in a lung cavity that has healed from a previous lung disease or infection.

KEY TERMS

allergic bronchopulmonary aspergillosis: an allergic reaction to the presence of *Aspergillus* components (e.g., spores or hyphae) in the lower respiratory tract

aspergillus: a genus of fungus commonly found indoors and outdoors and a wide range of climates

CAUSES

ABPA is caused by an allergic reaction to inhaled AF, which is a common fungus. AF grows and flourishes in decaying vegetation and soil, certain foods, dust, and water. The allergic reaction worsens respiratory symptoms in people with asthma or cystic fibrosis. The inhaled AF colonizes mucus in the lungs, causing sensitization to AF. Further AF exposure causes recurring allergic inflammation of the lungs. Such chronic lung inflammation packs the alveoli (tiny air sacs in the lungs) with eosinophils (a type of white blood cell involved in specific allergic reactions and infections with parasites).

RISK FACTORS

Risk factors for ABPA include asthma; cystic fibrosis; tuberculosis; sarcoidosis; human immunodeficiency virus (HIV); acquired immunodeficiency syndrome (AIDS); lowered immune resistance, as occurs with certain cancers or chemotherapy, or after organ transplants; use of steroid or antimicrobial medications; and hospitalization.

SYMPTOMS

Symptoms of ABPA are usually those of progressive asthma. These include shortness of breath, wheezing, weakness, malaise, unintended weight loss, and chest pain. As ABPA progresses, other symptoms may occur, including the production of thick, brownish, or bloody sputum and a low-grade fever. In severe, long-term cases, ABPA can cause bronchiectasis, the widening of areas of the bronchus usually caused by inflammation and scarring of the lungs.

SCREENING AND DIAGNOSIS

Screening includes a chest X-ray to check the lungs; sputum tests to check sputum for the presence of AF and high levels of eosinophils; blood tests for high levels of eosinophils and for antibodies suggesting an allergic reaction to AF; skin prick tests for allergic sensitivity by placing small amounts of AF in the skin; a biopsy of lung or sinus tissue; and pulmonary function tests to monitor the breathing capacity of the lungs.

Because ABPA can appear similar to non-ABPA-induced asthma, it is often difficult to determine to what extent ABPA contributes to symptoms. Therefore, ABPA diagnosis results after several repeatedly positive tests for ABPA over several months or years.

TREATMENT AND THERAPY

Treatment goals include suppressing the allergic reaction to AF, minimizing lung inflammation, and preventing AF from colonizing the lungs. ABPA is usually treated with two medications: prednisone (an oral corticosteroid medication) and antifungal drugs, such as itraconazole (Sporanox), amphotericin B, or voriconazole.

PREVENTION AND OUTCOMES

Avoiding exposure to AF is the best way to prevent ABPA. However, this is difficult, because AF is so prevalent in the environment. Guidelines to help prevent exposure to AF include avoiding areas with decaying vegetation and standing water; keeping the home as dust-free as possible; and remaining in air-filtered, air-conditioned environments whenever possible. Measures to avoid symptoms and prevent permanent lung damage caused by ABPA include ongoing testing and monitoring of ABPA and early and continuing medical treatment for the disease.

—*Rick Alan*

Further Information

Barnes, Penelope D., and Kieren A. Marr. "Aspergillosis: Spectrum of Disease, Diagnosis, and Treatment." *Infectious Disease Clinics of North America*, vol. 20, 2006, pp. 545-61.

Ferri, Fred F., editor. *Ferri's Clinical Advisor 2011: Instant Diagnosis and Treatment*. Mosby/Elsevier, 2011.

Patterson, Thomas F. "*Aspergillus* Species." *Mandell, Douglas, and Bennett's Principles and Practice of Infectious Diseases*, edited by Gerald L. Mandell, John F. Bennett, and Raphael Dolin, 7th ed., Churchill Livingstone/Elsevier, 2010.

Porter, Robert S., et al., editors. *The Merck Manual Home Health Handbook*. 3rd ed., Merck Research Laboratories, 2009.

Richardson, Malcolm D., and Elizabeth M. Johnson. *Pocket Guide to Fungal Infection*. 2nd ed., Blackwell, 2006.

ALLERGIES

Category: Diseases/Disorders
Anatomy or system affected: Gastrointestinal system, immune system, lungs, nose, skin, stomach
Specialties and related fields: Dermatology, family medicine, immunology, internal medicine, otorhinolaryngology, pediatrics, pharmacology
Definition: Exaggerated immune reactions to materials that are intrinsically harmless; the body's release of pharmacologically active chemicals during allergic reactions may result in discomfort, tissue damage, or, in severe responses, death.

KEY TERMS

allergen: any substance that induces an allergic reaction

anaphylaxis: an immediate immune reaction, triggered by mediators that cause vasodilation and the contraction of smooth muscle

basophil: a type of white blood cell that contains mediators associated with allergic reactions; represents 1 percent or less of total white cells

histamine: a compound released during allergic reactions that cause many of the symptoms of allergies

IgE: a type of antibody associated with the release of granules from basophils and mast cells

mast cell: a tissue cell with granules containing vasoactive mediators such as histamine, serotonin, and bradykinin; the tissue equivalent of basophil

CAUSES AND SYMPTOMS

Allergies represent inappropriate immune responses to intrinsically harmless materials or antigens. Most allergens are common environmental antigens. Approximately one in every six Americans is allergic to material such as dust, molds, dust mites, animal dander, or pollen. The effects range from a mere nuisance, such as rhinitis, or nasal irritation, associated with hay fever allergies or the itching of poison ivy, to the life-threatening anaphylactic shock that may follow a bee sting. Allergies are most often found in children, but they may affect any age group.

Allergy is one of the hypersensitivity reactions generally classified according to the types of effector molecules that mediate their symptoms and according to the time delay that follows exposure to the allergen. P. G. H. Gell and Robin Coombs defined four types of hypersensitivities. Three of these, types 1 through 3, follow minutes to hours after the exposure to an allergen. Type 4, or delayed-type hypersensitivity (DTH), may occur anywhere from twenty-four to seventy-two hours after exposure. People are most familiar with two of these forms of allergies: type 1, or immediate hypersensitivity, commonly seen as hay fever or asthma; and type 4, most often following an encounter with poison ivy or poison oak.

Type 1 hypersensitivities have much in common with any normal immune response. A foreign material, an allergen, comes in contact with the host's immune system, and an antibody response results. The response differs according to the type of molecule produced. A special class of antibody, IgE, is secreted by the B lymphocytes. IgE, when complexed with the specific allergen, can activate several types of mediator cells, mainly basophils and mast cells.

Mast cells are found throughout the skin and tissue. The mucous membranes of the respiratory and gastrointestinal tract, in particular, have high concentrations of these cells, as many as ten thousand cells per cubic millimeter. Basophils, the blood cell equivalents of the mast cells, represent 1 percent or less of the total white cell count. Though the cells are not identical, they do possess features related to the role that they play in an allergic response. Both basophils and mast cells contain large numbers of

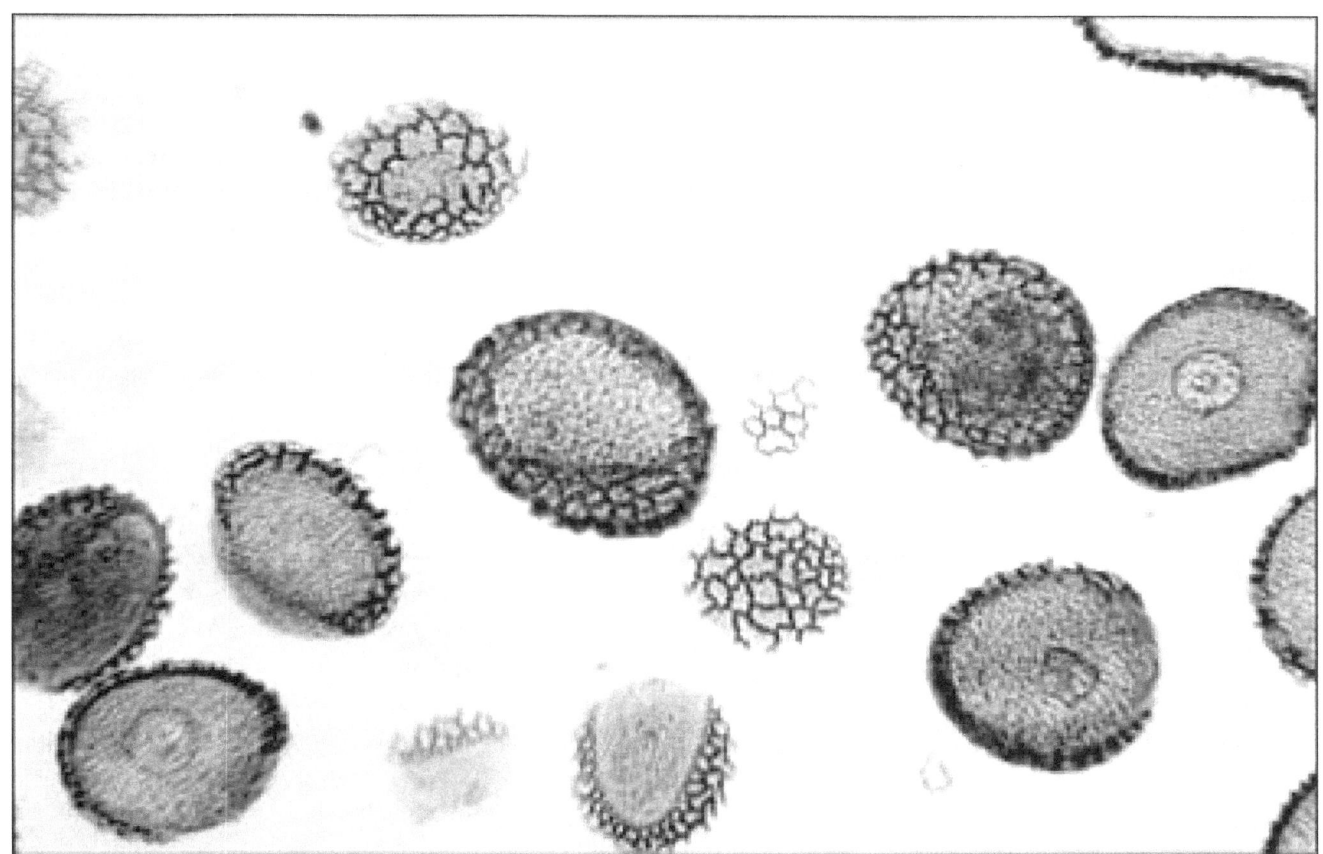

Microscopic pollens, which are responsible for many allergic reactions. [PhotoDisc.]

granules composed of pharmacologically active chemicals. Both also contain surface receptors for IgE molecules. The binding of IgE/allergen complexes to these cells triggers the release of the granules.

Many common antigens can cause allergies. These include plant pollens (as are found in ryegrass or ragweed), foods such as nuts or eggs, bee or wasp venom, mold, or animal dander. A square mile of ragweed may produce as much as 16 tons of pollen in a single season. Almost any food or environmental substance could serve as an allergen. The most important defining factor as to whether an individual is allergic to any particular substance is the extent and type of IgE production against that substance.

Type 1 allergic reactions begin as soon as the sensitized person is exposed to the allergen. In the case of hay fever, this results when the person inhales the pollen particle. The shell of the particle is enzymatically dissolved, and the specific allergens are released in the vicinity of the mucous membranes in the respiratory system. If the person has had prior sensitization to the materials, his/her immune system recognizes it as a foreign matter and IgE molecules are secreted by localized B lymphocytes. IgE antibodies bind to specialized receptors (called "FceRI receptors") on the surfaces of mast cells and basophils. When these cell surface-bound IgE molecules bind to allergens, they form an antibody/antigen complex.

The formation of IgE-allergen complexes on the surfaces of mast cells and basophils initiates the cross-linking of FceRI receptors on the cell. Such cross-linking is necessary because, in its absence, no granules are released. On the other hand, artificial cross-linking of the receptors in laboratory experiments, even in the absence of IgE, results in the release of vasoactive granules.

Following the activation of the cell surface, a series of biochemical events occur, the key is an influx of calcium into the cell. Two events rapidly follow: The cell begins synthesizing prostaglandins and leukotrienes, two mediators that play key roles in allergic reactions, and preexisting granules move toward the cell surface. When they reach the cell surface, the granules fuse with the cell membrane, releasing their contents into the tissue.

The contents of the granules mediate the clinical manifestations of allergies. These mediators can be classified as either primary or secondary. Thus, clinical responses are divided into immediate and late-phase reactions. Primary mediators are those found in preexisting granules and released initially following the activities at the cell surface. They include substances such as histamine and serotonin, associated with increased vascular permeability and smooth muscle contraction. Histamine itself may constitute 10 percent of the weight of the granules in these cells. The results are a runny nose, irritated eyes, and bronchial congestion. These substances include the leukotrienes (also called "slow reactive substances of anaphylaxis," or SRS-A) and prostaglandins. Pharmacological effects from these chemicals include vasodilation, increased capillary permeability, contraction of smooth muscles in the bronchioles, and, more important, a group of chemotactic activities that attract many different white cells in the site to magnify the inflammatory reaction. This is why an allergic reaction is divided

---

INFORMATION ON ALLERGIES

Causes: Antigens such as pollen, mold, certain foods (nuts, eggs, seafood), drugs (penicillin), bee or wasp venom, animal dander, dust mites, etc.

Symptoms: Sneezing, runny nose, coughing, itching, breathing difficulties, hives, inflammation, vomiting, diarrhea, shock

Duration: Chronic, with acute episodes

Treatments: Antihistamines, mast cell stabilizers, steroids (cortisone), desensitization

into two phases and the late reaction may last for days.

Foods to which one is allergic may trigger similar reactions in the gut. Mast cells in the gastrointestinal tract also contain receptors for IgE, and contact with food allergens results in the release of mediators similar to those in the respiratory passages. The result may be vomiting or diarrhea. The allergen may also pass from the gut into the circulatory system or other tissues, triggering asthmatic attacks or hives.

In severe allergic reactions, the response may be swift and deadly. The venom released during a bee sting may trigger a systemic response from circulating basophils or mast cells, resulting in the contraction of pulmonary muscles and rapid suffocation, a condition known as anaphylactic shock. The leukotrienes, platelet-activating factor, and prostaglandins play key roles in these reactions.

DTHs, also known as contact dermatitis reactions, are most commonly manifested following the presentation of a topical allergen. These may include the catechol-containing oils of poison oak, the constituents of hair dyes or cosmetics, environmental contaminants such as nickel or turpentine, or any of a wide variety of environmental agents. Rather than being mediated by antibodies, as are the other types of hypersensitivities, DTH is mediated through a specific cellular response. These cells appear to be a special class of T (for thymus-derived) lymphocytes.

DTH reactions are initiated following the exposure to the appropriate antigen. Antigen-presenting cells in the skin bind and "present" the allergen to the specific T lymphocytes. This results in the secretion by these T cells of a variety of chemicals mediating inflammation. These mediators, or cytokines, include gamma interferon, interleukin-2, and tumor necrosis factor. The result, developing over twenty-four to seventy-two hours, is a significant inflammatory response with subsequent localized damage to tissue.

IN THE NEWS: PEANUT ALLERGIES

In the United States alone, between fifty and one hundred fifty people die each year from serious allergic reactions to peanuts. One and a half million Americans have a demonstrated allergic sensitivity that puts them at risk for life-threatening reactions to peanut protein exposure. Reactions can be so severe to minute amounts of airborne peanut protein that some schoolchildren must eat lunch in peanut-free rooms, and many airlines have stopped serving peanuts to passengers. Because peanuts and peanut oil can be ingredients in a diverse range of food items such as chili, potato chips, and egg rolls, peanut allergy sufferers live under a constant threat of having an adverse reaction despite their best efforts to avoid the allergen.

In the March 13, 2003, issue of the *New England Journal of Medicine*, Hugh A. Sampson and his colleagues of Mount Sinai School of Medicine in New York reported the results of a study that show the first successful preventive treatment for peanut allergy. In a double-blind study, eighty-four volunteers with peanut allergy were given either placebo shots or injections of various doses of the experimental drug TNX-901 once a month over four months. At the end of the study, participants were given capsules of peanut flour in increasing amounts until they exhibited an allergic reaction. The results showed that those given placebos reacted when given the equivalent of half a peanut. People who received low doses of the drug could ingest a bit more before reacting. Those receiving the highest doses could ingest, on average, the equivalent of nine peanuts (and for some, twenty-four peanuts) before developing an allergic response.

TNX-901 is a genetically engineered antibody that prevents allergic response by binding to potentially harmful immune cells that are produced in response to allergen exposure. Binding these immune cells interrupt the series of events that lead to an allergic reaction.

While TNX-901 is not a cure for peanut allergy, its preventive potential makes the required monthly shot appealing to those afflicted with the disorder. Since accidental exposure to peanut protein is estimated to be equivalent to one or two peanuts, TNX-901 could provide sufferers with confidence that accidental peanut exposure would not lead to a life-threatening reaction. Legal disputes have hampered its development, however, and a similar drug called "Xolair" is being researched. Other researchers are examining oral immunotherapy as a treatment for peanut allergy.

—*Karen E. Kalumuck, PhD*

The other classes of hypersensitivity reactions, types 2 and 3, are less commonly associated with what most people consider to be allergies. Yet they do have much in common with type 1, immediate hypersensitivity. Type 2 reactions are mediated by a type of antibody called "IgG." Clinical manifestations result from the antibody-mediated destruction of target cells, rather than through the release of mediators. One of the most common forms of reaction is blood transfusion reactions, either against the A or B blood group antigen or as a result of an Rh incompatibility. For example, if a person with type O blood is accidentally transfused with type A, an immune reaction will occur. The eventual result is the destruction of the incompatible blood cells. Rh incompatibilities are most commonly associated with a pregnant woman who is lacking the Rh protein in her blood (that is, Rh-negative) carrying a child who is Rh-positive (a blood type obtained from the father's genes). The production of IgG directed against the Rh protein in the child's blood can set in motion events that destroy the baby's red blood cells, a condition known as hemolytic disease of the newborn. This is usually not problematic during a woman's first pregnancy but becomes a problem in later pregnancies when her immune system can recognize the baby's Rh factor as a foreign body.

Type 3 reactions are known as immune complex diseases. In this case, sensitivity to antigens results in the formation of IgG/antigen complexes, which can lodge in the kidney or other sites in the body. The complexes activate what is known as the complement system, a series of proteins that include vasoactive chemicals and lipolytic compounds. The result can be a significant inflammation that can lead to kidney damage. Type 3 reactions can include

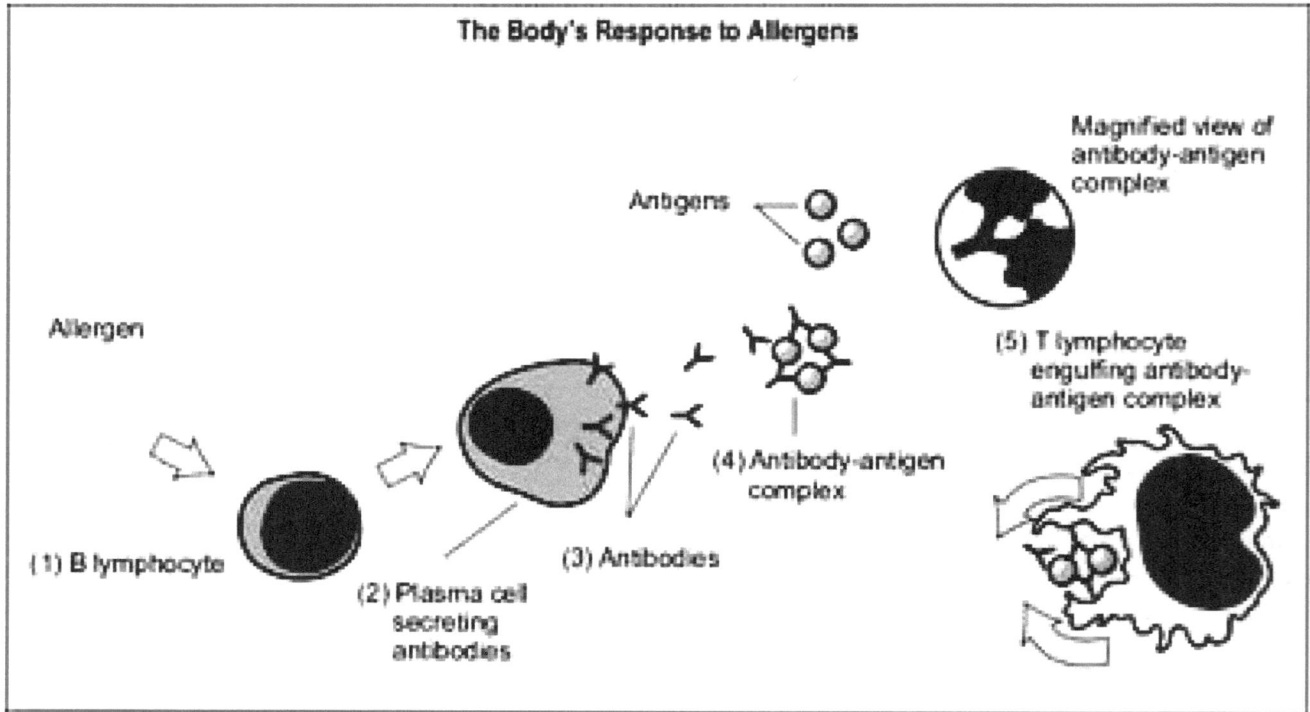

An allergic reaction is caused when foreign material, or antigens, enter the immune system, which produces B lymphocytes (1) that cause blood plasma cells to secrete antibodies (2). The antibodies (3) link with antigens to form antigen-antibody complexes (4), which then are engulfed and destroyed by a T lymphocyte (5).

autoimmune diseases such as arthritis or lupus, or drug reactions such as some forms of penicillin allergies (some penicillin allergies are type 1).

It should be kept in mind, however, that none of these reactions is inherently abnormal. Under normal circumstances, these same reactions mediate an inflammatory defense against foreign pathogens. For example, the normal role of IgE appears to be associated with the destruction of parasites such as are found in helminthic infections (such as parasitic worms). The release of mediators under these conditions is important as a defensive reaction leading to the expulsion or destruction of worms. It is only during the inappropriate release of these same mediators that one observes the symptoms of allergies.

Most individuals are familiar with immediate hypersensitivity reactions involving a localized area. The most common form of allergy is rhinitis, known as hay fever, which affects approximately 10 percent of the population. When a person inhales an environmental allergen such as ragweed pollen, the result is a release of pharmacologically active mediators from mast cells located in the upper respiratory tract. If the release occurs in the lower respiratory tract, the condition is known as asthma. In both instances, the eyes and nose are subject to inflammation and the release of secretions. In mild cases, the person suffers from watery discharges, coughing, and sneezing. In more severe asthma attacks, the bronchioles may become constricted and obstruct the air passages.

TREATMENT AND THERAPY
Three methods for dealing with allergies exist: avoidance of the allergen, palliative treatments, and desensitization. Ideally, one can attempt to avoid the allergen. For example, cow's milk, a common allergen, should not be given to a child at too young an age, and one can stay away from patches of poison ivy or avoid eating strawberries if one is allergic to them.

Avoidance, however, is not always possible or desirable, as the problem may be the fur, for example, from the family cat. Pets are problematic because their bodily secretions, such as urine or saliva, dry on household objects. When an object, such as a pillow, is used, the molecules become disturbed and the airborne molecules create a pool of allergens that are hard to get rid of since so many household objects are usually contaminated.

It is sometimes difficult to identify the specific substance causing the symptoms. This is particularly true when dealing with foods. Various procedures exist to identify the irritating substance, skin testing being the most common. In this procedure, the patient's skin is exposed to small amounts of suspected allergens. A positive test is indicated by the formation of hives or reddening within about twenty to thirty minutes. If the person is hypersensitive to a suspected allergen and finds a skin test too risky, then a blood test, a radioallergosorbent test (RAST) may be substituted. In addition to running a battery of tests, a patient's allergy history (including family history, since allergies are in part genetic) or environment may give clues as to the identity of the culprit.

The most commonly used method of dealing with allergies is a palliative treatment that treats the symptoms. Antihistamines act by binding to histamine receptors on target cells, interfering with the binding of histamine. There are four types of histamine receptors: H1, H2, H3, and H4. H1 histamine receptors play the most significant role in allergies. The smooth muscle surrounding blood vessels, endothelial cells that line blood vessels, neurons in the brain have H1 receptors on their surfaces. Histamine binding to H1 receptors results in relaxation of vascular smooth muscles, shrinkage of endothelial cells, increased mucus secretion on the upper and lower respiratory passages, and increased alertness.

Binding to H2 receptors results in increased vasopermeability and swelling, and increased stomach acid production. Histamine II blockers such as cimetidine are used primarily to control gastric secretions and treat peptic ulcers. Occasionally they are used as adjunctive therapy or in the prevention of severe allergic reactions. The brain contains H3 receptors and activation of H3 receptors decreases neurotransmitter release from specific neurons. Leukocytes in the bone marrow and circulating blood contain H4 receptors and activation of these receptors provides attracts leukocytes toward areas of tissue damage (chemotaxis).

Antihistamines for allergies inhibit H1 receptors. Antihistamines include alkylamines (e.g., chlorpheniramine, brompheniramine), ethanolamines (e.g., diphenhydramine), piperazines (e.g., hydroxyzine, fexofenadine), and miscellaneous drugs (e.g., loratadine, desloratadine). Antihistamine classification depends on when each drug was developed. For example, "first-generation" antihistamines include the older antihistamines, such as diphenhydramine, brompheniramine, chlorpheniramine, doxylamine, clemastine, and others. Because first-generation antihistamines cross the blood-brain barrier, they inhibit H1 receptors in the brain and cause sedation. For this reason, some first-generation antihistamines, such as the piperazines cyclizine and meclizine, effectively treat motion sickness. Some first-generation antihistamines also inhibit muscarinic receptors that bind the neurotransmitter acetylcholine. This antimuscarinic activity may cause urine retention, blurred vision, and, especially in elderly patients, confusion and worsening dementia. Consequently, everyone should use over-the-counter antihistamines with some modicum of caution. Second-generation antihistamines include loratadine, cetirizine, fexofenadine, olopatadine, azelastine, and others. Second-generation antihistamines have longer half-lives, and, therefore, people only need to take them once a day. Additionally, they do not cross the blood-brain barrier and do not cause drowsiness. Both types of antihistamines effectively treat the symptoms of acute allergies such as hay fever, atopic dermatitis and atopic urticaria (allergic rash).

IN THE NEWS: "BIG 8" ALLERGENS ON FOOD LABELS

On December 20, 2005, the Food and Drug Administration (FDA) announced that effective January 1, 2006, it would enforce regulations established by the Food Allergen Labeling and Consumer Protection Act of 2004. The FDA edict requires manufacturers to list in clear language on product labels the presence of any of the eight most important food allergens—milk, eggs, fish, crustacean shellfish such as shrimp, tree nuts, peanuts, wheat, and soybeans—and protein derived from them. Thus, if a product contains casein, a milk-derived protein, then the label will have to say "contains milk," in addition to listing casein among the ingredients.

The FDA estimated that these eight allergens were responsible for 90 percent of all allergic reactions to food, requiring complete avoidance of the allergy-producing substances to prevent severe or even life-threatening reactions. The clear language provisions were designed to be particularly useful to children and teenagers who could not be expected to recognize technical names of all possible derivatives of allergens that they needed to avoid. About 11 million Americans—2 percent of adults and 5 percent of infants and young children—are affected by food allergies. Some 300,000 people end up in emergency rooms each year, and 150 die as a result of extreme reactions.

Consumer advocates welcomed the new rules, but, by the summer of 2006, they complained that some manufacturers confused purchasers by using "may contain" declarations on their labels rather than the specific language preferred by the FDA and consumers. Larger food companies rarely used "may contain" statements, and smaller manufacturers, either uncertain about the regulations or fearful of product liability lawsuits, were major offenders. The ambiguous language was particularly perplexing to teenagers, unsure how seriously to take the warnings, who might either risk severe reactions or unnecessarily limit their choice of food.

—*Milton Berman, PhD*

Improper use of over-the-counter antihistamines can cause serious side effects. Overuse may result in toxicity, particularly in children, and overdoses in children can be fatal. Because first-generation antihistamines can depress the central nervous system, side effects include drowsiness, nausea, constipation, and drying of the throat or respiratory passage. Over-the-counter second-generation antihistamines are long-acting and free of the sedative effect of other antihistamines.

Other symptomatic treatments include the use of cromolyn sodium, which blocks the influx of calcium into the mast cell and thus is called a "mast cell stabilizer." It acts to block steps leading to degranulation and the release of mediators. In more severe cases, the administration of steroids (cortisone) may prove useful in limiting symptoms of allergies.

Anaphylaxis is the most severe form of immediate hypersensitivity, and unless treated promptly, it may be fatal. It is often triggered in susceptible persons by common environmental substances: bee or wasp venom, drugs such as penicillin, foods such as peanuts and seafood, or latex protein in rubber. Symptoms include labored breathing, rapid loss of blood pressure, itching, hives, and/or loss of bladder control. Sudden and massive release of mast cell or basophil mediators such as histamine, leukotrienes, or prostaglandin derivatives trigger these symptoms. Treatment consists of immediate injection of epinephrine with an epinephrine autoinjector or *EpiPen*. Epinephrine prevents constriction of the bronchial tubes and helps maintain open air passage into the lungs. Corticosteroids and antihistamines are also administered. If cardiac arrest occurs, cardiopulmonary resuscitation must be undertaken. Persons in known danger of encountering such a triggering allergen often carry with them an emergency kit containing an EpiPen and antihistamines.

Contact dermatitis is a form of DTH, developing several days after exposure to the sensitizing allergen. Rather than resulting from the presence of IgE antibody, the symptoms of contact dermatitis resulting from a series of chemicals released by sensitized T lymphocytes in the area of the skin on which the allergen (often poison ivy or poison oak) is found. Treatments generally involve the application of topical corticosteroids and soothing or drying agents. In more severe cases, systemic use of corticosteroids may be necessary.

In some persons, the relief of allergy symptoms may be achieved through desensitization. This form of immunotherapy involves the repeated subcutaneous injection of increasing doses of the allergen. In a significant number of persons, such therapy leads to a decrease in symptoms. The idea behind such therapy is that repeated injections of the allergen may lead to the production of another class of antibody, the more systemic IgG. These molecules can serve as blocking antibodies, competing with IgE in binding to the allergen. Because IgG/allergen complexes can be phagocytosed (destroyed by phagocytes) and do not bind receptors on mast cells or basophils, they should not trigger the symptoms of allergies. Unfortunately, for reasons that remain unclear, not all persons or all allergies respond to such therapy.

The type 1 immediate hypersensitivity reactions commonly run in families. This is not so surprising if one realizes that the regulation of IgE production is genetically determined. Thus, if both parents have allergies, there is little chance that their offspring will escape the problem. On the other hand, if one or both parents are allergy-free, the odds are at least even that the offspring will also be free from such reactions.

PERSPECTIVE AND PROSPECTS

Though allergies in humans have probably existed since humans first evolved from ancestral primates, it was only in the nineteenth century that an understanding of the process began to develop. Type 1 hypersensitivity reaction was first described in 1839 through experiments in which dogs were repeatedly injected with egg albumin and developed an immediate fatal shock. The term "anaphylaxis" was coined for this phenomenon in 1902 when Paul Portier and Charles Richet observed that dogs repeatedly immunized with extracts of sea anemone tentacles suffered a similar fate. Richet was awarded the 1913 Nobel Prize in Physiology or Medicine for his work on anaphylaxis.

In the 1920s, Sir Henry Dale established that at least some of the phenomena associated with immediate hypersensitivity were caused by the chemical histamine. Dale sensitized guinea pigs against various antigens. He then observed that when the muscles from the uterus were removed and exposed to the same antigen, histamine was released and the muscles underwent contraction (known as the Schultz-Dale reaction).

The existence of a component in human serum, which mediates hypersensitive reactions, was demonstrated by Otto Prausnitz, a Polish bacteriologist, and Heinz Kustner, a Polish gynecologist, in 1921. Kustner had a severe allergy to fish. Prausnitz removed a sample of serum from his colleague and injected it under his own skin. The next day, Prausnitz injected fish extract in that same region. Hives immediately appeared, indicating that the serum contained components that mediated the allergy. For some time, the Prausnitz-Kustner test, or P-K test, remained a means of testing for allergens under circumstances in which a person could be tested for sensitivity. (It is no longer in use because of safety concerns.) In this test, a serum sample from the test subject was injected under the skin of a surrogate (usually a relative) and later followed with test allergens. The presence of a wheal and flare reaction (hives) indicated sensitivity to the allergen. The serum component responsible for this sensitivity was later identified as the antibody IgE by K. and T. Ishizaka and S. G. O. Johansson in 1967. The target cells to which the IgE bound were later identified as mast cells and basophils.

The discovery of IgE allowed scientists to develop a blood test called a radioallergosorbent test (RAST) that could measure a specific IgE antibody to an allergic substance. RAST is fully as sensitive as a skin test and is a substitute in some clinical circumstances. Furthermore, discoveries of numerous mediators from mast cells and other white cells such as cytokines, chemokines, interleukins, growth factors, and interferon have helped scientists understand the pathology of allergy at the molecular level. It helps clinically to divide the allergic reaction into immediate reaction (onset within a few minutes after exposure to allergens) and delayed or late-phase reaction (onset hours after exposure to antigens and a reaction that may last for days). The definition of allergy has now expanded from the traditional, immediate allergic reaction to the inclusion of chronic inflammatory processes in the tissues. With a better understanding of how allergies develop, better treatments can be offered to patients who suffer from this disorder.

The eventual goal of the research is to understand the molecular defects that result in allergies and ultimately to find a means to eliminate the problem, rather than simply offer palliative measures. For example, it is now known that interleukin-4 (one of the mediators of T cells) raises IgE production, while interferon (another mediator of T cells) lowers IgE production. By understanding the regulation of IgE production, it may become possible to inhibit IgE production in allergic persons selectively, without affecting the desired functions of the immune response.

—*Richard Adler, PhD and Catherine Avelar, BS*

Further Information
Adelman, Daniel C., et al., editors. *Manual of Allergy and Immunology.* 4th ed., Lippincott Williams & Wilkins,

2002. Examines research developments and the clinical diagnosis and treatment of allergies and immune disorders. Topics include asthma, disorders of the eye, diseases of the lung, anaphylaxis, insect allergies, drug allergies, rheumatic diseases, transplantation immunology, and immunization.

Brostoff, Jonathan, and Linda Gamlin. *Food Allergies and Food Intolerance: The Complete Guide to Their Identification and Treatment*. Inner Traditions, 2000. Examines the role of food allergies in chronic health conditions such as migraines and persistent fatigue and gives a step-by-step process for identifying and treating food allergies.

Cutler, Ellen W. *Winning the War against Asthma and Allergies*. Delmar, 1998. This clearly written book provides practical information on all aspects of allergies-what they are, their causes, testing, diagnosis, and treatment, including nontraditional therapies. Preventive measures are covered, as are scenarios for various allergy elimination therapies.

Delves, Peter J., et al. *Roitt's Essential Immunology*. 11th ed., Blackwell, 2006. Written by a leading author in the field, the text provides a fine description of immunology. The section on hypersensitivity is clearly presented and profusely illustrated. Though too detailed in places, most of the material can be understood by individuals who have taken high school biology.

Eggleston, P. A., & Wood, R. A. "Management of Allergies to Animals." *Allergy and Asthma Proceedings*, vol. 13, no. 6, Nov. 1992, pp. 289-92.

Joneja, Janice M. V., and Leonard Bielory. *Understanding Allergy, Sensitivity, and Immunity*. Rutgers UP, 1990. The authors provide an extensive discussion of allergies and the roles played by the immune system. They describe how one can learn to cope with allergies and discuss various testing methods for the identification of allergens.

Kindt, Thomas J., Richard A. Goldsby, and Barbara A. Osborne. *Kuby Immunology*. 6th ed., W. H. Freeman, 2007. The section on hypersensitivity in this immunology textbook is well written and includes a mixture of detail and an overview of the subject. Particularly useful are discussions of the various types of hypersensitivity reactions. Some knowledge of biology is useful.

Life, Death, and the Immune System. W. H. Freeman, 1994. This comprehensive collection of articles from Scientific American provides basic information and research directions on AIDS, autoimmune disorders, and allergies as well as an excellent discussion of the immune system in general.

Ring, J., U. Krämer, T. Schäfer, and H. Behrendt. "Why Are Allergies Increasing?" *Current Opinion in Immunology*, vol. 13, no. 6, 2001, pp. 701-8. This article shows evidence, and gives possible explanations, for the increasing prevalence of allergies in Western countries.

Skoner, D. P. "Allergic Rhinitis: Definition, Epidemiology, Pathophysiology, Detection, and Diagnosis." *Journal of Allergy and Clinical Immunology*, vol. 108, no. 1, 2001, pp. S2-S8.

Walsh, William. *The Food Allergy Book*. J. Wiley, 2000. In this excellent guide to one highly prevalent form of allergy, the author presents useful background information on food allergies and a pragmatic guide to identifying and eliminating food allergens from one's diet.

Young, Stuart, Bruce Dobozin, and Margaret Miner. *Allergies*. Rev. ed., Plume, 1999. In addition to discussing the diagnosis and treatment of allergies, the authors evaluate the various remedies on the market at the time of publication. Also useful are lists of organizations to contact for @REF = Further Information.

ALLERGIST AND IMMUNOLOGIST

Category: Health-care career
Anatomy or system affected: All systems
Specialties and related fields: Immunology, internal medicine, ophthalmology, otorhinolaryngology, pharmacology, pulmonary medicine
Definition: A physician specially trained to diagnose, treat and manage allergies, asthma, and immunologic disorders.

KEY TERMS

autoimmune disease: a condition in which the immune system mistakenly attacks the body in response to normally harmless substances, causing abnormally low activity or over-activity of the immune system

food allergy: an abnormal response to a food triggered by the body's immune system

Medical College Admission Test (MCAT): a standardized examination for prospective medical students in the United States, Australia, Canada, and Caribbean Islands designed to assess problem solving, critical thinking, written analysis and knowledge of scientific concepts and principles

sinus infection: inflammation or swelling of the tissue lining the sinuses resulting in nasal congestion, drainage, facial pain/pressure, and decreased sense of smell

OVERVIEW

Sphere of work. Allergists and immunologists are medical doctors who specialize in diagnosing, treating, and studying allergies, autoimmune deficiencies, and related diseases and conditions. Allergists and immunologists conduct extensive blood tests and skin patch tests to determine the causes of patient symptoms. They diagnose food allergies, medication allergies, bronchitis, asthma, sinus infections, and autoimmune and immunodeficiency diseases. They work with patients to develop effective treatments and implement lifestyle and dietary changes to prevent complications.

Work environment. Allergists and immunologists work in medical offices, hospitals, clinics, university medical centers, and similar medical environments. These locations are immaculate, highly organized, and very busy. Allergists and immunologists, along with other staff, must adhere to strict patient records and safety protocols. Allergists work long hours, averaging about fifty hours a week. They must spend some of their time on-call, answer patient phone calls from home, and, when necessary, travel to the office or hospital after hours. Many allergists and immunologists also teach at medical schools.

Occupation interest. Allergists and immunologists treat patients from different backgrounds. Diagnosis is similar to careful detective work, as allergists and immunologists test potential causes for symptoms one clue at a time. Like other physicians, allergists and immunologists are well compensated. The market for these medical professionals continues to show strong growth. Different career options available to allergists and immunologists include private practice, specialization in a subfield, medical research, and teaching at a medical school.

A day in the life—duties and responsibilities. Allergists and immunologists meet with and examine patients, listening to their symptoms and reviewing their patient histories. They then order and conduct diagnostic tests designed to assess the causes of allergies and other symptoms. Some of these tests include skin pricks, patches, scratch tests, and delayed hypersensitivity tests. Among the allergies for which these physicians search are airborne, medicinal, food, pet, and environmental allergens affecting the nose, eyes, throat, and lungs. They may also draw blood to investigate if an immune deficiency or disorder exists.

When the nature and extent of the patient's condition have been established, allergists and immunologists formulate a course of treatment. They assess the benefits and risks that may develop during treatment and create individualized patient treatment plans. These plans consider patient preferences, clinical data, and the information provided by other doctors, nurses, and associated medical professionals. Allergists and immunologists frequently work with their patients over long periods, enabling them to develop working relationships. They must stay current on the most effective approaches to addressing these conditions by studying clinical data and reviewing the scholarly medical literature.

In addition to patient care, many immunologists and allergists research immune disorders and allergens and treatment options. Many physicians also teach at medical schools and similar institutions.

WORK ENVIRONMENT

Immediate physical environment. Allergists and immunologists work primarily in medical settings, such as hospitals and medical centers, clinics, private medical offices, and medical groups. Many also teach at medical schools. Due to needles employed in diagnosis and treatment, there is a risk of exposure to blood and other bodily fluids. In clinical settings, allergists and immunologists must follow strict safety guidelines that mandate the maintenance of a sterile environment.

Human environment. Allergists and immunologists interact with patients, families, other physicians, nurses, medical technicians and phlebotomists, medical students and interns, medical assistants, and nursing assistants. They also work with hospital administrators, pharmaceutical sales representatives, and medical device sales representatives.

Technological environment. Allergists and immunologists work with basic and specialized medical instruments, including thermometers, hypodermic needles, stethoscopes, nebulizers, spirometers, and blood pressure cuffs. They also use blood- and skin-testing kits: medical diagnosis software and medical databases aid doctors with diagnosis, treatment, and recordkeeping.

EDUCATION, TRAINING, AND ADVANCEMENT

High school/secondary. High school students interested in pursuing a career in this field should take biology, chemistry, physics, physiology, calculus, algebra, and psychology courses. Training in nutrition, first aid, and CPR are helpful as well. Additionally, social studies and communications courses are beneficial for aspiring allergists and immunologists.

Postsecondary. Allergists and immunologists must complete four years of undergraduate study in a premedical discipline. They then must pass the Medical College Admission Test (MCAT) and complete a four-year medical school program, followed by three to eight years of internships and residencies. Their residency programs must include two or more years of allergy and immunology training.

—*Michael Auerbach*

Further Information

"About Allergists/Immunologists." www.aaaai.org/About/About-Allergists-Immunologists. Accessed 2 Sept. 2021.

"About Careers in Allergy/Immunology." *American Academy of Allergy, Asthma, and Immunology*, www.aaaai.org/Professional-Education/careers-in-a-i. Accessed 2 Sept. 2021.

"Physicians and Surgeons." *Occupational Outlook Handbook*, Bureau of Labor Statistics, 11 Jun. 2018, www.bls.gov/ooh/healthcare/physicians-and-surgeons.htm. Accessed 25 Oct. 2018.

BITES AND STINGS

Category: Diseases/Disorders
Anatomy or system affected: Heart, immune system, skin
Specialties and related fields: Emergency medicine, immunology, toxicology
Definition: Injuries from animals or insects.

KEY TERMS

bites: when an animal uses its teeth to inflict an injury

stings: a small sharp-pointed organ at the end of the abdomen of some arthropods, including bees, wasps, ants, and scorpions, that can inflict a painful or dangerous wound by injecting poison.

venom: a poisonous substance secreted by animals such as snakes, spiders, and scorpions that is injected into prey or aggressors by biting or stinging.

BITES AND STINGS

Bites and stings cause four major types of damage to the victim's body: physical damage, the introduction of disease-causing organisms, the introduction of poisons (toxins, venoms), and allergic responses, including anaphylactic shock. Often, more than one form of damage is associated with a bite or sting. Alone or in combination, they can be life-threatening, but usually, the damage from a bite or sting is minor. A wide variety of organisms can bite or sting, but the most important among them are mammals, reptiles (snakes and lizards), some fish (sharks, rays, moray eels), arthropods (including insects, centipedes, spiders, mites, ticks, and scorpions), and cnidarians (jellyfish, Portuguese man-of-war, and their relatives).

BITES CAUSING PHYSICAL DAMAGE

Bites delivered by a mammal (most often a dog or cat) are likely to cause the most extensive physical damage. The specialized teeth of mammals, especially carnivores, in combination with powerful jaw muscles, can produce a serious wound. If wounding is in a vulnerable spot or is very extensive, or if the bleeding is not stopped, the physical damage can be fatal. A bite that causes physical damage is almost

> **INFORMATION ON BITES AND STINGS**
>
> **Causes**: Bite or wound from an organism
>
> **Symptoms**: Bleeding, swelling, infection, allergic response
>
> **Duration**: Temporary or acute
>
> **Treatments**: Immunization, drug therapy (antivenin, adrenaline, antihistamines)

certain to introduce bacteria, viruses, or other infectious agents. An important example is the rabies virus, but many kinds of organisms are dangerous if introduced into the bloodstream, or the bone marrow of bones broken by the bite. Most mammalian bites do not introduce toxins into the victim. Some shrews have venom in their saliva, but their small size and secretive habits minimize their threat to human health. Bites from mammals are also of minimal concern concerning dangerous allergic responses. Physical damage is also the most serious problem in shark and moray eel bites.

Prevention, by avoiding animals prone to bite, is usually readily accomplished. Treatment involves stopping the bleeding, repairing the damage, and preventing infection.

BITES INTRODUCING INFECTIOUS AGENTS

Bites that cause serious physical damage are not the only ones that can introduce infectious agents. Any bite or sting can introduce infection to the victim because it penetrates the first line of defense, the skin. The arthropods are the most important disease vectors. Malaria is caused by a parasitic protozoan (single-celled, animal-type organism) transferred from one host to another by mosquitoes. Lyme disease is caused by a bacterium and is transported between hosts by ticks. Viruses cause yellow fever, and mosquitoes transport the virus to new hosts. Insects and ticks are vectors for several other diseases, most of which are introduced to the victim by a bite (includ-

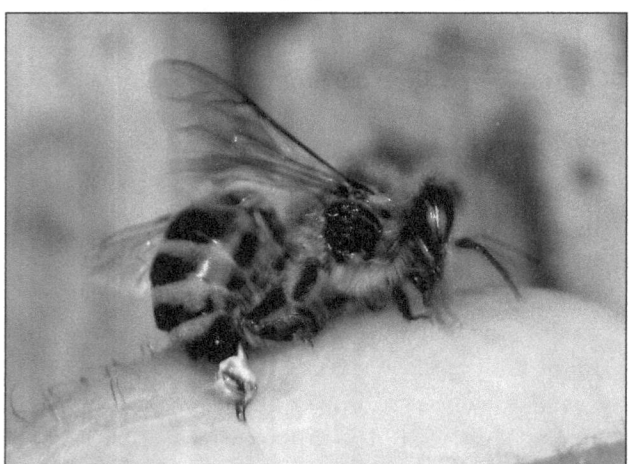

Bee sting. The stinger is torn off and left in the skin. Photo by Waugsberg, via Wikimedia Commons.

ing the stabs of blood-sucking arthropods such as mosquitoes).

Prevention of these diseases involves avoiding and/or eliminating the vectors; neither is always possible. Active immunization (stimulating the host to form antibodies against the disease-causing organism) is also used when available. Treatment involves drugs that destroy the disease organism or the use of passive immunization (the injection of preformed antibodies against the disease organism).

BITES AND STINGS INTRODUCING TOXINS

Toxins or poisons are introduced to the victim most often by arthropods (scorpion stings, spider bites), cnidarians (stings), or reptiles (bites). Some mollusks—the cone shell snails, for example—can also inject toxins into a victim. The chemicals involved include enzymes that destroy tissue, neurotoxins that interfere with appropriate nerve cell responses (blocking or stimulating nerve cell signals), and others that interfere with the normal functions of the victim's body chemistry. Rattlesnakes and their relatives, coral snakes, and the Gila monster (a large lizard) are examples of poisonous reptiles. The brown recluse and black widow spiders are dangerous examples of their group. The sea wasp (a jellyfish) and the Portuguese man-of-war are the best known but by no means the only, dangerous cnidarians in coastal waters off North America.

Prevention involves avoiding the animals that inject the toxin, which is easily accomplished much but not all, of the time. Treatment involves the injection of antivenin, a solution of antibodies that neutralize a specific toxin. Research on snake antivenin indicates that it might be possible to create a single antivenin that inactivates several snake venoms.

BITES AND STINGS CAUSING ALLERGIC REACTIONS

Any bite or sting can cause an allergic response in the victim because all introduce large foreign mole-

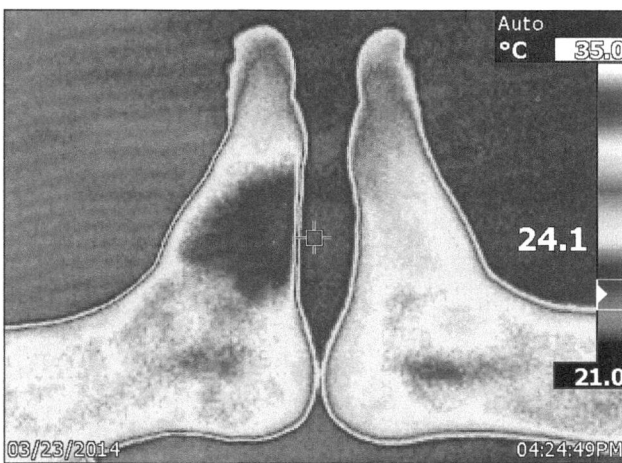

The left side of the image shows the ˉ4 °C (7 °F) temperature increase (saturated red zone) caused by a bee sting after about 28 hours. Photo by Volkan Yuksel, via Wikimedia Commons. [CC 3.0.]

cules, called "antigens." These are often proteins, and they stimulate a response in the victim's immune system. If the response is more than that needed to destroy the antigen, it is called an "allergic response," and the foreign protein is called an "allergen." The allergic response may simply be a nuisance causing minor inflammation, but it is exceptionally dangerous if it escalates into anaphylaxis. Anaphylaxis is a hyperreaction to a foreign substance in which the heart rate increases; bronchioles in the lungs constrict, making breathing difficult; and blood pressure drops. If symptoms continue, the victim may go into shock and even die. The toxins introduced by venomous arthropods, reptiles, cnidarians, and mollusks are often allergenic, even causing anaphylaxis but even nonpoisonous or minimally toxic materials such as the venom introduced in a bee or wasp sting can cause life-threatening anaphylactic shock in sensitive people. A painful sting for people not sensitized to foreign material becomes a threat to the life of a sensitized, hypersensitive person.

Prevention, by avoiding the allergen, is the preferred defense against allergic reactions. If avoidance is not possible or cannot be assured, the injection of small amounts of the substance to which an individual is hypersensitive, followed by increasingly larger doses, is sometimes effective in desensitizing the individual. Treatment of severe anaphylactic reactions involves the injection of adrenaline (epinephrine). Antihistamines, taken orally or injected, are used in less severe situations.

—*Carl W. Hoagstrom, PhD*

Further Information

Dossenbach, Hans D. *Beware! We Are Poisonous! How Animals Defend Themselves.* Blackbirch Press, 1999. Dossenbach examines some of the world's most poisonous animals and shatters some myths about creatures long perceived as dangerous. Includes a bibliography.

Foster, Steven, and Roger A. Caras. *A Field Guide to Venomous Animals and Poisonous Plants: North America, North of Mexico.* Houghton Mifflin, 1994. Containing excellent information and bright color pictures, and written for an easy understanding, this book should be in any nature enthusiast's library.

Halstead, Bruce W., and Paul S. Auerbach. *Dangerous Aquatic Animals of the World: A Color Atlas.* Darwin Press, 1992. Spectacular gallery of animals as diverse as polar bears and sea anemones. A natural history of the envenomation, or wounding apparatus, with slight detail on the range, and none on life cycles. The excellent color photos are augmented by fine drawings of the anatomy of the dangerous parts of animals.

Harvey, Alan L., editor. *Snake Toxins.* Pergamon Press, 1991. Discusses various topics, such as immunology of snake toxins, dendrotoxins, the structure and pharmacology of elapid cytotoxins, the influence of snake venom proteins on blood coagulation, and amino acid sequences and toxicities of snake venom components. Includes an index.

Krohmer, Jon R., editor. *American College of Emergency Physicians First Aid Manual.* 2nd ed., DK, 2004. A comprehensive guide that details the treatment and techniques, in-text and photographically, of a range of emergencies. Bites and stings are covered specifically.

Nagami, Pamela. *Bitten: True Medical Stories of Bites and Stings.* St. Martin's Press, 2004. Nagami describes strange and often gruesome true cases of bites and stings, resulting infections, and treatments.

Silverstein, Alvin, et al. *Bites and Stings.* Scholastic, 2002. A young adult book that covers information about bites and stings from insects, pets, wild animals, sea creatures, and plants. Body reactions, transmittable diseases, treatment, and protection are also covered.

Spiders and Other Arachnids, spiders.ucr.edu. The site provides links to information about the spider, scorpion, bee, wasp, and ant species worldwide whose bites cause morbidity and mortality.

Tu, Anthony T., editor. *Reptile Venoms and Toxins.* Marcel Dekker, 1991. In twenty-four contributed chapters, thirty-seven international specialists describe the latest developments in research on snake venom-including different types of venoms and toxins, actions, antidotes, and applications-and summarize what is known to date on the Gila monster and frog toxins.

Wilcox, Christie. *Venomous: How Earth's Deadliest Creatures Mastered Biochemistry.* Scientific American/Farrar, Straus and Giroux, 2016. A molecular biologist turned science writer takes the reader on an engrossing journey into the world of poisonous animals and the scientists who study them.

COUGHING

Category: Diseases/Disorders
Anatomy or system affected: Chest, immune system, lungs, respiratory system
Specialties and related fields: Family medicine, internal medicine, pulmonary medicine
Definition: A physiological act in which air is forcibly expelled from the lungs.

KEY TERMS

bronchial tubes: delicate hoses connecting the throat to the lungs

diaphragm: a muscular partition separating the thorax from the abdomen; plays a major role in breathing as its contraction increases the volume of the thorax and so inflates the lungs

hemoptysis: the expectoration of blood, alone or mixed with mucus, from the lower respiratory tract

glottis: the part of the larynx consisting of the vocal cords and the opening between them; affects voice modulation through expansion or contraction

larynx: the hollow muscular organ forming an air passage to the lungs and holding the vocal cords

respiratory tract: the passage formed by the mouth, nose, throat, and lungs, through which air passes during breathing

sputum: a mixture of saliva and mucus coughed up from the respiratory tract, typically because of infection

trachea: the airway that leads from the larynx to the bronchi; also called the windpipe

CAUSES AND SYMPTOMS

The energy consumed during the breathing process stretches the chest cavity and allows air to flow into the lungs. Breathing amounts to about 1 percent of the basic energy requirements of the body. Still, it increases considerably during periods of exercise or respiratory system illness.

When the respiratory tract is invaded by irritants (such as smoke, perfume, and pollen) or there is an excessive accumulation of secretions in the lungs, coughing occurs. It arises via a reflex mechanism that stimulates the nerves that supply the larynx, trachea (windpipe), and bronchial tubes. The pressure within the chest cavity is increased by the action of chest muscles and the diaphragm. The glottis, the opening of the windpipe at the back of the mouth, remains closed, allowing the pressure to rise. The

> ### INFORMATION ON COUGHING
> **Causes**: Various diseases, allergens, lung infection, environmental factors
> **Symptoms**: Breathlessness, chest and lung pain
> **Duration**: Ranges from short term to chronic
> **Treatments**: Antibiotics, anti-inflammatory drugs

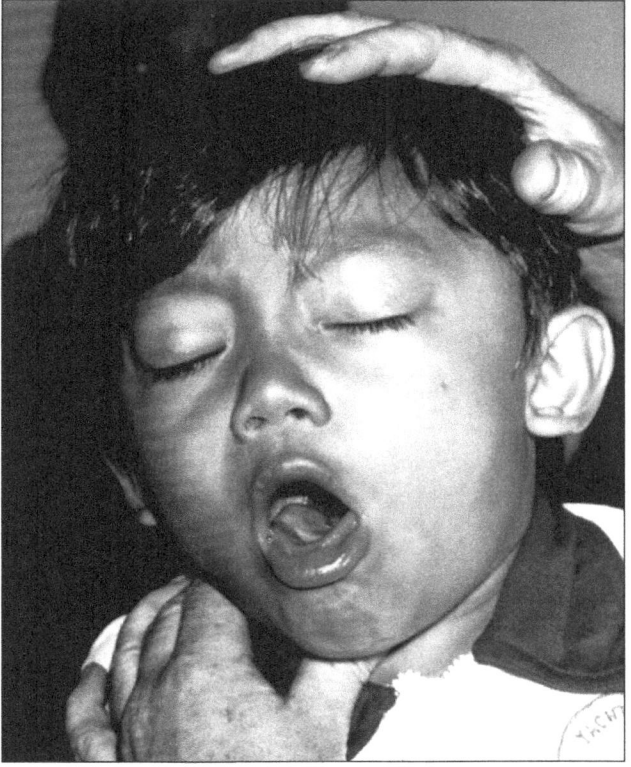

A young boy coughing. Photo via Wikimedia Commons. [Public domain.]

glottis opens again within a few seconds, and a rapid, noisy release of air is allowed through the bronchial tubes and the windpipe. Any foreign substance is expelled through the mouth.

TREATMENT AND THERAPY

Coughing is an important symptom of diseases that affect any part of the respiratory system, such as the nasal cavities, the pharynx (throat), the larynx, the trachea, the bronchi, and the lung tissue. By coughing, foreign matter called "sputum," which is chiefly composed of mucus, that accumulated in the respiratory system is expectorated. Sputum formation during coughing is important evidence of a disease, such as bronchitis. In this case, the lining of the bronchi enlarges dramatically, and sputum production may increase to 60 milliliters per day. An irritative cough without sputum may be due to the

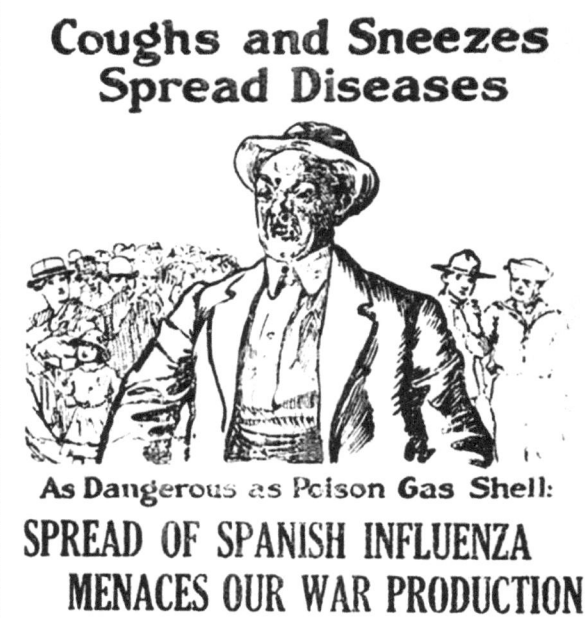

U.S. Public Health ad on dangers of Spanish Flu epidemic during World War I. Photo via Wikimedia Commons. [Public domain.]

extension of the disease to the bronchial tube and eventually to nearby organs. The use of antibiotics and anti-inflammatory agents to reduce discomfort is part of the standard treatment.

The presence of blood in the sputum (called "hemoptysis") is important. It should alert patients or their caregivers to call a doctor. This symptom often arises from an existing infection, inflammation, or tumor. It is also a sign of tuberculosis. In this case, extensive and reliable tests will identify the real cause of the bleeding.

Polluted air increases the possibility of chronic bronchitis. Common air pollutants include vehicle exhaust, chemical fumes, smoke, smog, molds, and pollen. They are all responsible for a decrease in arterial oxygen and increased carbon dioxide tension in the lungs. The use of air-conditioning, air filters, and inhalers, and an increased oxygen environment can provide relief for people with respiratory problems.

—*Soraya Ghayourmanesh, PhD*

Further Information

Adelman, Daniel C., et al., editors. *Manual of Allergy and Immunology.* 5th ed., Lippincott Williams & Wilkins, 2012.

Braga, Pier Carlo, and Luigi Allegra, editors. *Cough.* Raven Press, 1989.

Chung, Kian Fan, John G. Widdicombe, and Homer A. Boushey, editors. *Cough: Causes, Mechanisms, and Therapy.* Blackwell, 2008.

"Cough." *Mayo Clinic,* 24 May 2013.

Glenn, Jim. *Colds and Coughs.* Springhouse, 1986.

"How Is Cough Treated?" *National Heart, Lung, and Blood Institute,* 1 Oct. 2010.

Kimball, Chad T. *Colds, Flu, and Other Common Ailments Sourcebook.* Omnigraphics, 2001.

Korpás, Juraj, and Z. Tomori. *Cough and Other Respiratory Reflexes.* S. Karger, 1979.

"What Is Cough?" *National Heart, Lung, and Blood Institute,* 1 Oct. 2010.

Woolf, Alan D., et al., editors. *The Children's Hospital Guide to Your Child's Health and Development.* Perseus, 2002.

DERMATITIS

Category: Diseases/Disorders
Also known as: Eczema
Anatomy or system affected: Hair, skin
Specialties and related fields: Dermatology
Definition: A wide range of skin disorders, some resulting from allergy, some caused by contact with a skin irritant, and some attributable to other causes.

KEY TERMS

allergen: a substance that excites an immunologic response; also called an "antigen"

crusting: the appearance of slightly elevated skin lesions made up of dried serum, blood, or pus; they can be brown, red, black, tan, or yellowish

immunoglobulin E (IgE): ordinarily, a relatively rare antibody; in patients with atopic dermatitis, levels can be significantly higher than in the general population

lesion: any pathologic change in tissue
scaling: a buildup of hard, horny skin cells
secondary infection: a bacterial, viral, or other infection that results from or follows another disease
wheal: a small swelling in the skin

CAUSES AND SYMPTOMS

"Dermatitis" does not refer to a single skin disease but a variety of skin-based disorders. Dermatitis and eczema are often used interchangeably. The two most common dermatitides are contact dermatitis and atopic (allergic) dermatitis. People appear to inherit a preference for these dermatitides. The individual's skin reacts immediately to contact with a substance or develops sensitivity to it.

Atopic dermatitis often occurs in individuals with a family history of allergies, such as hay fever or asthma. Between 50 and 70 percent of children with severe atopic dermatitis develop asthma. This rate is more than five times higher than for the general population. These people often have elevated serum levels of a particular antibody, immunoglobulin E (IgE), which may be associated with their skin's tendency to break out. However, a specific antigen-antibody reaction has not been demonstrated.

There are many distinct characteristics of atopic dermatitis, some of which depend on the patient's age. The disease usually starts early in childhood. It is often first discovered in infants in the first months of life when redness and weeping crusted lesions appear primarily on the face. However, the scalp, arms, and legs may also be affected. There is intense itching. Papules (pimples), vesicles (small, blisterlike lesions filled with fluid), edema (swelling), serous exudation (discharge of liquid), and scaly crusts may appear. At one year of age, oval, scaly lesions appear on the arms, legs, face, and torso. Older children and adults usually have lesions in the crook of the elbow and the back of the knees, and the face and neck may be involved. The course of the disease is variable. It usually subsides by the third or fourth year of life. Still, periodic outbreaks may occur throughout childhood, adolescence, and adulthood. Cases persisting past the patient's middle twenties, or beginning then, are the most difficult to treat.

Dryness and itching are always present in atopic dermatitis. People with atopic dermatitis seem to lose skin moisture more readily than ordinary people: Rather than soft, pliable skin, they develop dry, rough, sensitive skin that is particularly prone to chapping and splitting. The skin becomes itchy, and the individual's tendency to scratch significantly aggravates the condition in what is called the "itch-scratch-itch" cycle or the "scratch-rash-itch" cycle: the individual scratches to relieve the itching, which causes a rash, which in turn causes increased itching, which invites increased scratching and increased irritation. After years of itching and scratching, the skin of older children and adults with atopic dermatitis develops red, lichenified (rough, thickened) patches in the crook of the arm and behind the knees as well as on the eyelids, neck, and wrists.

Constant chafing of the affected area invites bacterial infection and lymphadenitis (inflammation of lymph nodes). Furthermore, patients with atopic dermatitis seem to have altered immune systems. They appear to be more susceptible than others to skin infections, warts, and contagious skin diseases. *Staphylococcus aureus* and certain streptococci are common infecting bacteria in these patients. Pyoderma refers to any skin disease that causes pus-filled lesions, and bacterial infections can cause pyoderma in atopic dermatitis. This condition features redness, oozing, scaling, crusting, and the formation of small pustules (pus-filled pimples).

Patients with atopic dermatitis are also susceptible to herpes simplex and vaccinia viruses. Exposure to either can cause a severe skin disease called "Kaposi's varicelliform eruption." Preparation of the smallpox vaccine utilizes the vaccinia virus, the agent that causes cowpox. Therefore, patients with atopic dermatitis must not receive the smallpox vac-

> **INFORMATION ON DERMATITIS**
>
> **Causes**: Allergies, infection, contact irritation, altered immune system
>
> **Symptoms**: Dry and itchy skin, rashes, inflammation, pain
>
> **Duration**: Short term to chronic
>
> **Treatments**: Topical corticosteroids or antihistamines, antibiotics, dietary changes, and specialized lotions, soaps, or shampoos

cination. Furthermore, they must be isolated from patients with active herpes simplex and those recently vaccinated against smallpox.

Patients with atopic dermatitis may also develop contact dermatitis, which can significantly exacerbate their condition. They are also sensitive to a wide range of allergens, which can bring on outbreaks and low humidity (such as in centrally heated houses in winter), contributing to dry skin. They may not be able to tolerate woolen clothing.

A condition called "keratosis pilaris" often develops in the presence of atopic dermatitis. Young infants do not suffer from keratosis, but it does appear in childhood. Hair follicles on the torso, buttocks, arms, and legs become plugged with horny matter and protrude above the skin, giving the appearance of goosebumps or "chicken skin." The palms of patients with atopic dermatitis have significantly more fine lines than those of ordinary people. In many patients, there is a tiny "pleat" under the eyes. They are often prone to cold hands and may have pallor, seen as blanching of the skin around the nose, mouth, and ears.

Rubbing normal skin with a pointed object almost immediately causes a red line, followed by a red flare, and finally, a wheal or slight elevation of the skin along the line. However, there is an entirely different reaction in patients with atopic dermatitis: The red line appears, but it instantly becomes white. The flare and the wheal do not appear.

About 4 to 12 percent of patients with atopic dermatitis develop cataracts at an early age (some estimates range as high as nearly 40 percent). Usually, cataracts do not appear until the fifties and sixties; those with atopic dermatitis may develop them in their twenties. These cataracts typically affect both eyes simultaneously and grow quickly.

Psychologically, children with atopic dermatitis often show distinct personality characteristics. They are usually bright, aggressive, energetic, and prone to fits of anger. Children with severe, unmanageable cases of atopic dermatitis may become selfish and domineering, and some develop significant personality disorders.

What causes the itching and dry skin that are the fundamental signs of atopic dermatitis and the root of many of its complications remains unknown. It is by definition an allergic disorder, but the allergens that are specifically involved and how they produce the signs of atopic dermatitis are unknown. Theories suggest various origins. One of the most exciting theories consists of the antibody IgE. Theoretically, the union of IgE with an antigen causes specific cells called "mast cells" to release pharmacologic mediators, such as histamine, bradykinin, and slow-reacting substance (SRSA, also known as "leukotrienes"), that cause itching and thus begin the cycle of scratching and irritation characteristic of atopic dermatitis. The fact that patients with atopic dermatitis have higher than normal levels of IgE and that there is a relationship between IgE levels and the severity of atopic dermatitis seems to lend support to this theory.

Contact dermatitis resembles atopic dermatitis at certain stages, but the dry skin of atopic dermatitis may not appear. Contact dermatitis is usually characterized by a rash with small bumps, itchiness, blisters, and general swelling. Exposure of the skin to substances to which it is allergic or sensitive causes contact dermatitis. If contact with a caustic substance causes contact dermatitis, it is called "irritant contact dermatitis." The causative agents are primary irritants that cause inflammation at first contact. Some obvious irritants are acids, alkalis, and other harsh chemicals or substances. An example is fiberglass dermatitis, in which fine glass particles from fiberglass fabrics or insulation enter the skin and cause redness and inflammation.

If allergic sensitivity to a substance causes dermatitis, it is called "allergic contact dermatitis." Agents that may cause allergic contact dermatitis include soaps, acetone, skin creams, cosmetics, poison ivy, and poison sumac. In this case, it may take hours, days, weeks, or years for the patient to develop sensitivity to the point where exposure to these substances causes allergic contact dermatitis.

Allergic contact dermatitis comprises the most extensive variety of contact dermatitides, many of them named for the allergens that cause them. Hence, there is pollen dermatitis; plant and flower dermatitides, such as poison ivy or poison oak; clothing dermatitis; shoe, and even sandal strap, dermatitis; metal and metal salt dermatitis; cosmetic dermatitis; and adhesive tape dermatitis, among others. They all have one thing in common: exposure of the skin to an allergen from any source. It becomes so sensitive to it that further exposure causes a rash, itching, and blistering.

The development of sensitivity to an allergen is an immunological response to exposure to that substance. With many allergens, the first contact elicits no immediate immunological reaction. Sensitivity develops after allergen presentation to those T lymphocytes that mediate the immune response.

Because it often takes a long time to develop sensitivity, patients are surprised to discover they have become allergic to substances they have used for years. For example, a patient who has been applying a topical medication to treat a skin condition may one day find that the drug causes an outbreak of dermatitis. Ironically, some medicines commonly used to treat skin conditions are among the major allergens that cause allergic contact dermatitis. These include antibiotics, antihistamines, topical anesthetics, antiseptics, and the inactive ingredients used in formulating the medications, such as stabilizers.

Other substances to which the patient may develop sensitivity include the chemicals used in making fabric for clothing, tanning chemicals used in making leather, dyes, and ingredients in cosmetics. Many patients develop sensitivity to allergens found in the workplace. The list of potential allergens in the industrial setting is virtually endless. It includes solvents, petroleum products, chemicals commonly used in manufacturing processes, and coal tar derivatives.

In some cases, the allergen requires sunlight or other forms of light to precipitate an outbreak of contact dermatitis. This sun-induced skin condition is called "photoallergic contact dermatitis." Another light reaction termed "phototoxic contact dermatitis" can be caused by exposure to sunlight after exposure to perfumes, coal tar, certain medications, and various chemicals. Such agents may cause it as aftershave lotions, sunscreens, topical sulfonamides, and other preparations applied to the skin.

A different form of dermatitis involves the sebaceous glands, which secrete sebum, a fatty substance that lubricates the skin and helps retain moisture. Sebaceous dermatitis usually occurs in areas of the body with high concentrations of sebaceous glands, such as the scalp or face, behind the ears, the chest, and in areas where skin rubs against skin, like the buttocks and the groin. It is seen most often in infants and adolescents, although it may persist into adulthood or start at that time.

In infants, sebaceous dermatitis can begin within the first month of life and appears as a thick, yellow, crusted lesion on the scalp called "cradle cap." There can be yellow scaling behind the ears and red pimples on the face. Diaper rash may be persistent in these infants. In older children, the lesion may appear as thick, yellow plaques in the scalp. When sebaceous dermatitis begins in adulthood, it starts slowly, and usually, its only manifestation is scaling on the scalp (dandruff). In severe cases, yellowish-red scaling pimples develop along the hairline and on the face and chest. Its cause is unknown, but a yeast commonly found in the hair follicles, *Pityrosporum ovale*, may be involved.

There are many other kinds of dermatitis. Diaper dermatitis, or diaper rash, is a complex skin disorder that involves irritation of the skin by urine and feces, irritation by constant rubbing, and secondary infection by *Candida albicans*. Nummular dermatitis consists of crusting, scaly, disc-shaped papules, and vesicles filled with fluid, often pus. Pityriasis alba is a common dermatitis with pale, scaly patches. In lichen simplex chronicus, there is intense itching, with lesions caused and perpetuated by scratching and rubbing. Stasis dermatitis occurs at the ankles; brown discoloration, swelling, scaling, and varicose veins are common. Extremely high IgE levels characterize Hyperimmunoglobulin E (Hyper IgE) syndrome, ten to one hundred times higher than expected, and a family history of allergy; the patient has frequent skin infections, suppurative (pus-forming) lymphadenitis, pustules, plaques, and abscesses. Pompholyx occurs on the hands and soles of the feet; there is excessive sweating, with eruptions of deep vesicles accompanied by burning or itching.

Friction can also cause dermatitis. In intertrigo, the friction of skin rubbing against the skin causes inflammation that can become infected. In frictional lichenoid dermatitis or sandbox dermatitis, the abrasive action of sand or other gritty material on the skin causes the characteristic lesions. Winter eczema seems to be caused by the skin-drying effects of low humidity, harsh soaps, and overfrequent bathing; dry skin and itching are common. Acrodermatitis diseases usually children and may be limited to the hands and feet. However, acrodermatitis enteropathica may erupt in other body parts, such as around the mouth and on the buttocks. In fixed-drug eruption, lesions appear in direct response to the administration of a drug; the lesions are generally in the same parts of the body, but they may spread. Swimmer's itch is a parasitic infection from an organism that lives in freshwater lakes and ponds. At the same time, sea bather's eruption seems to be caused by a similar saltwater organism.

TREATMENT AND THERAPY

Many dermatitides resemble one another, and a physician must precisely identify the patient's complaints to treat them effectively. The physician confirms the identity of the condition through a process known as differential diagnosis. This method allows them to rule out all similar conditions, pinpoint the exact nature of the patient's problem, and develop a therapeutic regimen to treat it.

In treating atopic dermatitis, one of the first goals is to relieve dryness and itching. Wet compresses can bring relief to patients with atopic dermatitis. Skin hydration with a daily bath followed by emollient lotions improves the signs and symptoms of atopic dermatitis. Emollients reduce the need for topical anti-inflammatory medications. Excessive bathing, however, dries the skin. Scratching can break the skin and invite infection and is discouraged. The patient should avoid any known offending agents and not apply any medication to the skin without their doctor's knowledge.

Topical corticosteroids, the first-line treatment when nonpharmacological therapies fail, help resolve acute flare-ups. However, topical corticosteroid use is only for short-term treatment because prolonged use can produce undesirable side effects. High-potency corticosteroids should be used on the trunk and appendages, not on the face, groin, or armpits. Low-potency corticosteroids, however, are safe for use in these places, but only once or twice weekly. Long-term topical corticosteroid use causes thinning of the skin, bruising, stretch marks, and "spider veins." If applied to the eyelids, they cause cataracts and glaucoma. If used over large areas of the body, particularly in children, corticosteroids can suppress adrenal gland function.

Alternative medications for atopic dermatitis include topical tacrolimus (Protopic and generics) and pimecrolimus (Elidel and generics). These Food and Drug Administration (FDA)-approved medications inhibit the cell signaling protein calcineurin. Calcineurin inhibitors work as well as corticosteroids, and switching someone to a calcineurin inhibitor decreases their use of corticosteroids. Calcineurin inhibitors also can be used on the face, groin, and armpits. The adverse effects of calcineurin inhibitors include mild itching, burning, stinging, and redness. However, they do not cause thinning of the skin. Both drugs seem to increase susceptibility to viral skin infections such as herpes simplex and varicella-zoster.

Another topical agent for atopic dermatitis is crisaborole (Eucrisa). This drug inhibits an enzyme called "phosphodiesterase type-4," which increases cyclic adenosine monophosphate (cAMP) levels in skin cells. Increased cAMP staunches inflammatory processes in the skin. Stinging and burning at the application are the main adverse effects. Crisaborole is safe in infants.

If drugs do not provide satisfactory relief, then ultraviolet phototherapy may prove effective. Narrowband ultraviolet type B (UVB) phototherapy is the safest and most frequently recommended. Phototherapy is usually administered two to three times per week but is discontinued if the patient shows no improvement within four to eight weeks. Narrowband UVB phototherapy is safe during pregnancy. Though safe while breastfeeding, women should avoid breastfeeding for at least twenty-four hours after treatment.

If topical treatments fail to provide adequate treatment, then systemic therapies often are effective. Oral antihistamines, such as loratadine, desloratadine, cetirizine, levocetirizine, and fexofenadine relieve itching and help the patient sleep. There is no evidence that antihistamines effectively treat atopic dermatitis. Short courses of oral corticosteroids, including prednisone, methylprednisolone, and dexamethasone, provide relief. However, symptoms often rebound soon after stopping the drugs.

Immunosuppressants including azathioprine, methotrexate, cyclosporine, and mycophenolate mofetil effectively ameliorate atopic dermatitis symptoms. However, these drugs have significant side effects and are not appropriate for long-term use. A newer medication called "dupilumab" (Dupixent) shows excellent activity against atopic dermatitis. Dupilumab is a monoclonal antibody that binds to the alpha subunit used by the receptors of two cytokines, IL-4 and IL-13. By inhibiting these receptors, dupilumab inhibits signaling by these inflammatory cytokines. This drug is injected subcutaneously, is very well tolerated, and is safe for pregnant women. Unfortunately, it is costly: one prefilled syringe costs $1423.

Diet may play a role in atopic dermatitis in infants; some pediatric dermatologists and other physicians recommend eliminating milk, eggs, tomatoes, citrus fruits, wheat products, chocolate, spices, fish, and nuts from the diets of these patients. Other recommendations include dressing the child in soft cotton clothing and avoiding pets or fuzzy toys that might be allergenic. For secondary infections that arise from atopic dermatitis, the physician prescribes appropriate antibiotic therapy. Probiotic supplements are popular among dermatitis patients, but clinical trials have not established any efficacy for them.

In primary irritant contact dermatitis, the offending agent is eliminated or avoided. In allergic contact dermatitis, one of the main goals is to discover the offending agent so that the patient can avoid contact with it. Sometimes a patient interview reveals this, and it becomes necessary to conduct a series of patch tests. In this procedure, known allergens are applied to the patient's skin to find those that irritate it. Avoidance of the offending agent can cause the patient some difficulty if the agent happens to be something that is found everywhere. An example is the metal nickel in coins, jewelry, and hundreds of other objects. Patients who insist on wearing nickel jewelry are advised to periodically paint it with clear nail polish to avoid contact of the metal with the skin. Similarly, many other allergens are in everyday use. Patients are advised to read cosmetics labels and food and medical ingredients lists to avoid contact with agents to which they are sensitive.

Because there is such a wide range of allergic contact dermatitides, treatments vary considerably. Topical and oral steroids are used, as well as antihistamines. Sometimes the physician finds it necessary to drain large blisters and apply drying agents to weeping lesions. Sometimes the condition calls for wet compresses to relieve itching and soothe the patient. Specialized lotions, soaps, and shampoos treat dryness and, as in sebaceous dermatitis, remove scales and ease oiliness.

Allergen immunotherapy, also known as desensitization or hyposensitization, is a clinical treatment for allergies, including asthma or other environmental allergies. Allergen immunotherapy involves exposing patients to minuscule amounts of the allergen and then gradually increasing the dose over time. The goal is to increase the tolerance of the immune system to the allergen. Patients receive allergens orally, subcutaneously, sublingually, or transdermally. Because allergic individuals respond to allergens by synthesizing IgE, constant exposure to slightly increased amounts of allergens reduces the tendency to induce IgE synthesis. Constant allergen exposure causes more T-regulatory cells that secrete two cytokines, interleukin-10 (IL-10) and transforming growth factor-beta (TGF-ß). These two cytokines turn the immune response away from IgE production. In some clinical trials, allergy immunotherapy significantly reduces atopic dermatitis symptoms, but other trials were unsuccessful. Therefore, the efficacy of this technique for atopic dermatitis remains currently undetermined.

Other treatments depend on the type of dermatitis from which the patient suffers. Patients with photoallergic or phototoxic dermatitis are advised to avoid light. Acrodermatitis enteropathica results from a zinc deficiency; in addition to palliative therapy to relieve the symptoms, these patients take zinc sulfate, which results in the complete remission of the disease. As with atopic dermatitis, bacterial infections resulting from a flare-up of allergic contact dermatitis are treated with appropriate antibiotic therapy.

PERSPECTIVE AND PROSPECTS
The skin is the largest organ of the human body. It is subject to an extraordinary range and number of diseases, with atopic dermatitis and contact dermatitis among the most common. They may afflict patients of all ages, but they are particularly prevalent in children. Many of the dermatitides start in the first weeks of life and continue through childhood. In many cases, the disease resolves by the time the child reaches adolescence. Still, in some, it continues into adulthood.

Although disorders of the skin are readily apparent, understanding of them has been imperfect throughout history. For example, physicians did not understand the allergic nature of many dermatitides until the twentieth century. In addition, because their symptoms are similar to one another and diseases not correctly classified as dermatitides, there has been much confusion in identifying them. For example, many of the biblical lepers were suffering only from a form of dermatitis. With prolonged exposure, however, they probably contracted leprosy in time.

The dermatitides are often highly complex diseases involving genetic, allergic, metabolic, and immune, and infective factors, among many others. They are not usually life-threatening, but they take an enormous toll in pain, discomfort, and disfigurement, with an equal toll in psychological distress that patients can suffer.

Future medications in the testing stages include the Janus kinase inhibitors tofacitinib (Xeljanz, Xeljanz XR), baricitinib (Olumiant), upadacitinib (Rinvoq), and abrocitinib (an investigational drug). Although no Janus kinase inhibitor is FDA-approved for atopic dermatitis, clinical trials have established that these drugs significantly relieve symptoms in atopic dermatitis. Several biologics under investigation for atopic dermatitis include:
- the IL-12/-23 antagonist ustekinumab
- the investigational monoclonal antibody and IL-13 antagonist, lebrikizumab
- the investigational anti-IL-31 receptor monoclonal antibody nemolizumab

Understanding of these disorders improves constantly, and with knowledge comes new methods of treating them. Nevertheless, progress will probably be limited. Allergy immunotherapy effectively desensitizes a patient's immune system. Patients can tolerate those allergens that previously caused their eruptions. However, it is unlikely that there will ever be vaccines to immunize against this group of diseases, nor can many of them be cured.

—*C. Richard Falcon and Michael A. Buratovich, PhD*

Further Information

Adelman, Daniel C., et al., editors. *Manual of Allergy and Immunology*. 4th ed., Lippincott Williams & Wilkins, 2002.

"Atopic Dermatitis." *MedlinePlus*, 5 Aug. 2021, medlineplus.gov/ency/article/000853.htm. Accessed 24 Aug 2021.

Bair, Brooke, et al. "Cataracts in Atopic Dermatitis: A Case Presentation and Review of the Literature." *Archives of Dermatology*, vol. 147, no. 5, 2011, pp. 585-88.

Chan, Lawrence S., and Vivian Y. Shi. *Atopic Dermatitis: Inside Out or Outside In?* Elsevier, 2022.

"Contact Dermatitis." *MedlinePlus*, 5 Aug. 2021, medlineplus.gov/ency/article/000869.htm. Accessed 24 Aug. 2021.

"Eczema Types: Atopic Dermatitis Overview." www.aad.org/public/diseases/eczema/types/atopic-dermatitis. Accessed 24 Aug. 2021.

Kalb, Robert E., and Jeffery M. Weinberg. *Atopic Dermatitis: New Perspectives on Managing a Chronic Inflammatory Disease*. ?Integritas Communications, 2018.

Lumann, Paula, "What Is Contact Dermatitis?" 14 Dec. 2020, www.aad.org/public/diseases/eczema/types/contact-dermatitis/causes. Accessed 24 Aug. 2021.

Mancini, Anthony J., and Daniel P. Krowchuk, editors. *Pediatric Dermatology: A Quick Reference*. 4th ed., American Academy of Pediatrics, 2020.

Middlemiss, Prisca. *What's That Rash? How to Identify and Treat Childhood Rashes*. Hamlyn, 2002.

Parker, James N., and Philip M. Parker, editors. *The Official Patient's Sourcebook on Atopic Dermatitis*. Icon Health, 2002.

Rietschel, Robert L., and Joseph F. Fowler, editors. *Fisher's Contact Dermatitis*. 6th ed., Marcel Decker, 2008.

EAR INFECTIONS AND DISORDERS

Category: Diseases/Disorders
Anatomy or system affected: Ears
Specialties and related fields: Audiology, neurology, otorhinolaryngology
Definition: Infections or disorders of the outer, middle, or inner ear, which may result in hearing impairment or loss.

KEY TERMS

conductive loss: a hearing loss caused by an outer-ear or middle-ear problem that results in reduced transmission of sound

frequency: the number of vibrations per second of a source of sound, measured in hertz; correlates with perceived pitch

intensity of sound: the physical phenomenon that correlates approximately with perceived loudness; measured in decibels
otitis: any inflammation of the outer or middle ear
sensorineural loss: a hearing loss caused by a problem in the inner ear; this impairment is caused by a hair cell or nerve problem and is usually not amenable to surgical correction

CAUSES AND SYMPTOMS

The hearing mechanism, one of the most intricate and delicate structures of the human body, consists of three sections: the outer ear, the middle ear, and the inner ear. The outer ear converts sound waves into the mechanical motion of the eardrum (tympanic membrane), and the middle ear transmits this mechanical motion to the inner ear, where it is transformed into nerve impulses sent to the brain.

The outer ear consists of the visible portion, the ear canal, and the eardrum. The middle ear is a small chamber containing three tiny bones—the auditory ossicles, termed "malleus" (hammer), "incus" (anvil), and "stapes" (stirrup)—which transmit the vibrations of the eardrum (attached to the hammer) into the inner ear. The chamber is connected to the back of the throat by the Eustachian tube, which allows equalization with the external air pressure. The inner ear, or cochlea, is a fluid-filled cavity containing the complex structure necessary to convert the mechanical vibrations of the cochlear fluid into nerve pulses. The cochlea, shaped something like a snail's shell, is divided lengthwise by a slightly flexible partition into upper and lower chambers. The upper chamber begins at the oval window, to which the stirrup is attached. When the oval window is pushed or pulled by the stirrup, vibrations of the eardrum are transformed into cochlear fluid vibrations.

The lower surface of the cochlear partition, the basilar membrane, is set into vibration by the pressure difference between the fluids of the upper and lower ducts. Lying on the basilar membrane is the organ of Corti, containing tens of thousands of hair cells attached to the nerve transmission lines leading to the brain. When the basilar membrane vibrates, the cilia of these cells are bent, stimulating them to produce electrochemical impulses. These impulses travel along the auditory nerve to the brain, where they are interpreted as sound.

Although well protected against normal environmental exposure, the ear, because of its delicate nature, is subject

Depiction of the middle ear. Image by Bruce Blaus, via Wikimedia Commons. [CC 3.0.]

to various infections and disorders. These disorders, which usually lead to some hearing loss, can occur in any of the three parts of the ear.

The ear canal can be blocked by a buildup of waxy secretions or by infection. Although earwax serves the useful purpose of trapping foreign particles that might otherwise be deposited on the eardrum, if the canal becomes clogged with an excess of wax, less sound will reach the eardrum, and hearing will be impaired.

Swimmer's ear, or otitis externa, is an inflammation caused by contaminated water that has not been completely drained from the ear canal. A moist condition in a region with little light favors fungal growth. Symptoms of swimmer's ear include an itchy and tender ear canal and a small amount of foul-smelling drainage. If the canal is allowed to become clogged by the concomitant swelling, hearing will be noticeably impaired.

A perforated eardrum may result from a sharp blow to the side of the head, an infection, the insertion of objects into the ear, or a sudden change in air pressure (such as a nearby explosion). Small perforations are usually self-healing, but larger tears require medical treatment.

Inflammation of the middle ear, acute otitis media, is one of the most common ear infections, especially among children. Infection usually spreads from the throat to the middle ear through the Eustachian tube. Children are particularly susceptible to this problem because their short Eustachian tubes afford bacteria in the throat easy access to the middle ear. When the middle ear becomes infected, pus begins to accumulate, forcing the eardrum outward. This pressure stretches the auditory ossicles to their limit and tenses the ligaments so that vibration conduction is severely impaired. Untreated, this condition may eventually rupture the eardrum or permanently damage the ossicular chain. Furthermore, the pus from the infection may invade nearby structures, including the facial nerve, the mastoid bones, the inner ear, or even the brain. The most common symptom of otitis is a sudden severe pain and an impairment of hearing resulting from the reduced mobility of the eardrum and the ossicles.

Secretory otitis media is caused by occlusion of the Eustachian tube as a result of conditions such as a head cold, diseased tonsils and adenoids, sinusitis, improper blowing of the nose, or riding in unpressurized airplanes. People with allergic nasal

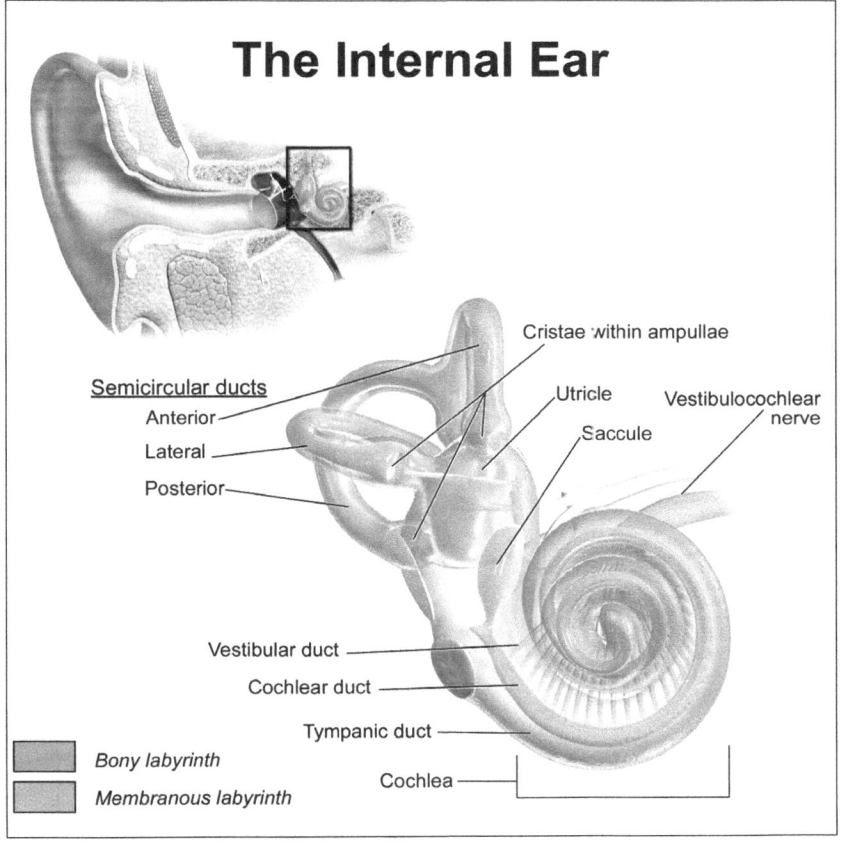

The internal ear. Image by Bruce Blaus, via Wikimedia Commons. [CC 3.0.]

blockage are particularly prone to this condition. The blocked Eustachian tube causes the middle-ear cavity to fill with a pale yellow, noninfected discharge which exerts pressure on the eardrum, causing pain and impairment of hearing. Eventually, the middle-ear cavity is completely filled with fluid instead of air, impeding the movement of the ossicles and causing hearing impairment.

A mild, temporary hearing impairment resulting from airplane flights is termed "aero-otitis media." This disorder results when a head cold or allergic reaction does not permit the Eustachian tube to equalize the air pressure in the middle ear with atmospheric pressure when a rapid change in altitude occurs. As the pressure outside the eardrum becomes greater than the pressure within, the membrane is forced inward, while the opening of the tube into the upper part of the throat is closed by the increased pressure. Symptoms are a severe sense of pressure in the ear, pain, and hearing impairment. Although the pressure difference may cause the eardrum to rupture, more often the pain continues until the middle ear fills with fluid or the tube opens to equalize pressure.

Chronic otitis media may result from inadequate drainage of pus during the acute form of this disease or from a permanent eardrum perforation that allows dust, water, and bacteria easy access to the middle-ear cavity. The main symptoms of this disease are fluids discharging from the outer ear and hearing loss. Perforations of the eardrum result in hearing loss because of the reduced vibrating surface and a buildup of fibrous tissue that further induces conductive losses. In some cases, an infection may heal but still cause hearing loss by immobilizing the ossicles. There are two distinct types of chronic otitis, one relatively harmless and the other quite dangerous. An odorless, stringy discharge from the mucous membrane lining the middle ear characterizes the harmless type. The dangerous type is characterized by a foul-smelling discharge coming from a bone-invading process beneath the mucous lining. If neglected, this process can lead to serious complications, such as meningitis, paralysis of the facial nerve, or complete sensorineural deafness.

The ossicles may be disrupted by infection or by a jarring blow to the head. Most often, a separation of the linkage occurs at the weakest point, where the anvil joins the stirrup. A partial separation results in a mild hearing loss, while complete separation causes severe hearing impairment.

Disablement of the mechanical linkage of the middle ear may also occur if the stirrup becomes calcified, a condition known as "otosclerosis." The normal bone is resorbed and replaced by very irregular, often richly vascularized bone. The increased stiffness of the stirrup produces conductive hearing loss. In extreme cases, the stirrup becomes completely

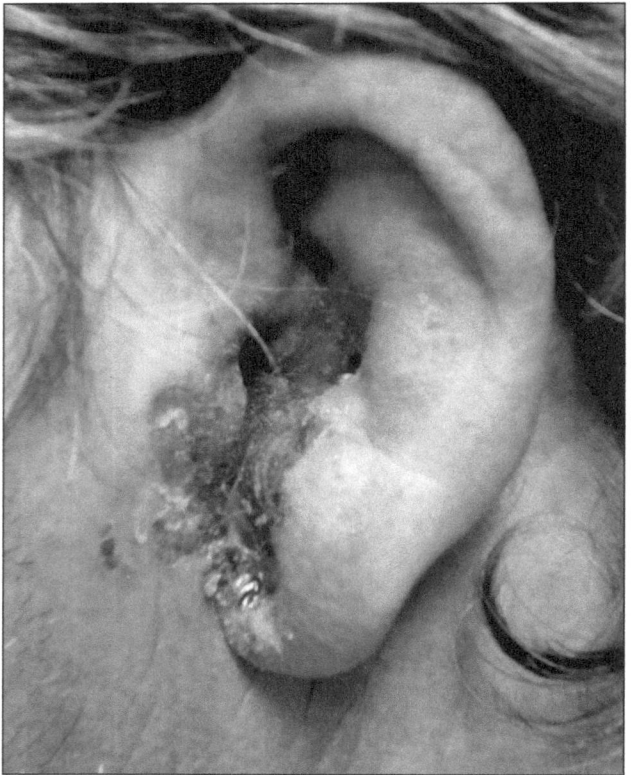

A severe case of Otits Externa (Swimmer's Ear). Photo by James Heilman, MD, via Wikimedia Commons. [CC 3.0.]

immobile and must be surgically removed. Although the exact cause of this disease is unknown, it seems to be hereditary. About half of the cases occur in families in which one or more relatives have the same condition, and it occurs more frequently in females than in males. There is also some evidence that the condition may be triggered by a lack of fluoride in drinking water and that increasing the intake of fluoride may retard the calcification process.

Tinnitus is characterized by ringing, hissing, or clicking noises in the ear that seem to come and go spontaneously without any sound stimulus. While tinnitus is not a disease of the ear, it is a common symptom of various ear problems. Possible causes of tinnitus are earwax lodged against the eardrum, a perforated or inflamed eardrum, otosclerosis, high aspirin dosage, or excessive use of the telephone. Tinnitus is most serious when caused by an inner-ear problem or by exposure to very intense sounds, and it often accompanies hearing loss at high frequencies.

Ménière's disease is caused by production of excess cochlear fluid, which increases the pressure in the cochlea. This condition may be precipitated by allergy, infection, kidney disease, or a number of other causes, including severe stress. The increased pressure is exerted on the walls of the semicircular canals as well as on the cochlear partition. The excess pressure in the semicircular canals (the organs of balance) is interpreted by the brain as a rapid spinning motion, and the victim experiences abrupt attacks of vertigo and nausea. The excess pressure in the cochlear partition has the same effect as a very loud sound and rapidly destroys hair cells. A single attack causes a noticeable hearing loss and could result in total deafness without prompt treatment.

Of all ear diseases, damage to the hair cells in the cochlea causes the most serious impairment. Cilia may be destroyed by high fevers or from a sudden or prolonged exposure to intensely loud sounds. Problems include destroyed or missing hair cells,

> **INFORMATION ON EAR INFECTIONS AND DISORDERS**
>
> **Causes**: Infection, buildup of earwax, fluid retention, injury, fungal growth, allergies, exposure to loud noise, sudden change in air pressure, certain drugs
>
> **Symptoms**: Hearing impairment or loss, itchiness, pain, inflammation, discharge, tinnitus
>
> **Duration**: Temporary to chronic
>
> **Treatments**: Wide ranging; can include flushing ear with a warm solution under pressure, antibiotics, surgery

hair cells that fire spontaneously, and damaged hair cells that require unusually strong stimuli to excite them. At the present time, there is no means of repairing damaged cilia or of replacing those that have been lost.

Viral nerve deafness is a result of a viral infection in one or both ears. The mumps virus is one of the most common causes of severe nerve damage, with the measles and influenza viruses as secondary causes.

Ototoxic (ear-poisoning) drugs can cause temporary or permanent hearing impairment by damaging auditory nerve tissues, although susceptibility is highly individualistic. A temporary decrease of hearing (in addition to tinnitus) accompanies the ingestion of large quantities of aspirin or quinine. Certain antibiotics, such as those of the mycin family, may also cause permanent damage to the auditory nerves.

Repeated exposure to loud noise (in excess of 90 decibels) will cause a gradual deterioration of hearing by destroying cilia. The extent of damage, however, depends on the loudness and the duration of the sound. Rock bands often exceed 110 decibels; farm machinery averages 100 decibels.

Presbycusis (hearing loss with age) is the inability to hear high-frequency sounds because of the increasing deterioration of the hair cells. By age thirty, a perceptible high-frequency hearing loss is present. This deterioration progresses into old age, often resulting in severe impairment. The problem is accelerated by frequent unprotected exposure to noisy environments. The extent of damage depends on the frequency, intensity, and duration of exposure, as well as on the individual's predisposition to hearing loss.

TREATMENT AND THERAPY
The simplest ear problems to treat are a buildup of earwax, swimmer's ear, and a perforated eardrum. A large accumulation of wax in the ear canal is best removed by having a medical professional flush the ear with a warm solution under pressure. One should never attempt to remove wax plugs with a sharp instrument. A small accumulation of earwax may be softened with a few drops of baby oil left in the ear overnight and then washed out with warm water and a soft rubber ear syringe. Swimmer's ear can usually be prevented by thoroughly draining the ears after swimming. The disease can be treated with an application of antibiotic ear drops after the ear canal has been thoroughly cleaned. A small perforation of the eardrum will usually heal itself. Larger tears, however, require an operation, tympanoplasty, that grafts a piece of skin over the perforation.

Fortunately, the bacteria that usually cause acute otitis respond quickly to antibiotics. Although antibiotics may relieve the symptoms, complications can arise unless the pus is thoroughly drained. The two-part treatment—draining the fluid from the middle ear and antibiotic therapy—resolves the acute otitis infection within a week. Secretory otitis is cured by finding and removing the cause of the occluded Eustachian tube. The serous fluid is then removed by means of an aspirating needle or by an incision in the eardrum so as to inflate the tube by forcing air through it. In some cases, a tiny polyethylene tube is inserted through the eardrum to aid in reestablishing normal ventilation. If the Eustachian tube remains inadequate, a small plastic grommet may be inserted. The improvement in hearing is often immediate and dramatic. The pain and hearing loss of aero-otitis is usually temporary and disappears of its own accord. If, during or immediately after flight, yawning or swallowing does not allow the Eustachian tube to open and equalize the pressure, medicine or surgical puncture of the eardrum may be required. The harmless form of chronic otitis is treated with applied medications to kill the bacteria and to dry the chronic drainage. The eardrum perforation may then be closed to restore the functioning of the ear and to recover hearing. The more dangerous chronic form of this disease does not respond well to antibacterial agents, but careful X-ray examination allows diagnosis and surgical removal of the bone-eroding cyst.

Ossicular interruption can be surgically treated to restore the conductive link by repositioning the separated bones. This relatively simple operation has a very high success rate. Otosclerosis is treated by operating on the stirrup in one of several ways. The stirrup can be mechanically freed by fracturing the calcified foot plate or by fracturing the foot plate and one of the arms. Although this operation is usually successful, recalcification often occurs. Alternatively, the stirrup can be completely removed and replaced with a prosthesis of wire or silicon, yielding excellent and permanent results.

Since tinnitus has many possible, and often not readily identifiable, causes, few cases are treated successfully. The tinnitus masker has been invented to help sufferers live with this annoyance. The masker, a noise generator similar in appearance to a hearing aid, produces a constant, gentle humming sound that masks the tinnitus.

Ménière's disease, usually treated with drugs and a restricted diet, may also require surgical correction to relieve the excess pressure in severe cases. If this procedure is unsuccessful, the nerves of the inner ear may be cut. In drastic cases, the entire inner ear may be removed. To treat the vertigo caused by Ménière's disease, motion sickness drugs such as meclizine (Antivert) and diazepam (Valium) can diminish the spinning sensation that causes nausea and vomiting. Prochlorperazine (Compazine) effectively quells nausea associated with vertigo is the other medications fail to do so. Finally, diuretics, such as triamterene/hydrochlorothiazide (Dyazide or Maxzide) reduce the excessive fluid buildup in the ear, decreasing the vertigo.

Presently there is no cure for damaged hair cells; the only treatment is to use a hearing aid. It is more advantageous to take preventive measures, such as reducing noise at the source, replacing noisy equipment with quieter models, or using ear-protection devices. Recreational exposure to loud music should be severely curtailed, if not completely eliminated.

PERSPECTIVE AND PROSPECTS

For many centuries, treatment of the ear was associated with that of the eye. In the nineteenth century, the development of the laryngoscope (to examine the larynx) and the otoscope (to examine the ears) enabled doctors to examine and treat disorders such as croup, sore throat, and draining ears, which eventually led to the control of these diseases. As an offshoot of the medical advances made possible by these technological devices, the connection between the ear and throat became known, and otologists became associated with laryngologists.

The study of ear diseases did not develop scientifically until the early nineteenth century, when Jean-Marc-Gaspard Itard and Prosper Ménière made systematic investigations of ear physiology and disease. In 1853, William R. Wilde of Dublin published the first scientific treatise on ear diseases and treatments, setting the field on a firm scientific foundation. Meanwhile, the scientific investigation of the diseased larynx was aided by the laryngoscope, invented in 1855 by Manuel Garcia, a Spanish singing teacher who used his invention as a teaching aid. During the late nineteenth century, this instrument was adopted for detailed studies of larynx pathology by Ludwig Türck and Jan Czermak, who also adapted this instrument to investigate the nasal cavity, which established the link between laryngology and rhinology. Friedrich Voltolini, one of Czermak's assistants, further modified the instrument so that it could be used in conjunction with the otoscope. In 1921, Carl Nylen pioneered the use of a high-powered binocular microscope to perform ear surgery. The operating microscope opened the way for delicate operations on the tiny bones of the middle ear. With the founding of the American Board of Otology in 1924, otology (later otolaryngology) became the second medical specialty to be formally established in North America.

Prior to World War II, the leading cause of deafness was the various forms of ear infection. Advances in technology and medicine have now brought ear infections under control. Today the leading type of hearing loss in industrialized countries is conductive loss, which occurs in those who are genetically predisposed to such loss and who have had lifetime exposure to noise and excessively loud sounds. In the future, protective devices and reasonable precautions against extensive exposure to loud sounds should reduce the incidence of hearing loss to even lower levels.

—*George R. Plitnik, PhD*

Further Information

Canalis, Rinaldo, and Paul R. Lambert, editors. *The Ear: Comprehensive Otology.* Lippincott Williams & Wilkins, 2000.

Dugan, Marcia B. *Living with Hearing Loss.* Gallaudet UP, 2003.

Ferrari, Mario. *PDxMD Ear, Nose, and Throat Disorders.* PDxMD, 2003.

Friedman, Ellen M., and James M. Barassi. *My Ear Hurts! A Complete Guide to Understanding and Treating Your Child's Ear Infections.* Diane, 2004

Greene, Alan R. *The Parent's Complete Guide to Ear Infections. Reprint.* People's Medical Society, 2004.

Jerger, James, editor. *Hearing Disorders in Adults: Current Trends.* College-Hill Press, 1984.

Kemper, Kathi J. *The Holistic Pediatrician: A Pediatrician's Comprehensive Guide to Safe and Effective Therapies for the Twenty-five Most Common Ailments of Infants, Children, and Adolescents.* Rev. ed., Quill, 2002.

"Lack of Consensus About Surgery for Ear Infections." *Health News*, vol. 18, no. 3, June/July 2000, p. 11.

MedlinePlus. "Ear Disorders." *MedlinePlus*, 1 Apr. 2013.

MedlinePlus. "Ear Infections." *MedlinePlus*, 1 Apr. 2013.

National Center for Immunization and Respiratory Diseases, Division of Bacterial Diseases. "Ear Infections." *Centers for Disease Control and Prevention*, 23 May 2011.

Pender, Daniel J. *Practical Otology.* J. B. Lippincott, 1992.

Roland, Peter S., Bradley F. Marple, and William L. Meyerhoff, editors. *Hearing Loss.* Thieme, 1997.

EOSINOPHILIC ESOPHAGITIS

Category: Diseases/Disorders

Anatomy or system affected: Blood, gastrointestinal system, immune system, lymphatic system, mouth, skin, throat

Specialties and related fields: Allergist, dermatology, epidemiology, gastroenterology, hematology, immunology, internal medicine, otorhinolaryngology, pathology, rheumatology

Definition: A chronic inflammatory disorder in which a type of white blood cell called "eosinophils" accumulate in the esophageal mucosa, damaging it.

KEY TERMS

atopy: a tendency to develop allergic diseases and aberrantly respond to common allergens such as inhaled and food allergen

dysphagia: difficulty or discomfort when swallowing

eosinophil: a type of white blood cell responsible for combating multicellular parasites and plays a significant role in allergies

gastroesophageal reflux disease (GERD): a chronic disease that results from stomach acid or bile flowing into the esophagus, irritating and damaging it

lower esophageal sphincter (LES): a bundle of muscles at the bottom of the esophagus, where it meets the stomach that closes to prevent acid and stomach contents from refluxing into the esophagus

WHAT WE KNOW

Eosinophilic esophagitis (EE) is a chronic inflammatory disorder in which eosinophils (i.e., a type of white blood cell that promotes inflammation) accumulate in the esophageal mucosa, causing it to become inflamed. Mucosal injury often develops. Researchers believe EE is an allergic disorder. Many persons with EE develop dysphagia (i.e., difficulty swallowing), food impaction (i.e., food becomes stuck in the esophagus), gastroesophageal reflux disease (GERD), and conditions that result from food and respiratory allergies (e.g., asthma, eczema). Effective treatment for EE is often challenging to determine. It involves assessing allergies through skin prick testing, patch testing, and following a food elimination diet. Identifying and eliminating foods

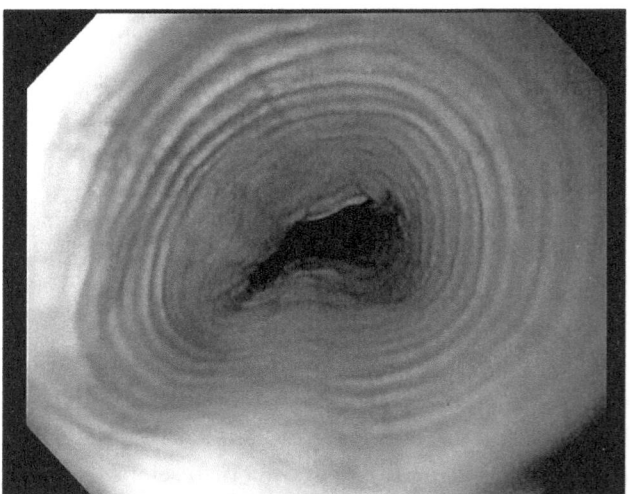

Endoscopic image of esophagus in a case of eosinophilic esophagitis. Concentric rings are termed trachealization of the esophagus. Photo by Samir via Wikimedia Commons. [CC 3.0.]

that cause allergic reactions combined with corticosteroids can improve the signs and symptoms of EE.

SIGNS AND SYMPTOMS OF EE

The signs and symptoms of EE vary. Most patients complain of dysphagia, which means that they have trouble swallowing. EE patients may have a disease that mainly affects the upper part of the esophagus and others that mainly affect the lower part of the esophagus. Some of those EE patients whose condition affects the lower esophagus suffer from GERD, which is colloquially known as "acid reflux." The damage caused by EE compromises the function of the lower esophageal sphincter (LES). Typically, the LES contracts while the stomach is working to prevent the stomach's acid contents from backwashing into the esophagus, damaging it. Damage to the LES causes stomach acid to wash into the lower esophagus, further damaging it. As the lower esophagus undergoes this constant cycle of damage and incomplete healing, it thickens. The thickening of the upper part of the stomach decreases the stomach's ability to hold food, and patients often feel a sensation of fullness.

Those EE patients whose disease affects the upper part of the esophagus can have so much trouble swallowing that food particles go into their respiratory tract. This phenomenon, aspiration, causes choking but can also cause aspiration pneumonia. Aspiration also predisposes patients to asthma, wheezing, and coughing.

Because the esophagus of EE patients does not work properly, they do not want to eat since it is too painful to do so. This self-induced anorexia causes weight loss and iron deficiency anemia. EE causes bleeding, further exacerbating the anemia. Food also gets stuck in the malfunctioning esophagus; a phenomenon called "food impaction" is another feature of EE.

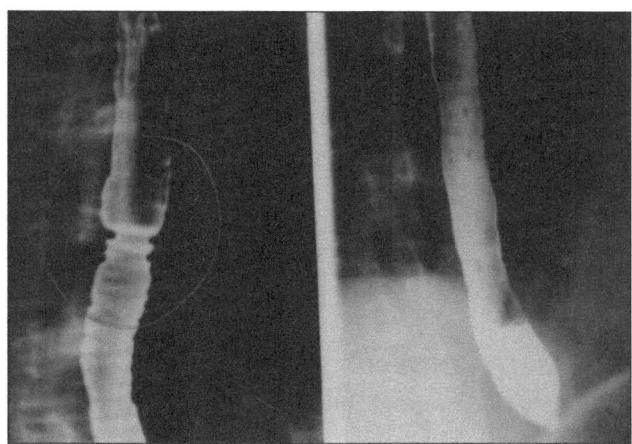

The barium swallow of the esophagus on the left side shows multiple rings associated with eosinophilic esophagitis. Photo by Runder, via Wikimedia Commons. [CC 2.0.]

RISK FACTORS FOR EE

EE tends to develop early in life. Therefore, being younger is a risk factor for EE. Interestingly, EE is most prevalent in Caucasians and males. Consequently, being a white male younger than 45 years of age increases your risk for developing EE. EE also tends to run in families, which argues for a genetic cause for EE as well. EE also has a definite connection with GERD, and GERD patients have a higher risk for EE. Because EE is a condition of the immune system, people with food, respiratory, or atopic allergies also have a higher risk of developing EE.

MEDICAL NUTRITION THERAPY FOR EE

Specific foods induce EE. What foods cause an EE flare-up differs between patients. Identifying and eliminating causal foods from the diet can reliably EE-related manifestations. The most common foods that cause allergic reactions are milk and milk products, eggs, wheat, soy, peanuts, other tree nuts, and shellfish.

Following an elemental diet, which consists of consuming a formula of amino acids in a predigested form that is easily absorbed and provides total nutrition, helps reduce signs and symptoms of EE. However, the elemental diet is not very palatable, making it a less effective dietary option for long-term treatment.

Pharmacological interventions for EE involve episodic use of corticosteroids to diminish esophageal inflammation. Oral or swallowed corticosteroids can calm the inflammation in EE patients.

RESEARCH FINDINGS
Although challenging, following an elimination diet is valuable for identifying causative agents in persons with EE. It can take months to identify the causal foods, significantly reducing the quality of life. The registered dietician (RD) must work closely with patients and their families throughout an elimination diet. Researchers found that RDs play an important role in providing extensive education and emotional support throughout the process of dietary elimination, which is vital to the successful identification of allergens and the reestablishment of a dietary plan that is effective in reducing allergic reactions and improving the patient's quality of life (QOL).

SUMMARY
Individuals diagnosed with EE (and their family members) should become knowledgeable about EE and diet to assess personal characteristics and health needs accurately. These patients should be aware of the most common food allergens and meet with an RD to receive education, guidance, and support for an elimination diet. It is important to report any health-related changes to the treating clinician as soon as possible to prevent further damage. Patients and their family members should adhere to prescribed treatment regimens and continue medical surveillance to monitor health status. Research suggests that although it is difficult to follow an elimination diet, it is the most effective way to figure out the cause of EE.

—*Cherie Marcel, BS and Michael A. Buratovich, PhD*

Further Information
Almansa, C., K. R. Devault, and S. R. Achem. "A Comprehensive Review of Eosinophilic Esophagitis in Adults." *Journal of Clinical Gastroenterology*, vol. 45, no. 8, pp. 658-64, doi:10.1097/MCG.0b013e318211f95b.

de Leon, L. M., and E. Feller. "Eosinophilic Esophagitis." *The 5-Minute Clinical Consult*, edited by F. J. Domino, pp. 440-41, 21st ed., Wolters Kluwer Health/Lippincott Williams & Wilkins, 2013.

DynaMed. "Eosinophilic Esophagitis in Adults." *EBSCO Information Services*, 13 Jun. 2014, search.ebscohost.com/login.aspx?direct=true&db=dme&AN=435297. Accessed 17 Mar. 2015.

DynaMed. "Eosinophilic Esophagitis in Children." *EBSCO Information Services*, 13 Jun. 2014, search.ebscohost.com/login.aspx?direct=true&db=dme&AN=435298. Accessed 17 Mar. 2015.

Feuling, M. B., and R. J. Noel. "Medical and Nutrition Management of Eosinophilic Esophagitis in Children." *Nutrition in Clinical Practice*, vol. 25, no. 2, 2010, pp. 166-74, doi:10.1177/0884533610361608.

Greenberger, N. J. "Eosinophilic Esophagitis." *Current Diagnosis & Treatment Gastroenterology, Hepatology, & Endoscopy*, edited by N. J. Greenberger, pp. 183-86, 2nd ed., McGraw-Hill Medical, 2012.

Klinnert, M. D. "Psychological Impact of Eosinophilic Esophagitis on Children and Families." *Immunology & Allergy Clinics of North America*, vol. 29, no. 1, 2009, pp. 99-107, doi:10.1016/j.iac.2008.09.011.

McQuaid, K. R. "Gastrointestinal Disorders." *2013 Current Medical Diagnosis & Treatment*, edited by M. A. Papadakis, S. J. McPhee, and M. W. Rabow, p. 600, 52nd ed., McGraw-Hill Medica, 2013.

Santangelo, C. M., and E. McCloud. "Nutritional Management of Children Who Have Food Allergies and Eosinophilic Esophagitis." *Immunology & Allergy Clinics of North America*, vol. 29, no. 1, 2009, pp. 77-84, doi:10.1016/j.iac.2008.09.009.

Spergel, J. M., and M. Shuker. "Nutritional Management of Eosinophilic Esophagitis." *Gastrointestinal Endoscopy Clinics of North America*, vol. 18, no. 1, pp. 179-94, 2008, doi:10.1016/j.giec.2007.09.008.

Food Allergies

Category: Diseases/Disorders
Anatomy or system affected: Circulatory system, gastrointestinal system, immune system, respiratory system, skin
Specialties and related fields: Gastroenterology, immunology, nutrition
Definition: An abnormal response by the immune system to some foods, causing mild to severe symptoms that may become life-threatening.

KEY TERMS

allergen: any substance that causes an allergic reaction

anaphylaxis: a severe allergic reaction involving the circulatory and respiratory systems; often fatal without immediate treatment

biphasic reaction: delayed allergic reaction to an allergen, between one to four hours after the initial reaction

EpiPen: a device that administers a prescribed dose of injectable epinephrine

epinephrine: a hormone that acts as a vasoconstrictor and cardiac stimulant

food allergy action plan: a care plan that outlines lifesaving strategies when experiencing a food allergy reaction

immunoglobulin antibody: a protein activated during allergic reactions by the immune system

radioallergosorbent test (RAST): the most accurate blood test available to diagnose allergies

CAUSES AND SYMPTOMS

Allergic reactions occur when the immune system is stimulated to protect the body from foreign organisms known as allergens. Allergens, usually proteins, are perceived by the body as potentially harmful. When the immune system is activated, two types of white blood cells respond phagocytes and lymphocytes. Phagocytes destroy bacteria, viruses, and parasites. Lymphocytes destroy other types of harmful organisms. These white blood cells respond when a portion of food is perceived as dangerous. Therefore, when an allergen is encountered, white blood cells respond and attach an immunoglobulin (Ig) antibody to it. Five different immunoglobulin antibodies can be activated, and each has a different responsibility. Immunoglobulin E (IgE) is the antibody that responds to most food allergy reactions. Marking an allergen with an Ig antibody distinguishes it from healthy tissue and cells. Items marked with antibodies induce white blood cells called "mast cells" to release a chemical spray, usually histamine, which targets and destroys only the harmful allergen.

Food is essential for life and good health. The exact reason a food substance is identified as harmful is still inconclusive. Genetics provides the strongest link to food allergy incidence. Research studies show that a family history of allergies increases the chance of developing all allergies, including those to food. If both parents have an allergy, there is a 70 to 80 percent chance that their children will develop an allergy. Even those with no family history of allergies can still develop them, indicating that other factors play a role. Many theories have been proposed. The hygiene hypothesis suggests that the Western world's habit of cleanliness causes the immune system to become bored and attack itself. Introducing foods at too early an age may overstimulate an immature gastrointestinal tract and trigger an allergic reaction. The leaky gut theory, in which an unhealthy gastrointestinal tract leaks allergens into the bloodstream, is also theorized to promote allergies. Many foods also contain proteins, and it is thought the body confuses food proteins with an allergenic protein from another source. Frequent use of antacids, food additives, vaccines, genetic manipulations of food crops, and exposure to environmental toxins are also linked to an abnormal immune system response to foods.

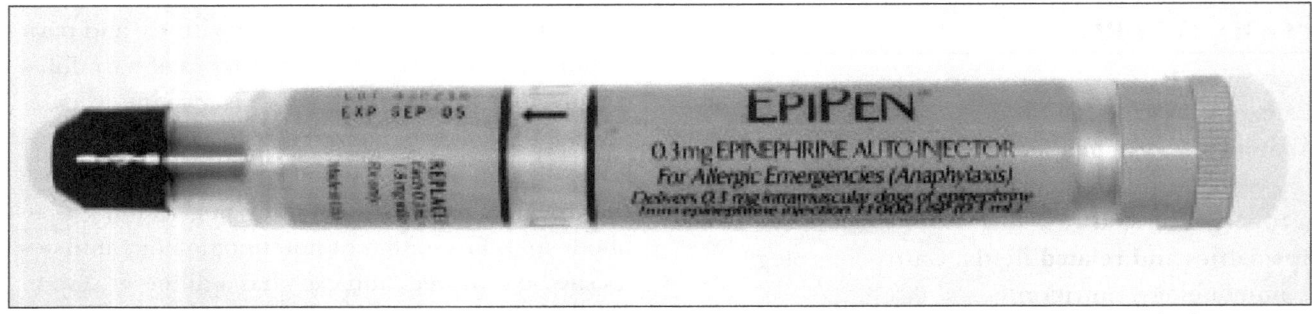

An epinephrine autoinjector is a medical device for injecting a measured dose or doses of epinephrine by means of autoinjector technology. It is most often used for the treatment of anaphylaxis. Photo by Sean William, via Wikimedia Commons. [CC 3.0.]

Food allergies differ from food intolerances. Food allergies result from an immunological response against a component in the food. The symptoms of food allergies, such as hives, itching, vomiting, diarrhea, or difficulty breathing, occur every time the offending food is ingested. Suppose you have an allergy to cow's milk, for example. In that case, you will experience symptoms every time you drink cow's milk or eat anything that contains cow's milk, such as yogurt, ice cream, cream cheese, cheese, cake, or cheese pizza. A medical history, coupled with blood tests and skin prick tests, can diagnose such a food allergy. Food intolerances result from an inability to digest and assimilate one or more components in foodstuffs. The best example of food intolerance is the inability to digest the milk sugar lactose. So-called lactose intolerance results from the microorganisms of the gastrointestinal tract fermenting the undigested lactose. Lactose fermentation causes flatulence, bloating, diarrhea, and stomach pain. The immune system does not cause food intolerances, and blood and skin prick tests play no role in diagnosing them.

More than two hundred foods, some food additives, and foods naturally high in histamine have been reported to cause adverse food reactions. However, not all adverse food reactions are diagnosed as food allergies. An estimated 3 to 4 percent of adults and 6 to 8 percent of children worldwide are diagnosed with food allergies. Approximately 90 percent of food allergies are to cow's milk, eggs, fish, peanuts, shellfish, soybeans, tree nuts, and wheat. Frequently, food allergy symptoms mimic food intolerances, sensitivities, and other medical disorders, making diagnosis difficult. In general, an actual food allergy reaction occurs anywhere from minutes to two hours after eating a specific food. Symptoms range from mild to severe, life-threatening anaphylaxis. The severity of reactions is unpredictable, no matter how mild or severe the previous response was. Most symptoms involve the circulatory and respiratory systems. Common symptoms include difficulty breathing, facial swelling, heart arrhythmias, runny or stuffy nose, and fainting. Mild symptoms often affect the skin, causing angioedema, eczema, and hives. The gastrointestinal system may be affected, causing abdominal pain, bloating, diarrhea, metallic taste in the mouth, difficulty swallowing, and vomiting. Children may experience weight loss or poor growth. Eliminating one or more food groups from the diet may cause malnutrition and eating disorders if there is a fear of experiencing a reaction.

Contact dermatitis with certain foods is uncommon but is observed in children and adults. Atopy testing (skin testing) effectively diagnoses it. Avoiding food allergens is the best way to manage food contact dermatitis.

Many individuals assume, without a medical evaluation, that they have a food allergy. If a food allergy is suspected, then a food allergist and a gastroenterologist should be consulted when indicated. A combination of medical and family history, blood and skin tests, and an elimination diet are the tools used to make a firm diagnosis of food allergies. Blood tests include checking serum IgE antibody concentrations and the radioallergosorbent test (RAST), which tests if a reaction to a specific food allergen occurs. The RAST is considered to be one of the most reliable tests in use to diagnose food allergies. However, between 50 and 60 percent of positive RAST scores are false positives, and 10 to 30 percent are false negatives. Skin tests involve scratching the skin with food extracts and monitoring for allergic reactions, such as hives. Still, these tests also have a large percentage of false positives. Therefore, an elimination diet, in which suspected food allergens are eliminated from the diet for two to four weeks, is often prescribed and symptom changes evaluated.

Non-IgE food allergies result from cellular reactions to food-based proteins. These conditions do not correlate with serum IgE levels. Food protein-induced enterocolitis syndrome (FPIES), food protein-induced allergic proctocolitis (FPIAP), and food protein-induced enteropathy (FRIE) are three non-IgE food allergies that occur mainly in infants but can arise in adults.

FPIES tends to occur in three- to six-month-old infants upon the introduction of formula or at four to seven months with the introduction of solid foods. The symptoms of FPIES include vomiting one to three hours after eating, with or without diarrhea. The gastrointestinal irritation results from reactions to soy- or cow-based proteins. However, other foods can also elicit a reaction, such as rice, wheat, oats, eggs, fruit, and poultry. The symptoms are always associated with feeding and do not last long. Children with FPIES may experience dehydration and failure to thrive and may require intravenous fluids. FPIES rarely occurs in exclusively breast-fed infants.

> **INFORMATION ON FOOD ALLERGIES**
>
> **Causes**: Substance found in food (usually a protein), histamine, some food additives; often cow's milk, eggs, fish, peanuts, shellfish, soybeans, tree nuts, or wheat
>
> **Symptoms**: Anaphylaxis, angioedema, asthma, abdominal pain, low blood pressure, difficulty breathing, diarrhea, gastrointestinal bloating, difficulty swallowing, dizziness, faintness, headache, hives, itchy mouth, metallic taste in the mouth, tightness in chest, vomiting, wheezing
>
> **Duration**: Minutes to hours; may be fatal without immediate treatment
>
> **Treatments**: Epinephrine injection or oral antihistamine medications, intravenous or oral steroids, topical hydrocortisone ointments; often immediate emergency medical care

The only known treatment is to withdraw the offending food. Fortunately, children tend to outgrow this condition within a year or two.

FPIAP usually presents in infants who are about six months old. The symptoms include blood-streaked and mucous-filled stools. Infants with FPIAP do not look sick and typically grow. Cow's milk protein is the most common culprit in FPIAP. Switching to a different formula usually resolves this condition. FPIAP is a relatively benign condition that usually disappears by 12 months of age.

FPIE occurs within the first months of life and produced copious diarrhea and poor nutrient absorption. Many infants with FPIAP have failure to thrive. Cow's milk protein is the most common cause of FPIE, but other foods can also cause it. Elimination diets are the best way to manage it. Children outgrow this condition within the first one to two years of age.

Eosinophilic esophagitis (EoE) is related to the ingestion of certain foods, but it also has a strong genetic component. Males suffer from EoE at a 3:1 ratio over women. EoE can occur in adults or children.

The presentation of EoE differs in children and adults. Children tend to experience stomach pain, nausea, vomiting, and failure to thrive. Adults tend to have heartburn, trouble swallowing, and food impaction in the esophagus. Milk is the leading cause of EoE, but eggs and wheat can cause it too. Symptoms plus an esophagus biopsy that reveals eosinophils in tissue samples with inflammation. Management of EoE involves dietary avoidance, proton pump inhibitors, or swallowed corticosteroids. The prognosis of EoE varies from person to person.

TREATMENT AND THERAPY
Food allergy symptoms can escalate from minor to life-threatening in a matter of minutes. Individuals with asthma are at the highest risk for severe food reactions. Epinephrine injection and emergency medical treatment must be administered as quickly as possible when a severe food reaction occurs. Mild reactions may require an oral/intravenous antihistamine or steroid medication or topical hydrocortisone ointment. Food allergy patients must be continually monitored for four to six hours after the initial reaction, even when their symptoms seem to be over or under control. Allergy food symptoms can progress rapidly to life-threatening due to a delayed reaction known as a biphasic reaction.

The only way to prevent a food allergy reaction is by strictly avoiding the food. Allergic individuals must be careful about every food they eat because food allergens can go airborne or be used in the processing or cooking of food. Reading food ingredient labels (disclosures by food processing manufacturers are required by law) and questioning food preparers about prepared foods are critical prevention steps that anyone with a food allergy must take. However, accidental exposures can still occur no matter how careful an individual is. Therefore, persons with food allergies should carry an EpiPen or its equivalent and a food allergy action plan with them at all times.

An EpiPen is a device that administers a prescribed dose of injectable epinephrine during severe allergic reactions; quick treatment with it can mean the difference between life and death. Surveys of health-care providers show that EpiPens are underused. Food allergy action plans are also necessary because they identify the problem and outline a quick and appropriate lifesaving plan of care when an individual is unconscious. A food allergy action plan lists allergenic foods, symptoms, medications, and dose prescribed, a sequence of steps to follow during an emergency, emergency contact information, and the name and phone number of the treating physician. Wearing medical alert jewelry is also advised.

While adults can develop food allergies as they age, young children frequently outgrow them. However, this is not always true for fish, peanut, shellfish, and tree nut allergies. Therefore, the American Academy of Allergy, Asthma, and Immunology recommends that children undergo food challenges periodically to evaluate if they remain allergic to a specific food. Food challenges reintroduce an allergenic food into the diet under strict medical supervision only since the potential for a severe and fatal allergic reaction is high.

PERSPECTIVE AND PROSPECTS
It has long been recognized that surviving an illness often protects against that illness in the future. This connection between immunity and disease was particularly apparent during the ancient plagues of smallpox. Smallpox, an infectious virus, has killed three hundred to five hundred million people worldwide in just the twentieth century. Ancient Egyptian mummies show the ravages of this disease, and Greek historians record the decimated population during the Athenian plague (430-426 BCE). Historians have recorded efforts to increase popula-

tion survival rates, namely the inhaling of crushed smallpox scabs (early immunization technique) and inoculations using pus from smallpox lesions (early vaccination technique) to prevent the disease.

During the eighteenth and nineteenth centuries, naturalists made many lifesaving advances in science and medicine. They explored the body's defense mechanisms, the immune system and successfully eradicated many diseases over time. Preventative vaccines to protect and increase life span were developed and are now accepted medical practice. However, understanding the mechanism of food allergies has taken much longer. In the twentieth century, Carl Prausnitz-Giles, a bacteriologist/immunologist, was the first to discover that food allergies are intimately tied to the immune system. Scientists Kimishige Ishizaka and Terako Ishizaka found that IgE is the principal agent for food allergy reactions.

Research in food allergies has dramatically expanded in recent years since many countries are experiencing increases in food allergy incidence. In 2008, the United States implemented the Exploratory Investigations in Food Allergy program to focus on research into the origin and epidemiology of food allergies and the discovery of more reliable testing methods and effective treatments. The EuroPrevall Project includes European countries and Australia, China, Ghana, India, and New Zealand. The program was initiated in 2005 to improve the quality of life for those who live and struggle with food allergies and discover breakthroughs in clinical research.

Progress is being made in developing more reliable diagnostic methods and treatment options. Promising areas include using pure allergens rather than extracts for skin and blood tests and improved technologies to measure IgE antibodies and the immune response to foods. Also promising are the development of safe injectable and sublingual immunotherapies as preventive treatments, along with anti-IgE medicines that may block allergic reactions.

—*Alice C. Richer, RD, MBA, LD and Michael A. Buratovich, PhD*

Further Information

FARE: Food Allergy Research & Education. n.d., www.foodallergy.org/. Accessed 26 Aug. 2021.

"Food Allergy." *MedlinePlus*, 5 Aug. 2021, medlineplus.gov/ency/article/000817.htm. Accessed 26 Aug. 2021.

"Food Allergy." *National Institute of Allergy and Infectious Diseases*, 29 Oct. 2019, www.niaid.nih.gov/diseases-conditions/food-allergy. Accessed 26 Aug. 2021.

"Food Protein-Induced Enterocolitis Syndrome (FPIES)." *American Academy of Allergy, Asthma, and Immunology*. 28 Sept. 2020, www.aaaai.org/tools-for-the-public/conditions-library/allergies/food-protein-induced-enterocolitis-syndrome-(fpies. Accessed 26 Aug. 2020.

Melina, Vesanto, Jo Stepaniak, and Dina Aronson. *Food Allergy Survival Guide*. Healthy Living, 2004.

Richer, Alice C. *Food Allergies*. Greenwood Press, 2009.

Sicherer, Scott H. *Understanding and Managing Your Child's Food Allergies*. Johns Hopkins UP, 2006.

Stukus, David R., and Irene Mikhail. "Pearls and Pitfalls in Diagnosing IgE-Mediated Food Allergy." *Current Allergy and Asthma Reports*, vol. 16, no. 5, 2016, p. 34, doi:10.1007/s11882-016-0611-z.

Wood, Robert A. *Food Allergies for Dummies*. Wiley, 2007.

Food Allergy Testing Panels

Category: Laboratory test

Anatomy or system affected: Blood, immune system, intestines, lymphatic system, mouth, respiratory system, skin, throat

Specialties and related fields: Allergist, dermatology, gastroenterology, hematology, immunology, internal medicine, pulmonary medicine, rheumatology

Definition: Blood tests that measure the levels of antibodies against specific allergens found in foods.

KEY TERMS

anaphylaxis: a severe and potentially life-threatening allergic reaction that occurs within seconds or minutes of exposure to an allergen

histamine: an amino acid-derived bioactive amine released from mast cells when the body encounters an allergen that causes smooth muscle constriction and blood vessel leakiness

immunoglobulin G (IgG): the most common type of antibody in the body, made by B lymphocytes in response to a repeated bacterial, fungal, or viral infection

immunoglobulin E (IgE): a type of antibody made by B lymphocytes in response to allergies or worm infections

mast cells: cells found throughout connective tissue in the body that contains histamine and other mediators of inflammation that release in response to allergies

CAUSES AND SYMPTOMS

Food allergies are adverse responses to foods resulting from immunologic reactions. Food allergies and food hypersensitivities often refer to the same phenomena. Food allergies are either immunoglobulin E (IgE)-mediated or non-immunoglobulin E-mediated. Food protein-induced enterocolitis (FPIES) and cell-mediated contact dermatitis to foods are two non-non-IgE-mediated food allergies. IgE-mediated food allergies are "immediate" because the signs and symptoms develop rapidly after someone ingests the offending food, usually within seconds to minutes. Some people have uncommon food allergies that take up to two hours and beyond to experience symptoms. The pathophysiology of food allergies involves the sudden and widespread activation of mast cells and basophils, leading to massive histamine release within the digestive system.

Food allergies differ from food intolerances that result from nonimmunologic mechanisms. Examples of food intolerances include lactose intolerance or fructose malabsorption. Lactose intolerance results from deficiencies in the lactase enzyme that degrades the milk sugar lactose. Ingestion of milk products causes the intestinal microorganisms to ferment lactose into gases and organic acids that cause bloating, flatulence, abdominal cramping, and diarrhea in some cases. Fructose malabsorption results from poor absorption of the plant-based sugar fructose. Large quantities of undigested fructose in the intestines invite resident microorganisms to feast on fructose, causing bloating, flatulence, and diarrhea after eating fruit or fruit-based sweeteners. Neither of these conditions depends on the immune system and do not constitute food allergies but food intolerances.

Former estimates of food allergy prevalence were up to five percent of adults and about eight percent of children. However, more recent studies have documented higher food allergy rates double that in adults.

The most typical symptoms of IgE-based food allergies include itching, hives, swelling of the lips, face, or throat, nausea, vomiting, cramping, diarrhea, wheezing, light-headedness, fainting, and low blood pressure. An acute case of hives (urticaria) is the most common manifestation of IgE-mediated food allergies. Hives usually appear within minutes of ingesting the causative food. Several factors can worsen food allergy symptoms, including:

- Having asthma—people with asthma are at higher risk for food-induced anaphylaxis
- Eating things that increase intestinal permeability (e.g., aspirin and alcohol)
- Drugs that interfere with epinephrine activity, such as angiotensin-converting-enzyme (ACE) inhibitors and beta-blockers
- Stress, exertion, or exercise
- Lack of sleep
- Illness
- Menstruation

The severity of IgE-mediated food allergies varies wildly and is unpredictable. Someone who is allergic to peanuts may develop hives one day and then experience life-threatening anaphylaxis the next.

The most common foods people are allergic to are fish or other seafood, peanuts, or tree nuts. Other causative foods infrequently include meat products, such as beef, pork, and lamb.

DIAGNOSIS

The most important aspect of diagnosing food allergies is the patient's history. The primary focus is the symptoms that occurred after ingestion of the offending food. The allergist must note the type of symptoms the patient reports, the timing of symptoms onset, and what foods elicited the reported symptoms.

When a patient's history supports a diagnosis of IgE-mediated food allergy, there are three different tests to confirm the diagnosis. The gold standard test is an in-office oral food challenge. In this test, the patient is given small quantities of the presumptively causative food in the doctor's office. If symptoms appear soon after that, the test confirms the diagnosis. Other tests include the skin prick test or blood IgE tests.

Skin prick, or scratch tests, introduce tiny amounts of food allergens into the skin. The allergist scratches the skin with a needle dipped in a dilute solution of different food allergens. Allergies to specific food allergens should elicit a "wheal and flare" response as the mast cells in the skin coated with IgEs specific for the food allergen respond to the allergen by releasing copious quantities of histamine. Vast histamine release by mast cells causes local blood vessels to dilate and leak, causing the tissue to swell and turn red. The skin prick test cannot properly diagnose food allergies in the absence of the patient's history. Instead, they confirm a diagnosis draw from the patient's history. A licensed physician with experience in skin prick tests should interpret all skin prick tests. Without proper experience and training, skin prick tests are easily misread or misinterpreted.

A third test to confirm an IgE-mediate food allergy diagnosis is the IgE blood test. This test measures the concentration of IgE molecules in the patient's blood. Patients with food allergies should have detectable levels of specific IgE molecules that bind to food allergens. The concentration of these IgE molecules varies extensively from person to person. IgE concentration in the blood ranges from approximately 2 to 150 kilounits per liter in people without food allergies. However, studies have demonstrated that about thirty percent of the population has detectable IgE against specific foods in their blood but can ingest them without any food allergy symptoms. Therefore, the presence of IgE in a patient's blood does not necessarily mean that they are allergic. Furthermore, the quantity of IgE in the patient's blood does not correlate to the severity of their reaction against the causative food. The presence of specific IgE molecules in a patient's blood confirms an IgE-mediate food allergy diagnosis when the patient's history supports it. IgE blood tests are meant to confirm the diagnosis surmised from the patient's history. They cannot, on their

---

INFORMATION ON IgE-MEDIATED FOOD ALLERGIES

Causes: Massive histamine release after ingesting food to which the person is allergic

Symptoms: Itching, rash, flushing; swelling of the lips, face, or throat; nausea; vomiting; cramping; diarrhea; wheezing; light-headedness; fainting; or low blood pressure.

Duration: Chronic, but children sometimes outgrow food allergies

Treatments: Avoidance of the offending food; epinephrine injections for emergencies; second-generation antihistamines for hives or itching

own, effectively diagnose an IgE-mediated food allergy. According to the Food Allergy Research and Testing site: "About 50 to 60 percent of all blood tests and skin prick tests will yield a 'false positive' result. This means that the test shows positive even though you are not really allergic to the food being tested."

IgE blood tests are sometimes overused to diagnose IgE-mediated food allergies. This overuse underscores the importance of using IgE blood tests to confirm a diagnosis based on the patient's history rather than using them in isolation. A dependence on IgE testing apart from a patient history can cause overdiagnosis of IgE-based food allergies.

When commercially available food allergy panels bundle food allergens together for IgE blood tests, overuse becomes a particularly acute problem. Many laboratories offer IgE blood tests for several different foods to determine if patients are allergic to them. Studies have shown that IgE testing with food panels is overused and woefully misinterpreted. Patients initially diagnosed with IgE-mediated food allergies to certain foods based on IgE blood tests were later shown by in-office food challenges not to be allergic to that food. Overdependence on IgE blood tests with food panels led to overdiagnosis of IgE-mediated food allergies and a good deal of patient anxiety and suffering. If an IgE-mediate food allergy is suspected, then using an IgE blood test for those specific foods to confirm the diagnosis is the best way to proceed.

Worse still, commercially available home tests use panels of bundled food allergens that people can purchase over the counter to test their blood for the presence of food allergen-specific IgE molecules. The clinical value of such tests is highly dubious, and no licensed allergist would accept the results of such tests. These tests bundle foods allergen together and fail to use it in collaboration with a patient's history as meant to be used.

Other home blood tests measure the levels of a different immunoglobulin, immunoglobulin G (IgG), against specific food allergens. IgG is made by the immune system when it experiences an infection the second, third, or fourth time. In other words, IgG is a memory antibody that has nothing to do with allergies. These IgG detection tests, therefore, are medically worthless for assessing food allergies.

Anyone who suspects that they have a food allergy should see a licensed allergist.

TREATMENT AND THERAPY
Identifying the causative food with an oral food challenge is the best way to know which food or foods cause the patient's symptoms. Once the causative food is identified, avoiding it will prevent the appearance of symptoms.

Should the patient consume the causative food allergen by accident or unknowingly, second-generation antihistamines, such as loratadine, fexofenadine, cetirizine, or others help with hives and itching. Diphenhydramine (Benadryl), though less well tolerated, is heavily used, even though better alternatives exist. In emergency cases, if ingestion of the causative food causes severe wheezing, tightness in the throat, or fainting, the preferred treatment is epinephrine, not diphenhydramine (Benadryl). Epinephrine delivery by intramuscular injection quells the harmful effects of anaphylaxis. Any food allergy patient who has ever experienced tightness of the throat or difficulty breathing should carry at least two epinephrine autoinjectors.

To use an epinephrine autoinjector, remove it from its case, hand it without covering either end with your fingers, remove the safety cap, and press the autoinjector firmly into the thigh and hold it in place for two to three seconds. If symptoms do not improve or worsen after five minutes, give yourself another dose. After you use the autoinjector, call an ambulance (911) or go to the hospital because the effects of epinephrine do not last long.

The commercially available epinephrine injectors include EpiPen and EpiPen Jr for children. These come as two per package. Canadian autoinjectors are marketed as Auvi-Q and come in three doses for adults and older children, another for children, and a third for infants and toddlers who weigh less than 33 pounds. Auvi-Q epinephrine autoinjectors are about the size of a cell phone. Generic epinephrine autoinjectors are cheaper versions of these devices that deliver the same medicine.

PERSPECTIVE AND PROSPECTS
Allergy testing remains a fertile source of companies that sell medically useless tests. Educated consumers should be mindful of attempts to market these products to the unaware. The public waste money every year on products that will bring them to closer to understanding their health status.

Surveys of companies that make and sell food panel tests reveal that food sensitivity kits are a multibillion-dollar industry. Executives from such companies have been interviewed for entrepreneurial publications, business shows, and podcasts and have even appeared on television shows. The monetary success of these businesses does not change the fact that many of their products are often neither clinically validated nor valuable.

The internet is filled with food allergy and food sensitivity blood tests that have no recognized medical usefulness. Other companies market IgG blood tests that generate data unrelated to food allergies and border on fraud. Other tests that have no usefulness for food allergies include:
- Applied kinesiology (allergy testing by testing muscle strength or weakness)
- Cytotoxicity testing for food allergy
- Rinkel skin titration method
- Provocative neutralization testing
- Sublingual provocation

None of these tests have any scientific backing and should be summarily avoided.

—*Michael A. Buratovich, PhD*

Further Information
"Allergy Testing." *American Academy of Allergy, Asthma, and Immunology*, www.aaaai.org/tools-for-the-public/conditions-library/allergies/allergy-testing. Accessed 6 Sept. 2021.
Barrett, Stephen M., et al. *Consumer Health: A Guide to Intelligent Decisions*. 9th ed., McGraw-Hill, 2013.
Bond, Allison. "A 'Shark Tank'-Funded Test for Food Sensitivity Is Medically Dubious, Experts Say." *STAT*, 23 Jan. 2018, www.statnews.com/2018/01/23/everlywell-food-sensitivity-test/. Accessed 6 Sept. 2021
Food Allergy Research & Education. Blood Tests. 2021, www.foodallergy.org/resources/blood-tests. Accessed 6 Sept. 2021.
"Measurement of IgE to Ara h 2 & Diagnostics for Peanut Allergy." *American Academy of Allergy, Asthma, and Immunology*, 19 Jan. 2021, www.aaaai.org/Tools-for-the-Public/Latest-Research-Summaries/The-Journal-of-Allergy-and-Clinical-Immunology/2021/ara. Accessed 6 Sept. 2020.
"The Myth of IgG Food Panel Testing." *American Academy of Allergy, Asthma, and Immunology*, 28 Sept. 2020, www.aaaai.org/tools-for-the-public/conditions-library/allergies/igg-food-test. Accessed 6 Sept. 2021.
Stukus, David. "The Pitfalls of Food Allergy Panel Testing." *YouTube*, American Academy of Allergy, Asthma, and Immunology, 7 Nov. 2017, www.youtube.com/watch?v=22I-9JkRyU4.

HAY FEVER

Category: Diseases/Disorders
Also known as: Seasonal allergic rhinitis
Anatomy or system affected: Eyes, immune system, lungs, lymphatic system, nose, respiratory system, throat
Specialties and related fields: Immunology, otorhinolaryngology

Definition: A damaging immune response to otherwise harmless foreign substances such as pollen grains and mold spores.

KEY TERMS

allergy: a harmful immune response by the body to a substance, especially pollen, fur, food, or dust, to which it has become hypersensitive.

histamine: a bioactive amine released by cells in response to injury, during allergies, and inflammatory reactions, causing contraction of smooth muscle and dilation of capillaries

immunoglobulin E (IgE): a type of antibody made in response to worm infections and allergies

mast cells: cells found in numbers in connective tissue and filled with basophil granules that release histamine and other substances during inflammatory and allergic reactions

CAUSES AND SYMPTOMS

Allergic rhinitis, popularly known as hay fever, represents the most common allergic disorder, affecting approximately 10 percent of the population; the most common source of the allergy is wind-dispersed pollen. Trees, grasses, and certain forbs (especially the ragweeds) are the most common culprits. These tiny grains are produced in phenomenal numbers to ensure the transfer of the pollen (which contains the plant's sperm) to other flowers of the same plant species. The first time that a susceptible person is exposed, the pollen acts to sensitize the immune system. On second and subsequent exposures, the pollen triggers an allergic response.

This response is triggered by forming a specific class of antibody known as IgE against the proteins on the pollen grains (generally called "antigens" and, in this case, "allergens"). Immunoglobulin E (IgE) attaches to mast cells at one end and the pollen grains at the other end. This attachment causes the mast cells to release defensive substances, the best known of which is histamine. These substances cause increased permeability of capillaries and the production and release of mucous and watery substances from the nasal passages and eyes. Itching and sneezing accompany the release. The tendency to produce IgE against pollen allergens is an inherited trait; persons with one or both parents who have allergies to certain substances are more likely to exhibit the same allergies than persons whose parents do not show such responses.

TREATMENT AND THERAPY

It is generally agreed that avoidance of the allergen is the most effective therapy for hay fever. Staying inside a building with air conditioning or well-filtered air during the worst allergy season helps. However, avoiding an allergen altogether, such as ragweed pollen during ragweed's flowering season, is essentially impossible.

The most common treatments employed are desensitization and drugs. Desensitization involves a series of oral therapies that slowly increase concentrations of the allergen in the hope of turning the patient's immune system from the production of IgE to the production of immunoglobulin G (IgG), which does not trigger the mast cells. Products exist for allergies to peanuts (Palforzia), timothy grass pollen (Grastek), house dust mites (Odactra), mixed grass pollens (Oralair), and short ragweed pollen (Ragwitek).

Commonly recommended drugs such as antihistamines block the action of histamine and the other

---

INFORMATION ON HAY FEVER

Causes: Allergic reaction to pollen

Symptoms: Itchy eyes and nose, sneezing

Duration: Chronic

Treatments: Avoidance of allergens, desensitization, antihistamines

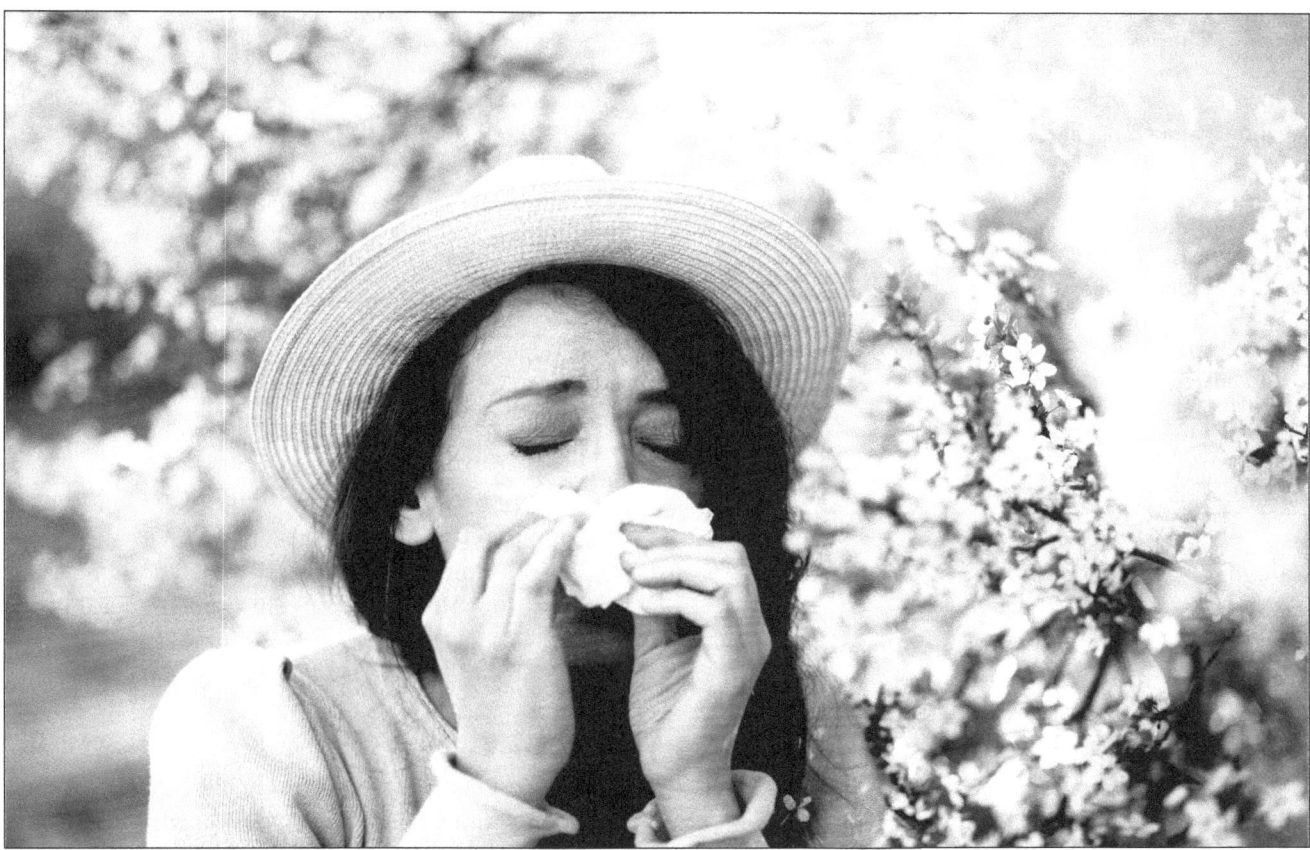

Hay fever. Photo via iStock.com/Goxy89. [Used under license.]

substances released by mast cells. Antihistamines come in prescription-strength or over-the-counter formulations. Mast cell stabilizers, like cromolyn sodium, prevent histamine release from mast cells and prevent allergies from occurring. Cromolyn sodium, however, cannot arrest allergic reactions after they have occurred. Steroid and decongestant nasal sprays are also successful in relieving the symptoms of hay fever in some individuals. Antihistamine or mast stabilizing eye drops treat eye itching caused by allergic conjunctivitis.

PERSPECTIVE AND PROSPECTS

For many persons, long-term avoidance of allergens such as pollen may be difficult. Current drugs such as antihistamines are directed primarily at relieving symptoms without removing the cause: the binding of IgE to the allergen. Future drugs may address the variety of steps involved in the allergic response while causing fewer side effects such as sleepiness. Other treatments may include augmentation of IgG production in response to immunization with the allergen since IgG competes with IgE in binding to the allergen.

—*Carl W. Hoagstrom, PhD and Richard Adler, PhD*

Further Information

Abbas, Abul K., Andrew H. Lichtman, and Shiv Pillai. *Basic Immunology: Functions and Disorders of the Immune System.* 6th ed., Saunders/Elsevier, 2019.

"Hay Fever." *Mayo Clinic*, www.mayoclinic.org/diseases-conditions/hay-fever/symptoms-causes/syc-20373039. Accessed 27 Aug. 2021.

Janeway, Charles A., Jr., et al. *Immunobiology: The Immune System in Health and Disease.* 6th ed., Garland Science, 2005.

Martin, Seamus J., et al. *Roitt's Essential Immunology.* 13th ed., Blackwell, 2017.

Moore, Kristeen, "Allergic Rhinitis." 7 Mar. 2019, www.healthline.com/health/allergic-rhinitis. Accessed 27 Aug. 2021.

Punt, Jenni, et al. *Kuby Immunology.* 8th ed., W. H. Freeman, 2018.

Rabson, Arthur, et al. *Really Essential Medical Immunology.* 2nd ed., Blackwell Science, 2005.

HIVES

Category: Diseases/Disorders
Also known as: Urticaria
Anatomy or system affected: Immune system, skin
Specialties and related fields: Dermatology, family medicine, immunology, internal medicine, pediatrics
Definition: Pink swellings called "wheals" that may occur in groups on any part of the skin.

KEY TERMS

allergies: a harmful immune response by the body to a substance, especially pollen, fur, food, or dust, to which it has become hypersensitive

histamine: a bioactive amine released by cells in response to injury, during allergies, and inflammatory reactions, causing contraction of smooth muscle and dilation of capillaries

urticaria: a rash consisting of round, red welts on the skin that itch and are often swollen, caused by an allergic reaction, usually to specific foods

CAUSES AND SYMPTOMS

Hives are produced by blood plasma leaking through tiny gaps between the cells lining small vessels in the skin. Mast cells, which lie along the blood vessels in the skin, release a chemical called "hista-

> **INFORMATION ON HIVES**
>
> Causes: Allergic reactions, foods, drugs, environmental toxins, infections, insect bites, internal diseases, physical stimuli (e.g., heat, cold)
>
> Symptoms: Inflammation, itchiness
>
> Duration: Acute or chronic
>
> Treatments: Antihistamines

mine." Allergic reactions, foods, drugs, or other chemicals can cause histamine release.

Hives, or urticaria, vary in size from as small as a pencil eraser to as large as a dinner plate, and they may join together to form larger swellings. When hives form, they are usually very itchy and may also burn or sting. Nearly 20 percent of the general population will have at least one episode of hives in their lifetime. Acute hives may last for a few days to weeks. If they last for more than six weeks, they are called "chronic hives."

The most common causes of acute hives are foods, drugs, infections, insect bites, and internal diseases. Other causes include physical stimuli, such as pressure, cold, and sunlight.

TREATMENT AND THERAPY

The best treatment for hives is to find the cause and then eliminate it. Unfortunately, this is not always an easy task. Even if a reason for hives is not apparent, antihistamines are usually prescribed to provide some relief. Antihistamines work best if taken on a regular schedule. It may be necessary to try more than one or use different combinations of antihistamines to find out what works best. In severe hives, an injection of epinephrine (adrenalin) or a cortisone preparation can bring dramatic relief.

PERSPECTIVE AND PROSPECTS

In 1927, Sir Thomas Lewis reported the association between wheals and slight blood vessel dilation,

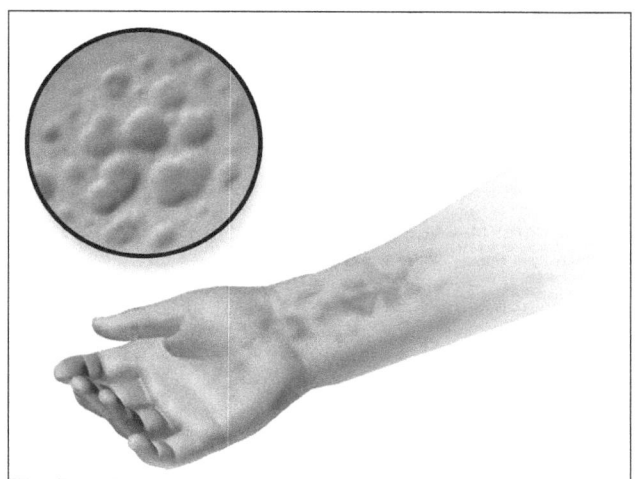

Drawing of hives. Image by Bruce Blaus, via Wikimedia Commons. [Public domain.]

which later confirmed the importance of histamine as a cause of hives. Years of research showed that in addition to allergy, nonimmunological stimuli cause hives as well. A 1993 report in the *New England Journal of Medicine* found that 30 to 40 percent of patients with idiopathic chronic hives have anti-IgE receptor antibodies in their systems, suggesting that the causes of hives could be multifactorial.

—*Shih-Wen Huang, MD*

Further Information

Adelman, Daniel C., Thomas B. Casale, and Jonathan Corren, editors. *Manual of Allergy and Immunology*. 5th ed., Lippincott Williams & Wilkins, 2012.

"Chronic Hives." Mayo Clinic, 9 Jun. 2020, www.mayoclinic.org/diseases-conditions/chronic-hives/symptoms-causes/syc-20352719. Accessed 27 Aug. 2021.

Healthline Editorial Team. "Hives." *Health Library*, 8 Mar. 2019, www.healthline.com/health/hives. Accessed 27 Aug. 2021.

Hide, Michihiro, et al. "Autoantibodies against the High-Affinity IgE Receptor as a Cause of Histamine Release in Chronic Urticaria." *New England Journal of Medicine*, vol. 328, no. 22, 1993, pp. 1599-1604.

"Hives." *MedlinePlus*, 28 Jul. 2021, medlineplus.gov/hives.html. Accessed 27 Aug. 2021.

Kau, Andrew, et al. *The Washington Manual Allergy, Asthma, and Immunology Subspecialty Consult*. 3rd ed., Lippincott Williams & Wilkins, 2021.

Martin, Seamus J., et al. *Roitt's Essential Immunology*. 13th ed., John Wiley & Sons, 2017.

Middlemiss, Prisca. *What's That Rash? How to Identify and Treat Childhood Rashes*. Hamlyn, 2002.

Punt, Jenni, et al. *Kuby Immunology*. 8th ed., W. H. Freeman, 2018.

Young, Stuart H., Bruce S. Dobozin, and Margaret Miner. *Allergies: The Complete Guide to Diagnosis, Treatment, and Daily Management*. Rev. ed., Plume, 1999.

ITCHING

Category: Diseases/Disorders
Also known as: Pruritus
Anatomy or system affected: Skin
Specialties and related fields: Dermatology, otorhinolaryngology, pharmacology, psychiatry
Definition: An unpleasant sensation on or in the skin that causes a desire to scratch or rub the affected area.

KEY TERMS

antihistamine: medications that nullify the effects of histamine, including itching

drying agent: astringents or water-based products that remove excess oil from the skin and tighten pores

emollient: preparations that smooth and soften the skin

CAUSES AND SYMPTOMS

Itching is elicited by the physical or chemical stimulation of nerve receptors in the skin. It can be caused by a wide variety of problems in a variety of different organ systems.

Nearly any skin lesion may itch; skin-related causes include such varied problems as eczema, psoriasis, contact dermatitis, insect bites, bacterial infections, fungal infections, sunburn, and exposure to wool. Viral infections such as chickenpox can cause intense itching. Itching of the eyes and nose is commonly associated with allergies. Itching without a skin rash may be caused by several internal problems. In children, various endocrine problems associated with itching include liver disease, kidney failure, thyroid disease, and diabetes. Some malignancies, particularly lymphomas, may cause itching. Hookworms and pinworms are both internal causes of itching, as are certain drugs. Finally, some women experience generalized itching during pregnancy.

Some psychiatric issues are associated with itching. Patients may scratch hard enough to create deep ulcers. The intensity of the itching seems to be related to the degree of nervous tension. In addition, patients who suffer from certain psychotic states or those who abuse drugs such as cocaine may experience a deep itching sensation that they describe as bugs crawling beneath the skin.

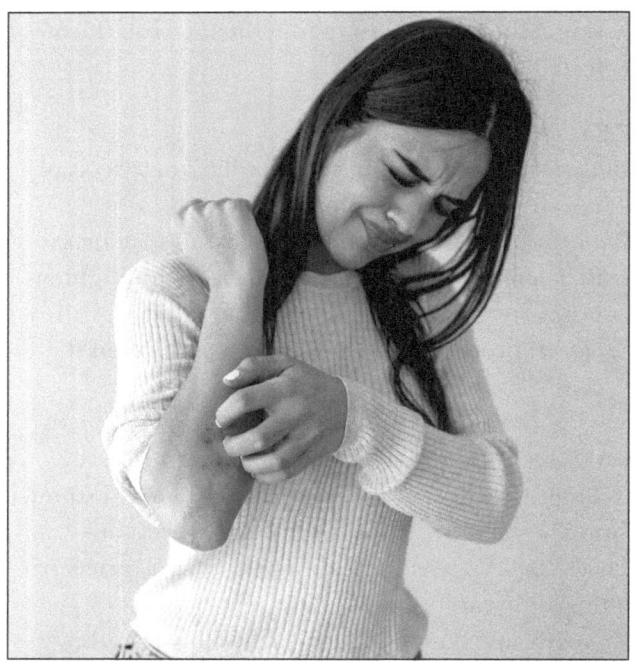

Itching, also known as pruritus, is an irritating sensation that makes people want to scratch. Photo via iStock.com/dragana991. [Used under license.]

> **INFORMATION ON ITCHING**
>
> **Causes**: Eczema, psoriasis, contact dermatitis, insect bites, bacterial or viral infections, fungal infections, sunburn, exposure to wool, allergies, malignancies, parasites, reaction to certain drugs
>
> **Symptoms**: Vary; can include dry, red, or flaky skin; rashes; hives; pain and inflammation
>
> **Duration**: Acute to chronic
>
> **Treatments**: Hydration, moisturizing lotion, various medications (primarily antihistamines)

Itching may rarely be associated with neurologic disease in which the patient interprets changes in sensation as itching. Occasionally, circulatory problems will cause itching, primarily on the legs. Both of these conditions are more common in older adults than in children or young adults.

TREATMENT AND THERAPY

Treatment should be directed toward the cause of the itching. Hydration (bathing followed by moisturizing lotion) or emollient lotions may help provide relief. However, drying agents like witch hazel, apple cider vinegar, or baking soda paste and water palliate itching caused by poison ivy. Various medications, such as antihistamines) may relieve itching, but first-generation antihistamines, like diphenhydramine, can cause significant sleepiness. Second-generation antihistamines, including fexofenadine, loratadine, and cetirizine, relieve itching without causing significant drowsiness.

—*Rebecca Lovell Scott, PhD, PA-C*

Further Information

Adelman, Daniel C., et al., editors. *Manual of Allergy and Immunology*. 4th ed., Lippincott Williams & Wilkins, 2002.

Bernhard, Jeffrey D., editor. *Itch: Mechanisms and Management of Pruritus*. McGraw-Hill, 1994.

Fleischer, Alan B., Jr. *The Clinical Management of Itching*. Parthenon, 2000.

Litin, Scott C., editor. *Mayo Clinic Family Health Book*. 4th ed., HarperResource, 2009.

Middlemiss, Prisca. *What's That Rash? How to Identify and Treat Childhood Rashes*. Hamlyn, 2002.

Turkington, Carol, and Jeffrey S. Dover. *The Encyclopedia of Skin and Skin Disorders*. 3rd ed., Facts On File, 2007.

Weedon, David. *Skin Pathology*. 3rd ed., Churchill Livingstone/Elsevier, 2010.

MOLD AND MILDEW

Category: Biology; Diseases/Disorders
Anatomy or system affected: Immune system, lungs, nose, respiratory system, skin
Specialties and related fields: Environmental health, microbiology, pediatrics, pulmonary medicine, toxicology
Definition: Mold is a generalized term describing nonfruiting fungi, often microscopic and living in moist areas outdoors and inside buildings, which consume nutrients and produce spores. Mold, which thrives in humid and closed spaces, has contributed to the development of effective pharmaceuticals but has also been blamed for various health problems and diseases.

KEY TERMS

conidiophore: a spore-creating area on hyphae in fungi
conidium: spores
hyphae: thin tubes in fungi that secure food and grow, expanding mold size
mycelium: mold colonies consisting of numerous meshed hyphae
mycologists: scientists who study the biological field specializing in fungi and similar spore producers that do not undergo photosynthesis
mycotoxins: poisons released by fungi

STRUCTURE AND FUNCTIONS

Although mycologists consider "mildew" an outdoor fungal plant disease, that term is popularly used to designate mold found indoors on cloth and wooden objects. Thousands of mold species and millions of strains exist. Scientists have found molds both on Earth and in space. Mold grows in wet environments where abundant food, primarily organic materials such as cellulose, provides nourishment. Mold spores are always present in the air, moving with currents and surrounding humans, and cannot be eliminated inside buildings.

Fungi release enzymes to digest food in hyphae to create cells and energy. Mold eats dust, paper, and leather products, living in basements and cooling and heating systems. It can be found in walls, in insulation, and on ceilings. Flooding intensifies mold growth. Mold perishes if food sources are completely devoured or if mites that eat mold spores are present.

Mold hyphae have conidiophores that make conidium. Mold spores can be barbed or smooth and shaped like spirals, ovals, or spheres. Suppose spores have access to nutrients, moisture, air, and sufficiently warm temperatures. In that case, germination starts within twelve to forty-eight hours of being discharged from the conidiophore. An initial hyphae emerges from the spore. As the hyphae consume food, a mycelium forms in a period ranging from several days to almost two weeks later for *Stachybotrys chartarum*, also called "black mold."

Although some molds such as penicillin are helpful, many molds are toxic. In their spores usually,

---

INFORMATION ON MOLD AND MILDEW

Causes: Exposure to parasitic fungi

Symptoms: Allergies, runny nose, sinus problems, coughing, rashes, asthma attacks, headaches, nausea, memory loss

Duration: Acute to chronic

Treatments: Frequent household cleaning, allowing air to circulate, keeping moisture levels in check

but sometimes in hyphae, molds create mycotoxins, which protect them from bacteria and cause sickness in other organisms. The access of molds to food and water affects their production of mycotoxins, not created by every mold. Molds do not discharge mycotoxins every place they grow, nor do they always create toxic quantities of mycotoxins. Molds are primarily benign when outdoors because mycotoxins frequently scatter in the air. Inside, however, mycotoxins can accumulate in dangerous amounts.

DISORDERS AND DISEASES
Scientists have proven that outdoor molds can cause many human, plant, and animal illnesses. Some researchers have considered inside molds detrimental to human health, associating them with weakened immune systems and various ailments because people have suspected that exposure to indoor molds intensified their allergies and asthma. Some have blamed mold contact in their homes and other buildings for triggering headaches, skin rashes, nosebleeds, and fevers.

Based on animal testing and cases of humans exposed to moldy agricultural products, medical researchers recognize known mold dangers. For example, black mold produces satratoxin, which can attack and destroy brain cells, particularly neurons,

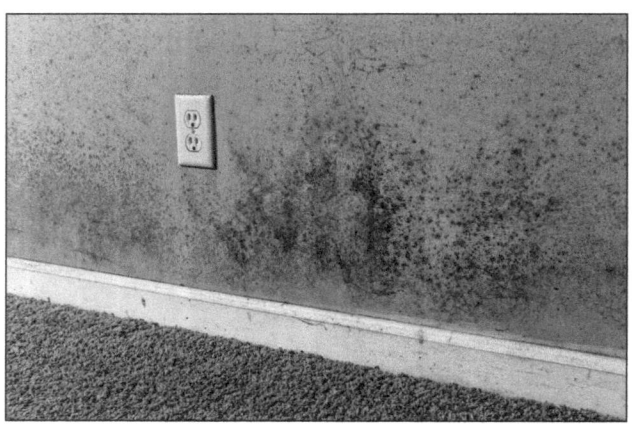

Mold and mildew. Photo via iStock.com/cmannphoto. [Used under license.]

impeding the ability to smell and detect odors. *Trichothecenes* mycotoxins created by *Stachybotrys* and *Fusarium* molds can cause sore throats, blistered skin, and excessive bleeding. *Aspergillus flavus* produces aflatoxins, which can be carcinogenic. Aspergillosis, a disease affecting the lungs, is triggered by mycotoxins created by *Aspergillus* molds. *Claviceps purpurea*, referred to as ergot, produces mycotoxins that can be hallucinogenic. Some forms of that mycotoxin are helpful, however, in soothing migraines or inducing childbirth.

Although individual mold mycotoxins might be harmless, mixtures of mycotoxins can be potentially damaging as their adverse effects combine. The degree to which molds might cause health problems depends on the concentration of mycotoxins and how they invade body systems, specifically whether humans breathe or ingest spores and where the spores settle within their bodies. The size of spores influences their impact on people's health. Researchers hypothesize that some mycotoxins might reach vulnerable lung tissues because they are too tiny to be stopped by nasal defenses that block other harmful microorganisms.

PERSPECTIVE AND PROSPECTS
In 1837, scientists initially discovered black mold in wallpaper in a Prague, Czechoslovakia, residence. By 1986, William Croft, B. B. Jarvis, and C. S. Yatawara presented the first scientific paper, published in *Atmospheric Environment*, discussing the toxicity of indoor mold. They suggested that black mold spores located in a Chicago house, which later proved lethal to laboratory animals, might be linked to health issues that the residents experienced.

During 1993 and 1994, physicians treated infants whose lungs bled at a Cleveland, Ohio, children's hospital. An investigation by hospital physicians and Centers for Disease Control and Prevention (CDC) personnel revealed that the infants lived in homes containing black mold spores. The media printed stories blaming black mold for the infants' sickness. At the same time, hospital officials emphasized the complexity of the situation and the need for a thorough investigation to verify if mold had caused the medical conditions.

The possible dangers of indoor molds again became news in 1999, when *USA Weekend* magazine warned of health hazards allegedly attributed to black mold. Lawsuits resulting in several million dollars in damages increased public awareness of the mold health issue as the media sensationalized the topic. Litigation and mold-related services escalated; con artists took advantage of people's fears of toxic mold. Some legislation relevant to mold and health concerns required house sellers to reveal whether mold had ever existed in structures for sale.

In 2004, the Institute of Medicine of the National Academies in the United States published a consensus report on damp indoor spaces and health. The report concluded that an association exists between damp indoor environments and problems such as upper-respiratory tract symptoms, coughing, wheezing, and asthma symptoms in some human populations. However, the CDC notes that an association between acute idiopathic pulmonary hemorrhage among infants and *Stachybotrys chartarum* has not been proven. Further studies are needed to determine what causes acute idiopathic hemorrhage. Research in this area continues to lead to healthier work and home environments. Reductions in indoor spaces' dampness improve health and address known problems such as mold, bacteria, and dust.

—Elizabeth D. Schafer, PhD

Further Information

"Facts about *Stachybotrys chartarum*." Centers for Disease Control and Prevention, 16 Dec. 2019, www.cdc.gov/mold/stachy.htm. Accessed 3 Sept. 2021.

Lankarge, Vicki. *What Every Home Owner Needs to Know About Mold (And What to Do About It)*. McGraw-Hill, 2003.

May, Jeffrey C., and Connie L. May. *Mold Survival Guide for Your Home and for Your Health*. Johns Hopkins UP, 2004.

Money, Nicholas P. *Carpet Monsters and Killer Spores: A Natural History of Toxic Mold*. Oxford UP, 2004.

Shoemaker, Ritchie C. *Mold Warriors: Fighting America's Hidden Health Threat*. Gateway Press, 2007.

Prevention of Viral Infections

Category: Prevention
Anatomy or system affected: All tissues
Specialties and related fields: Dermatology, epidemiology, gastroenterology, hematology, immunology, internal medicine, microbiology, neurology, oncology, ophthalmology, otorhinolaryngology, public health, pulmonary medicine, virology
Definition: A viral infection is an infection caused by a virus, an intracellular parasitic organism that infects the cells of other organisms. Common viral infections include the common cold, influenza (the flu), chickenpox, and human immunodeficiency virus (HIV).

KEY TERMS

chickenpox: an infectious disease caused by herpes zoster virus that produces a mild fever and a rash of itchy inflamed blisters

human immunodeficiency virus (HIV): a type of lentivirus that infects humans and causes acquired immunodeficiency syndrome (AIDS), a condition resulting in progressive failure of the immune system

influenza: a highly contagious viral infection of the respiratory passages that causes fever, runny nose, and severe achiness

rhinovirus: a group of picornaviruses that cause some forms of the common cold

TYPES OF VIRAL INFECTION

The common cold is an infection of the upper respiratory tract. Several different types of viruses can cause it. Influenza is an upper respiratory tract infection caused by ribonucleic acid (RNA) viruses. Chickenpox is an infection that results in a skin rash. The varicella-zoster virus causes it. Acquired immunodeficiency syndrome (AIDS) is a chronic condition caused by human immunodeficiency virus (HIV), which attacks the immune system.

PREVENTION

Common cold. The common cold is spread through droplets in the air or by direct contact with infected surfaces. No vaccine exists for the prevention of the common cold. The best method of preventing the common cold is frequent handwashing, particularly before eating or preparing food.

Another way to help prevent the common cold is to periodically clean with antibacterial wipes jointly shared surfaces, such as telephones, computer keyboards, refrigerator handles, doorknobs, and toys. A third method for preventing the common cold is to teach children to drink from their own, rather than a shared drinking glass or cup. The fourth prevention method is to avoid close contact with people who have a cold or other respiratory tract infection.

Influenza. Influenza is spread through droplets in the air or by direct contact with infected surfaces. The best way to prevent the flu is to get a flu shot (influenza vaccination). The flu vaccine protects against the most common flu viruses: seasonal influenza and the H1N1 virus (swine flu). The Centers for Disease Control and Prevention (CDC) recommends that everyone six months of age or older be vaccinated, although there are some exceptions.

The following persons should not get a flu vaccine without first consulting a physician: those allergic to eggs, have had a previous allergic reaction to the flu vaccine, have Guillain-Barré syndrome, are younger than age six months, and are already sick and who have a fever. (Vaccination is okay after the person is no longer sick.)

In addition to being vaccinated, other preventive steps include frequent handwashing, using a tissue to cover the nose or mouth when coughing or sneezing, periodically cleaning shared surfaces, avoiding close contact with people who have symptoms of a cold or flu, not sharing drinking glasses, and not going to work when sick.

Chickenpox. The best method for preventing chickenpox is getting varicella (chickenpox) vaccine. The CDC recommends that all children and adults who do not have evidence of immunity to varicella be vaccinated. The CDC defines "evidence of immunity" as any of the following: documentation of two doses of varicella vaccine, blood tests that show immunity, laboratory confirmation of prior varicella disease, a diagnosis of chickenpox, or verification of a history of chickenpox from a qualified health-care provider, or a diagnosis of herpes zoster (shingles) or verification of a history of herpes zoster (shingles) from a qualified health-care provider.

Some people are given the chickenpox vaccine after exposure to help prevent them from contracting the disease. According to the CDC, the chickenpox vaccine is not recommended for persons who are allergic to gelatin, who have a moderate or severe illness (vaccination is okay after the illness), who are pregnant, who are immunocompromised because of illness (such as HIV infection) or treatment (such as chemotherapy) of an illness, who have received blood or blood products within the previous three to eleven months, or who have a family history of immune deficiency.

HIV. HIV is a sexually transmitted disease, but it also can be spread through contact with infected blood or from woman to fetus during childbirth. There is no vaccination for the prevention of HIV. The best way to prevent HIV is to avoid exposure to blood or body fluids of people who are or may be infected. One can do this by taking the following precautions: wash hands before and after eating, after using the toilet, and after contact with another person's blood or body fluids; wear disposable gloves when touching anything that may have come in contact with blood or body fluids, including wound dressings; avoid sharing personal items such as razors or toothbrushes; avoid sharing drug needles, and use latex condoms during sex. Health-care workers should use universal precautions to avoid exposure to blood or body fluid.

IMPACT
According to the National Institutes of Health, more than one billion cases of the common cold occur in the United States each year. The World Health Organization (WHO) estimates that there are between 3 million and 5 million cases of severe influenza illness each year during seasonal epidemics, resulting in 250,000 to 500,000 deaths.

According to the CDC, before developing the varicella vaccine in 1995, about 4 million cases of chickenpox occurred each year in the United States, averaging 10,600 hospitalizations and between 100 and 150 deaths. From 1995 to 2005, the United States saw a 90 percent decline overall in the incidence of chickenpox. In 2002, hospitalizations from chickenpox had decreased 88 percent from what they were in 1994 to 1995. Death rates dropped 66 percent from 1990 to 2001.

The WHO estimates that 33.3 million people worldwide are living with HIV infection. In 2009, 2.6 million people were newly infected, and 1.8 million people died from AIDS-related complications.

—*Julie Henry, RN, MPA*

Further Information
Centers for Disease Control and Prevention. "Seasonal Flu: What to Do if You Get Sick." www.cdc.gov/flu/whattodo.htm. Discusses influenza diagnosis, symptoms, medical treatment, recovery, and emergency warning signs.
Kane, Melissa, and Tatyana Gotovkina. "Common Threads in Persistent Viral Infections." *Journal of Virology*, vol. 84, 2010, pp. 4116-23. Examines how some viruses establish a permanent host relationship and recurrent infection by avoiding immune system actions.
Mayo Foundation for Medical Education and Research. "Common Cold." www.mayoclinic.com/health/common-cold/ds00056. A detailed description of the common cold that includes a definition of the common cold and its symptoms, risk factors, complications, prevention, and treatment.
Mayo Foundation for Medical Education and Research. "HIV/AIDS." www.mayoclinic.com/health/hiv-aids/ds00005. An overview of HIV and AIDS that includes definitions, risk factors, symptoms, diagnosis, treatment, complications, and prevention.
MedlinePlus. "Chickenpox." www.nlm.nih.gov/medlineplus/ency/article/001592.htm. An overview of chickenpox, including causes, symptoms, diagnosis, treatment, prevention, prognosis, and possible complications.

Immune System Diseases

This category is divided into two major types of immune system diseases—immunodeficiency and autoimmune response. Immunodeficiency occurs when the immune system does not adequately respond to an infection. This can be due to insufficient or lack of antibodies, immune cells, or both. Immunodeficiency can be inherited (as with severe combined immunodeficiency) or acquired through infection (as with HIV) or it can result from certain medical treatments (like chemotherapy). Autoimmune response is a misplaced reaction of the immune system that results in your body attacking healthy cells. The exact cause of autoimmune disease is not known, but many factors, genetic and environmental, affect autoimmunity. Not all individuals with immunodeficiency develop autoimmunity, and not all individuals with autoimmunity are immunodeficient. However, certain immune system defects increase the risk for developing autoimmunity. The forty-two essays in this two-part section include discussions of immune deficiencies such as AIDS/HIV, Kaposi's sarcoma, leukemia, and metabolic disorders, and autoimmune conditions like Addison's disease, Crohn's disease, Hashimoto's thyroiditis, juvenile idiopathic arthritis, and multiple sclerosis.

Immune Deficiencies
Acquired immunodeficiency syndrome (AIDS) 173
Human immunodeficiency virus (HIV) 179
HIV/AIDS-related cancers 183
Kaposi's sarcoma 187
Kawasaki disease 189
Leukemia 191
Leukopenia 200
Lymphocytosis 202
Ménière's disease 204
Metabolic disorders 205
Neutropenia 210
Purine nucleoside phosphorylase (PNP) deficiency 211
Severe combined immunodeficiency syndrome (SCID) 214
T-cell immunodeficiency syndrome 217

Autoimmune Diseases
Addison's disease 221
Autoimmune disorders 223
Autoimmune polyglandular syndrome 231
Congenital hypothyroidism 234
Crohn's disease 236
Cushing's syndrome 241

Diabetes mellitus 245
Eczema 254
Graft-versus-host disease (GVHD) 255
Guillain-Barré syndrome 259
Hashimoto's thyroiditis 264
Histiocytosis 266
Hyperthyroidism 267
Idiopathic thrombocytopenic purpura. 271
Juvenile idiopathic arthritis 273
Multiple sclerosis 276
Myasthenia gravis 282
Myositis. 285
Psoriasis and psoriatic arthritis. 287
Rheumatoid arthritis 296
Sjögren's syndrome 300
Spondylitis 302
Systemic lupus erythematosus (SLE) 304
Thyroid disorders. 310
Ulcerative colitis 313
Uveitis. 316
Vasculitis 318
Vitiligo 321

Immune Deficiencies

Acquired immunodeficiency syndrome (AIDS)

Category: Diseases/Disorders

Anatomy or system affected: Blood, brain, eyes, gastrointestinal system, immune system, intestines, liver, lungs, lymphatic system, mouth, psychic-emotional system, reproductive system, respiratory system, skin, throat

Specialties and related fields: Bacteriology, dermatology, epidemiology, gastroenterology, gynecology, hematology, immunology, internal medicine, microbiology, neurology, oncology, ophthalmology, osteopathic medicine, otorhinolaryngology, pathology, pharmacology, proctology, psychiatry, public health, pulmonary medicine, virology

Definition: A disease state caused by infection with human immunodeficiency virus (HIV), leading to a progressive deterioration of the immune system and characterized by the development of any of a large number of opportunistic infections.

KEY TERMS

highly active antiretroviral therapy (HAART): the use of a combination of three or four anti-HIV drugs in a human immunodeficiency virus (HIV)-positive individual to suppress replication of new HIV particles and slow the progression to full-blown acquired immunodeficiency syndrome (AIDS)

Kaposi's sarcoma: a form of blood vessel tumor that produces pink to purple splotches or plaques on the skin in about 25 percent of persons with AIDS and may also affect internal organs; caused by sexual transmission of human herpesvirus 8 (HHV8)

lentivirus: a classification of retroviruses characterized by a very long incubation period (ten to twenty years) before symptoms of a disease appear

opportunistic infection: an infection caused by any type of pathogen in individuals who have an impaired immune system

Pneumocystis pneumonia: a form of pneumonia caused by the fungus *Pneumocystis jirovecii* and commonly seen in persons with AIDS

protease inhibitors: any of several drugs that inhibit the assembly of HIV

retrovirus: a virus with ribonucleic acid (RNA) as its genetic material that produces a deoxyribonucleic acid (DNA) copy of the RNA to be integrated into a chromosome of the host cell, from which it will make new infectious copies of the RNA during the viral life cycle

seroconversion: the detection of anti-HIV antibodies in the blood of an HIV-infected person, who is then said to be HIV-positive

syndrome: a collection of symptoms associated with a particular disease state; an individual patient may show some, but not necessarily all, of these symptoms

T4 cells: also called "CD4 cells" or "T-helper cells"; a specific type of white blood cell (lymphocyte) which regulates the entire immune system and is the preferred target for HIV infection, resulting in immunodeficiency

viral load: a measurement of the amount of HIV present in the blood; often used to monitor the effectiveness of anti-HIV therapy

CAUSES AND SYMPTOMS

Acquired immunodeficiency syndrome (AIDS) is caused by the human immunodeficiency virus (HIV), a member of the lentivirus family of retroviruses.

This virus is thought to have arisen in Africa in the early to mid-twentieth century from related viruses in the chimpanzee and the sooty mangabey monkey. The virus cannot survive long in the air and cannot be transmitted by casual contact. Individuals can be infected only by the exchange of certain body fluids, including semen, vaginal fluid, blood, and human milk. Other body fluids such as sweat, tears, saliva, urine, and feces may contain HIV, but the virus exists in such low concentrations that these fluids are completely ineffective in transmitting an infection. The most common mode of transmission is through sexual contact in which semen or vaginal fluid is exchanged. The presence of another sexually transmitted disease (STD), such as gonorrhea, syphilis, chlamydia, genital herpes, or human papillomavirus, increases dramatically the risk of acquiring an HIV infection through sexual contact.

The second most common mode of transmission is through the sharing of needles contaminated with HIV-positive blood by intravenous (IV) drug users. A pregnant HIV-positive woman may transmit the virus to her child in utero, or more commonly during childbirth. Mother-to-child transmission may also occur through breastfeeding in which the virus is present in the milk. Early in the AIDS epidemic and before a blood test for HIV was available, blood and blood products from blood banks were sometimes contaminated with HIV that subsequently infected recipients. Indeed, more than 90 percent of hemophiliacs became HIV-positive through injections of HIV-contaminated clotting factor VIII. Because of the development of a heat treatment for clotting factor VIII and the screening of the blood supply, hemophiliacs are no longer at high risk for HIV infection. Although the blood supply is relatively safe today, a very low probability of acquiring HIV through a transfusion of contaminated blood still exists, as a recently infected donor may not yet test positive for HIV.

Although HIV can infect virtually all cells of the body, it has a strong affinity for cells of the immune system. The virus uses a cell surface receptor called "CD4" to bind to the membrane of a cell. The CD4 receptor is found on many cells in the body but is in relatively high concentrations on the surface of a class of T lymphocytes called "T4 or CD4 cells." The virus uses a coreceptor called "CXCKR4," also found on the membrane, that promotes the fusion of the membrane of the virus particle with the membrane of the cell, thereby allowing entry of the virus. Persons who lack the coreceptor on their cells appear to resist infection by the virus. The T4 cells are also known as T-helper cells, as they produce a series of chemical signals called "lymphokines" that are needed for the development and maintenance of the entire immune system. While the body constantly makes new T4 cells, HIV has a very small edge in the rate at which these T4 cells are infected and destroyed. Thus, there is a slow but progressive decrease in T4 lymphocytes in the body and loss of immune function. This process may take ten or more years.

The clinical course of infection occurs in three stages. Initially, upon infection, HIV produces an

---

Information on Acquired Immunodeficiency Syndrome (AIDS)

Causes: HIV infection through the exchange of certain body fluids, then the destruction of T lymphocytes of the immune system

Symptoms: Initially, flu-like or mononucleosis-like symptoms, then none until opportunistic infections (candidiasis, cytomegalovirus, ulcers, *Pneumocystis carinii* pneumonia, histoplasmosis, toxoplasmosis) and cancers (Kaposi's sarcoma, Burkitt's lymphoma) become common

Duration: Chronic, eventually fatal

Treatments: Surgery, chemotherapy, and radiation for cancers; antibiotics for bacterial and fungal infections; anti-HIV drugs (nucleoside analogs, reverse transcriptase inhibitors, protease inhibitors, fusion inhibitors)

acute retroviral syndrome referred to as the prodromal stage, beginning about three to four weeks after initial infection and lasting for two to three weeks. During a retroviral syndrome, the patient experiences flu-like or mononucleosis-like symptoms. The patient will believe that he or she simply has a moderate-to-severe case of influenza or if the symptoms are prolonged mononucleosis. During this period, HIV is rapidly proliferating, disseminating throughout the body, and infecting lymphoid tissues. Viral load is high at this stage, and the patient is highly infectious. At the same time, the T4 cell count, which normally is about 1,000 per cubic millimeter, drops by about half. The patient's immune system will mount an antibody response against HIV, but these antibodies are ineffective in stopping the infection. When such antibodies are detectable, the patient is then said to have seroconverted. Anti-HIV antibody detection by a simple blood test is the basis for assigning HIV-positive status. In most cases, seroconversion occurs between six to eighteen weeks after initial infection, although, in rare cases, antibodies may not be detectable until later. By three months, 95 percent of patients will have seroconverted; by six months, more than 99 percent will have detectable circulating antibodies to HIV.

The second stage is called the "clinical latency period" or "asymptomatic stage." Without anti-HIV therapy, this period may last ten or more years. It is during this time that the patient usually has no AIDS symptoms. Early in the latent period, T4 cell counts usually recover somewhat during the first year of infection, averaging approximately 700 per cubic millimeter. After that, there is a very slow decline. In the meantime, viral loads, which were high during the acute retroviral syndrome stage, drop by several orders of magnitude as the T4 count rises. At about one year into the infection, the viral load very slowly increases as the latent period progresses.

The third phase is full-blown AIDS. AIDS usually occurs when the T4 count drops below 200 per cubic millimeter. Opportunistic infections and cancers become common, and patients may have several infections simultaneously. Many of these diseases are rare in healthy individuals. Most common is *Pneumocystis carinii* pneumonia, a form caused by a fungus that is virtually unseen in individuals with a functional immune system. Indeed, the fungus is present in most of the population yet seldom causes pneumonia unless the immune system is compromised. As one of the functions of the immune system is to destroy cancer cells when they arise, immune impairment leads to the development of cancer in about 40 percent of those with AIDS. One of these cancers is Kaposi's sarcoma, a very rare tumor of blood vessels characterized by pink to purple spots or slightly raised areas on the skin. These lesions may also arise on internal organs, where they can impair function. Kaposi's sarcoma is caused by human herpesvirus 8 (HHV8) and is sexually transmitted. It is primarily found in gay men with AIDS and not often seen in IV drug users or girls and women with AIDS. Another cancer commonly associated with AIDS is non-Hodgkin's lymphoma, often in the brain.

In 1987, the Centers for Disease Control and Prevention (CDC) published the criteria for the diagnosis of AIDS, including the appearance of one or more opportunistic infections or cancers. Twenty-three different conditions were listed in the definition: candidiasis of the bronchi, trachea, or lungs; esophageal candidiasis; disseminated or extrapulmonary coccidiomycosis; extrapulmonary cryptococcosis; chronic intestinal cryptosporidiosis (greater than one month in duration); cytomegalovirus disease (other than liver, spleen, or lymph nodes); cytomegalovirus retinitis (with loss of vision); HIV encephalopathy; herpes simplex causing chronic ulcers (greater than one month in duration) or bronchitis, pneumonitis, or esophagitis; disseminated or extrapulmonary histoplasmosis; chronic intestinal cystoisosporiasis (greater than one month in duration); Kaposi's sarcoma; Burkitt's lymphoma; immunoblastic lymphoma; primary lymphoma of the brain; *Mycobacterium avium* complex or *M. kansasii*; extrapulmonary infection due to *Mycobacterium tuberculosis*; other or unidentified *Mycobacterium* species; *Pneumocystis jiroveci* pneumonia; progressive multifocal leukoencephalopathy (PML); recurrent *Salmonella* septicemia; toxoplasmosis of the brain; and wasting syndrome caused by HIV. In 1993, three conditions were added to the criteria: pulmonary tuberculosis, recurrent pneumonia, and invasive cervical carcinoma. Moreover, the definition was expanded to include any HIV-positive person whose T4 count had dropped to 200 per cubic millimeter or lower or whose level of T4 lymphocytes had fallen to 14 percent or less of total lymphocytes.

TREATMENT AND THERAPY
As of 2021, no effective vaccine had been developed to prevent HIV infection. While some candidate vaccines have been under development and in clinical trials, none has proven successful. The usual strategies used with most antiviral vaccines in the past, immunization with attenuated or inactivated viruses, have so far proven ineffective for HIV given its significant rate of mutation. Control of the epidemic has shifted significantly toward preventing exposure and decreasing infectivity by treating to reduce viral load, a measure of the number of viruses in blood and body fluids.

AIDS treatment and therapy fall into two categories: prophylaxis and treatment of opportunistic infections to slow progression to full-blown AIDS. Treatment of opportunistic infections must follow established guidelines for the individual disease. Thus, in the treatment of Kaposi's sarcoma, surgery, chemotherapy, and radiation treatment singly or in combination are utilized. Bacterial and yeast or other fungal infections are treated with antibiotics or antifungal agents. Although some medications may reduce the severity of viral infections, such infections are not easily treated. Because a person with AIDS might suffer from more than one opportunistic infection and/or cancer at the same time, simultaneous treatments often take a severe toll on the patient. The life expectancy for an individual who has progressed to full-blown AIDS is about two years. Death results from an opportunistic infection or cancer.

The second strategy for HIV treatment involves interfering with the viral life cycle to slow viral replication. Anti-HIV drugs target several steps in the life cycle, primarily at the levels of reverse transcription or assembly. In 1987, the first generation of drugs was developed to treat HIV. The first effective treatment utilized zidovudine (ZDV; Epivir), commonly called "azidothymidine" (AZT), a drug originally developed for cancer chemotherapy. ZDV competitively inhibits the virally encoded enzyme, reverse transcriptase, which copies the RNA viral genome into a DNA copy. It also inserts a nucleoside analog into the growing DNA, terminating further synthesis of the DNA copy. Zidovudine is the founding member of the nucleoside and nucleotide reverse transcriptase inhibitors (NRTIs). Other NRTIs that have similar effects include abacavir (Ziagen), emtricitabine (Emtriva), lamivudine (Epivir), and tenofovir (Viread). The side effects of NRTIs include muscle toxicity, liver toxicity, and, in the case of tenofovir, decrease bone density and acute renal failure. Non-nucleoside reverse transcriptase inhibitors (NNRTIs) are noncompetitive inhibitors of the viral reverse transcriptase enzyme. NNRTIs include nevirapine (Viramune), delaviridine (Rescriptor), rilpivirine (Edurant), and efavirenz (Sustiva). NNRTIs cause gastrointestinal distress, liver toxicity (especially nevirapine), and skin rashes.

The final step in HIV replication involves the cleavage of a large precursor protein into smaller structural proteins, an event taking place at the cell surface and followed by the release of the completed virus. The cleaving enzyme is called a "protease" and is encoded by the virus. The second generation of anti-HIV drugs, developed in the 1990s, were protease inhibitors (PIs). PIs interfere with the cleavage of the precursor and prevent viral assembly. As a result, functional virions cannot be made. Food and Drug Administration (FDA)-approved drugs in this class include ritonavir, nelfinavir, lopinavir, fosamprenavir, atazanavir, tipranavir, and darunavir.

Other types of anti-HIV drugs called "fusion inhibitors" interfere with the entry of HIV into cells. The first of these drugs, enfuvirtide (Fuzeon), binds to and inhibits gp41 on HIV virions and is given as a subcutaneous injection every 12 hours. This drug causes pain and the development of cysts or nodules at the injection site and increases the risk of bacterial infections like pneumonia. The small molecule maraviroc (Selzentry) binds to the coreceptor CCR5 on the surfaces of macrophages and T-cells to prevent HIV from binding. This drug is ineffective against HIV strains that use CXCR4 as a coreceptor rather than CCR5. Maraviroc comes as a tablet or solution taken orally twice a day. Though generally well tolerated, maraviroc can cause diarrhea, joint and muscle pain, liver damage (jaundice and elevated liver enzymes). A third HIV entry inhibitor includes a monoclonal antibody called "ibalizumab" (Trogarzo). Clinicians administer ibalizumab intravenously and use it to treat multidrug-resistant HIV-1 (MDR-HIV) infection in patients who have failed with other treatments. This drug blocks entry of HIV-1 into CD4+ cells and prevents HIV transmission via cell-cell fusion by binding to the second extracellular domain of the CD4+ receptor. However, it does not interfere with CD4+ cell activity. Ibalizumab causes diarrhea, dizziness, nausea, and rash and a condition called "severe immune reconstitution inflammatory syndrome". Finally, a very new medication called "fostemsavir" (Rukobia) comes as an extended-release tablet taken twice a day. The FDA approved this medication in June of 2020. It causes nausea, diarrhea, headache, severe immune reconstitution syndrome, heart arrhythmias, and hepatotoxicity.

Integrase inhibitors prevent the DNA copy of the virus from inserting itself into one of the host cell's chromosomes. These highly effective drugs form an essential component of contemporary highly active antiretroviral therapy (HAART). Integrase inhibitors include bictegravir (Biktarvy), dolutegravir (Tivicay), elvitegravir (Viteka), and raltegravir (Isentress). Common side effects of integrase inhibitors include nausea, diarrhea, headache, and fever. Therefore, the anti-HIV arsenal includes drugs that act at different sites or stages in the HIV life cycle.

The HIV reverse transcriptase makes numerous mutations during the synthesis of DNA. Consequently, resistance to individual anti-HIV drugs arises easily and frequently. In 1995, a new strategy for anti-HIV therapy called "HAART," also known as AIDS cocktail therapy, was developed. HAART consists of using a combination of three or more anti-HIV drugs, and the most effective combinations consist of at least three anti-HIV medications from at least two different drug classes. These combinations usually include:

- two NRTIs and one integrase inhibitor;
- two NRTIs and a boosted protease inhibitor;
- two NRTIs and one non-nucleoside reverse transcriptase inhibitor (NNRTI.

Examples include:
- Bictegravir/tenofovir alafenamide/emtricitabine;
- Dolutegravir/abacavir/lamivudine;
- Dolutegravir plus (emtricitabine or lamivudine) plus (tenofovir alafenamide [TAF] or tenofovir disoproxil fumarate;
- Dolutegravir/lamivudine.

HAART therapy is very effective, as it has been estimated that it prolongs the life expectancy of a person with AIDS by three to ten years. Moreover, many patients with full-blown AIDS and in terminal stages of the disease have made remarkable recoveries when placed on HAART. In many cases, HAART dramatically reduced viral loads, T4 cells made some recovery, and the incidence of opportunistic infections diminished. Another advantage of multiple drug therapy is that the probability of HIV developing simultaneous resistance to three or four different drugs is very low, extending the useful therapeutic life of the individual drugs.

The long-term effectiveness of HAART is underscored by an examination of the AIDS deaths in the United States. In 1981, the CDC began to track the number of AIDS deaths. Each year, the number of deaths climbed steadily, reaching a peak of 50,610 in 1995. In 1996, the first full year of widespread HAART therapy, AIDS deaths dropped by 25 percent, and they have continued to decrease every year since. In 2011, an estimated 1.7 million people died of the disease worldwide, down from approximately 2.3 million in 2005. While these statistics are encouraging, about half of all persons with AIDS cannot tolerate the drugs. Moreover, those taking anti-HIV drugs often experience mild to serious side effects.

PERSPECTIVE AND PROSPECTS
AIDS was first recognized as a new disease in the United States in late 1980. Michael Gottlieb at the University of California, Los Angeles (UCLA) diagnosed gay men with *Pneumocystis carinii* pneumonia and Kaposi's sarcoma, diseases that in the past were extremely rare. In June 1981, the CDC alerted doctors in a report on this new epidemic for the first time in the *CDC Weekly Morbidity and Mortality Report*. Shortly afterward, the *New York Times* reported on the new "gay cancer." At first, the disease was called "gay-related immunodeficiency" (GRID). The name was changed to acquired immunodeficiency syndrome, or AIDS, in an August 8, 1982, article in the *New York Times*, representing the first time that the term was used in a publication. The change reflected the fact that this new disease was not restricted to gay men; cases involving intravenous drug users, hemophiliacs, and infants were being diagnosed. In January 1983, Luc Montagnier and colleagues at the Pasteur Institute in Paris were the first to isolate the virus causing AIDS. It was given the name human immunodeficiency virus, or HIV, in 1985; previously, the virus had been given several names by different researchers. With the isolation of the virus, researchers developed a blood test for HIV.

Testing of blood and blood products started in March 1985. A test called "enzyme-linked immunosorbent assay" (ELISA) screens for the presence of anti-HIV antibodies. Results once took weeks, but the test is now automated, takes less than four hours, and costs fewer than ten dollars at publicly supported laboratories.

HIV has been confirmed in the United States since at least 1969. At that time, a physician in St. Louis, Missouri, had a young male patient with several AIDS symptoms. After the patient died, the pathologist took samples of his tissues and froze them. Later, when tests to detect HIV became available, the tissue samples were tested and found positive for HIV. The oldest positively identified HIV sample came from blood collected from a male patient by a Belgian physician in Kinshasa, Democratic Republic of the Congo. The doctor had saved many blood samples taken between 1959 and 1982; thus, the earliest confirmation of HIV infection in Africa dates from 1959. The virus has probably been present in the human population for much longer, but without blood or tissue samples, this cannot be confirmed.

There are two major classes of HIV: HIV-1, which arose in Central Africa, and HIV-2, which arose in Western Africa. HIV-1 and HIV-2 are genetically similar to viruses know as simian immunodeficiency viruses (SIV) in chimpanzees (SIVcmp) and the sooty mangabey monkey (SIVsm). In 2006, scientists determined that in all likelihood, HIV-1 originated in chimpanzees from regions of the nation of Cameroon; as many as one-third of chimpanzees from some colonies were found to carry SIV. The first confirmed human infection was that of a man from the nearby Congo, who developed AIDS in 1959. However, evidence suggests that HIV may have emerged in humans as early as 1930.

The statistics associated with the AIDS epidemic are startling. In the United States by the end of 2007, an estimated 1.1 million persons were living with AIDS; approximately 14,000 persons died from AIDS during the year. Worldwide numbers only begin to illustrate the extent of the epidemic. The World Health Organization (WHO) estimates that in 2011, more than 2.5 million persons became infected with the virus, with nearly 2 million deaths. Over 3 million newly infected persons are under the age of 15. Nearly 34 million persons worldwide were estimated to be living with AIDS. In the absence of effective treatment, most of those persons will die, often after infecting others with the virus and leave behind a generation of orphans.

It is hoped that several new medications in development will enlarge the arsenal of anti-HIV drugs. The success of HAART promises to extend the life of persons with AIDS by many years. Current studies are testing whether it is better to start HAART therapy early after infection or to wait until T4 counts are declining. Additional studies will determine whether the therapy may be interrupted for varying periods. A significant issue is the high financial burden of such therapy. A typical HAART regimen may cost $1,500 to $2,000 per month. Although many people in affluent countries can purchase these drugs through insurance providers or government subsidies, this financial burden precludes the use of HAART or indeed almost any anti-HIV drug in the developing world, where HIV prevalence is so high. Thus, effective prevention of HIV infections, through vigorous public education about HIV and AIDS, is critical. Such a program in Uganda dramatically reduced the incidence of HIV infections, showing the effectiveness of public education campaigns. In 2009, WHO reported that since the 2001 United Nations Declaration of Commitment on HIV/AIDS, treatment and education have reduced the rate of new infections by 17 percent worldwide. In 2011, the UN General Assembly adopted a new declaration, setting new targets in the global fight against HIV/AIDS.

—*Ralph R. Meyer, PhD, Richard Adler, PhD, and Michael A. Buratovich, PhD*

Further Information

Behrman, Greg. *The Invisible People: How the U.S. Has Slept Through the Global AIDS Pandemic, the Greatest Humanitarian Catastrophe of Our Time*. Free Press, 2004.

Cichocki, Mark. *Living with HIV: A Patient's Guide*. McFarland, 2009.

Ezzell, Carol. "Hope in a Vial: Will There Be an AIDS Vaccine Anytime Soon?" *Scientific American*, vol. 186, June 2002, pp. 38-45.

Fan, Hung Y., Ross F. Conner, and Luis P. Villarreal. *AIDS: Science and Society*. 5th ed., Jones and Bartlett, 2007.

Friedman-Kien, Alvin, and Clay J. Cockerell. *Color Atlas of AIDS*. 2nd ed., Elsevier Health Sciences, 1996.

Matthews, Dawn D., editor. *AIDS Sourcebook*. 3rd ed., Omnigraphics, 2003.

U.S. Department of Health and Human Services. "AIDSInfo, 2013." *MedlinePlus*. "HIV/AIDS." *MedlinePlus*, 30 Apr. 2013

Human immunodeficiency virus (HIV)

Category: Diseases/Disorders
Anatomy or system affected: Immune system
Specialties and related fields: Immunology, microbiology, virology
Definition: A retrovirus that attacks cells of the immune system, leading to a loss of immune function and the development of acquired immunodeficiency syndrome (AIDS).

Key terms

highly active antiretroviral treatment (HAART): a treatment with two or more drugs that stops human immunodeficiency virus (HIV) replication in infected persons

retrovirus: a virus with a ribonucleic acid (RNA) genome that makes a deoxyribonucleic acid (DNA) copy it when it infects cells and inserts it into the host cell's genome

reverse transcriptase: a polynucleotide polymerase that utilizes an RNA template to synthesize a DNA copy of it

CAUSES AND SYMPTOMS

Human immunodeficiency virus (HIV) is a human retrovirus containing two copies of a 9,749-base ri-

> INFORMATION ON
> HUMAN IMMUNODEFICIENCY VIRUS (HIV)
>
> **Causes**: Transmission through the exchange of body fluids (semen, vaginal fluid, blood, human milk)
>
> **Symptoms**: Flulike or mononucleosis-like symptoms upon initial transmission; later, various opportunistic infections
>
> **Duration**: Chronic, eventually fatal
>
> **Treatments**: Highly active antiretroviral therapy (HAART) with nucleoside or nucleotide analogs, reverse transcriptase inhibitors, protease inhibitors, inhibitors of cellular entry

bonucleic acid (RNA) molecule as its genetic material. Among the proteins carried by retrovirus particles is an enzyme called "reverse transcriptase," which transcribes the RNA genome into a deoxyribonucleic acid (DNA) copy upon infection of the cell. The DNA copy then integrates into a human chromosome and is maintained in a form called a "provirus." The provirus acts as a template to produce copies of the HIV RNA genome. Once the provirus has integrated, the infection is irreversible.

HIV falls into the subgroup of lentiviruses called "slow viruses" that do not cause a disease state until many years after infection. For example, the time between HIV infection and the development of disease averages between five and ten years in untreated persons. Despite the absence of symptoms, the person may be infectious during this period.

There are two forms of HIV: HIV-1, which arose in central Africa, is the predominant form throughout most of the world, including the United States; HIV-2, a less common form found in western Africa, is less harmful and reproduces more slowly. These viruses evolved from related agents called "simian immunodeficiency viruses" (SIV) in apes and monkeys. HIV-1 is believed to have arisen from SIV found in chimpanzees in either the Republic of the Congo or Cameroon. In contrast, HIV-2 is believed

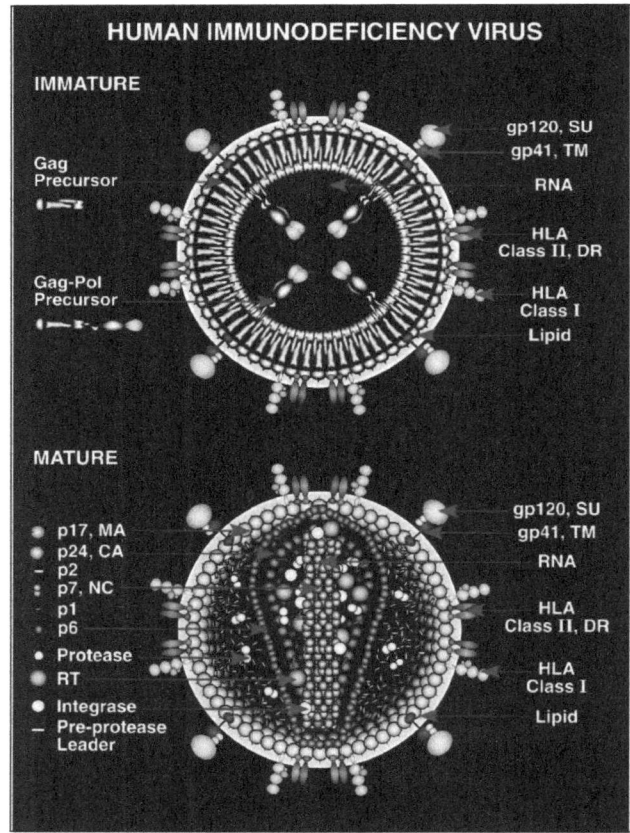

Diagram of the immature and mature forms of HIV. Image via Wikimedia Commons. [Public domain.]

to have arisen from SIV of the Sooty Mangabey monkey of western Africa.

HIV is transmitted only through exchanging body fluids, including semen, vaginal fluid, blood, and human milk. Therefore, the primary routes are sexual transmission, the use of dirty needles by intravenous drug users, and HIV-positive mother-to-child transmission during childbirth or from HIV-contaminated breast milk. Transmission through dirty needles used in body piercing or tattooing may occur. Early in the acquired immunodeficiency syndrome (AIDS) epidemic, infection was also acquired through the transfusion of contaminated blood or blood products, leading to a very high transmission rate to hemophiliacs. Today, such transmission is infrequent, as the blood supply is routinely tested for HIV.

TREATMENT AND THERAPY

The lack of fidelity associated with replication of HIV results in a high number of mutations, making it difficult for the immune system of the infected host to respond as it would to infections by other viruses. Consequently, no effective vaccine to prevent infection with HIV has been developed. The Food and Drug Administration (FDA) has approved some two dozen drugs to treat HIV infection; more are in clinical trials. These drugs fall into four categories: nucleoside or nucleotide analogs, which act as direct inhibitors of reverse transcriptase; inhibitors that in-

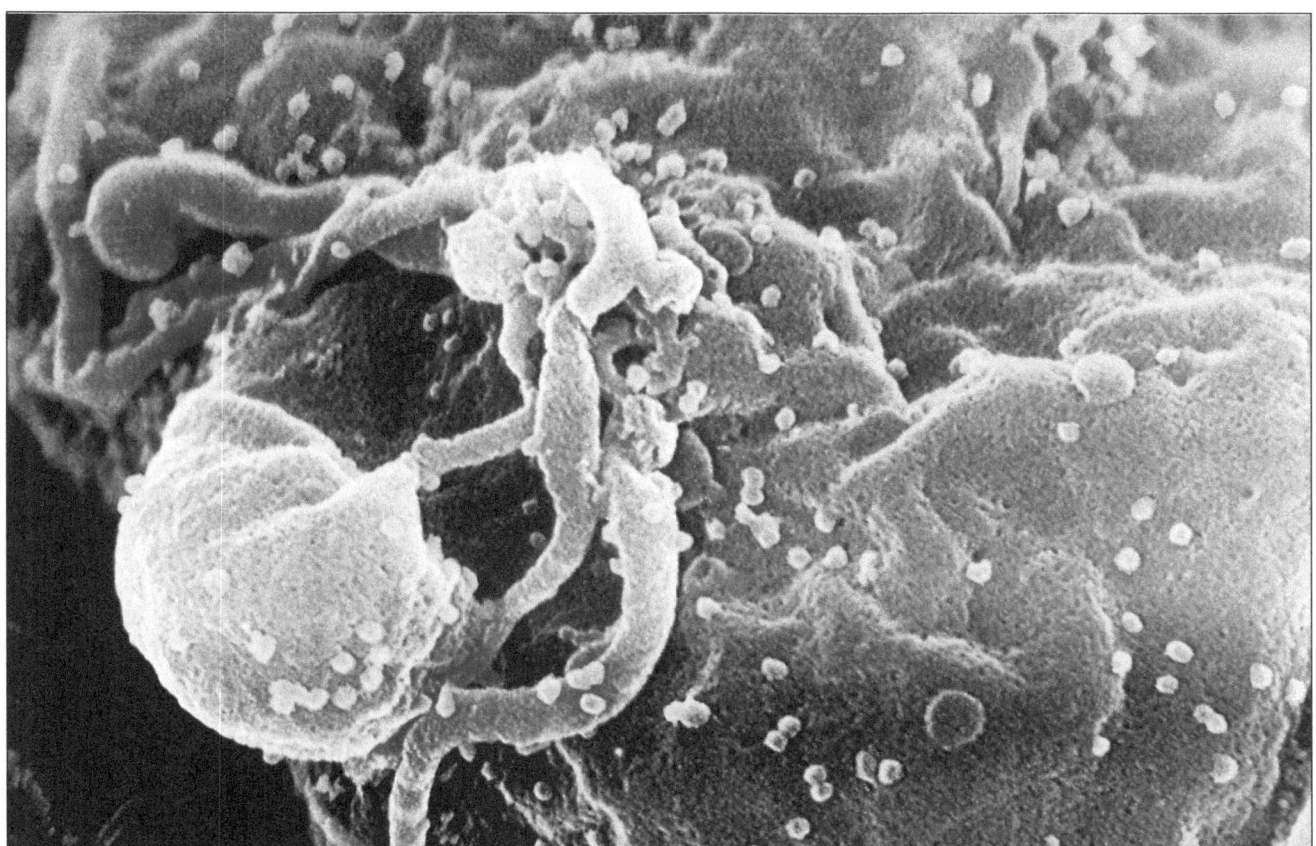

Scanning electron micrograph of HIV-1 (in green) budding from cultured lymphocyte. Multiple round bumps on cell surface represent sites of assembly and budding of virions. Photo via Wikimedia Commons. [Public domain.]

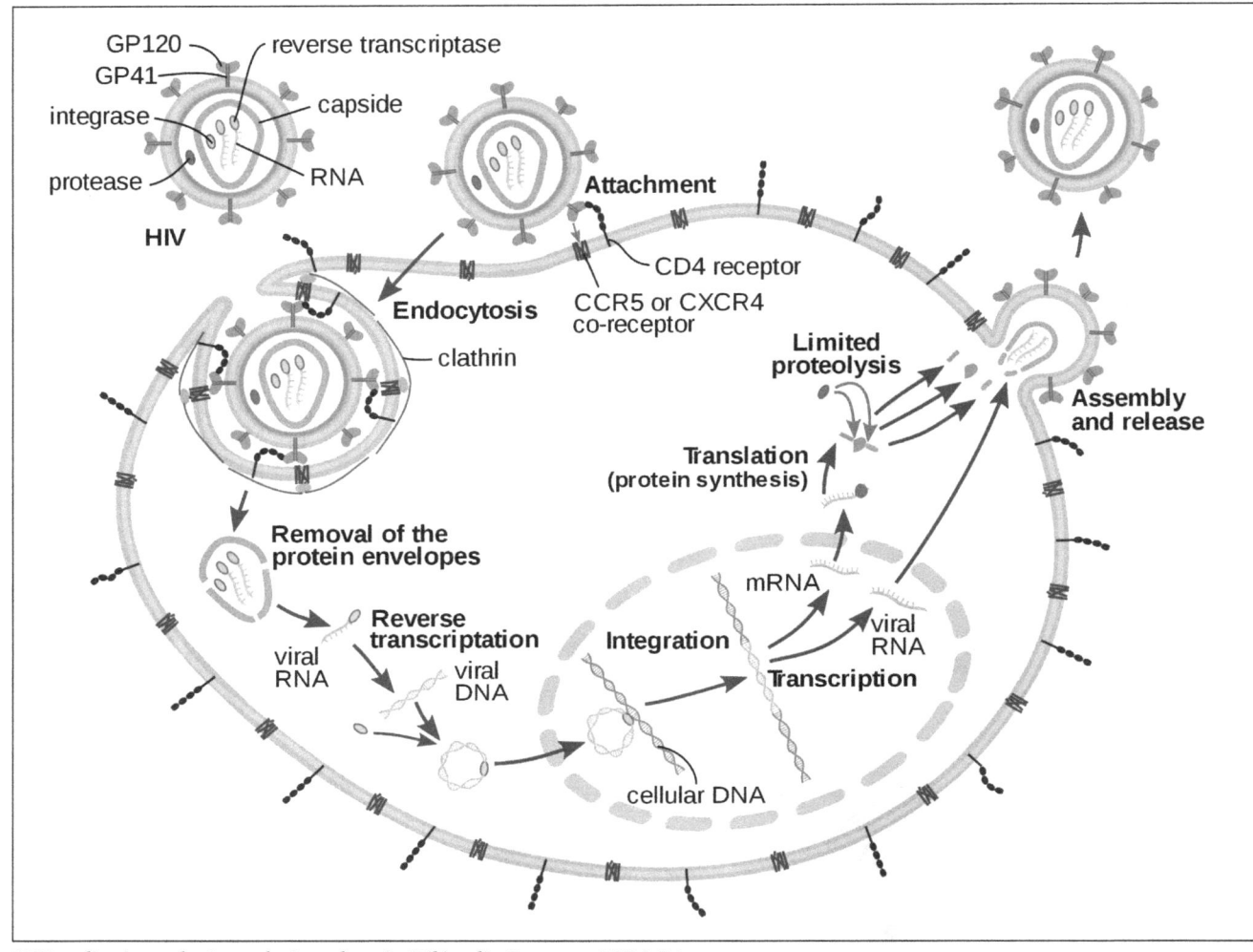

HIV replication cycle. Image by Jmarchn, via Wikimedia Commons. [CC 3.0.]

directly inhibit reverse transcriptase by binding to the enzyme; protease inhibitors that interfere with the processing of HIV proteins and assembly of progeny viruses; and inhibitors of HIV entry into cells.

Because the virus has a very high rate of mutation, resistance to individual anti-HIV drugs may appear quickly. Current therapy, called "highly active antiretroviral therapy" (HAART), involves using three or four anti-HIV drugs simultaneously. HAART therapy also termed "cocktail therapy," increases efficacy and reduces the probability of developing simultaneous resistance of HIV to all three or four drugs being used.

—*Ralph R. Meyer, PhD and Richard Adler, PhD*

Further Information

Fan, Hung, Ross F. Conner, and Luis P. Villarreal. *The Biology of AIDS*. 4th ed., Jones and Bartlett, 2000.

Farnan, Rose, and Maithe Enriquez. *What Nurses Know: HIV/AIDS*. Demos Health, 2012.

Matthews, Dawn D., editor. *AIDS Sourcebook*. 3rd ed., Omnigraphics, 2003.

Sande Merle A., et al. *Sande's HIV/AIDS Medicine: Medical Management of AIDS, 2013*. Elsevier Saunders, 2012.

> **IN THE NEWS:
> EXPERIMENTAL HIV VACCINE**
>
> Despite more than twenty-five years of intensive research—and a global expenditure of more than $6 billion—a vaccine that prevents HIV infection has remained elusive. One notorious trial was halted early when vaccinated subjects suffered an increased risk of infection.
>
> There are many complex reasons that candidate vaccines have proven ineffective. One reason is that the molecules on the virus's surface to which the immune system's antibodies can bind are much more variable than in typical pathogens. The HIV genome, composed of RNA, can accumulate mutations at frequencies up to 100 times higher than genomes composed of DNA like the human genome. Thus, selection pressure due to an immune response against one set of HIV surface molecules will rapidly evolve resistant strains displaying distinct sets of surface molecules. Indeed, multiple highly divergent strains are found in patients in different regions of the globe.
>
> Finally, in September 2009, a U.S.-Thai team of investigators announced the first demonstration of reduced risk of HIV infection after immunization. The study employed a combination of two vaccines that had individually failed to be effective in previous experiments. Low-to-moderate risk HIV-negative volunteers aged eighteen to thirty were given vaccine or placebo injections and subsequently tested for infection every six months for three years. In the control group, 74 of 8,198 subjects were infected by the end of the study; in the vaccinated group, only 51 of 8,197 subjects became infected. Those figures reflect a statistically significant 31.2 percent reduction in the probability of infection after vaccination.
>
> Although the observed effect was encouraging, the results include some caveats. The vaccine combination targets the HIV strain encountered most frequently in Thailand and therefore would not be expected to provide immunity to the strains responsible for most infections in Africa, Europe, North America, and elsewhere. Vaccination had no apparent effect on the severity of infection in subjects who contracted HIV during the study. Lastly, the vaccine's efficacy is far below the 80 percent threshold required for approval for public distribution.
>
> —*Carina Endres Howell, PhD*

Stine, Gerald J. *AIDS Update 2013*. McGraw-Hill Higher Education, 2013.
Strauss, James, and Ellen Strauss. *Viruses and Human Disease*. 2nd ed., Academic Press/Elsevier, 2008.
Weeks, Benjamin S., and Teri Shors. *AIDS: The Biological Basis*. 6th ed., Jones and Bartlett Learning, 2013.

HIV/AIDS-RELATED CANCERS

Category: Diseases, Symptoms, and Conditions; Carcinogens/Suspected Carcinogens
Also known as: acquired immunodeficiency syndrome (AIDS)-associated Kaposi's sarcoma (KS)
Related conditions: Kaposi's sarcoma lymphoma, progressive multifocal leukoencephalopathy (PML)
Anatomy or system affected: All tissues
Specialties and related fields: Dermatology, epidemiology, hematology, immunology, internal medicine, microbiology, neurology, oncology, ophthalmology, otorhinolaryngology, pathology, pharmacology, proctology, pulmonary medicine, virology
Definition: The immunodeficiency associated with advanced human immunodeficiency virus (HIV) disease can give rise to various cancers. HIV infection does not appear to cause cancer directly. However, some researchers have suggested HIV can alter the regulation of certain types of oncogenes.

KEY TERMS

antiretroviral therapy (ART): combinations of drugs that inhibit replication of the human immunodeficiency virus (HIV) and the infection from transitioning to full-blown acquired immune deficiency syndrome (AIDS)
acquired immune deficiency syndrome (AIDS): a chronic, life-threatening condition caused by HIV characterized by the functional collapse of the immune

system and the overwhelming of the human body by opportunistic infections and tumors.

human herpesvirus-8 (HHV-8): a small herpes virus common to human populations that plays a role in the development of Kaposi's sarcoma

intralesional chemotherapy: treatment of small, localized tumors in the skin with focused radiation, the injection of anticancer directly into the tumor, or the application of antitumor gels of the tumor

non-Hodgkin's lymphoma: cancer that starts in the lymphocytes and is most commonly appears in adults

INTRODUCTION

The most common cancer related to acquired immunodeficiency syndrome (AIDS) is Kaposi's sarcoma, a disease that arises from cells of mucous membranes or tissues lining lymphatic vessels. Other cancers observed more frequently among human immunodeficiency virus (HIV)-positive individuals include progressive multifocal leukoencephalopathy (PML), which results from the activation of a human papovavirus; non-Hodgkin's lymphoma; and squamous cell carcinomas. A variety of other forms of tissue-specific cancers, including liver and lung cancers, are also observed with greater frequency among AIDS patients.

RISK FACTORS

The type of HIV-related cancer most likely to develop is a function of the transmission of the virus. Kaposi sarcoma is associated with transmission through sex and is found primarily in gay men. Other forms of AIDS-related cancers result from immunosuppression, particularly the reduced level of CD4+ T-lymphocyte helper cells. Intravenous drug users, hemophiliacs, and those who engage in unprotected sex (especially with multiple partners) are at high risk of contracting HIV. They are not limited to those infected with HIV through sexual means.

ETIOLOGY AND THE DISEASE PROCESS

Both Kaposi's sarcoma and progressive multifocal leukoencephalopathy have a viral etiology. Since Kaposi's sarcoma is most commonly found in gay men rather than among HIV-positive hemophiliacs or in populations of intravenous drug abusers, HIV researchers long suspected it was a sexually transmitted disease with a viral etiology. In 1994, a newly discovered agent, later termed "human herpesvirus-8" (HHV-8), was determined to cause HIV-related Kaposi's sarcoma. While the virus is relatively common, it appears to replicate in the white cell population of immunosuppressed individuals, eventually triggering the development of Kaposi's sarcoma. The increased diagnosis of Kaposi's sarcoma in people with an immune system weakened by mechanisms other than AIDS lends support to the hypothesis.

The induction of Kaposi's sarcoma in AIDS patients results from an interaction between the two viruses,

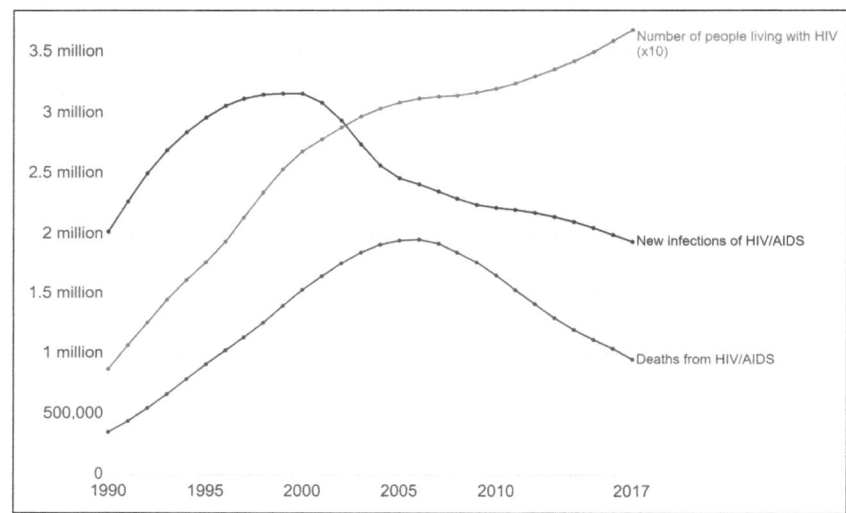

HIV/AIDS new cases and deaths per year, 1990–2017. By Our World in Data, via Wikimedia. [CC4.0.]

HIV and HHV-8. Among the gene products produced by HIV is a transactivation protein, TAT, which acts to induce endothelial cell growth. HHV-8, in turn, encodes several cytokines that likewise stimulate cell division within the skin. At the same time, angiogenesis factors are produced that induce blood-vessel production within the developing tumor. The result is a substantial blood supply that produces the purplish lesions common in Kaposi's sarcoma. Kaposi's sarcoma is more common in men than in women, suggesting that hormonal factors may also play a role in the process.

Several forms of lymphomas, either non-Hodgkin's lymphomas (NHL) or, less commonly, Hodgkin's disease, represent the second most common type of AIDS-related cancers. Although viruses cause some lymphomas, including Hodgkin's disease, the actual cause of most lymphomas remains unknown. In some cases, the underlying cause is mutations within specific oncogenes.

A member of the human papovirus family, the Jamestown Canyon (JC) virus, carried by many individuals within the central nervous system, causes PML. PML resulting from JC infection is rare, limited almost entirely to persons with a defective immune system. The mechanism of JC virus activation remains unclear, but immune system suppression increases PML risk. Treatments for multiple sclerosis, including natalizumab, cause "iatrogenic PML." It seems that persistent surveillance by the immune system prevents JC reactivation and inhibiting aspects of immune surveillance reactivates it.

INCIDENCE

Approximately 40 percent of persons with advanced HIV disease will develop cancer. The most common form is Kaposi's sarcoma, developing in some 20 percent of HIV-infected persons. Before the AIDS epidemic in the 1970s, the Kaposi's sarcoma incidence within the population of the United States was about 0.3 per 100,000 people. The incidence peaked nationally at 8.9 per 100,000 by the end of the 1980s, as high as 32 per 100,000 in cities such as San Francisco. Since then, Kaposi's sarcoma numbers have decreased, the result of the introduction of antiretroviral therapy and the decrease in numbers of individuals newly infected with HIV. In San Francisco, for example, the incidence of Kaposi's sarcoma had dropped to a level of 2.8 per 100,000 by the year 2000. The number of people affected by Kaposi's sarcoma remains high in Africa and Asia, where HIV infection remains common and treatment is minimal.

As with Kaposi's sarcoma, the incidence of lymphomas showed a significant increase in the 1980s due to the AIDS epidemic. The incidence of non-Hodgkin's lymphomas rose from a level of 10.7 per 100,000 in the mid-1970s to a peak of 31.4 per 100,000 in the mid-1990s. The introduction of antiretroviral therapy and a leveling and reduction in the numbers of new cases of HIV infection resulted in a decline of such lymphomas to 21.6 per 100,000 by the end of the twentieth century.

A study examined the Kaposi's sarcoma rates of more than 375,000 AIDS patients from 1980 to 2002. During this period, the Kaposi's sarcoma rates in AIDS patients declined sixfold. The advent of improved ART drove the incidence of Kaposi's sarcoma even lower. Other extensive epidemiologic studies discovered similar decreases that strongly correlate with the introduction of improved ART.

About 5 percent of HIV-positive persons are estimated to develop progressive multifocal leukoencephalopathy. The actual incidence is unclear because diagnosis is often made during the autopsy, resulting in a likely underreporting of the precise number.

SYMPTOMS

Kaposi's sarcoma, associated with AIDS, is a particularly aggressive form of the disease. A spreading purplish lesion is often the first indication of

Kaposi's sarcoma, mainly if the individual is HIV-positive. Lymphomas usually begin as lumps or tumors in lymph nodes, with confirmation based on biopsy. Evidence for progressive multifocal leukoencephalopathy is symptomatic, based on evidence of neurological deterioration: mental disturbances, ataxia, and loss of speech, sight, and other senses.

SCREENING AND DIAGNOSIS
A preliminary diagnosis of Kaposi's sarcoma depends on the appearance of purplish lesions. A histological examination of biopsy material confirms the diagnosis. The staging system for Kaposi's sarcoma differs from that for other cancers that define a stage based on cancer metastasis. Staging of Kaposi's sarcoma attempts to consider the extent of immunosuppression as well as the characteristics of the sarcoma by using three criteria: the size or extent of the tumor (T), the level of CD4 cells (I), and the extent of illness (S). Each category has two subgroups, 0 (good risk) or 1 (poor risk).

Diagnosis of the type of non-Hodgkin's lymphoma requires the pathologist to identify the "appropriate" cell from biopsy material. To stage the tumor, pathologists use the Ann Arbor system:
- Stage I: Cancer is limited to a single site or organ and has not spread.
- Stage II: Cancer is limited to two lymph node groups or organs in the same region but has begun to spread.
- Stage III: Cancer is in two lymph node groups with possible involvement of an organ.
- Stage IV: Cancer has spread beyond the initial site.

TREATMENT AND THERAPY
Since the development of AIDS-related cancer results from the immunosuppression that follows HIV infection, any form of chemical treatment is carried out in conjunction with reversal, even if temporary, of the immunosuppressive state. Treatment of the immunosuppressive state involves a combination of drug cocktails—highly active antiretroviral therapy (HAART)—that do not cure the disease but may inhibit replication of the virus for varying periods.

Treatment of Kaposi's sarcoma depends on the extent of cancer, including whether metastasis has taken place. The combination of HAART with anticancer treatments significantly increases treatment success rates. Intralesional chemotherapy causes regression of small, localized tumors. Intralesional chemotherapy involves the injection of vinblastine into the lesion, radiation therapy for larger local lesions, and topical alitretinoin gel for broad skin surfaces with many lesions. However, Kaposi's sarcoma frequently develops at multiple sites or has already spread by the time of diagnosis, requiring the initial use of anticancer chemotherapeutic agents such as pegylated liposomal doxorubicin or liposomal daunorubicin. These so-called liposomal anthracyclines reliably shrink tumors, diminish swelling, and cause the color of lesions to fade. Response rates range from 30 to 60 percent depending on the trial. After the initial chemotherapeutic treatment, the preferred drug is paclitaxel. This drug, though more toxic than the liposomal anthracyclines, is highly effective against Kaposi's sarcoma tumors. Other agents used to treat systemic Kaposi's sarcoma cases include bleomycin, vinblastine, vincristine, and etoposide. Some agents that hold some future promises are the platelet-derived growth factor and C-kit receptor inhibitor imatinib, the mTOR pathway inhibitors rapamycin and temsirolimus, and the antiangiogenic monoclonal antibody bevacizumab. Combinations of therapy that include drugs to enhance the immune response are also under investigation.

Treatment of non-Hodgkin's lymphoma also depends on reducing the viral load and restoring a level of immune function. Following HAART, radiation or chemotherapy is the preferred treatment.

Generally, chemotherapy uses a combination of drugs—cyclophosphamide, hydroxydoxorubicin/doxorubicin, vincristine (Oncovin), and prednisone (CHOP protocol)—as well as selective combinations. Other treatments have adapted forms of immunotherapy in conjunction with chemotherapy, including the use of monoclonal antibodies, such as the antiCD20 monoclonal antibody, rituximab (Rituxan). A new drug for non-Hodgkin's lymphoma, copanlisib (*Aliqopa*), and a related medicine, idelalisib *(Zydelig),* may change treatment strategies for this condition. These drugs inhibit an enzyme called "phosphatidylinositol 3-kinase" (PI3K) that promotes malignant B cells' proliferation, survival, and motility in non-Hodgkin's lymphoma. Blocking PI3K activity prevents the survival and localization of malignant B cells in lymph nodes. These drugs treat non-Hodgkin's lymphoma after patients failed with standard treatment regimens and may extend the survival of AIDS patients with non-Hodgkin's lymphoma.

Treatment of progressive multifocal leukoencephalopathy is problematic and historically has involved the direct infusion of drugs into the brain. However, HAART treatment, if successful, frequently results in the spontaneous remission of the disease.

PROGNOSIS, PREVENTION, AND OUTCOMES

The prognosis for AIDS-related Kaposi's sarcoma patients is a function of the extent of spread. If caught early and immune function has improved, the recovery rate is high. Once the disease has spread, however, the chances for recovery become increasingly poor. However, Kaposi's sarcoma is a very treatable cancer and, today, few people die from it. Kaposi's sarcoma responds to the available treatments. The National Cancer Institute reports that the five-year relative survival is about 72 percent.

The likely prognosis of non-Hodgkin's lymphoma is based on the International Prognostic Index, which considers factors such as age, the stage of the disease, and the extent of overall general health, including the state of immunosuppression. If all factors are optimal, especially the level of immune function, approximately 75 percent of patients survive five years or more.

Prognosis in progressive multifocal leukoencephalopathy patients remains poor. Before the development of HAART, 90 percent of patients died within three months of diagnosis. Even in the presence of therapy, the mortality rate remains approximately 50 percent within several months of diagnosis.

—*Richard Adler, PhD and Michael A. Buratovich, PhD*

Further Information
Cockerell, Clay, and Alvin Friedman-Kien. *Color Atlas of AIDS*. W. B. Saunders, 1996.
"Copanlisib (*Aliqopa*) for Relapsed Follicular Lymphoma." *Medical Letter on Drugs and Therapeutics*, vol. 60, no. 1545, 2018, pp. 74-75.
Engels E. A., et al. "Trends in Cancer Risk Among People with AIDS in the United States 1980-2002." *AIDS*, vol. 20, no. 12, 2006, p. 1645.
Feigal, Ellen, et al., editors. *AIDS-Related Cancers and Their Treatment*. Marcel Dekker, 2000.
"Global HIV & AIDS Statistics—Fact Sheet." *UNAIDS*, 2021, www.unaids.org/en/resources/fact-sheet. Accessed 5 Sept. 2021
Pelengaris, Stella, and Michael Khan, editors. *The Molecular Biology of Cancer*. Blackwell, 2006.
Stine, Gerald. *AIDS Update: 2007*. McGraw-Hill, 2007.

KAPOSI'S SARCOMA

Category: Diseases/Conditions
Anatomy or system affected: Blood, lymphatic system, mouth, nose, skin, throat
Specialties and related fields: Dermatology, hematology, immunology, internal medicine, microbiology, oncology, otorhinolaryngology, pathology, virology

Definition: A cancer that develops from cells that line lymph or blood vessels. Tumors typically appear on the skin or mucosal surfaces such as inside the mouth, but they can also develop in other parts of the body, such as in the lymph nodes, lungs, or digestive tract.

KEY TERMS

human herpesvirus-8 (HHV-8): The virus that causes Kaposi's sarcoma
iatrogenic: a condition caused by healthcare-based interventions
titer: antibody or viral particle concentration

INTRODUCTION

Kaposi's sarcoma (KS), first described by the Hungarian dermatologist Moritz Kaposi in 1872, is a cancer of the endothelium of lymphatic and blood vessels. It commonly manifests as a series of lesions under the skin and in the lining of the mouth, nose, and throat. The lesions appear as purple, red, or brown blotches. KS can also result in lesions of the gastrointestinal tract, lungs, and liver.

There are several types of KS, which are defined by the population affected: classic KS, which is seen primarily in older men of Mediterranean, Eastern European, or Middle Eastern origin; epidemic KS, which is seen in persons with acquired immunodeficiency syndrome (AIDS); African KS, which is endemic to equatorial Africa and affects mostly men under age forty years; Iatrogenic or transplant-associated KS, which is seen in immune-suppressed persons who have had transplants; and nonepidemic-related KS, a rarer type of KS that is seen in men who test negative for human immunodeficiency virus (HIV) and who have sex with men.

CAUSES

Kaposi's sarcoma is caused by the human herpesvirus-8 (HHV-8), which is also known as Kaposi's sarcoma-associated herpesvirus (KSHV). Approximately 1 to 5 percent of the U.S. population carries the virus.

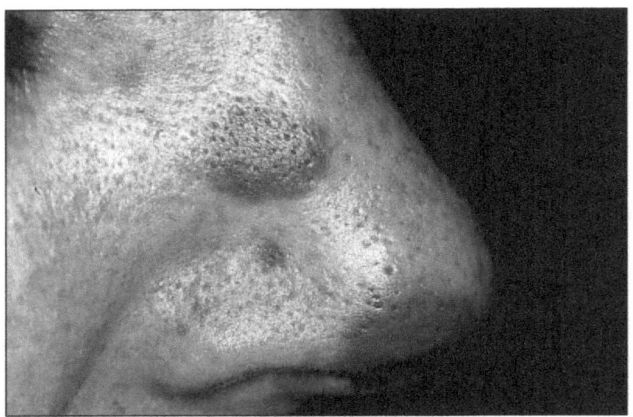

An HIV+ woman with characteristic lesions on the alar and tip of nose, signifying Kaposi's sarcoma. Photo by M. Sand, D. Sand, C. Thrandorf, V. Paech, P. Altmeyer, F. G. Bechara, via Wikimedia Commons.

RISK FACTORS

The greatest risk factor in developing KS is being HHV-8 positive (and, thus, immunosuppressed). Most cases do not progress to KS unless the carrier is also immunosuppressed because of HIV infection (persons who are HIV-positive have about a 50 percent chance of developing KS), organ transplantation (iatrogenic KS), or aging (classic KS). The HHV-8 virus is sexually transmitted, but virus titers are highest in saliva and may be transmitted through deep kissing.

SYMPTOMS

The appearance of colored skin blotches is the typical KS symptom. The skin form may cause edema, especially of the legs, because of lymphatic blockage. Shortness of breath is found in cases involving the lungs. Cases involving the gastrointestinal (GI) system will show weight loss, nausea, vomiting, and rectal bleeding.

SCREENING AND DIAGNOSIS

A skin examination for typical KS lesions and asexual history is the most common method of diagnosis. Cytological examination of a skin biopsy can confirm diagnosis. For lung involvement, a doctor will order X rays and a bronchoscopy with biopsy. Suspected GI cases are checked through occult blood testing and a rectal examination, followed by an endoscopy and a biopsy to confirm the GI diagnosis.

TREATMENT AND THERAPY

Treatment for KS focuses on the underlying immune deficiency. In persons with HIV/AIDS, treatment will include highly active antiretroviral therapy (HAART), in which three or more anti-HIV drugs are used simultaneously. KS skin lesions are reduced and may disappear. In persons who have received a transplant, an effective treatment is to reduce the level of immune suppressive drugs already being taken by the transplant recipient. Surgery is possible when only a few small lesions are present, and often, the doctor will order cryosurgery.

Local treatment with alitretinoin has good results for some persons. Intralesion injection of chemotherapy agents, such as vinblastine, has also been used. When widespread lesions are present, systemic chemotherapy can be employed with liposomal anthracyclines (doxorubicin or daunorubicin). Other agents (bleomycin, etoposide, vincristine, vinblastine, paclitaxel, and etoposide) may also be used. Electron-beam radiation therapy has been effective on facial lesions. Experimental treatments include angiogenesis inhibitors and interferon alpha.

PREVENTION AND OUTCOMES

Avoiding HIV infection is the most effective way to prevent the development of KS. Preventive methods include maintaining a strong and healthy immune system, practicing safer sex (such as using condoms during sexual intercourse) or abstaining from sex, and avoiding intravenous drug use, especially if it involves using shared needles.

—*Ralph R. Meyer, PhD*

Further Information
Brown, Elizabeth E., et al. "Virologic, Hematologic, and Immunologic Risk Factors for Classic Kaposi Sarcoma." *Cancer*, vol. 107, no. 9, 2006, pp. 2282-90.
Di Lorenzo, Giuseppe, et al. "Management of AIDS-Related Kaposi's Sarcoma." *Lancet Oncology*, vol. 8, 2007, pp. 167-76.
Galanda, Claudia D., editor. *AIDS-Related Opportunistic Infections*. Nova Biomedical Books, 2009.
Ganem, Don. "KSHV Infection and the Pathogenesis of Kaposi's Sarcoma." *Annual Review of Pathology*, vol. 1, 2006, pp. 273-96.
Murphy, Kenneth, Paul Travers, and Mark Walport. *Janeway's Immunobiology*. 7th ed., Garland Science, 2008.
Parker, James N., and Philip M. Parker, editors. *The Official Patient's Sourcebook on Kaposi's Sarcoma*. Icon Health, 2003.

KAWASAKI DISEASE

Category: Diseases/Disorders
Also known as: Kawasaki syndrome, mucocutaneous lymph node syndrome (MLNS)
Anatomy or system affected: Brain, blood vessels, circulatory system, heart, immune system, lymphatic system, mouth, skin
Specialties and related fields: Cardiology, family medicine, immunology, pediatrics
Definition: An inflammatory disease that affects numerous organs and systems in the body and typically occurs in children under five.

KEY TERMS

electrocardiogram: a test that measures the electrical activity of the heart
gamma-globulin: a fraction of human blood that contains antibodies that protect against disease

CAUSES AND SYMPTOMS

The exact cause of Kawasaki disease is unknown. Approximately 80 percent of the victims are aged five and under. Some doctors believe that the disease

> **INFORMATION ON KAWASAKI DISEASE**
>
> **Causes**: Unknown; possibly allergic reaction, viral or bacterial infection, or immune system response
>
> **Symptoms**: High fever; patchy rash; red lips, mouth, tongue, and throat; swollen lymph nodes in the neck; swollen hands and feet; diarrhea; vomiting; stomach pain; joint pain; irritability; peeling skin on fingers and toes
>
> **Duration**: Two weeks to three months; long-term heart damage possible
>
> **Treatments**: Aspirin, gamma-globulin

may be an allergic reaction to certain types of infection. Others think that a virus or bacterium produces it. Some researchers believe that the source is an interaction of T cells, white blood cells that help regulate the immune system's response to infections, with toxins produced by bacteria.

Kawasaki disease begins abruptly with a fever that persists for five days or longer and can reach 104 degrees Fahrenheit. A red, patchy rash typically spreads over the chest and genital area and may cover the entire body. The lips, mouth, tongue, and throat become very red. The lymph nodes in the neck may be swollen, as well as the hands and feet. The hands, feet, eyes, and mucous membrane linings of the eyelids turn red. These symptoms may be accompanied by diarrhea, vomiting, stomach pain, joint pain, and irritability. As the fever subsides, there is a characteristic peeling of the skin from the fingers and toes. The symptoms associated with Kawasaki disease may last for two weeks up to three months.

TREATMENT AND THERAPY

A patient diagnosed with Kawasaki disease should seek treatment as soon as possible. Their doctor can prescribe several different valuable medications. Aspirin can reduce fever, ease joint pain, and relieve the rash. Parents should consult their family physician about the risk of Reyes syndrome before giving aspirin to children and teens. Gamma-globulin, purified antibodies found in blood, is administered intravenously to help fight infection and reduce the risk of developing coronary artery abnormalities or damage to the heart muscle. Suppose the disease is treated within ten days of its onset. In that case, less than 20 percent of the patients experience any heart problems.

A doctor may order an electrocardiogram (ECG or EKG), chest radiograph, and echocardiogram to monitor heart functions. If liver or gallbladder malfunction occurs, then ultrasonic imaging of those organs may be necessary.

PERSPECTIVE AND PROSPECTS

Tomisaku Kawasaki first identified Kawasaki disease in 1967 when he reported the symptoms in fifty children in cases occurring between 1961 and 1967. Epidemics occurred in Japan in 1979, 1982, and 1985. In children under five, the disease has become the leading cause of acquired heart disease in the United States. About three thousand children are hospitalized with Kawasaki disease annually in the

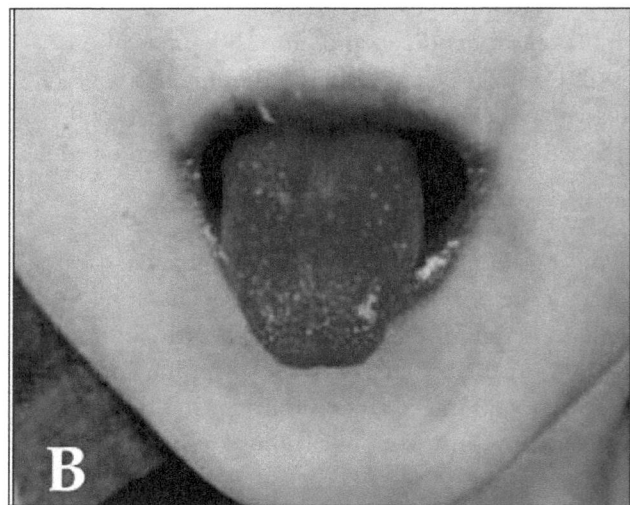

Kawasaki disease: Strawberry tongue and bright red, swollen lips with vertical cracking and bleeding. Photo by Dong Soo Kim, via Wikimedia Commons. [CC 2.0.]

United States. Death from heart-related problems related to Kawasaki disease occurs in less than 2 percent of the victims. Less than 2 percent of children who experience Kawasaki disease have a reoccurrence.

—*Alvin K. Benson, PhD*

Further Information
Hawker, Jeremy, et al. *Communicable Disease Control Handbook.* 2nd ed., Blackwell, 2006.
MedlinePlus. "Kawasaki Disease." *MedlinePlus,* 19 May 2013.
Parker, James N., and Philip M. Parker. *Kawasaki Disease: A Bibliography, Medical Dictionary, and Annotated Research Guide to Internet References.* ICON Health, 2004.
Powell, Michael, and Oliver Fischer. *101 Diseases You Don't Want to Get.* Thunder's Mouth Press, 2005.
Safer, Diane A. "Kawasaki Disease." *Health Library,* 26 Nov. 2012.

Leukemia

Category: Diseases/Disorders
Anatomy or system affected: Blood, bone marrow, circulatory system, lymph nodes, spleen
Specialties and related fields: Hematology, internal medicine, oncology, serology, toxicology
Definition: A family of cancers that affect the blood, characterized by an increased number of, often abnormal, white blood cells.

KEY TERMS

anthracyclines: a class of anticancer drugs that are effective against a broad range of different types of cancer and derived from molecules synthesized by members of the bacterial genus *Streptomyces*
blast cell: an immature dividing cell
bone marrow: the tissue within bones that produces blood cells; in children, all bones have active marrow, but in adults, blood cell production occurs only in the trunk
bone marrow transplant: the removal of bone marrow from an immunologically matched individual for infusion into a patient whose bone marrow has been destroyed
chemotherapy: the use of drugs to kill rapidly growing cancer cells; this treatment will also kill some normal cells, producing undesirable side effects
cytopenia: a condition in which the production of one or more types of blood cells either stops or is significantly reduced
granulocytes: white blood cells that generally help to fight bacterial infection; these cells can pass from the blood capillaries into damaged tissues
hematopoiesis: the process by which blood cells develop in the bone marrow; this maturation is regulated by specific molecules called growth factors
immune system: the cells and organs of the body that fight infection; destruction of these cells leaves the body vulnerable to numerous diseases
lymphocytes: white blood cells that specifically target a foreign organism for destruction; the two classes of lymphocytes are B cells, which produce antibodies, and T cells, which kill infected cells
oncogenes: genes found in every cell that can cause cancer if activated or mutated
Philadelphia chromosome: a translocation, or swap of parts, between nonhomologous chromosomes 9 and 22 that generates a fusion between the *ABL* and *BCR* genes; the resultant BCR-ABL gene product is an unregulated protein kinase that drives cells to divide uncontrollably.
T cells: one of the two subclasses of lymphocytes, distinguished by the exacting developmental program they undergo within the thymus gland before their release into the bloodstream, where they actively participate in the immune response

CAUSES AND SYMPTOMS

Blood is essential for all the physiological processes of the body. It is composed of red cells called "erythrocytes," white cells called leukocytes, and platelets, each of which has distinct functions. Erythrocytes, which contain hemoglobin, are essential for transporting oxygen from the lungs to all the cells and organs of the body. Leukocytes are essential for protecting the body against infection by bacteria, viruses, and other parasites. Platelets play a role in the formation of blood clots; therefore, these cells are critical in the process of wound healing.

Blood cell formation, or hematopoiesis, begins in the bone marrow with immature stem cells that can produce all three types of blood cells. Under the influence of particular proteins called "growth factors," and other small proteins called "cytokines," these stem cells divide rapidly and form blast cells that differentiate into one of the three blood cell types. After several further divisions, these blast cells ultimately mature into fully functional erythrocytes, leukocytes, and platelets. In a healthy individual, each type of blood cell remains relatively constant within a specific range. For example, the normal number of leukocytes in blood cell range from 4,300 to 10,800 cells per cubic millimeter, and the normal number of erythrocytes ranges from 4.2 to 5.9 million cells per cubic millimeter. Thus, the rate of new cell production is approximately equivalent to the rate of old cell destruction and removal.

Mature leukocytes are the key players in defending the body against infection. There are three types of leukocytes: monocytes, granulocytes, and lymphocytes. In leukemia, leukocytes multiply at an increased rate, resulting in an abnormally high number of white cells, a significant proportion of which

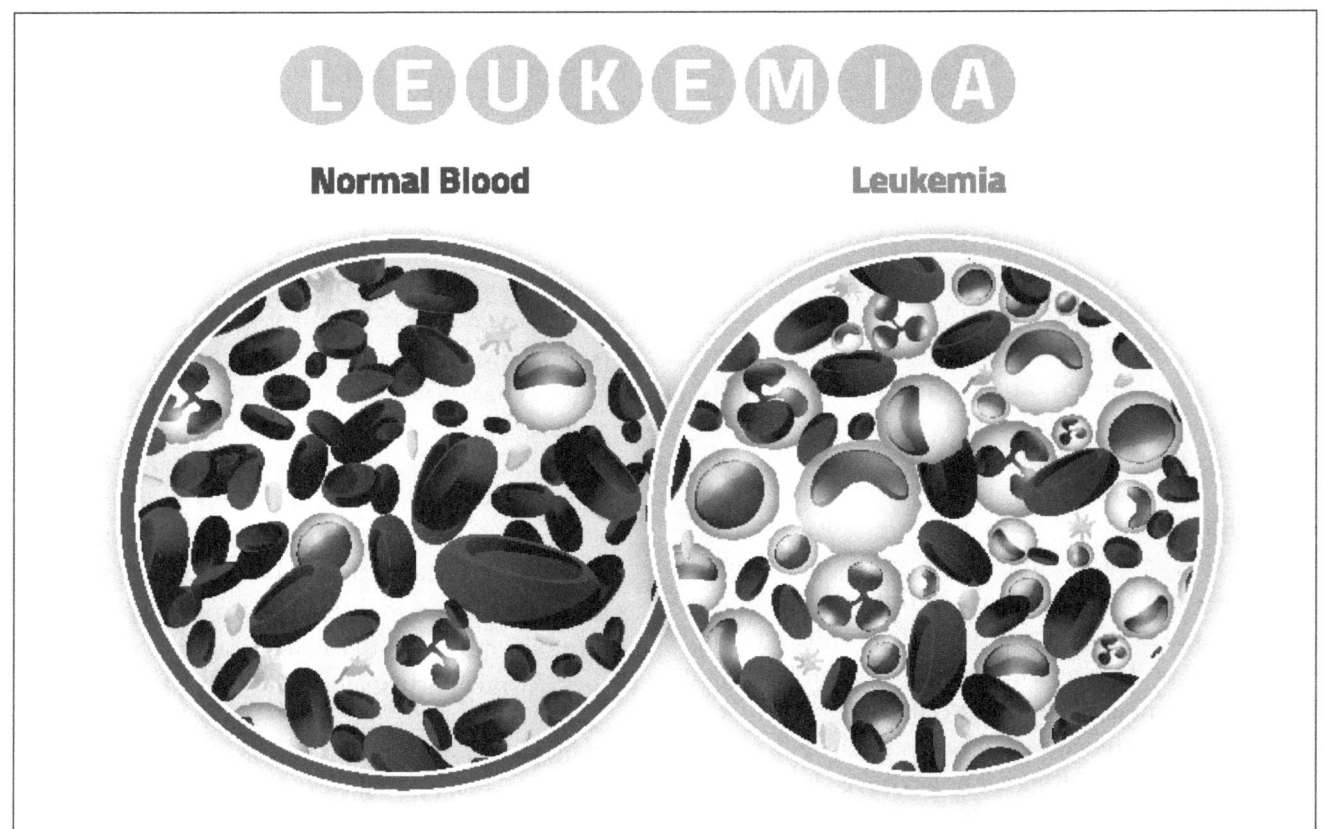

Leukemia. Image via iStock.com/newannyart. [Used under license.]

are immature. This abnormally regulated growth characterizes all forms of leukemia; therefore, leukemia is cancer, even though tumor masses typically do not form. The cancerous cells live longer than the normal leukocytes and accumulate first in the bone marrow and then in the blood. These abnormal cells crowd the bone marrow, preventing normal hematopoiesis in a person with leukemia. The patient will usually become weak because of the lack of oxygen-carrying red cells and susceptible to bleeding because of platelet deficiencies. The abnormal leukocytes do not function effectively in defending the body against infection, and they prevent normal leukocytes from developing; therefore, the patient is immunologically compromised. In addition, once the abnormal cells accumulate in the blood, they may hinder the functioning of other organs, such as the liver, kidney, lungs, and spleen.

There are four main types of leukemia, and they are classified according to the type of leukocyte they affect and the maturity of the leukocytes observed in the blood and the bone marrow. Both lymphocytes and granulocytes can be affected. When the cells are mainly immature blasts, the leukemia is termed "acute," and when the cells are primarily mature, the leukemia is termed "chronic." Therefore, the four types of leukemia are acute lymphocytic (ALL), acute myelogenous (AML), chronic lymphocytic (CLL), and chronic myelogenous (CML). The myelogenous leukemias are also known, less commonly, as granulocytic leukemias (AGL, CGL) or nonlymphoid leukemias (ANLL, CNLL). These are the main types of leukemia, although there are additional rarer forms. These four forms of leukemia account for about 5 percent of the cancer cases in the United States. The incidence of acute and chronic forms is approximately equivalent, but specific forms are more common at different stages of life. The major form of leukemia in children is ALL, but after puberty, there is a higher incidence of AML. Chronic leukemia occurs in the adult population af-

> **INFORMATION ON LEUKEMIA**
>
> **Causes**: Unclear; possibly environmental and genetic factors
>
> **Symptoms:** Mild cold symptoms; fever; enlargement of lymph nodes, spleen, and liver; fatigue; paleness; weight loss; repeated infections; increased susceptibility to bleeding and bruising
>
> **Duration:** Acute or chronic with recurrent episodes
>
> **Treatments:** Chemotherapy, bone marrow transplantation

ter the fourth or fifth decade of life, and men are twice as likely to be affected as women.

The causes of leukemia are still not completely understood, but scientists have put together many pieces of the puzzle. Several environmental factors increase the risk of developing leukemia. Among these are exposure to radiation, chemicals such as chloramphenicol and benzene, and possibly viruses. In addition, there is a significant genetic component to this disease. Siblings of patients with leukemia have a higher risk of developing the disease, and chromosomal changes occur in the cells of most patients. However, they disappear when the patient is in remission. For example, the genetic basis of certain forms of CML is an exchange of chromosomal material (translocation) between chromosome 22 and chromosome 9; the shortened chromosome 22 is the "Philadelphia chromosome." These different "causes" can be linked by understanding how oncogenes function. As part of their genome, every person has several protooncogenes that drive cell proliferation and, if altered, can cause cancer. In a healthy person, these protooncogenes function carefully to drive cell growth under tightly controlled conditions. After exposure to an environmental or genetic influence that causes mutations or gross chromosomal abnormalities, alteration in protooncogenes may become activate or deregulate them so that they become oncogenes. Oncogenes encode unregulated proteins that drive cell growth in an uncontrolled manner. The expression of oncogenes in blood cells drives uninhibited cell growth, which results in the abnormally high number of blood cells observed in leukemia. The translocation that creates the Philadelphia chromosome makes an abnormal oncogene (*BCR-ABL*) that encodes a protein that upregulates cell division.

Leukemia is often challenging to diagnose early because more common or less severe diseases cause the symptoms. "Flu-like" symptoms, sometimes accompanied by fever, may be the earliest evidence of acute leukemia; in children, the first symptoms may be less pronounced. The symptoms quickly become more pronounced as white cells accumulate in the lymph nodes, spleen, and liver, causing these organs to become enlarged. Fatigue, paleness, weight loss, repeated infections, and increased susceptibility to bleeding and bruising are associated with leukemia. As the disease progresses, the fatigue and bleeding increase, various skin disorders develop, and the joints become painfully swollen. If untreated, the afflicted individual will die within a few months. Chronic leukemia has a more gradual progression and may be present for years before symptoms develop. When symptoms are present, they may be vague feelings of fatigue, fever, or energy loss. There may be enlarged lymph nodes in the neck and armpits and a feeling of fullness in the abdomen because of an increase in the size of the spleen as much as tenfold. Loss of appetite and sweating at night may be initial symptoms. Often, chronic leukemia eventually leads to a syndrome resembling acute leukemia, which is ultimately fatal.

If these symptoms are present, a doctor will diagnose the presence of leukemia in two stages. First, blood will be drawn, and a blood smear will be analyzed microscopically. The blood smear may show fewer erythrocytes, leukocytes, and platelets than usual and the presence of abnormal cells. However, a blood smear may show only slight abnormalities, and the number of leukemic cells in the blood may not correspond to the extent of the disease in the bone marrow. Further analysis requires a bone marrow biopsy to examine the bone marrow itself. Bone marrow tissue can be obtained by inserting a needle into a bone such as the hip and aspirating a small sample of cells. This bone marrow biopsy, done under local anesthetic on an outpatient basis, is the definitive test for leukemia. Visual examination of the marrow usually reveals many abnormal cells, and biochemical and immunological tests confirm this finding. After a positive diagnosis, a doctor will also examine the cerebrospinal fluid to see if leukemic cells have invaded the central nervous system.

TREATMENT AND THERAPY

The treatment and life expectancy for leukemic patients varies significantly for each of the four types of leukemia. Treatment is designed to destroy all the abnormal cells and produce a complete remission. Complete remission is the phase of recovery when the symptoms of the disease disappear, and no abnormal cells appear in the blood or bone marrow. Unfortunately, a complete remission may be only temporary since a small number of abnormal cells may still exist even though the pathologist cannot find them under the microscope. These can, with time, multiply and repopulate the marrow, causing a relapse of the disease. With repeated relapses, the response to therapy becomes poorer, and the duration of the remissions that follow become shorter. However, most oncologists generally believe that a remission that lasts five years in ALL, eight years in AML, or twelve years in CML may be permanent. Therefore, the goal of leukemia research is to develop ways to prolong remission.

When acute leukemia has been diagnosed, abnormal cells have often spread throughout the bone marrow and into several organs; therefore, surgery and radiation are usually not effective. Treatment programs include chemotherapy or bone marrow transplants, or both. Chemotherapy is usually divided into several phases. In the first, or induction, phase, combinations of drugs destroy all detectable abnormal cells and induce clinical remission. The patient's age and health, and type of cancer all factor into the chemotherapeutic regimen chosen for the patient.

For patients with AML who are younger than 60 years of age, induction involves treatment with two drugs; usually, a seven-day continuous infusion of cytarabine (Cytosar-U) and one to three days of an anthracycline such as daunorubicin (Cerubidine) or idarubicin (Idamycin PFS); this treatment regimen is called the "7 + 3" regimen. Anthracyclines intercalate into deoxyribonucleic acid (DNA) and damage it. Therefore, these drugs kill cells indiscriminately and are somewhat toxic to the heart. If the patient has a weak heart, then fludarabine is substituted for anthracyclines. Sometimes a third drug called cladribine (Leustatin) is included in the induction treatment. If the patient's leukemia results from cells that have a mutation in the *FLT3* gene, then a targeted therapy drug called "midostaurin" (Rydapt) is included.

For child or adolescent patients with ALL, the typical induction cocktail depends upon the type of cancer. For ALL patients whose cancer cells do not have the Philadelphia chromosome, induction therapy includes weekly administration of vincristine (Marqibos/Vincasar PFS) for three to four weeks, daily treatments with corticosteroids (dexamethasone, prednisone, or prednisolone), and L-asparaginase. L-asparaginase is an enzyme made from genetically engineered bacteria that degrades the amino acid asparagine, which starves cancer cells for a critical component of protein synthesis. For high-risk patients, an anthracycline is added. For ALL patients whose cancer cells possess the Philadelphia chromosome (5 percent), tyrosine kinase inhibitors (TKIs) such as imatinib (Gleevec) or dasatinib (Sprycel) are included in their induction regimens. During induction, the patient may need intrathecal chemotherapy (chemotherapeutic agents injected directly into the spinal fluid) to prevent the spread of leukemic cells into the central nervous system. Methotrexate (Trexall, Rasuvo, Otrexup) is typically used, but cytarabine is a potential alternative agent.

Most chemotherapy induction regimens for adult patients with Philadelphia chromosome-negative ALL contain vincristine, a corticosteroid, and an anthracycline. Multiple chemotherapeutic regimens exist. Some protocols add cyclophosphamide (Cytoxan, Neosar), cytarabine, methotrexate, 6-mercaptopurine (Purixan), etoposide (Etopophos, Toposar), teniposide (Vumon) or L-asparaginase. The anti-CD20 monoclonal antibody rituximab (Rituxan) is added to some ALL induction regimens to treat younger adult patients whose cancers possess a cell surface protein called "CD20." Rituximab is a monoclonal antibody that binds the CD20 protein and facilitates the destruction of cells with the CD20 protein on their cell surfaces. Adult patients with Philadelphia chromosome-positive ALL are treated with the same induction regimens as patients with Philadelphia chromosome-negative ALL, except that TKIs are added to the regimen. Remissions induced by TKIs alone are almost always short-lived, and for that reason, standard chemotherapy is used in combination with TKIs. Central nervous system prophylaxis with intrathecal methotrexate with or without cranial radiation is used in adult ALL patients.

Treatment of CML exploits the presence of the Philadelphia chromosome in CML cells, which encodes the BCR-ABL fusion protein. Therefore, first- and second-generation TKIs are the drugs of choice for CML. In younger patients (2 years old), bone marrow transplantation from properly matched bone marrow donors is an option that cures the cancer (see below).

Treatment of CLL presents unique challenges because it is a highly heterogeneous disease. Some CLL patients show survival rates without treatment that are similar to the average population. Furthermore, current treatment options do not cure CLL, and clinical trials have produced no evidence that early treatment of CLL causes any improvement in long-term survival. Bone marrow transplantations can cure CLL but are only an option in younger patients. Therefore, in most cases, the initial response to CLL is a "wait and see" strategy that routinely monitors the patient's health and holds treatment until the disease worsens.

CLL patients become candidates for treatment if they show signs of rapidly progressing disease. The signs of progressive CLL include weight loss of more than 10 percent over six months, extreme fatigue, leukemia-related fever, night sweats, bone marrow failure, anemia, low numbers of platelets (thrombocytopenia), enlargement of the spleen, enlarged lymph nodes, too many white blood cells in the blood (lymphocytosis). Chemotherapeutic regimens for rapidly progressive CLL include: (1) fludarabine (Fludara), cyclophosphamide, and rituximab; (2) pentostatin (Nipent), cyclophosphamide, and rituximab; (3) fludarabine, cyclophosphamide, and mitoxantrone (Novantrone); (4) cyclophosphamide, vincristine, and prednisone; (5) cyclophosphamide, doxorubicin (Adriamycin), vincristine, and prednisone; (6) cladribine or fludarabine, in combination with cyclophosphamide; and (7) bendamustine (Treanda) and rituximab. The specific regimen employed depends on the genetic nature of the cancer. For example, some cases of CLL consist of tumor cells that have a small piece of chromosome 17 missing (del17p13.1), and such cells lack a gene called "*TP53*" that encodes a protein called "p53." Since the p53 protein plays a critical role in controlling cell growth, tumors with no p53 are much more aggressive and much harder to kill. Some chemotherapeutic regimens, such as cladribine or fludarabine, in combination with cyclophosphamide, are ineffective against p53-negative tumors. Therefore, the genetic characteristics of the tumor must be taken into consideration when choosing a chemotherapeutic regimen.

Although the induction phase achieves clinical remission in more than 80 percent of patients, a second phase, called "consolidation therapy," is essential to prevent relapse. Oncologists employ different combinations of anticancer drugs to kill any remaining cancer cells resistant to the drugs in the induction phase. Once the patient is in remission, the patient tolerates higher doses of chemotherapy. Sometimes, additional intensive treatments further reduce the number of leukemic cells so that they cannot repopulate the tissues. During these phases of treatment, patients must be hospitalized. The destruction of their normal leukocytes along with the leukemic cells makes them very susceptible to infection. Their low numbers of surviving erythrocytes and platelets increase the probability of internal bleeding, and transfusions are often necessary. The oncologists must carefully calculate dosages of chemotherapeutic agents to kill as many leukemic cells as possible without destroying so many normal cells that they cannot repopulate the marrow. In general, children handle intensive chemotherapy better than adults.

For ALL, standard consolidation regimens usually consist of Ara-C in combination with an anthracycline or epipodophyllotoxin (i.e., etoposide or teniposide). In AML, four cycles of high-dose cytarabine is a standard option for consolidation therapy in younger patients. Alternative consolidation regimens include four courses of fludarabine plus cytarabine. CML tends to show three distinct clinical phases: (1) an initial chronic phase during which TKIs easily control the cancer; (2) an accelerated phase during which the disease transitions to an unstable condition; and (3) a more aggressive blast crisis, which is typically fatal. If a patient's CML is still in the chronic phase, consolidation therapy is not needed. TKIs can drive CML into remission. Even though the present consensus is that patients should continue taking TKIs indefinitely, in a significant number of cases, patients suffered no ill effects when they stopped taking TKIs. Consolidation treatment for patients with CLL includes: (1) the monoclonal antibody alemtuzumab (Campath-1H); (2) ibrutinib (Imbruvica) or idelalisib (Zydelig) plus an anti-CD20 antibody (rituximab, obinutuzumab, ofatumumab); or (3) venetoclax (Venclexta) plus an anti-CD20 antibody.

Leukemia patients may suffer from enlargement of the spleen, a condition called "splenomegaly." The enlarged spleen may chew up lots of blood cells, and the patient may experience "cytopenia" or low numbers of specific types of blood cells. Typically, treatment can alleviate cytopenia, but in some patients, their cytopenia resists treatment, and the best option is to remove the patient's spleen (splenectomy). Patients with CLL may also experience large, bulky masses of tumor cells that may compress other organs and impede their function. Since CLL lymphocytes are susceptible to radiation, focused radiation therapy can shrink these masses.

Following the induction and consolidation phases, maintenance therapy is sometimes used. In ALL, maintenance therapy lasts for two to three years; however, its benefit in other forms of leukemia is a matter of controversy. The second form of therapy is sometimes indicated for patients who have not responded to chemotherapy or are likely to relapse. Bone marrow transplantation has been increasingly used in leukemic patients to replace diseased marrow with normally functioning stem cells. This procedure treats the patient with intensive chemotherapy and whole-body irradiation to destroy all leukemic and normal cells. Then the patient received an infusion of a small amount of marrow from a normal donor. The donor could be the patient himself if they had marrow removed during a previous remission or an immunologically matched donor, usually a sibling. If a sibling is not available, it may be possible to find a matched donor from the National Marrow Donor Program, with approximately ten million donors on file. Marrow is removed from the donor, broken up into small pieces, and given to the patient intravenously. The stem cells from the transplanted marrow circulate in the blood, enter the bone marrow, and multiply. The first signs that the transplant is functioning occur in two to four weeks as the numbers of circulating granulocytes and platelets in the patient's blood increase. Eventually, in a successful transplant, normal cells will repopulate the bone marrow cavity.

Bone marrow transplantation is a dangerous procedure that requires highly trained caregivers. During this process, the patient is utterly vulnerable to infection since there is no functional immune system. The patient is in an isolation unit with special food-handling procedures. There is little chance that the patient will reject the transplanted marrow because the patient's immune system is suppressed. However, a more significant problem remains because it is possible for immune cells that exist in the donor's marrow to reject the tissues and organs of the patient. This graft-versus-host disease (GVHD) affects between 50 and 70 percent of bone marrow transplant patients. Even though the donor is immunologically matched, the match is not perfect, and the recently transplanted cells regard the cells in their new host as a "foreign" threat. Twenty percent of the patients who develop GVHD will die. Therefore, physicians prescribe immune-suppressing drugs like cyclophosphamide and cyclosporine to minimize this response. GVHD is not a problem if the donor is the patient. In 2012, Health Canada approved the stem-cell-based drug remestemcel-L (formerly known as Prochymal, but now is Ryoncil) for children with GVHD. Since the availability of matching bone marrow cells exceeds the need, recent studies have involved testing hematopoietic umbilical cord cells from unrelated donors. The incidence of relapse and GVHD was similar to that when using matched bone marrow cells, suggesting that cord blood cells have the potential to serve as an alternative to conventional transplants.

Aggressive chemotherapy and bone marrow transplantation have dramatically increased the number of long-lasting remissions. For those who survive the therapy, it appears that, in ALL, approximately 40 percent of adults are cured of leukemia. The outlook for permanent remission is 10 to 20 percent in AML and 65 percent for CML patients. Statistics for chronic lymphocytic leukemia have been challenging to predict because individual cases that were similarly treated have had very different outcomes. The average lifespan after a diagnosis of CLL is three to four years; however, some patients live longer than fifteen years.

PERSPECTIVE AND PROSPECTS
As the number of deaths from infectious diseases has decreased, cancer has become the second most common cause of disease-related death. It is estimated that one in three people in the United States will develop a form of cancer and that the disease will kill one in five people. The search for causes and treatments of various cancers is perhaps the most active area of biological research today. Multiple lines of experimentation are being pursued, and significant advances have been made.

Leukemia is one of the cancers that scientists understand reasonably well, but many unanswered questions remain. Leukemia research bifurcates into two broad approaches. In the first, the researcher seeks to modify and improve the current methods for treatment: chemotherapy and bone marrow transplantation. In the second, an effort is being made to understand more about the disease itself, hoping that completely different treatment strategies might present themselves.

The risks involved in current therapy for leukemia have been discussed in the previous section. Treatment schedules, individually designed for each patient, will add to the understanding of how other physiological characteristics affect treatment outcomes. Significant advances in reducing the risk of GVHD are likely to come quickly. In marrow transplants in which the donor is the patient, research is in progress to screen out abnormal cells, even if they are present at very low levels before they are infused back into the patient. In addition, for transplants in which the donor is not the patient, techniques that remove the harmful components of the bone marrow are being developed. Bone marrow cells can be partially purified, resulting in an enriched population of stem cells. Administering these to the leukemic patient should significantly reduce the risk of GVHD. Since bone marrow can be stored easily, the day may come when healthy people will store a bone marrow stem cell sample if they contract a disease that would require a transplant.

The Food and Drug Administration (FDA) has recently approved a new treatment for leukemia called "chimeric antigen receptor T cells" or CAR T cells. CAR T cells are made by genetically engineering the patient's T cells. Briefly, T cells are isolated from the patient's peripheral blood by a procedure called "apheresis" that samples circulating blood cells and takes a selection of the white blood cells. These collected white blood cells undergo density gradients that isolate the T cells (a process called "enrichment"). Then these T cells are genetically modified with genetically engineered lentiviruses that transfer genes into the genome of the T cells. These viral vectors insert genes that encode a synthetic version of the T-cell antigen receptor that can bind to a cell surface protein on the surface of the tumor cells linked to an intracellular protein that activates the T cell when the receptor binds its target. This chimeric, or mixed T-cell receptor, is a chimeric antigen receptor or CAR. The genetically engineered T cells are activated and grown in culture to larger numbers, after which they are tested for safety and efficacy. Only then are these CAR T cells reintroduced into the patient. CAR T cells recognize the tumor and stimulate and mobilize the immune system against it. To date, patients with refractory leukemia who had failed chemotherapy are entirely cancer-free. Furthermore, their cancer has not relapsed because a fraction of the CAR T cells become memory cells reactivate if new or previously hidden tumors cells arise. CAR T cells represent the new frontier in tumor treatment. Based on the success of CAR T cells, it may be possible to use similar strategies to "teach" the patient's immune system to destroy abnormal cells that it previously ignored. Similar forms of immunotherapy have shown promise in treating forms of cancer such as melanoma.

Cell biologists are seeking to understand the normal hematopoietic process to determine which steps of the process go awry in leukemia. Some of the growth factors involved in hematopoiesis are known, but it appears that the process is quite complex, and scientists do not yet have a clear picture of normal hematopoiesis. When the understanding of the normal process becomes complete, it may be possible to localize the defect in a leukemic patient and provide the missing growth factors. Employing the right cocktail of hematopoietic growth factors might drive abnormal, immature cells to complete the developmental process and relieve the symptoms of the disease. Geneticists are studying the chromosomal changes that underlie the onset of leukemia. As the oncogenes that are involved are identified, the reasons for their activation will also be determined. Once the effects of these genetic abnormalities are understood, it may be possible to intervene by genetically engineering stem cells so that they can develop normally.

These areas of research will likely converge to provide the leukemia treatments of the future. Leukemia is a cancer for which there is already a significant cure rate. It is not unreasonable to expect that this rate will approach 100 percent soon.

—*Katherine B. Frederich, PhD, Richard Adler, PhD, and Michael A. Buratovich, PhD*

Further Information

Bellenir, Karen, editor. *Cancer Sourcebook: Basic Consumer Health Information about Major Forms and Stages of Cancer.* 6th ed., Omnigraphics, 2012.

Dollinger, Malin, et al. *Everyone's Guide to Cancer Therapy.* 5th ed., Andrews McMeel, 2008.

Eyre, Harmon J., Dianne Partie Lange, and Lois B. Morris. *Informed Decisions: The Complete Book of CancerDiagnosis, Treatment, and Recovery.* 2nd ed., American Cancer Society, 2002.

Goldman, John, and Junia Melo. "Chronic Myeloid Leukemia: Advances in Biology and New Approaches to Treatment." *New England Journal of Medicine*, vol. 349, no. 15, 9 Oct. 2003, pp. 1451-64.

Henderson, Edward S., T. A. Lister, and M. F. Greaves. *Leukemia.* 7th ed., Saunders, 2002.

Keene, Nancy. *Childhood Leukemia: A Guide for Families, Friends and Caregivers.* 4th ed., O'Reilly, 2010.

Kimball, Chad T. *Childhood Diseases and Disorders Sourcebook: Basic Consumer Health Information about Medical Problems Often Encountered in Pre-adolescent Children.* Omnigraphics, 2003.

Levine, Bruce L., Miskin, James, Wonnacott, Keith, and Christopher Keir. "Global Manufacturing of CAR T Cell Therapy." *Molecular Therapy*, vol. 4, 2017, pp. 92-101.

Rattue, Petra. "Prochymal—First Stem Cell Drug Approved." *Medical News Today*, 22 May 2012, www.medicalnewstoday.com/articles/245704#1. Accessed 3 Sept. 2021.

Rennie, Ed. *Beginning of the End of My Life*. Xlibris, 2005. Leukemia and Lymphoma Society of America, www.leukemia.org.

Wapner, Jessica, and Robert A. Weinberg. *The Philadelphia Chromosome: A Mutant Gene and the Quest to Cure Cancer at the Genetic Level.* Workman, 2013.

Westcott, Patsy. *Living with Leukemia.* Raintree-Steck-Vaughn, 1999.

Wiernik, Peter H., et al. *Neoplastic Diseases of the Blood.* Springer, 2013.

Leukopenia

Category: Diseases, Symptoms, and Conditions
Also known as: Neutropenia, low white blood cell count, leucopenia
Related conditions: Neutropenia, which is a subset of leukopenia
Anatomy or system affected: Blood, brain, gastrointestinal system, immune system, intestines, liver, lungs, lymphatic system, mouth, respiratory system, skin, throat
Specialties and related fields: Bacteriology, dermatology, gastroenterology, hematology, immunology, internal medicine, microbiology, neurology, oncology, otorhinolaryngology, pathology, pharmacology, pulmonary medicine, virology
Definition: Leukopenia is an abnormally low number of white blood cells, or leukocytes. The laboratory standard measurement of leukocytes ranges from approximately $(4.0$ to $11.0) \times 10^9$ per liter.

KEY TERMS

agranulocytosis: an extremely low number of granulocytes in the blood
granulocytes: a white blood cell with secretory granules in its cytoplasm, including neutrophils, basophils, and eosinophils
granulocytopenia: a reduced absolute number of all circulating cells of the granulocyte series, including neutrophils, eosinophils, and basophils
neutropenia: abnormally few neutrophils in the blood that leads to increased susceptibility to infection and is an undesirable side effect of some cancer treatments

RISK FACTORS

Leukopenia may be related to use of certain drugs (such as barbiturates and chemotherapeutics), radiation therapy, bone marrow or stem cell transplant, severe infections, or bone marrow diseases such as leukemia, myelodysplastic syndromes, acquired immunodeficiency syndrome (AIDS), aplastic anemia, or lupus. Patients older than the age of seventy and those with comorbid diseases, such as diabetes, are at great risk for leukopenia during chemotherapy.

ETIOLOGY AND THE DISEASE PROCESS

Chemotherapy and radiation therapy for cancer target the rapidly dividing cancer cells as well as other rapidly dividing cells, that is, hematopoietic stem cells. It takes about ten days for a new leukocyte to differentiate and mature from a hematopoietic stem cell, which means that a patient receiving chemotherapy or radiation therapy can have a low number of leukocytes for days. The role of leukocytes is to safeguard against infection by destroying bacteria. Leukopenia and its associated impaired immunity make a patient more susceptible to infections and may lead to septicemia. Untreated, leukopenia may require hospitalization and use of intravenous anti-infective drugs.

Some drugs show an established association with agranulocytosis.

Major medications with a definite association with agranulocytosis:

Antibiotics
- Macrolides
- Trimethoprim/sulfamethoxazole
- Chloramphenicol
- Sulfonamides
- Semisynthetic penicillins
- Vancomycin
- Cephalosporin
- Dapsone

Anticonvulsants
- Carbamazepine
- Phenytoin
- Ethosuximide
- Valproate

Antifungal agents
- Amphotericin B
- Flucytosine

Anti-inflammatory drugs
- Sulfasalazine
- Nonsteroidal anti-inflammatory drugs
- Gold salts
- Penicillamine
- Antipyrine
- Dipyrone
- Phenacetin

Antimalarial drugs
- Amodiaquine
- Chloroquine
- Quinin

Antithyroid drugs
- Methimazole
- Carbimazole
- Propylthiouracil

Antiviral agents
- Oseltamivir
- Ganciclovir
- Acyclovir

Cardiovascular drugs
- Antiarrhythmic agents (tocainide, procainamide, flecainide)
- Ticlopidine
- ACE inhibitors (enalapril, captopril)
- Propranolol
- Dipyridamole
- Digoxin

Dermatologic drugs
- Dapsone
- Isotretinoin

Diuretics
- Thiazides
- Acetazolamide
- Furosemide
- Spironolactone

Gastrointestinal drugs
- Sulfasalazine
- Histamine type 2 receptor agonists

Iron Chelating agents
- Deferiprone

Miscellaneous
- Chlorpheniramine
- Sulfonylureas
- Chlorpropamide
- Tolbutamide

Psychotropic Drugs
- Clozapine
- Phenothiazines
- Tricyclic and tetracyclic antidepressants
- Meprobamate
- Cocaine/heroin (adulterated with levamisole)

INCIDENCE
Most patients who are receiving chemotherapy, radiation therapy, or a bone marrow transplant experience leukopenia, and very often chemotherapy must be delayed because of it.

SYMPTOMS
Symptoms include recurrent infections, high-grade fever and chills, and diarrhea.

SCREENING AND DIAGNOSIS
Leukopenia is defined as a leukocyte count less than approximately 4.0×10^9 per liter. Mild leukopenia is defined as a leukocyte count of $(1.0$ to $2.0) \times 10^9$ per liter, and severe as a leukocyte count less than 0.5×10^9 per liter. Leukopenia is determined by a blood test.

TREATMENT AND THERAPY

At this time, white blood cell transfusions are not a treatment option, primarily because of the abbreviated life span of a leukocyte, which is estimated to be between twenty-four and forty-eight hours. Most patients with leukopenia receive bone marrow stimulants such as recombinants granulocyte colony-stimulating factor (G-CSF) mimics such as filgrastim (Neupogen) and lenograstim (Granocyte). Pegfilgrastim (Neulasta) is a long-lasting G-CSF that is a preferred under some conditions. Sargramostim (Leukine) is a recombinant granulocyte-macrophage colony-stimulating factor (GM-CSF) that increases the number of circulating white blood cells. It reconstitutes blood cells after bone marrow transplantation, and treats neutropenia caused by chemotherapy during the treatment of acute myeloid leukemia. Sargramostim also regenerates the bone marrow of those who were exposed to sufficient radiation to suppress bone marrow function.

PROGNOSIS, PREVENTION, AND OUTCOMES

Hematopoietic growth factors are the standard for treatment of severe leukopenia at many cancer centers and can rapidly, within hours in some cases, increase leukocyte counts. Left untreated, the patient is at risk for serious and possibly life-threatening infections.

—*MaryAnn Foote, MS, PhD*

Further Information

Andersohn, Frank, et al. "Systematic Review: Agranulocytosis Induced by Nonchemotherapy Drugs." *Annals of Internal Medicine* vol. 146, no. 9, 2007, pp. 657-65, doi:10.7326/0003-4819-146-9-200705010-00009.

Andrès, Emmanuel, et al. "State of Art of Idiosyncratic Drug-Induced Neutropenia or Agranulocytosis, with a Focus on Biotherapies." *Journal of Clinical Medicine*, vol. 8, no. 9, 2019, p. 1351, doi:10.3390/jcm8091351.

Segel, George B., and Jill S. Halterman. "Neutropenia in Pediatric Practice." *Pediatrics in Review*, vol. 29, no. 1, 2008, pp. 12-23, doi:10.1542/pir.29-1-12.

Wei R., et al. "Pediatric Drug Safety Signal Detection of Non-chemotherapy Drug-induced Neutropenia and Agranulocytosis Using Electronic Healthcare Records." *Expert Opinion on Drug Safety*, vol. 18, no. 5, 2019, p. 435.

LYMPHOCYTOSIS

Category: Diseases, Symptoms, and Conditions
Also known as: Raised lymphocyte count
Related conditions: Lymph symptoms, absolute lymphocytosis, hematological malignancy, lymphoma, leukemia, lymphoproliferative disorders
Anatomy or system affected: Blood, immune system, lymphatic system
Specialties and related fields: Hematology, immunology
Definition: Lymphocytosis is an abnormal excess of lymphocytes in the blood. Lymphocytes are a type of white blood cell that helps fight infections. A healthy adult has an absolute lymphocyte count (ALC) of 1,300 to 4,000 per microliter of blood. ALC over 4,000 indicates lymphocytosis; however, this number may be higher in children up to six years of age, as their ALC is significantly higher than in adults.

KEY TERMS

leukemia: a malignant, progressive disease caused by bone marrow production of abnormal, immature white blood cells that inhibit the production of normal blood cells, leading to anemia and other symptoms.

lymphocyte: small white blood cells that have a single, round nucleus and inhabit the lymphatic system and bloodstream

lymphoma: cancer of the lymphatic system

RISK FACTORS

More than thirty medical conditions may underlie lymphocytosis. The most common causes include viral and bacterial infections, such as mononucleosis (glandular fever), influenza, pertussis (whooping cough), or tuberculosis. Malignant blood diseases, such as chronic lymphocytic leukemia, follicular lymphoma, hairy cell leukemia, and leukopenia, may also cause lymphocytosis.

ETIOLOGY AND THE DISEASE PROCESS

Lymphocytosis indicates an underlying problem, but it is not a disease in itself. The lymph nodes are the most commonly affected organs. Transient stress lymphocytosis may also occur after trauma or extensive psychological or physical stress. It typically resolves within two days of diagnosis. Transient stress lymphocytosis may be mediated by the modulation of catecholamine and steroid hormones and cell adhesion molecules.

INCIDENCE

Lymphocytosis is common and occurs in most people throughout life, usually associated with viral infections.

SYMPTOMS

Symptoms of lymphocytosis may include sore throat, fever, and fatigue. However, lymphocytosis typically causes no symptoms and is often discovered incidentally via a routine blood test.

SCREENING AND DIAGNOSIS

A complete blood count will identify lymphocytosis. Further investigation assesses the major lymphocyte subsets, such as T cells, B cells, and natural killer cells. The subgroups of T cells are CD4 T cells (helper cells) and CD8 T cells (cytotoxic cells). Approximately 75 percent of lymphocytes are T cells in a healthy person, with a 2:1 ratio of CD4 to CD8. About equal proportions of the remainder, cells are B cells and natural killer cells. A marked increase in lymphocytes may indicate a severe condition, such as the presence of chronic lymphocytic leukemia. Many types of blood cancer are often identified after diagnosing lymphocytosis.

> **INFORMATION ON LYMPHOCYTOSIS**
>
> **Causes**: Specific infectious diseases, lymphomas and leukemias, stress, drug hypersensitivities, thymomas (thymus tumors), the absence of a spleen, monoclonal B cell lymphocytosis, and syndrome of persistent polyclonal B cell lymphocytosis
>
> **Symptoms**: By itself, lymphocytosis causes no symptoms
>
> **Duration**: Acute or chronic
>
> **Treatments**: Depends on the underlying condition causing it

TREATMENT AND THERAPY

It is necessary to address the underlying issue that caused lymphocytosis for the best therapy. If a malignant blood disease is detected, the patient may require cancer treatments.

PROGNOSIS, PREVENTION, AND OUTCOMES

Depending on the cause of lymphocytosis, it may spontaneously resolve or need medical interaction to relieve its symptoms.

—*Anita Nagypál, PhD*

FURTHER READING

Delgado, Julio, et al. "Chronic Lymphocytic Leukemia: From Molecular Pathogenesis to Novel Therapeutic Strategies." *Haematologica*, vol. 105, no. 9, 2020, pp. 2205-17, doi:10.3324/haematol.2019.236000.

Hamad, Hussein, and Ankit Mangla. "Lymphocytosis." *StatPearls*, StatPearls Publishing, 21 Jul. 2021.

Justiz Vaillant, Angel A., and Christopher M. Stang. "Lymphoproliferative Disorders." *StatPearls*, StatPearls Publishing, 30 Dec. 2020.

Ménière's disease

Category: Diseases/Disorders
Anatomy or system affected: Brain, ears, nervous system
Specialties and related fields: Neurology
Definition: A disease state caused by infection with human immunodeficiency virus (HIV), leading to a progressive deterioration of the immune system and characterized by the development of any of many opportunistic infections.

KEY TERMS
tinnitus: ringing or buzzing in the ears
vestibular system: a sensory system that contributes to balance and spatial orientation to coordinate movement with balance

WHAT WE KNOW
Ménière's disease is a chronic condition affecting the inner ear that manifests as recurring episodes of vertigo (i.e., having a sensation of imbalance, spinning, and dizziness). Other symptoms include experiencing periods of hearing loss, tinnitus (i.e., ringing in the ears), and pressure in the ear. Ménière's disease and migraine headache can cause similar symptoms and are thought to be associated conditions.

RISK FACTORS FOR MÉNIÈRE'S DISEASE
The etiology of Ménière's disease is unclear. Researchers suggest that the cause is most likely due to a combination of factors, including the following: allergies, genetic predisposition, dysfunction of the immune system, infection, trauma to the head or ear, migraine, and fluctuation in electrolyte levels.

Commonly reported triggers of an episode of Ménière's disease include the following: changes in barometric pressure, an allergy attack, hormonal changes, stress, sleep deprivation, high sodium intake, consumption of caffeine or alcohol, and excessive sweating.

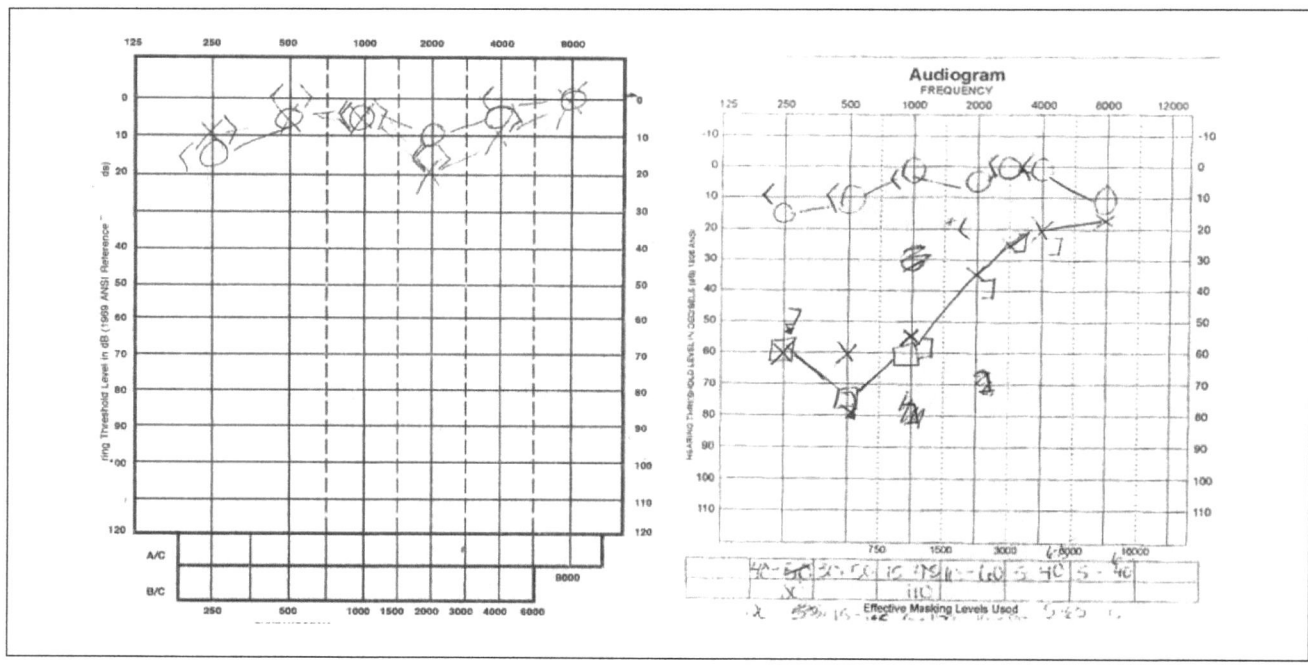

Audiograms illustrating normal hearing (left) and unilateral low-pitch hearing loss associated with Ménière's disease (right). Image via Wikimedia Commons. [Public domain.]

MEDICAL NUTRITION THERAPY FOR MÉNIÈRE'S DISEASE

When Ménière's disease is associated with food allergy, eliminating the food causing the allergic reaction can reduce symptomatic episodes. The use of an elimination diet can help to identify food allergies.

Patients have reported worsening episodes of Ménière's disease with sodium, caffeine, and alcohol. Restricting foods that contain these elements helps reduce the frequency and/or severity of symptomatic episodes in some cases.

Chocolate contains caffeine and should be avoided if following a diet that restricts caffeine. Researchers recommend restricting sodium to 1.53 grams/day. Because diuretics are relatively safe, they are frequently prescribed for symptomatic relief in patients with Ménière's disease. Research results are inconclusive regarding the use of diuretics as an effective treatment for Ménière's disease.

SUMMARY

Individuals diagnosed with Ménière's disease should learn about dietary considerations based on personal characteristics and health needs.

Individuals with Ménière's disease should be assessed for food-related allergies. The elimination of certain foods might be appropriate for the relief of symptomatic episodes. It is recommended that individuals with Ménière's disease restrict sodium, caffeine, and alcohol intake to reduce symptomatic episodes potentially. Individuals with Ménière's disease are encouraged to eat a nutrient-dense diet that includes fatty fish and lean proteins, unsaturated fats (including omega-3), complex carbohydrates (e.g., whole, unrefined grains), legumes, and a variety of fruits and vegetables.

—*Cherie Marcel, BS*

Further Information

Derebery, M. J., and K. I. Berliner. "Allergy and Its Relation to Meniere's Disease. *Otolaryngologic Clinics of North America*, vol. 43, no. 5, 2010, pp. 1047-58, doi:10.1016/j.otc.2010.05.004.

Greenberg, S. L., "Medical and Noninvasive Therapy for Meniere's Disease." *Otolaryngologic Clinics of North America*, vol. 43, no. 5, 2010, pp. 1081-90, doi:10.1016/j.otc.2010.05.005.

Hamid, M. A. "Meniere's Disease." *Practical Neurology*, vol. 9, no. 3, 2009, pp. 157-62, doi:10.1136/jnnp.2009.176602.

Mayo Clinic Staff. "Meniere's Disease." *Mayo Clinic*, 2012, www.mayoclinic.org/diseases-conditions/menieres-disease/basics/definition/con-20028251. Accessed 10 Jul. 2015.

Sajjadi, H., and M. M. Paparella. "Meniere's Disease." *The Lancet*, vol. 372, no. 9636, 2008, pp. 406-14, doi:10.1016/S0140-6736(08)61161-7.

METABOLIC DISORDERS

Category: Diseases/Disorders
Anatomy or system affected: All
Specialties and related fields: Biochemistry, endocrinology, genetics, nutrition, pediatrics, perinatology
Definition: Disorders resulting from alterations in the pathways by which the body derives energy and synthesizes other molecules from carbohydrates, lipids, and proteins in food; usually caused by genetic defects that result in a missing or faulty enzyme.

KEY TERMS

anabolic: the metabolic processes by which small molecules are combined to produce larger molecules; used for energy storage or growth of the organism

catabolic: the metabolic processes by which food and stored products are broken down to release energy for use by the cell

enzyme: a protein whose job is to enable chemical reactions to occur in the cell promptly; a biological catalyst

essential: referring to an amino acid, lipid, or vitamin that is necessary for proper cell functioning, but which the human body is ordinarily unable to produce on its own; must be supplied through the diet

metabolism: the process of extracting energy that can be used to power the cells of the body; includes both anabolic and catabolic processes

prenatal/neonatal screening: a tool whereby small volume fluid samples (prenatal) or blood samples (neonatal) are drawn and studied to determine the genetic traits carried by the child; neonatal screening is often mandated by law and used to find metabolic diseases as early in life as possible

CAUSES AND SYMPTOMS

Metabolic disorders of all types are usually inherited from one or both parents who carry a defective gene; the gene codes for an enzyme responsible for a part of the metabolic pathway (either anabolic or catabolic). Much like an assembly line that takes raw material and produces a final product through multiple steps, the metabolism of proteins, lipids, and carbohydrates in the human body requires multiple steps, each with its enzyme. In some cases, there are multiple pathways to metabolize a particular starting product. In this case, the lack of one enzyme may not have a dramatic effect. Other pathways are exclusive, however, and any disruption of an enzyme will lead to disease. In addition to the loss of a particular product, some enzyme defects lead to the accumulation of precursor molecules that may be toxic or interfere with the cell's normal function.

When the deoxyribonucleic acid (DNA) coding for a particular gene is altered, one of three outcomes may be seen: no change (silent mutation), partial loss of the ability of the enzyme to do its job (mild disease), or complete loss of enzyme function (mild to severe disease). Diseases in humans are not known for all enzymes that could potentially be lost; this is most likely because disruption of an enzyme necessary for the fetus's early development will lead to early (and undetected) loss of the fetus.

> **INFORMATION ON METABOLIC DISORDERS**
>
> **Causes:** Missing or faulty enzymes
>
> **Symptoms:** Depends on enzyme affected; may include mental retardation, seizures, rashes, nausea, vomiting, coma, delayed development, organ damage, paralysis, dementia, blindness
>
> **Duration:** Chronic and often fatal
>
> **Treatments:** Ranges from none to dietary restrictions to enzyme therapy

Disorders of metabolism may be classified according to the pathways that are disrupted. Disorders associated with protein/amino acid metabolism may be seen when amino acids cannot be effectively broken down or when they cannot be transported into the body's cells for use in building new proteins. Most of these disorders are seen early in life since many proteins are essential for the growth and development of the body. Examples of amino acid metabolism disorders are phenylketonuria (PKU) and maple syrup urine disease (MSUD). Other amino acid/protein disorders are homocystinuria, citrullinemia, alkaptonuria, and tyrosinemia.

Phenylalanine is an essential amino acid involved in the production of tyrosine, which in turn is converted to dopamine and serotonin. In PKU, the absence of this conversion means that phenylalanine accumulates in the body, causing toxic reactions within the brain and other organs. Mental retardation is the most apparent effect of this toxicity; other symptoms may include seizures, skin rashes, nausea and vomiting, and aggressive behavior. Phenylacetate (a byproduct of excess phenylalanine) is secreted in sweat and urine, giving a distinctive odor to the child.

Leucine, isoleucine, and valine are amino acids that have a branched side chain. As a result of this unique shape, an enzyme that can convert these enzymes is needed to metabolize food containing them. In MSUD, that enzyme is absent or deficient.

These amino acids accumulate in the urine, giving a distinctive smell for which the disorder is named. If left untreated, this can lead to vomiting, staggering, confusion, coma, and eventual death from degeneration of the developing nerves early in life. A total of six different genes are responsible for producing the branched-chain alpha-ketoacid dehydrogenase enzyme complex, thus leading to some variation in the severity of the disease. While this disease is rare in the general population, the Mennonite community of Pennsylvania has a high rate of carriers for these mutations and thus is particularly affected.

Lipids (fats) are used in numerous ways in the human body, including for energy, temperature regulation, cell membrane structure, and nerve function. A variety of enzymes are responsible for breaking down and processing both stored and dietary lipids. In the absence of efficient processing of lipids, accumulations occur that can be highly harmful to the body's organs. Examples of lipid metabolism disorders are fatty acid oxidation disorders and Tay-Sachs disease. Other lipid metabolism disorders include Gaucher's disease, Refsum disease, Niemann-Pick disease, Tangier disease, carnitine uptake defect, and trifunctional protein deficiency.

Several enzymes are involved in pathways that help stored lipids to be broken down and turned into energy. In the most common fatty acid oxidation disorder, the enzyme deficient in this pathway is medium-chain acyl-coenzyme A dehydrogenase (MCAD). This is one of the most common errors of metabolism among people of northern European descent. A buildup of acyl-coenzyme A leads to delayed development, heart muscle weakness, and enlarged liver; death may occur. Symptoms develop shortly after birth and are most severe if the child goes without food for a prolonged period or following exercise and the need for more energy to the cells (thus triggering the lipid breakdown pathways).

Perhaps the best known of the lipid metabolism disorders, Tay-Sachs disease results from errors in the enzyme-hexosaminidase, which is responsible for breaking down the lipid GM2 ganglioside. The gene for this enzyme is known to reside on chromosome 15. The absence of this enzyme allows large amounts of the ganglioside to accumulate in neurons. This accumulation leads to neurodegeneration that often results in floppy muscle tone, paralysis, dementia, blindness, and death by age three or four. Less severe forms lead to long-term problems in the nervous system that progress throughout life. Tay-Sachs disease is most commonly seen in the Ashkenazi Jewish community. Still, it is also seen in the French Canadian population of Quebec and the Cajun population of Louisiana.

Carbohydrates (primarily glucose) are the principal fuels for the body. Carbohydrate metabolism requires a variety of intracellular enzymes and those responsible for transport and entry into the cell. Diseases or disorders of carbohydrate metabolism can be quite severe. Examples of carbohydrate metabolism disorders are type 1 diabetes mellitus and glycogen storage diseases.

The ability to get glucose (the primary carbohydrate) into the body's cells requires the hormone insulin. A lack of insulin production in the pancreas (type 1 diabetes) leads to hyperglycemia (high blood glucose levels) and a lack of glucose for energy within the cells. In addition to lack of cellular energy, this can lead to an increased risk of blindness, heart disease, kidney failure, neurological diseases, and problems with circulation in the extremities. Type 1 diabetes may result from several known mutations in DNA, the most common on chromosome 6. In type 1 diabetes, the body attacks either the insulin or the pancreatic cells that produce it, making this an autoimmune disease.

Glycogen is the branched-chain storage form of glucose in the liver and muscles of the body. Glycogen storage diseases are a group of eleven similar diseases that result in the inability of the body to produce sufficient glucose for the bloodstream to be used by cells of the body to produce energy. In addition to low blood sugar levels, children with these diseases often have enlarged livers, swollen abdomens, and weak muscles. Elevated levels of lipids in the blood (taking the place of glucose as an energy source) may lead to acidosis and stress on the heart and kidneys.

In addition to the transport, storage, and breakdown of proteins, lipids, and carbohydrates, metabolism involves alterations in the use of elements such as iron and copper and the synthesis, storage, and use of the components of DNA and ribonucleic acid (RNA). Diseases and disorders in each of these areas are known as well. Examples include Wilson disease, Menkes disease, hereditary hemochromatosis, and Lesch-Nyhan syndrome.

Copper is necessary in cells for energy metabolism, bone production, and nerve maturation. Wilson and Menkes disorders are disorders of copper transport and absorption that lead to a buildup of copper to toxic levels in the liver and the brain. Both liver disease and neurological damage can be present if they are not diagnosed early on; eventually, toxicity can be seen in many other organs. Menkes disease is usually fatal during infancy. Both diseases have been mapped to chromosome 13 and appear to be the result of proteins that are part of a transmembrane pump system. Menkes disease is transmitted as an X-linked recessive trait, while Wilson's disease is autosomal recessive.

Hereditary hemochromatosis is a disorder of iron metabolism seen predominantly in those of Northern European, Caucasian descent and traceable to a mutation on chromosome 6. Because iron is not adequately metabolized, the levels stored in the body grow over time, leading to cirrhosis of the liver, cardiomyopathy (heart muscle disease), alterations in skin pigmentation, joint damage, and decreased functioning of the gonads. Because men generally retain iron better than women do, symptoms often occur earlier in men. Symptoms also occur early in alcoholics, as alcohol consumption affects the uptake of dietary iron.

Both DNA and RNA are constructed from nitrogen-containing bases; these bases are chemically grouped as purines and pyrimidines. The body can both make and recycle these bases. One of the genes involved in recycling purines (*HPRT1*) is located on the X chromosome. In Lesch-Nyhan syndrome, several known mutations result in low enzyme levels and thus a lack of purine recycling. The resulting disease is seen almost exclusively in males. It causes the accumulation of uric acid (the starting point in purine synthesis). Uric acid leads to gout (painful deposits in the skin and joints) and kidney stones. For unknown reasons, this enzyme deficiency also leads to self-mutilation (biting the fingers and tongue). Severe muscle weakness and mental retardation generally occur.

TREATMENT AND THERAPY
The most important diagnostic tool available for metabolic disorders is routine neonatal genetic screening. In 2005, the American College of Medical Genetics report recommended a core panel of twenty-eight metabolic disorders that should be screened for in all newborn children. This list includes disorders of protein metabolism, carbohydrate metabolism, lipid metabolism, and a few multisystem disorders. Such screening does not prevent disorders but does allow early detection and therefore early intervention with diet, drugs, and other regimens that allow extended life spans for those afflicted. As of 2013, newborn screening in the United States varies from state to state, with most states testing for more than thirty disorders.

Once detected, the treatment of metabolic disorders is quite varied and related to the disorder's underlying cause. For protein/amino acid disorders, dietary restrictions are a vital element in treatment. For instance, in PKU, phenylalanine intake must be restricted starting in the first few weeks of life. This means the elimination of most forms of natural protein and substitution with phenylalanine-free foods. Patients with homocystinuria often improve with vitamin B_6 (pyridoxine) or vitamin B_{12} (cobalamin). In MSUD, restricting the dietary intake of the three branched-chain amino acids to the minimal amount required for growth and development allows for the best improvement. Vitamin B1 (thiamine) is helpful in those with mild disease; dialysis is used in those with severe disease. Gene therapy is a possibility in the future.

In lipid disorders, control of diet is also essential. With fatty acid oxidation disorders, patients must eat often, never skip meals, and consume a diet high in carbohydrates and low in lipids. Treatment with intravenous glucose is helpful during attacks. The long-term outcome is very good in those who follow a strict dietary regimen. Likewise, in Refsum disease, a diet with little or no phytanic acid (carefully controlled plant products that contain no chlorophyll) is the key; plasmapheresis may also be helpful. Other lipid disorders, including Gaucher's and Tay-Sachs, require drug intervention. Gaucher's type I patients (especially those without nervous system damage) can be treated with enzyme replacement therapy; the modified enzyme is given intravenously every two weeks. Enzyme therapy has been shown to stop and even reverse many of the symptoms of this disease. The late-onset (less severe) form of Tay-Sachs has seen some promise from treatment with a ganglioside synthesis inhibitor. Treatment of the infantile form has shown little promise since much of the neurological damage occurs before birth, and reversing neurological damage that has already occurred has proven to be extremely difficult.

Type 1 diabetes can usually be controlled well with daily insulin (artificial) and diet control (to match the amount of energy needed for daily activities). Although islet cell transplantation or immunosuppression has been on the drawing board for several years, no real success has yet been obtained.

Other metabolic disorders run the gamut from easy to impossible to treat. Hereditary hemochromatosis, for instance, is easy to control, with therapeutic phlebotomy (blood-letting) to remove excess iron that has built up. Early diagnosis and treatment lead to a normal life span. By contrast, there is no cure for Niemann-Pick disease. These children generally die of infection or degeneration of the central nervous system. For Menkes disease, the administration of copper histidinate has shown promise. Still, it only increases the patient's life span by a few years (less than ten). In Lesch- Nyhan syndrome, medications decrease uric acid levels; restraint against self-mutilation is commonly needed. Advances in gene therapy look promising for several of these conditions as well.

PERSPECTIVE AND PROSPECTS

Metabolic disorders have existed since the earliest humans roamed the earth. Still, it was not until the early twentieth century that the mechanism for these disorders was recognized. The term "inborn error of metabolism" was coined by Archibald Garrod, a British physician. He published a classic text on the subject in 1923, following a study of children with alkaptonuria. This was the first treatise to explain how symptoms often seen in sickly children could be explained based on enzyme defects. Many of these diseases, such as diabetes, had been well established and named years before but not yet understood in terms of their biochemistry. The genetic basis for these disorders was not determined until much later-the 1970s and beyond.

Another early pioneer in this field was the German pediatrician Albert Niemann, who in 1914 described in detail a child with nervous system impairment. This condition later became known as Niemann-Pick disease. After their deaths, Ludwick Pick took tissue samples from several such children and provided chemical evidence of a specific lipid storage problem.

The discovery of insulin in the 1920s provided the first opportunity to treat a metabolic disease, as insulin could be extracted and purified in a controlled laboratory setting. The availability of insulin has saved millions of lives since its discovery.

The hope for the future is gene therapy. There are many trials throughout the world to improve the chances of survival and healthy lives of those with similar metabolic disorders through correction of the genetic defect. The first gene therapy successes were recorded in children with enzyme deficiencies. In the future, such therapy might even be available in utero.

—*Kerry L. Cheesman, PhD*

Further Information

Gilbert, Hiram F. *Basic Concepts in Biochemistry*. 2nd ed., McGraw-Hill, 2002.

MedlinePlus. "Metabolic Disorders." *MedlinePlus*, 21 May 2013.

National Institute of General Medical Sciences (US). *The Structures of Life*. U.S. Department of Health and Human Services, Public Health Service, National Institutes of Health, National Institute of General Medical Sciences, 2007. NIH publication no. 07-2778.

National Newborn Screening and Global Resource Center. "Families: Newborn Screening." NNSGRC: *National Newborn Screening & Global Resource Center*, 22 Apr. 2013.

Nussbaum, Robert L., et al. *Thompson and Thompson Genetics in Medicine*. 7th ed., Saunders/Elsevier, 2007.

Scriver, Charles R., et al., editors. *The Metabolic and Molecular Bases of Inherited Disease*. 8th ed., McGraw-Hill, 2002.

Wheeler, Patricia G. "Newborn Screening Tests." *KidsHealth from Nemours*, Sept. 2012.

Neutropenia

Category: Immune response
Also known as: Agranulocytosis, granulocytopenia
Anatomy or system affected: All tissues
Specialties and related fields: All specialties
Definition: Neutropenia occurs when the peripheral blood contains an abnormally low number of circulating neutrophils, a type of white blood cell that helps the body fight bacterial infections. Diagnosis is made when a blood test, the absolute neutrophil count (ANC), is less than 1.5×10^9 per liter.

KEY TERMS

neutrophils: the most abundant type of white blood cells in the blood that form an essential part of the innate immune system

phagocytosis: a form of ingestion of bacteria or other foreign material by white blood cells

NEUTROPENIA AND THE IMMUNE SYSTEM

Neutrophils are essential to the immune system because they help to destroy bacteria. In homeostasis (physiologic health), the body maintains an equilibrium between neutrophil production and utilization. When this balance is disrupted, and more neutrophils are needed than are produced, neutropenia results.

Healthy adults produce about sixty billion neutrophils per day, but only a small percentage is usually expended. Neutrophils, sometimes called "granulocytes," are produced in the bone marrow and released through the bloodstream. Neutrophils contain microscopic granules (sacs of enzymes) that help them kill and digest invading microorganisms through a process known as phagocytosis. People with neutropenia cannot rid the body of these foreign organisms and thus become highly susceptible to infection.

SEVERE CHRONIC NEUTROPENIA (SCN)

SCN is characterized by abnormalities in neutrophil production and classified as congenital, cyclic, and chronic idiopathic neutropenia, the causes of which are thought to be a receptor signaling/postreceptor defect, a regulatory defect, and faulty immune mechanisms, respectively. SCNs affect the body's integumentary system and cause infections in the oropharyngeal (throat), respiratory, and gastrointestinal mucosa; the hair follicles; and the skin's glandular structures.

Kostmann's syndrome is an inherited disorder that causes significant fever and infection at birth and throughout life. Newborns typically have little evidence of mature neutrophil production and extremely low ANCs (0.1×10^9 per liter). People with cyclic neutropenia have recurring three to six-day episodes of neutropenia followed by recovery and are especially prone to fever and infection during extreme neutropenic periods when ANCs can fall as low as 0.1×10^9 per liter. In chronic idiopathic neutropenia, ANCs are normal at birth but become lower in time, thus predisposing patients to infection.

ACQUIRED OR SECONDARY NEUTROPENIA

Autoimmune neutropenia occurs when the immune system attacks the body's blood neutrophils; diagnosis requires that neutrophil-specific antibodies be present. Many drugs used to treat autoimmune disorders cause bone marrow suppression, compromising blood cell production and increasing the risk for neutropenia.

In some cases, neutropenia is linked to cancer. Chemotherapy-induced neutropenia (CIN) is a severe side effect of cancer treatment. In chemotherapy, cytotoxic agents destroy bone marrow cells and strip the body of its natural defenses against infection. Patients who become very neutropenic may need to halt chemotherapy or have their dosages lowered to prevent infection. CIN is called "febrile neutropenia" when fever develops in patients with ANCs below 500/cubic millimeters. Fever is the body's response to infection. These patients are especially troubling because they do not show the usual signs of redness, swelling, and pus associated with infection.

IMPACT

Neutropenia, particularly CIN, results in high morbidity and mortality, increases medical costs, and lowers the quality of life. The challenge is to minimize the incidence of infection with the judicious use of therapeutic interventions, such as granulocyte colony-stimulating factor (G-CSF) or hematopoietic growth factor, corticosteroids, and broad-spectrum antibiotics.

—*Barbara Woldin, BS*

Further Information
"Disorders of Phagocyte Function and Number." *Hematology: Basic Principles and Practice*, edited by Ronald Hoffman, et al., 5th ed., Churchill Livingstone/Elsevier, 2009.
Hadley, Andrew G., and Peter Soothill, editors. *Alloimmune Disorders of Pregnancy: Anaemia, Thrombocytopenia, and Neutropenia in the Fetus and Newborn*. Cambridge UP, 2002.
Holland, Steven, et al. "Immunodeficiencies." *Infectious Diseases*, edited by Jon Cohen, William Powderly, and Steven Opal, Mosby/Elsevier, 2010.
"Infectious Diseases: Neutropenia (Agranulocytosis; Granulocytopenia)." *The Merck Manual of Diagnosis and Therapy*, edited by Mark H. Beers, et al., 18th ed., Merck Research Laboratories, 2006.
Provan, Drew, and John Gribben, editors. *Molecular Haematology*. 2nd ed., Blackwell, 2005.

PURINE NUCLEOSIDE PHOSPHORYLASE (PNP) DEFICIENCY

Category: Diseases/Syndromes
Also known as: PNP-deficiency
Anatomy or system affected: All tissues
Specialties and related fields: Bacteriology, dermatology, gastroenterology, hematology, immunology, internal medicine, microbiology, neurology,

oncology, ophthalmology, otorhinolaryngology, pathology, pediatrics, pulmonary medicine, virology

Definition: Purine nucleoside phosphorylase (PNP) deficiency is a rare and severe, inherited primary immunodeficiency disease. PNP-deficiency destroys T-cell lymphocytes in the immune system, severely weakening the immune system and decreasing life expectancy.

KEY TERMS

enzymes: substances, usually proteins or ribonucleic acid (RNA) molecules, that act as catalysts to acceleration the rate of specific biochemical reactions

purines: nitrogen-containing, heterocyclic aromatic organic compounds with two rings fused that form one of the two main bases in deoxyribonucleic acid (DNA) and RNA

salvage pathway: enzyme-catalyzed reactions that form a biosynthetic pathway for purines and pyrimidines that use preformed purine or pyrimidine bases or nucleosides to form nucleotides.

severe combined immunodeficiency (SCID): a family of rare disorders caused by mutations in different genes that direct the development and function of infection-fighting immune cells

uric acid: an insoluble molecule that is a breakdown product of purine metabolism

RISK FACTORS

Family history is the only known risk factor for this disease. It is an autosomal recessive disorder, and symptomatic individuals inherit a defective purine nucleoside phosphorylase gene (*PNP*) gene at chromosomal location 14q11.2 from each parent. Carrier parents have a 25 percent chance of passing this genetic defect to their offspring. Neurological symptoms often accompany this disease, but the route by which they develop is still undiscovered. Risk is evenly distributed between males and females. PNP deficiency constitutes approximately 1 to 2 percent of all combined immunodeficiencies. In 2011, a literature review identified sixty-seven patients from forty-nine families. In 2014, a compilation of all PNP deficiency patients found that there were close to eighty patients.

ETIOLOGY AND GENETICS

This inherited genetic disease causes the absence or mutation of *PNP*. PNP deficiency is one of several severe combined immunodeficiency (SCID) diseases, which also include adenosine deaminase (ADA) deficiency and X-linked severe combined immunodeficiency (X-SCID). Individuals with X-SCID comprise the majority of SCID cases. PNP deficiency accounts for only about 4 percent of all combined immunodeficiency diseases (CID). It is differentiated by recurring symptoms of chronic and unusual infections resistant to drug therapies, neurological symptoms, lymphopenia, and increased incidences of lymphomas and autoimmune diseases at a young age.

Purines are components necessary in cellular energy systems and to produce deoxyribonucleic acid (DNA) and ribonucleic acid (RNA). Purines are often recycled during catabolism using the purine salvage pathway. PNP catalyzes the interconversion of adenosine plus phosphate to adenine and ribose 1-phosphate.

A PNP enzyme deficiency along this pathway elevates levels of deoxyguanosine triphosphate (dGTP) lymph tissues, whose primary function is immunity. Subsequently, ribonucleotide reductase activity is necessary for the synthesis of deoxynucleotides, which are used in the genetic code, and mitochondrial DNA repair is inhibited. As a result, T-cell lymphocyte and thymocyte sensitivity increases, leading to T-cell destruction and a decreased ability to fight infection. Unlike ADA deficiency, B-cell lymphocytes in the immune system are unaffected.

SYMPTOMS

PNP deficiency is often challenging to diagnose because of recurring sinopulmonary and urinary tract infections that may indicate other diseases, such as B-cell immunodeficiency, vitamin B_{12} deficiency, or interstitial cystitis. But PNP deficiency is distinguished from other diseases by neurological and autoimmune diseases coupled with unusual, recurring, and drug-resistant bacterial, fungal, mycobacterial, protozoal, and viral infections. Drug-resistant pneumonia and oral thrush before one year of age are usually the first indications of a PNP deficiency. Often neurological symptoms precede infections because T-cell immunity declines gradually, thus delaying the onset of infections. Ataxia, autoimmune hemolytic anemia, autoimmune neutropenia, behavioral issues, bronchiectasis, central nervous vasculitis, developmental and motor delays, diarrhea, failure to thrive, herpes infections, hypertonia, idiopathic thrombocytopenia, lupus, malabsorption, mental retardation, neurological symptoms, nodular lymphoid hyperplasia of the gastrointestinal tract, spasticity, recurrent sinopulmonary and urinary tract infections, thyroiditis, and tremors are all symptoms that have been associated with a PNP deficiency.

SCREENING AND DIAGNOSIS

When an immunodeficiency disease is suspected, family and patient history, physical exam, blood screening, and skin tests help make an accurate diagnosis. A physical exam usually finds absent or underdeveloped lymph glands and tissue. Blood screening tests include a complete blood count and manual differential, quantitative serum immunoglobulin levels, antibody response measurement, and complement response. Other blood tests include T-cell enumeration, evaluation of T-cell function (proliferative response to mitogens and antigens), and serum uric acid. Low uric acid (mg/dL) levels with a demonstrated T-cell deficiency strongly suggest PNP deficiency. In such cases, measuring PNP enzyme activity or *PNP* gene sequencing definitively confirms the diagnosis. Few laboratories perform PNP activity measurements, but several commercial vendors offer gene sequencing.

The U.S. National Library of Medicine's *Genetics Home Reference* reported in 2014 that approximately two-thirds of PNP deficient individuals present with neurological symptoms, including muscle spasticity and intellectual disability. Autoimmune hemolytic anemia, immune thrombocytopenia, neutropenia, thyroiditis, and lupus diseases are often found. Chest X-rays usually show an underdeveloped thymus gland. The average age of diagnosis is six and a half months.

TREATMENT AND THERAPY

PNP deficiency is fatal, but recent treatments can extend the life span. Treatment first involves treating any infections with appropriate antibiotic therapies. If failure to thrive is present, then appropriate nutrition interventions are also prescribed. In the case of anemia, red blood cell transfusions improve symptoms for a limited time. Successful bone marrow and stem cell transplantation from a compatible donor cure the underlying immunodeficiency and improve immune system function. However, accompanying neurological disorders or autoimmune diseases are not cured by bone marrow transplantation. Treatment of these disorders depends on the specific disease. Prophylactic precautions include avoiding situations where germs may spread and cause infections, using good hygiene and nutrition practices, avoiding live viral immunizations, and treatment with long-term, low-dose antibiotics to prevent and control infections.

In vitro studies show that gene and intracellular enzyme replacement therapies and infusing PNP fusion proteins may resolve PNP deficiency and offer promising treatments in the future. Nevertheless, gene therapy and enzyme replacement therapy for

PNP deficiency remain in the experimental stages. Transplants of stem cells from umbilical cord blood may also resolve neurological symptoms.

PREVENTION AND OUTCOMES

Genetic counseling to assess risk is recommended when there is a family history of PNP deficiency. Prenatal diagnosis is possible in families with a previously affected child.

However, the prognosis is generally poor for PNP deficiency. Life expectancy is usually not more than ten years of age currently.

—*Alice C. Richer, RD, MBA, LD
and Michael A. Buratovich, PhD*

Further Information

Allenspach, Eric, David J. Rawlings, and Andrew M. Scharenberg. "X-Linked Severe Combined Immunodeficiency." *Gene Reviews*, edited by Roberta A. Pagon, et al., U of Washington, Seattle, 1993-2014. *NCBI Bookshelf*. National Center for Biotechnology Information, 24 Jan. 2013. Accessed 20 Aug. 2014.

Brodszki, Nicholas, et al. "Novel Genetic Mutations in the First Swedish Patient with Purine Nucleoside Phosphorylase Deficiency and Clinical Outcome After Hematopoietic Stem Cell Transplantation with HLA-Matched Unrelated Donor." *JIMD Reports*, vol. 24, 2015, pp. 83-89, doi:10.1007/8904_2015_444.

Dror, Yigal, et al. "Purine Nucleoside Phosphorylase Deficiency Associated with a Dysplastic Marrow Morphology." *Pediatric Research*, vol. 55, no. 3, 2004, pp. 472-77.

Gates, Robert H. *Infectious Disease Secrets*. 2nd ed., Hanley, 2003.

Genetics Home Reference. "Purine Nucleoside Phosphorylase Deficiency." *Genetics Home Reference*. U.S. NLM, 18 Aug. 2014. Accessed 20 Aug. 2014.

Grunebaum, E., A. Cohen, and C. M. Roifman. "Recent Advances in Understanding and Managing Adenosine Deaminase and Purine Nucleoside Phosphorylase Deficiencies." Current Opinion in Allergy and Clinical Immunology, vol. 13, no. 6, 2013, pp. 630-38. *Medline*. Accessed 20 Aug. 2014.

Janeway, Charles A. *Immunobiology: The Immune System in Health and Disease*. 7th ed., Garland, 2007.

McKusick, Victor A., and Cassandra L. Kniffin. "#613179 Purine Nucleoside Phosphorylase Deficiency." *OMIM*. Johns Hopkins U, 8 Jan. 2013. Accessed 20 Aug. 2014.

MedlinePlus. "Immune System and Disorders." *MedlinePlus*. U.S. NLM/NIH, 20 Aug. 2014. Accessed 20 Aug. 2014.

Walker, P. L., et al. "Purine Nucleoside Phosphorylase Deficiency: A Mutation Update." *Nucleosides, Nucleotides & Nucleic Acids*, vol. 30, no. 12, 2011, pp. 1243-47. *Medline*. Accessed 20 Aug. 2014.

SEVERE COMBINED IMMUNODEFICIENCY SYNDROME (SCID)

Category: Diseases/Disorders
Also known as: Bubble boy disease
Anatomy or system affected: Immune system
Specialties and related fields: Biotechnology, genetics, immunology, pediatrics
Definition: A syndrome in which the immune system cannot produce T and B cells, resulting in catastrophic failure of the immune system. The underlying cause is a mutation in one of several key genes. Without specialized treatment, often with cells from a donor, death typically occurs before one.

KEY TERMS

B cell: a lymphocyte that synthesizes immunoglobulins (antibodies)

graft-versus-host disease (GVHD): a condition that occurs when transplanted organs or cells are recognized by the host's immune system as invaders, resulting in the donor cells being attacked by the host's immune system

leukemia: any of a variety of types of cancer involving the blood or bone marrow

reservoir: the host species in which a parasite is maintained in each area and from which it may infect other species, initiating an epidemic

T cell: a lymphocyte responsible for cell-mediated immune responses, including graft rejection

X-linked gene: a gene located on the X chromosome

CAUSES AND SYMPTOMS

Severe combined immunodeficiency syndrome (SCID) is a genetic defect in which one of several genes involved in the immune system has a mutation that either prevents gene expression or causes the production of faulty products. The most common cause of SCID, accounting for about half of cases, is mutations in the X-linked gene *IL2RG*, which codes for the third chain of the interleukin-2 (IL-2) receptor and a part of several other interleukin receptors. Interleukin receptors are proteins embedded in the plasma membrane of cells in the immune system that interact with interleukin molecules, carrying necessary immune system signals. This type of SCID is called "X-linked combined immunodeficiency" (XCID). The faulty interleukin receptors prevent the development of T cells and natural killer (NK) cells, both of which are required to prevent infections successfully. Because XCID is an X-linked defect, it is much more common in males.

The remaining cases of SCID are attributable to mutations in many different genes, with new defects being discovered every year. The genes involved range from those that code for proteins that interact with interleukin receptors and enzymes involved in purine metabolism to genes that code for enzymes involved in antigen receptor production. In addition, a variety of lesser-known defects and some genetic disorders show some, but not all, of SCID symptoms.

The most common of the remaining defects, accounting for about 20 percent of cases, is a deficiency in the enzyme adenosine deaminase (ADA), which is involved in purine degradation. Nucleotides are the building blocks of nucleic acids like deoxyribonucleic acid (DNA) and ribonucleic acid (RNA). These building blocks consist of phosphate, a five-carbon sugar, and a base. Nucleotides have a functional lifetime, and cells either degrade them into simpler components to either excrete or recycle them. ADA degrades the purine adenosine into inosine. The absence of functional ADA causes a form of SCID, called ADA SCID. Without ADA activity, a subunit of DNA, deoxyadenosine triphosphate or dATP, accumulates to toxic levels. dATP inhibits the enzyme ribonucleotide reductase, the enzyme responsible for making DNA subunits in the cell. Low levels of other deoxyribonucleotides (dNTPs) prevent lymphocytes from making DNA and proliferating in response to an infection or disease. No T or B cells are produced. Deficiency in another enzyme, purine nucleoside phosphorylase (PNP), although much rarer, acts similarly.

Regardless of the underlying causes, symptoms are similar for most types of SCID. The overwhelming clinical symptom is problems with repeated, persistent infections that do not respond to standard treatment. Severe infections such as meningitis or septic arthritis may occur. Infections with opportunistic pathogens such as *Pneumocystis carinii* also frequently occur. Symptoms of (GVHD) may occur in infants because of lymphocytes received from the mother or in patients following blood transfusion. A chest X-ray typically shows a lack of a thymic shadow, indicating that the thymus has not developed properly. There is often also a family history of

---

INFORMATION ON SEVERE COMBINED IMMUNODEFICIENCY SYNDROME (SCID)

Causes: Various genetic defects

Symptoms: Repeated, persistent infections that are unresponsive to standard treatments; may include meningitis, septic arthritis, opportunistic infections, graft-versus-host disease (GVHD)

Duration: Chronic

Treatments: Bone marrow transplantation, hormonal therapy, gene therapy

immunodeficiency and infant deaths caused by severe infection.

TREATMENT AND THERAPY
Left untreated, most infants die within the first year, so rapid identification of the symptoms is crucial. Prenatal diagnosis is possible and is recommended in families with a history of SCID or similar problems. If SCID is detected early enough, then several treatment options are available, even potential prenatal treatment.

For the majority of SCID cases, bone marrow transplantation is the standard treatment. To prevent GVHD, either the marrow must come from an identical twin or be depleted of T cells before transplantation. Although a close genetic match has the highest success rate, unmatched and T cell-depleted marrow can be used if matched marrow is unavailable. A more than 90 percent survival rate has been accomplished when the marrow is from a parent or full sibling. It has typically been routine to use chemotherapy to kill the recipient's bone marrow before transplanting donor marrow. However, in SCID patients, this has been found unnecessary (and seems to lower the survival rate) because the recipient has no T cells to cause rejection.

When transplantation is successful, donor stem cells in the marrow populate the recipient's marrow and establish a functioning immune system. Unfortunately, some residual GVHD may occur, and over time T-cell function seems to diminish in many cases, despite apparent initial success. The reasons for the latter problem are unknown.

Although transplantation may also work for ADA SCID, an alternative is polyethylene glycol (PEG)-bovine ADA replacement therapy. Attachment of PEG to the enzyme reduces its recognition by the immune system and prevents its degradation by plasma-based enzymes. PEG-ADA circulates throughout the blood, degrading adenosine and its metabolites, preventing their accumulation. This treatment must be administered on an ongoing basis by frequent intravenous injections of PEG-ADA to maintain appropriate enzyme levels. While PEG ADA does not enter cells, it does degrade those molecules whose buildup in cells caused them to spill into the bloodstream. More than 150 patients worldwide have received PEG-ADA treatment. It is usually administered weekly or twice a week by intramuscular injections. PEG-ADA treatment seems to be well tolerated and confers clinical benefits after the first month of therapy. Unfortunately, PEG-ADA is not always available and is extremely expensive, leaving transplantation the only option in some cases.

Still in the experimental stage is gene therapy to replace the defective genes. Experiments on this approach began in the early 1990s. Although the first attempts at curing ADA SCID showed partial success, the patients still required continued treatment with PEG-ADA. Since then, efforts have focused on better ways to insert the correct genes into the patient's stem cells. Stem cells from the bone marrow must be isolated, treated, and then returned to the patient.

The most promising results came from experiments begun in 1999 involving gene therapy for XCID. Following the procedure, the infants developed normal immune systems. Unfortunately, by the summer of 2002, one of the boys developed leukemia, and another developed it by the end of the same year. Some trials ceased as a result. The apparent cause of the leukemia was the insertion of the gene at an inappropriate location; a concern expressed early in the discussion of gene therapy for this disease. Gene therapy still holds great promise, but more work is needed to ensure its long-term safety and effectiveness.

—*Bryan Ness, PhD*

Further Information
Blaese, Michael R., et al. "T Lymphocyte-Directed Gene Therapy for ADA SCID: Initial Trial Results After Four

Years." *Science*, vol. 270, 1995, pp. 475-80. A research report on the long-term results of the first gene therapy trials involving SCID.

Cohen, Philip. "Fresh Blow for Gene Treatments as Safety of a Second Virus Is Questioned." *New Scientist*, vol. 178, 2003, p. 17. A brief article about some children treated for SCID using gene therapy who later developed leukemia.

Cooper, Max D., et al. "Immunodeficiency Disorders." *Hematology*, vol. 1, 2003, pp. 314-30. A thorough presentation on the cell biology behind immunodeficiency disorders with a detailed section on SCID.

Hawley, Robert G., and Donna A. Sobieski. "Of Mice and Men: The Tale of Two Therapies." *Stem Cells*, vol. 20, 2002, pp. 275-78. Discusses the experimental gene therapy trials for both XCID and ADA SCID.

Nelson, David L., and Michael M. Cox. *Lehninger Principles of Biochemistry*. 7th ed., W.H. Freeman, 2017. A standard biochemistry textbook that contains a superb explanation of the biochemical mechanisms behind several types of SCID.

Sauer, Aisha V., Immacolata Brigida, Nicola Carriglio, and Alessandro Aiuti. "Autoimmune Dysregulation and Purine Metabolism in Adenosine Deaminase Deficiency." *Frontiers in Immunology*, vol. 3, 2012, p. 265. www.frontiersin.org/article/10.3389/fimmu.2012.00265, doi:10.3389/fimmu.2012.00265. An excellent of the biochemical and clinical aspects of ADA-SCID.

Schwarz, Klaus, et al. "Human Severe Combined Immune Deficiency and DNA Repair." *Bioessays*, vol. 25, no. 11, 2003, pp. 1061-70. A current overview of the underlying causes of the various types of SCID and a discussion of the potential of gene therapy to cure it.

Scollay, Roland. "Gene Therapy: A Brief Overview of the Past, Present, and Future." *Annals of the New York Academy of Sciences*, vol. 953, 2001, pp. 26-30. Discusses the potential of gene therapy in curing single-gene diseases, with some mention of SCID.

T-CELL IMMUNODEFICIENCY SYNDROME

Category: Diseases/Syndromes
Anatomy or system affected: Blood, immune system, lymphatic system
Specialties and related fields: Hematology, immunology, internal medicine
Definition: T-cell immunodeficiency syndrome refers to the group of immunodeficiencies that increase susceptibility to infection as a result of an immune system with deficient, absent, or defective T cells. This immunodeficiency can be expressed as a primary (congenital) or a secondary (acquired) disorder. Primary T-cell immunodeficiency results from autosomal or X-linked genetic defects.

KEY TERMS

immunodeficiency: a condition, inherited or induced, in which the immune system fails to function normally, increasing the risk of life-threatening infections and cancers

severe combined immune deficiency (SCID): a group of rare disorders caused by mutations in various genes involved in the development and function of infection-fighting immune cells that cripples the immune system, increasing the risk of grave infections and tumors

T lymphocyte: a subtype of lymphocyte that matures in the thymus gland and plays a central role in the adaptive immune response

X-linked: a gene physically located on the X chromosome

RISK FACTORS

Secondary T-cell immunodeficiency is the most common and develops due to chronic infection, malnutrition, systemic disease, malignancy, or drug therapy. Although primary T-cell immunodeficiency is less common than secondary forms, they are rare genetic disorders. Generally, they develop in infancy or early childhood, accompanied by unusual recurrent infections.

ETIOLOGY AND GENETICS

Considering that T cells (a type of white blood cells) are the dominant type of lymphocytes in circulating blood, it is very likely that a significant T-cell deficiency usually may cause a decrease in the number of blood lymphocytes. Several genetic abnormalities may prevent T cells from identifying and destroying foreign or abnormal cells circulating in the body. An impaired T-cell immunity damages the immune system's ability to protect against bacterial, viral, fungal, or cancer cell attacks. The two general reasons contributing to the development of T-cell immunodeficiency syndrome are either autosomal or X-linked gene disorders resulting from mutations or deletions. These hereditary genetic disorders give rise to partial or absolute defects in T-cell function resulting in a defective immune system at birth or early in life. The most common forms of T-cell immunodeficiency disorders are severe combined immune deficiency (SCID), X-linked lymphoproliferative syndrome, X-linked hyper-immunoglobulin M (IgM) immunodeficiency, hyper-immunoglobulin E (IgE) syndrome, DiGeorge syndrome, ataxia-telangiectasia, Nijmegen breakage syndrome, Wiskott-Aldrich syndrome (WAS), and T-cell immunodeficiency, recurrent infections, and autoimmunity with or without cardiac malformations (TIIAC). SCID (or bubble boy syndrome) is the most severe immunodeficiency disorder. A mutation in the *IL2RG* gene of the X chromosome, responsible for making a protein that helps immune cells grow and mature, most commonly causes SCID. This results in low levels of antibodies (immunoglobulins) and no T cells. The severity of this deficiency results in the development of more severe infections with infants not growing or developing normally. Untreated children frequently die before the age of one. The X-linked disorder affects males more than females. Males only have one X chromosome, and therefore the mutation is enough to cause the disease. In contrast, females would need to inherit the

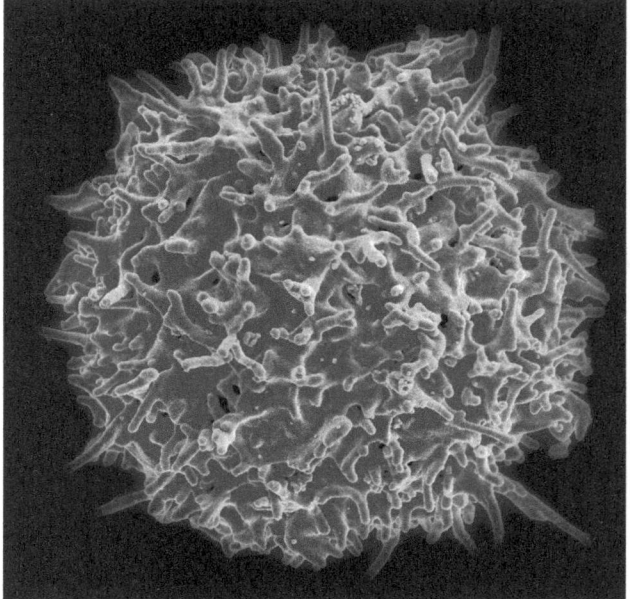

Human T-cell. Image via Wikimedia Commons. [Public domain.]

same mutation in both X chromosomes. Omenn syndrome is an example of an autosomal recessive form of SCID. In this case, both parents pass on the mutation typically to the *RAG1* or *RAG2* genes.

In DiGeorge syndrome, deletion of chromosome 22 (at 22q11.2) results in a thymus gland absent or underdeveloped at birth. The fetus has heart, face, thymus, and parathyroid gland abnormalities, leading to a mild to moderate T-cell deficiency. The X-linked lymphoproliferative (XLP) syndrome (Duncan disease) is caused by mutations in the *SH2D1A* (Type 1) and *XIAP* (Type 2) genes. It results in defective T cells and natural killer (NK) cells. It is characterized by extreme sensitivity to Epstein-Barr (mononucleosis) virus infection, resulting in liver failure, immunodeficiency, and malignant lymphoma.

Hyper-IgM syndrome is an antibody deficiency known by normal or elevated IgM levels and decreased levels or absence of other serum antibodies. It is caused by a mutation in the *CD40LG* gene of the X chromosome and leads to susceptibility to bacterial infections. The gene makes CD40 ligand protein necessary to make antibodies.

Hyper-IgE syndrome (Buckley or Job syndrome) is caused by a mutation in the *STAT3* gene of chromosome 17, which results in high levels of IgE and normal levels of the other antibody classes. These patients suffer from chronic eczema, recurrent lung infections, weak bones, coarse facial features, and pus abscesses.

The mutation in the ATM gene of chromosome 11 results in ataxia-telangiectasia (AT). AT is characterized by dilated capillaries, higher susceptibility to infections, body movement incoordination, and malignancy predisposition.

A mutation in the NBN gene located on chromosome 8 (at position 8q21.3) is responsible for the Nijmegen (Berlin) breakage syndrome, characterized by microcephaly and sinopulmonary infections immunodeficiency, and high risk for lymphoma cancer. People with Nijmegen breakage syndrome have abnormally low immunoglobulin G (IgG), immunoglobulin A (IgA), and T cells. Because Wiskott-Aldrich syndrome is caused by a mutation in the WAS gene on the X chromosome at Xp11.23, immunodeficiencies are characterized by thrombocytopenia, eczema, and recurrent respiratory infections. There is abnormal antibody production and impaired T-cell function, affecting boys only. There is a higher incidence of developing cancers such as lymphoma and leukemia.

Mutations in *STK4* on chromosome 20 have been identified as responsible for T-cell immunodeficiency, recurrent infections, and autoimmunity with or without cardiac malformations (TIIAC). TIIAC is a primary T-cell immunodeficiency syndrome causing recurrent infections, warts, abscesses, autoimmune diseases, and cardiac malformations, including atrial septal defect.

SYMPTOMS

A history of unusual recurrent infections might suggest T-cell immunodeficiency syndrome. Frequently, respiratory infections arise first and reappear, becoming severe and persistent and leading to complications. Generally, the earliest the symptoms in life arise in children, the more severe the T-cell immunodeficiency syndrome will be. Other different ailments may contrast or change based on the infections' severity and length. Due to weight loss, chronic diarrhea may cause infants or young children not to grow or develop (failure to thrive).

Type 1 diabetes, hypoadrenalism, hypothyroidism, glomerulonephritis, and autoimmune enteropathy often develop in children with immune disorders very early.

SCREENING AND DIAGNOSIS

Doctors suspecting a primary T-cell immunodeficiency will run a battery of tests to identify the specific genetic abnormality, immunoglobulin levels, white blood microscopic irregularities, skin tests, number of circulating B and T cells, and good B and T-cell function. Upon physical examination, rashes, weight loss, chronic cough, hair loss, and/or enlarged spleen or liver may suggest a particular disorder to doctors based on disease-specific clinical manifestations. Early-onset of recurring or unusual infections is a critical determinant in identifying the type of immunodeficiency disorder. Adverse prognosis follows a delayed diagnosis. The particular form of infection will also help healthcare professionals pinpoint the T-cell immunodeficiency variant.

TREATMENT AND THERAPY

Symptoms suggest the type of genetic disorder, and treatment strategies are tailored to meet specific immunodeficiencies needs. Many patients will require prompt aggressive treatment. General guidelines for these patients include periodic intravenous (IV) immunoglobulin replacement therapy, practicing excellent personal hygiene, avoiding undercooked food, drinking boiled water, routine non-live vaccines, and avoiding contact with infected people.

SCID patients are kept in protected environments, preventing exposure to pathogens, and are treated with antibiotics, antivirals, and antibodies. Bone marrow stem cell transplantation from an unaffected sibling matching the same tissue type is the only effective treatment for SCID and WAS. Thymus transplantation for DiGeorge syndrome patients can cure the immunodeficiency, and corrective heart surgery is done for severe heart conditions. Due to deoxyribonucleic acid (DNA) instability, chemotherapy for malignancy may need to be tailored to lower doses and more prolonged therapies.

Gene therapy is being studied for many of these diseases, particularly SCID and WAS.

PREVENTION AND OUTCOMES

Prevention and outcome strategies depend on the type of T-cell immunodeficiency disorder diagnosed and the time of diagnosis. Some T-cell immunodeficiency syndromes shorten their life span, while others can be managed throughout life. When the disorder does not impair antibody production, vaccination is recommended only with killed viral and bacterial vaccines since live vaccines might cause disease in immunodeficient patients. There is no effective form of prevention; therefore, genetic testing and counseling should be provided to people with a family history previously identified for these types of hereditary immunodeficiencies. Early diagnosis is critical in improving patient outcomes since many children die young if untreated. The role of alert healthcare professionals to recognize T-cell immunodeficiency clinical findings can play an essential part in confirming a rapid, accurate diagnosis, ultimately resulting in improved patient outcomes.

—*Ana Maria Rodriguez-Rojas, MS and Deanna M. Neff, MPH*

Further Information

Bonilla, F. A., et al. "Practice Parameter for the Diagnosis and Management of Primary Immunodeficiency." *Annals of Allergy, Asthma & Immunology*, vol. 94, no. 5 (Suppl 1), May 2005, pp. S1-63.

Boztug, K., et al. "Multiple Independent Second Site Mutations in Two Siblings with Somatic Mosaicism for Wiskott-Aldrich Syndrome." *Clinical Genetics*, vol. 74, 2008, pp. 68-74.

Conley, Mary Ellen. "Antibody Deficiencies." *The Metabolic and Molecular Bases of Inherited Disease*, edited by Charles Scriver, et al., 8th ed., McGraw-Hill, 2001.

Cooper, Megan A., Thomas L. Pommering, and Katalin Koranyi. "Primary Immunodeficiencies." *American Family Physician*, vol. 68, 2003, pp. 2001-8, 2011.

Edgar, J. D. "T Cell Immunodeficiency." *Journal of Clinical Pathology*, vol. 61, 2008, pp. 988-93.

Kingsmore, S. F., et al. "Identification of Diagnostic Biomarkers for Infection in Premature Neonates." *Molecular & Cellular Proteomics*, vol. 7, no. 10, Oct. 2008, pp. 1863-75.

Pachlopnik Schmid, J., T. Güngör, and R. Seger. "Modern Management of Primary T-Cell Immunodeficiencies." *Pediatric Allergy & Immunology*, vol. 25, no. 4, 2014, pp. 300-313.

Autoimmune Diseases

Addison's disease

Category: Diseases/Disorders
Also known as: Chronic adrenal insufficiency, hypoadrenocorticism
Anatomy or system affected: Endocrine system, glands, kidneys
Specialties and related fields: Endocrinology, nephrology
Definition: A failure of adrenal cortex function in which production of any or all of the hormones synthesized by the cortex is decreased.

KEY TERMS

adrenal cortex: the outer portion of the adrenal gland; produces a wide variety of regulatory hormones

adrenal gland: the gland located on top of each of the kidneys

androgenic hormones: any of several hormones that regulate the expression of male characteristics

corticosteroid: an adrenal cortex hormone that controls processes such as protein and carbohydrate metabolism and electrolyte balance

cortisol: a steroid hormone that regulates inflammation

glucocorticoid: an adrenal cortex hormone that regulates a variety of bodily functions, such as inflammation and the mobilization of fat

mineralocorticoid: an adrenal cortex hormone that regulates the retention of minerals such as potassium and sodium

CAUSES AND SYMPTOMS

Anything that results in damage to the adrenal gland can cause the development of Addison's disease. Most commonly, the disorder is the result of an autoimmune malfunction, in which the body begins to react against its own tissue. Addison's disease may also result from adrenal cancers or infections. The prevalence rate is approximately 1 per 100,000 people.

The specific cause of adrenal insufficiency may be either primary or secondary. In primary adrenal insufficiency, the disorder arises directly within the outer region of the adrenal gland, called the "adrenal cortex." Most of the time, primary adrenal insufficiency is associated with an autoimmune dysfunction in which the body produces antibodies against adrenal tissue. Over time, the immune system destroys the adrenal cortex. Consequently, the secretion of glucocorticoid, mineralocorticoid, and androgenic hormones, the products of the adrenal cortex, gradually ceases.

Another cause of primary adrenal insufficiency is bacterial infections, particularly those associated with tuberculosis. The first identification of the disease, described by Thomas Addison in 1855, was associated with a tuberculosis infection in his patient. Other less common causes include fungal infections and malignancies.

Information on Addison's Disease

Causes: Lack of hormone production by adrenal cortex from autoimmune dysfunction, cancer, or infection; abnormal regulation of adrenal hormone production by the pituitary gland

Symptoms: Extreme fatigue, low blood pressure, appetite loss, fainting, severe diarrhea and vomiting, craving for salty foods, skin darkening

Duration: Chronic, with acute episodes (Addisonian crises)

Treatments: Hormone replacement, dietary changes (such as increased salt content)

Secondary adrenal insufficiency does not originate with the adrenal glands but with abnormal regulation of adrenal hormone production, a function of the pituitary gland. Among the hormones produced within the pituitary gland is adrenocorticotropic hormone (ACTH), which stimulates glucocorticoid production by the adrenal cortex. Insufficient ACTH production results in a decrease in corticoid secretion. Any damage to the pituitary (or the hypothalamus, which regulates ACTH production by the pituitary) can affect ACTH production indirectly.

With Addison's disease, the onset of symptoms is gradual and can easily be overlooked or misdiagnosed during the early stages of the disease. Initially, the person may exhibit extreme fatigue, low blood pressure, and loss of appetite. The person may faint upon standing. Severe diarrhea and vomiting are also common. As a result of salt loss, the person may crave salty foods. Severe symptoms result in an Addisonian crisis; if untreated, it may be life-threatening. Because corticosteroid production regulates the ACTH secretion in a feedback mechanism, reduced adrenal function results in increased ACTH levels. Abnormally high ACTH levels can produce skin changes, particularly a darkening that mimics deep tanning. The presence of darkening equally over both exposed and unexposed skin can be indicative of Addison's disease, especially if other symptoms are also present.

A definitive diagnosis of Addison's disease requires a series of blood and urine tests. Patients may exhibit abnormally high potassium levels, a potentially life-threatening situation, or low sodium levels. More definitive tests measure the concentration of cortisol hormones in the urine. Because ACTH production is controlled by corticosteroid concentrations, an increase in blood ACTH may also be observed. The definitive test begins with the intravenous injection of ACTH. Cortisol levels in the blood are then measured over one hour. If cortisol levels do not change, this result is indicative of a likely adrenal insufficiency.

TREATMENT AND THERAPY

The treatment of Addison's disease generally involves replacing the hormones that the adrenal cortex is no longer manufacturing. Oral medication is available for most of these hormones, though dietary changes may also be necessary. For example, if the mineralocorticoid aldosterone is insufficient, resulting in a salt imbalance, then patients taking aldosterone supplements may also be advised to increase the salt content of their food.

Oral medications for Addison's disease include corticosteroid replacement medicines like hydrocortisone (Cortef), prednisone, or methylprednisolone. These hormones are given on a schedule to mimic the normal 24-hour fluctuation of cortisol levels. To replace aldosterone, physicians usually prescribe

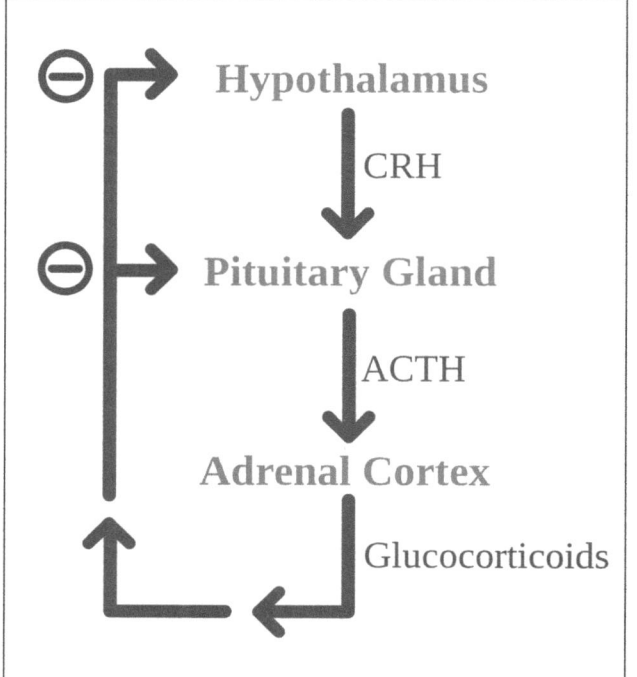

The negative feedback loop for glucocorticoids. Image by Drosenbach, via Wikimedia Commons.

fludrocortisone acetate. Patients may take fludrocortisone three times a week or daily as needed. When used at the prescribed dosages, these medications have few adverse effects.

Other forms of treatment may be symptomatic. If the patient suffers from low blood pressure or severe salt imbalances, potentially life-threatening conditions, then intravenous medication may be necessary.

As the monitoring of potassium and sodium levels is critical, it is generally recommended that patients routinely visit their physicians. It is important that a patient exhibiting symptoms of an Addisonian crisis (vomiting, diarrhea) receive an immediate salt replacement and probably hydrocortisone as well.

Because secondary adrenal deficiency most often originates in the pituitary gland, the primary result is decreased ACTH production. In turn, the adrenal cortex is deficient only in the production of cortisol. Treatment generally involves the oral replacement of cortisol, often in the form of synthetic prednisone.

PERSPECTIVE AND PROSPECTS

Addison's disease is a lifelong, chronic condition. While formerly a life-threatening disorder, proper monitoring, and hormone replacement can allow most people with the disease to live relatively normal lives with no restrictions. Because in most individuals the immediate cause is an autoimmune disorder, it is possible that eventually stem cell research, along with improved methods of controlling autoimmune phenomena will provide a means for replacing adrenal tissue.

—*Richard Adler, PhD*

Further Information
Bar, Robert, editor. *Early Diagnosis and Treatment of Endocrine Disorders*. Humana Press, 2003.
Besser, G. Michael, and Michael Thorner, editors. *Clinical Endocrinology*. 2nd ed., Gower-Mosby, 1994.
Greenspan, Francis S., Dolores M. Shoback, and David G. Gardner, editors. *Greenspan's Basic and Clinical Endocrinology*. 8th ed., McGraw-Hill, 2007.
Kronenberg, Henry M., et al., editors. *Williams Textbook of Endocrinology*. 11th ed., Saunders/Elsevier, 2008.
MedlinePlus. "Addison Disease." *MedlinePlus*, 8 Apr. 2013 (reviewed 3 May 2012).
Parker, James N., and Philip M. Parker, editors. *The Official Patient's Sourcebook on Addison's Disease*. Icon Health, 2002.
Rennert, Nancy J. "Addison's Disease." *MedlinePlus*, 11 Dec. 2011.

AUTOIMMUNE DISORDERS

Category: Diseases/Disorders
Anatomy or system affected: Circulatory system, lymphatic system, nervous system, skeletal system
Specialties and related fields: Immunology
Definition: Damage to the tissues or organs of the body caused by failure of the immune system to distinguish between "self" and "nonself," producing autoantibodies called "B cells" and "autoreactive cells" at the request of the T lymphocytes (cells).

KEY TERMS

alleles: a distinct form of a gene, inherited from either parent and present in pairs in each person
antibody: a molecule of the immune system, produced by B cells and targeted toward eliminating a specific antigen
antigen: a protein or related molecule that is seen as foreign and therefore induces antibody formation in an individual
autoantibody: an antibody that binds to a protein that is a normal part of the human body from which it originates, as opposed to part of a bacteria, virus, or another human being
B cells: also known as B lymphocytes; the antibody-producing cells of the immune system

haplotype: a group of genes within an organism inherited together from a single parent

human leukocyte antigen (HLA): highly polymorphic cell surface proteins that antigen-presenting cells use to present antigen to lymphocytes (class II HLAs) or are found on the surfaces of every nucleated cell in the body (class I HLAs) and act as identification tags by which the immune system distinguishes between self and nonself; also known as major histocompatibility complex (MHC) proteins

multigenic: referring to a trait or characteristic that requires the product of more than one gene to be expressed

polymorphic: genes that exist in multiple forms or alleles within a population; genes that show extensive variability within a population

selection: the process by which developing immune system cells are either allowed to continue to maturation or destroyed before they can enter the circulation

T cells: also known as T lymphocytes; the immune system cells involved in cellular immunity and regulation of the immune response

tolerance: the ability of the immune system to remain unresponsive to self-antigens

CAUSES OF AUTOIMMUNE DISORDERS

Autoimmunity refers to a group of widely varying diseases or disorders that include familiar examples (type 1 diabetes mellitus, myasthenia gravis, multiple sclerosis, rheumatoid arthritis) and many that are not as familiar (idiopathic thrombocytopenic purpura, Graves' disease, Felty syndrome, Hashimoto's thyroiditis). The list is long and growing as researchers continue to ferret out the root causes of many disorders that have been known for one hundred years or more. In many cases, environmental triggers or environmentally controlled flare-ups are common. All autoimmune disorders have one thing in common: the failure of the human immune system to distinguish between self (own) and nonself antigens, thus leading the body to attack itself and damage or destroy tissues or organs. Autoimmunity is not a rare event; it occurs in all people, and it does not necessarily give rise to disease. For instance, aged or damaged cells of the body are normally destroyed by autoantibodies (antibodies directed against the self). However, other autoantibodies, which arise by chance combinations of genes, are normally suppressed during development in the thymus gland. This is referred to as selection. If the thymus fails to do its job, then these autoantibodies may be released into the lymph nodes and the bloodstream, seeking out tissue or antigens to attack and destroy.

Autoimmune disorders can be classified in several ways. Some diseases affect only one organ system, and some affect multiple systems. Examples of organ-specific disorders are Addison's disease and Graves' disease; non-organ-specific disorders include systemic lupus erythematosus and scleroderma. Alternatively, one can classify autoimmune disorders by the type of immune system cells involved in their onset. Some diseases are caused by the antibody-secreting B cells; they include myasthenia gravis, multiple sclerosis, rheumatic fever, systemic lupus erythematosus, and Graves' disease. Other disorders result from the action of the sys-

---

INFORMATION ON AUTOIMMUNE DISORDERS

Causes: Unknown, possibly hereditary, environmental, or viral

Symptoms: Varies widely; may include pain, fatigue, joint and muscle inflammation, muscle weakness, sleep disturbances, headaches, numbness and tingling, central nervous system disturbances

Duration: Often chronic

Treatments: Alleviation of symptoms, strengthening the immune system

temic T cells, including Addison's disease and Hashimoto's thyroiditis.

The onset of an autoimmune disorder hinges on many factors, some of which are still being identified. It is well established, however, that autoimmunity is multifactorial and multigenic. In other words, many environmental factors and many genes are involved in determining susceptibility to autoimmune disorders. In addition, many environmental factors are thought to be involved in controlling remission and flare-ups of autoimmune disorders. Most autoimmune disorders are probably the result of the release of T or B cells that do not properly distinguish between self and nonself and should have been eliminated or suppressed by the body's immune system.

Autoimmune conditions are caused by hereditary, the environment, bacteria or viruses, fungi, or drugs, or some combination of these factors. Most autoimmune diseases have an unknown cause. Some rheumatologists postulate that some gene or group of genes must be activated for autoimmune diseases to develop.

SYMPTOMS

The symptoms of these diseases vary widely and depend on the specific autoimmune disease. Typical symptoms may include pain, fatigue, joint and muscle inflammation, muscle weakness, sleep disturbances, headaches, numbness and tingling, central nervous system disturbances, kidney damage, and liver damage. They can also affect the skin, red blood cells, connective tissue, blood vessels, nerves, and the endocrine glands. Most of them are chronic conditions.

ETIOLOGY OF VARIOUS AUTOIMMUNE DISEASES

Several studies have established genetic links in autoimmune diseases, but because most are multigenic, no simple Mendelian inheritance pat-

PARTIAL LIST OF AUTOIMMUNE DISEASES

Disease: Organ/Target
- Addison's disease: Adrenal glands
- Ankylosing spondylitis: Spine
- Antiphospholipid antibody syndrome: Blood clotting
- Celiac disease: Small intestine
- Crohn's disease: Gastrointestinal tract
- Dermatomyositis: Skeletal muscles and skin
- Diabetes mellitus type 1: (some forms) Pancreas islet cell
- Felty's disease: Joints and spleen
- Goodpasture's syndrome: Kidneys and lungs
- Graves' disease: Thyroid gland
- Guillain-Barré syndrome: Peripheral nervous system
- Hashimoto's thyroiditis: Thyroid gland
- Hemolytic anemia: Red blood cells, platelets
- Multiple sclerosis: Brain and spinal cord
- Myasthenia gravis: Junctions between nerves and muscles
- Pemphigus vulgaris: Skin and mucus membranes
- Pernicious anemia: Stomach parietal cells
- Polymyositis: Skeletal muscle
- Poststreptococcal glomerulonephritis: Kidneys
- Psoriasis: Skin
- Rheumatic fever: Heart
- Rheumatoid arthritis: Connective tissue and joints
- Scleroderma: Heart, lungs, kidney, gastrointestinal tract, and skin
- Sjögren's syndrome: saliva and tear glands
- Systemic lupus erythematosus: deoxyribonucleic acid (DNA), platelets, all organs
- Thrombocytopenic purpura: Platelets
- Ulcerative colitis: Colon
- Wegener's granulomatosis: Lungs and kidneys

tern is seen. Nonetheless, there seems to be a clear correlation between specific human leukocyte antigen (HLA) alleles and certain autoimmune disorders. The genes of the major histocompatibility complex (MHC) encode the HLAs. The MHC is a large cluster of tightly linked genes on chromosome six in human beings, but such genes are common to all vertebrates. MHC genes encode cell surface proteins essential for the adaptive immune response and they fall into two main classes, class I and class II MHC protein. Class I MHC proteins are found on the surfaces of all nucleated cells. Viral-infected cells use class I MHC proteins to present viral proteins on their surfaces. The immune system also uses class I MHC proteins to promote "tolerance" or an inability to attack its tissues and cells. Antigen-presenting cells use class II MHCs to present antigen to lymphocytes and other immune cells. Without class II MHC proteins, the immune system cannot recognize foreign substances and mount immune responses to them.

The MHC complex was named from its importance to transplanted tissue compatibility. MHC proteins mediate the interactions of antigen-presenting cells with lymphocytes and other white blood cells. MHC genes are highly polymorphic, meaning that they vary extensively within human populations. The array of alleles within someone's MHC genes determines their donor compatibility for organ transplants and susceptibility to specific autoimmune diseases. Therefore, the correlation between the susceptibility to specific autoimmune disorders and HLA alleles is unsurprising, since the class II HLA genes encode proteins that present antigens to lymphocytes. Specific alleles of class II HLA genes encode proteins that have a greater tendency to present self-peptides. Some examples should be illustrative.

For instance, those who have HLA allele B27 have a ninetyfold greater risk than the normal population of developing ankylosing spondylitis. Specific HLA-DRB1 alleles, especially those encoding amino acid sequence changes at positions 11 and 13, significantly increase the susceptibility to rheumatoid arthritis. Those with the HLA DR3 haplotype have a twelvefold greater risk of celiac disease and a tenfold greater risk of Sjögren's syndrome. In the case of insulin-dependent diabetes, the relative risk factor is fivefold. If someone has the DR3 and the DR4 haplotype, then the risk increases twentyfold. If the DR3 haplotype and DQw8 subtype of the DR4 haplotype are present, then the risk factor is one-hundredfold. Yet, these alleles themselves do not automatically cause autoimmune disease, as evidenced by several studies on identical twins in which the rate of disease in the twin of an affected person ranged from 25 to 50 percent. Environmental factors can change susceptibility to autoimmune disease into actual manifestation.

Autoimmune disorders are much more common in women than in men. In addition, they are usually more severe in women. This is likely because of estrogen, which has a role in enhancing the expression of HLA genes and activating macrophages, thus leading to higher tissue destruction. Some autoimmune conditions are noted to flare and subside throughout the menstrual cycle, in conjunction with the rise and fall of estrogen levels. Stress is likely a contributing factor that can cause an autoimmune disorder to flare. This response is likely mediated through the hypothalamus and pituitary glands, which release hormones that directly stimulate the immune system.

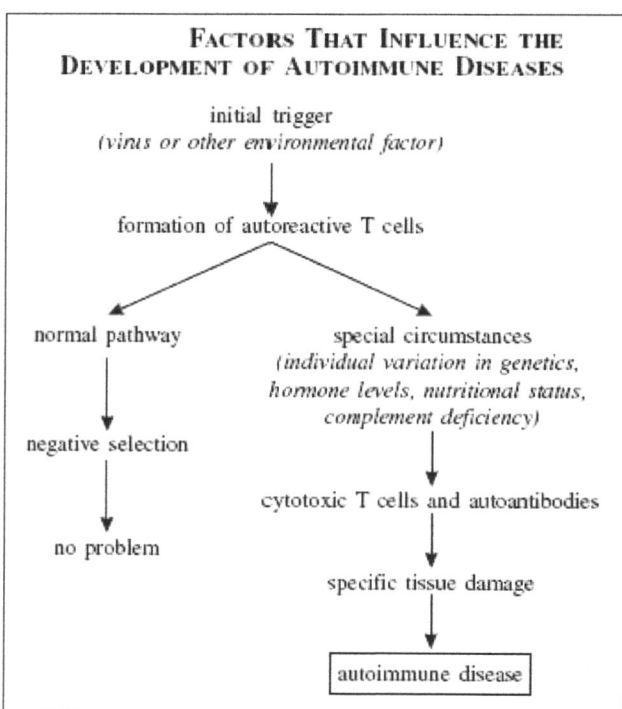

The expression of some autoimmune diseases is commonly preceded by infection by a virulent organism. Infections may contribute to autoimmunity in several ways. Some microbes produce antigens that are very close in structure to human antigens. When antibodies are produced against the invading organism, the antibodies also attack self-antigens because of the chemical similarity. Examples of this response are poststreptococcal glomerulonephritis and rheumatic fever. Other invaders may damage human cells and release proteins that are not normally seen by the immune system (sequestered proteins). These proteins are seen as foreign, and an immune response is set up against these self-antigens. A similar response may be seen when normally sequestered proteins are released through trauma or injury. An example is sympathetic ophthalmia, in which eye lens proteins that are normally not seen in the circulation are released, triggering antibodies that may then attack the opposite (uninjured) eye as well. The symptoms of autoimmune disorders are as varied as the disorders themselves. No one set of symptoms fits all disorders. Symptoms may be systemic or localized, progressive, or stable. Symptoms may also be life-threatening or simply annoying.

Multiple sclerosis (MS) is an autoimmune disorder involving the central nervous system. Nerve axons of the white matter of the brain are normally surrounded by myelin protein sheaths that protect the nerves and speed the process of transmission. In individuals with MS, these myelin sheath proteins are gradually attacked and destroyed, slowing nerve impulses so that patients develop a loss of control of motor function and vision. This disease often progresses irregularly and unpredictably and is irreversible. It appears to be the result of both B cells, producing antibodies against oligodendroglia, the cells that make myelin protein, and T cells, acting against a peptide product from the myelin protein. Although what triggers the initial response is unclear, it has been suggested that onset may follow infection with either Epstein-Barr or hepatitis B viruses. More than 2.1 million people worldwide are affected by MS. It is mostly women who are diagnosed between age twenty and fifty.

Systemic lupus erythematosus (SLE), known simply as lupus, is a generalized disorder that occurs predominantly in women. It is linked to B cells and the production of antibodies against parts of the DNA molecule. These DNA antibodies bind to free DNA and a subset of these DNA autoantibodies penetrate cells, translocate to nuclei, inhibit DNA repair, and directly damage DNA. DNA autoantibodies progressively injure cells and tissues and cells and accelerate the accumulated damage associated with the normal aging process. This may form immune complexes that are deposited in the kidneys and arterioles, leading to tissue destruction and fibrosis, and in the joints, leading to arthritis. Autoantibodies against red blood cells or platelets may also occur in SLE. Antibodies against muscles may be present and contribute to muscle inflammation, while the presence of antibodies against heart muscle may lead to myocarditis and endocarditis. Antibodies against skin components can lead to a characteristic "butterfly rash" on the bridge of the nose and the area around the eyes that is seen in many patients with SLE; this rash worsens in the presence of sunlight.

Rheumatoid arthritis is a common, crippling disease. It is controlled by B cells in the joints that are activated to produce several antibodies, including the rheumatoid factor. The result is the formation and deposition of immune complexes in the joint cartilage. Antibodies directed against cartilage may also be seen. The resulting destruction activates chemicals that stimulate T cells to come to the area, and they, in turn, release destructive enzymes, just as they would if bacteria were invading the joints. All these responses lead to joint damage, inflammation, and pain. As the disease progresses, the synovia swell and extend into the joints, causing further pain and discomfort along with disfigurement of the joints. The cause of antibody activation is unknown and may be quite variable.

Both Hashimoto's thyroiditis and Graves' disease are forms of autoimmune thyroiditis. In Hashimoto's disease, antibodies are formed against a protein within the thyroid cells, leading to immune attack of the thyroid cells and destruction of thyroid tissue. In Graves' disease, the immune system produces antibodies that bind to the receptors for thyroid-stimulating hormone (TSH), the pituitary hormone that stimulates the thyroid gland to produce thyroid hormone. The receptors in turn are stimulated. Thus, the thyroid gland is hyperstimulated, and excess thyroid hormone is turned out, a condition known as thyrotoxicosis.

An individual with myasthenia gravis experiences muscle fatigue and extreme weakness with only mild exercise, such as walking short distances. It is caused by autoantibodies that are directed against the acetylcholine (ACh) receptor molecule. In normal neural cells that control large muscles, ACh is stimulated to be released from the neuron and bind to receptors on the muscle fiber endplate. If that receptor is blocked or destroyed by an antibody, the ACh cannot bind, and therefore the muscle is not stimulated to respond (contract). If a few receptors are blocked, then the muscle may still respond weakly. If enough antibody is present to block many receptors, however, then the threshold limit for muscle response will not be achieved, and the muscle will not respond even in the presence of repeated stimulation from the neuron. Scleroderma, also known as progressive systemic sclerosis, predominantly affects middle-aged women and is caused by collagen deposition in a variety of tissues of the body. Antibodies may be found against the centromere portion of the DNA. Symptoms include calcium deposition in the skin, sensitivity to cold, and decreased esophageal motility. The lungs often experience fibrosis, as do the kidneys.

Most autoimmune disorders cannot be cured; they develop into chronic conditions that require a lifetime of care and monitoring. Treatment is quite varied and depends on the underlying cause and etiology of the disease. Overall, the goals of treatment are to reduce the symptoms and to control the disease or disorder while at the same time allowing the immune system to continue fighting the viruses and bacteria affecting the body daily. The drugs used to treat autoimmune disorders are listed below.

Corticosteroids. Prednisone and methylprednisolone are glucocorticoid analogs that suppress inflammatory mediator production and immune effector cells and promote T lymphocyte apoptosis (death). They are used during acute periods of the disease. Complications arise with high doses and prolonged therapy. Major adverse effects are bone marrow suppression, gastrointestinal complications, cataracts, and glaucoma.

Disease-modifying antirheumatic drugs (DMARDs). Azathioprine (AZA) is a purine analog (6-mercaptopurine) that inhibits the synthesis of deoxyribonucleic acid (DNA), ribonucleic acid (RNA), and proteins and interferes with purine metabolism and mitosis, suppressing delayed hypersensitivity responses and cell-mediated cytotoxicity. Common adverse effects include leukopenia, pancreatitis, hepatitis, bone marrow suppression, potential malignancies, and pulmonary disease.

Cyclophosphamide. Cyclophosphamide is a nitrogen-derived alkylating agent/cytotoxic immunosuppressant that cross-links DNA and RNA strands, inhibiting cell functions and protein synthesis. It has a dose-dependent effect on the immune system, and at high doses, it can induce an aberrant anti-inflammatory immune effect on lymphocyte activity, can affect regulatory T cells, and can cause a state of severe immunosuppression that includes significant bone-marrow suppression, leukopenia, anemia, and thrombocytopenia. There also can be adverse effects on the gastrointestinal or renal-genitourinary tracts and the cardiovascular system, and there can be an increased risk of malignancy and pulmonary toxicity.

Methotrexate (MTX). MTX is a dihydrofolate reductase inhibitor and antimetabolite approved for Crohn's disease, rheumatoid arthritis, and psoriasis. Despite its efficacy, MTX has severe toxic effects with prolonged use, including liver damage, cytopenias, and several pulmonary diseases, the most frequently reported is hypersensitivity pneumonitis.

Hydroxychloroquine. Hydroxychloroquine is an antimalarial agent with immunosuppressant properties and is used to treat systemic lupus erythematosus. The drug has cardiovascular effects that can cause toxic myopathy, cardiomyopathy, and peripheral neuropathy, but at prescribed doses is usually well tolerated.

Biological DMARDs. Adalimumab is a monoclonal antibody and tumor necrosis factor (TNF) inhibitor that binds TNF-alpha and blocks its interaction with cell surface receptors. Adverse events include renal-genitourinary effects and dyslipidemia. Other anti-TNF-alpha monoclonal antibodies include golimumab (Simponi) and certolizumab pegol (Cimzia).

Infliximab is a chimeric (part human/part synthetic) monoclonal antibody and anti-TNF agent that binds TNF-alpha and blocks its interaction with cell surface receptors. A twofold risk of infection is the most common adverse event, and the risk of developing tuberculosis may be greater than with other anti-TNF agents. Skin and subcutaneous tissue infections and apoptosis-inducing activity (cell death) can occur.

Etanercept is a TNF receptor antagonist that inhibits the binding of TNF-alpha and TNF-beta to cell surface receptors, preventing its interaction with TNF receptors and rendering it biologically inactive. Its use can cause infections of the respiratory tract, skin, or subcutaneous tissue.

Three biological DMARDs (infliximab, adalimumab, and golimumab) are Food and Drug Administration (FDA)-approved for severe ulcerative colitis that does not respond to other medications. Infliximab, adalimumab, and certolizumab pegol are FDA-approved for the treatment of moderate to severe Crohn's disease. Anti-TNF-alpha monoclonal antibodies also treat rheumatoid arthritis, psoriasis, psoriatic psoriasis, and ankylosing spondylitis.

Hormones, proteins, or other substances normally produced or secreted by the cells or organs damaged in autoimmune disease (such as thyroid hormone or insulin) can usually be supplemented to the point that they are within the proper physiologic range. Sometimes this works well. For instance, to effectively control Graves' disease, a surgeon removes the overactive thyroid gland, and the patient begins taking oral thyroid hormone supplements. Treating type 1 diabetes in children with insulin supplementation, however, is somewhat trickier. Insulin shots cannot duplicate the finely controlled release of insulin from the beta cells of the pancreas. However, with the advent of constant glucose monitors (CGMs) and insulin pumps, diabetic children can experience tight blood glucose control and normal growth and development. Cell phone-based glucose read-outs, such as the Dexcom System further simplify blood glucose monitoring and control.

Many investigators have worked on vaccinations for autoimmune disorders, using animal models of varying types. Some results have been promising, even if the mechanism of action is still mostly unexplained. Vaccinations against autoimmune thyroiditis, encephalitis, and arthritis have been successful in some animal models. Another experimental approach is oral tolerance therapy. Large quantities of the offending autoantigen are given to the patient to induce tolerance to the protein. This approach is like desensitization used with allergy sufferers. Oral doses of myelin, for instance, have shown some success as a treatment for patients with multiple sclerosis.

Miscellaneous medications. Other medications include rituximab, tocilizumab, and belimumab. Rituximab selectively deletes specific B cells that have a particular marker called "CD20." It treats rheumatoid arthritis, two types of vasculitis, MS, lupus, and other autoimmune diseases. Some patients have hypersensitivity reactions to rituximab. Tocilizumab is a monoclonal antibody that inhibits a cytokine from T cells called "interleukin-6" (IL-6). Tocilizumab treats rheumatoid arthritis, giant cell arteritis, and severe COVID-19. Sarilumab is a monoclonal antibody with similar activity to tocilizumab approved for rheumatoid arthritis. These drugs can cause infusion reactions, high blood pressure, low white blood cell counts, signs of liver damage, and elevated blood lipids.

Belimumab is a monoclonal antibody that inhibits B-cell activating factor and is used to treat lupus and Sjorgen's syndrome. Abatacept (Orencia) is a genetically engineered fusion protein that interferes with T-cell activation. This drug is used with other medicines to treat rheumatoid arthritis. Anakinra (Kineret) is a genetically engineered IL-1 receptor antagonist. It is the least commonly used biologic DMARD for rheumatoid arthritis because it is expensive since daily injections are required. A drug with a similar mechanism of action is a monoclonal antibody called "canakinumab" (Ilaris). This drug is FDA approved for systemic juvenile idiopathic arthritis and cryopyrin-associated periodic syndromes (CAPS) and effectively relieves gout pain and inflammation.

Ustekinumab (Stelara) is an anti-p40 antibody that blocks interleukin-12 and -23, two proinflammatory cytokines. It is FDA-approved for patients with moderately to severely active Crohn's disease after failure with other medications.

Oral medications that inhibit inflammation include JAK kinase inhibitors. JAK kinase is an integral part of lymphocyte activation, and its inhibition quells inflammation. JAK inhibitors include tofacitinib (Xeljanz), which is FDA-approved for the treatment of moderate to severe ulcerative colitis, baricitinib (Olumiant), useful for rheumatoid arthritis and severe COVID-19, and upadacitinib (Rinvoq), which is also FDA-approved for rheumatoid arthritis. These drugs can cause upper respiratory tract infections, headaches, diarrhea, and cold symptoms. More severe side effects include gastrointestinal bleeding, fatigue, rashes, sores, and urinary tract damage.

These mediations do not cure autoimmune diseases, but they can put them into remission. These medications are very potent and have significant side effects. However, they can permit a patient to live a relatively normal life.

PERSPECTIVE AND PROSPECTS

The history of human understanding of autoimmune disorders is quite short. Paul Ehrlich, early in the twentieth century, described a condition of "horror autotoxicus," the attack of the human immune system against the body's tissues. His studies set the stage for rapid advancement in the understanding of the human immune system. Understanding the genetic and molecular basis for autoimmunity, however, along with the realization that autoimmunity is a normal part of immune system development, began in the 1980s. Even where the cause was well established (such as with insulin-dependent diabetes, established in the 1920s), no significant changes in treatment were made until new genetic tools became available. Indeed, the entire field of immunology, which until the 1970s was in its infancy as a medical field, has grown exponentially as new molecular tools have enabled researchers to elucidate the pathways by which autoimmunity exacts its toll.

There is still plenty to do, both in terms of determining pathways and in developing new therapies aimed at specific targeting of these pathways. With the completion of the Human Genome Project, an incredible amount of new knowledge is available that will help researchers produce treatments that are much more targeted and specific than those used in the past. As more is learned about the immune system and pathways of inflammation, new therapies may be designed that may prevent the development of most autoimmune diseases. Stem cell treatments with mesenchymal stem cells and mesenchymal stem cell-derived products, while still experimental, may provide relief in several cases for patients who suffer from intractable autoimmune disorders.

—*Kerry L. Cheesman, PhD, Christine M. Carroll, RN, BSN, MBA, and Michael A. Buratovich, PhD*

Further Information

Abbas, Abul K., and Andrew H. Lichtman. Cellular and Molecular Immunology. 10th ed., Saunders/Elsevier, 2021.

"Autoimmune Conditions." Medline Plus, 31 Mar. 2021, medlineplus.gov/autoimmunediseases.html. Accessed 20 Aug. 2021.

Chatenoud, Lucienne. "Emerging Biological and Molecular Therapies in Autoimmune Disease." The Autoimmune Diseases, edited by Noel R. Rose and Ian R. Mackay, pp. 1437-57, 6th ed., Academic Press, 2020.

Dettmer, Philipp. Immune: A Journey into the Mysterious System That Keeps You Alive. Random House, 2021.

"Drugs for Psoriatic Arthritis." Medical Letter on Drugs and Therapy, vol. 61, no. 1588, 30 Dec. 2019, pp. 203-10.

Janeway, Charles A., Jr., et al. Immunobiology: The Immune System in Health and Disease. 6th ed., Garland Science, 2005.

Kahmini, Fatemeh Rezaei, and Shahab Shahgaldi. "Therapeutic Potential of Mesenchymal Stem Cell-Derived Extracellular Vesicles as Novel Cell-Free Therapy for Treatment of Autoimmune Disorders." *Experimental and Molecular Pathology*, vol. 118, 2011, p. 104566, doi:10.1016/j.yexmp.2020.104566.

Rose, Noel R., and Ian Mackay, editors. The Autoimmune Diseases. 6th ed., Academic Press, 2019.

Tsai, Sue, and Pere Santamaria. "MHC Class II Polymorphisms, Autoreactive T-Cells, and Autoimmunity." Frontiers in Immunology, vol. 4, no. 321, 2013, pp. 1-7.

Watson, Stephanie. "Autoimmune Diseases: Types, Symptoms, Causes, and More." Healthline, 26 Mar. 2019, www.healthline.com/health/autoimmune-disorders?print=true. Accessed 20 Aug. 2021.

Zack, Eric, "Emerging Therapies for Autoimmune Disorders". Journal of Infusion Nursing, vol. 37, no. 2, 2012, pp. 109-19.

Autoimmune polyglandular syndrome

Category: Diseases/Syndromes
Also known as: APS; polyglandular autoimmune syndrome (PGA); polyglandular failure syndrome
Anatomy or system affected: All tissues
Specialties and related fields: Endocrinology, gastroenterology, gynecology, hematology, immunology, internal medicine, neurology, oncology, ophthalmology, otorhinolaryngology, pathology, pharmacology, pulmonary medicine, rheumatology
Definition: As a set of multiple endocrine system failures or insufficiencies that result from an autoimmune attack on endocrine gland tissues.

KEY TERMS

Addison's disease: a condition characterized by insufficiency of the adrenal cortex, causing a drop in glucocorticoid and mineralocorticoid hormones, causing fatigue, low blood pressure, and other symptoms

autoimmune regulator (AIRE) gene: a transcription factor expressed in thymus gland cells that causes them to express an array of self-antigens; plays a critical role in self-tolerance

chronic atrophic gastritis: an autoimmune disease characterized by chronic inflammation of the stomach lining, leading to loss of stomach tissue and its replacement by intestinal-type epithelium, pyloric-type glands, and scar tissue

hypoparathyreosis: a state resulting from a malfunction of the parathyroid glands

INTRODUCTION

The term "autoimmune polyglandular syndrome" (APS), sometimes called "polyglandular autoimmune syndrome" (PGA), is best described as a set of multiple endocrine system failures or insufficiencies. It also is known as "polyglandular failure syndrome," and there are two further major classifications, denoted as type 1 and type 2. APS is an autoimmune disease that destroys endocrine gland tissues, shows multiple ectodermal disorders, and is responsible for a chronic case of "mucocutaneous candidiasis," which is the medical term for a yeast infection. The genetic mode of transmission is autosomal recessive inheritance.

RISK FACTORS

The incidence of APS depends significantly on location and ethnicity. The disease is rare, with an APS-1 prevalence of 1 in 80,000 in Norway and much of the world and an APS-2 prevalence of 8 per 100,000, as Pärt Peterson and Eystein S. Husebye reported in *The Autoimmune Diseases* (2014). There is an increased occurrence of APS-1 among specific populations, with Iranian Jews being the highest risk group at about 1 in 9,000. Sardinians have a ratio of 1 in 14,400, and the Finns have 1 in 25,000. Research has shown that it does affect both sexes, but with a slight female preponderance in APS-2.

ETIOLOGY AND GENETICS

Research on APS began as early as the mid-nineteenth century when Thomas Addison first started classifying the pathology behind adrenocortical failure with pernicious anemia. Since that time, the combined research of endocrinologists and immunologists has helped explain the pathophysiology and pathogenesis of APS. An autosomal recessive gene inheritance causes APS-1. The short arm of chromosome 21 near markers *D21s49* and *D21s171* on band *21p22.3* is the genetic locus. Mutations in the autoimmune regulator (*AIRE*) gene *AIRE* gene are to blame due to the mutated encoding of the AIRE protein, which acts as a transcription factor. The stop-codon mutation *R257X* is responsible for 83 percent of Finnish APS-1 cases. In contrast, *R139X* mutations are commonly found among Sardinians and *Y85C* mutations among Iranian Jews with the condition, as reported by Peterson and Husebye. APS-2 is associated with multiple genes, including human leukocyte antigen (HLA) genes on chromosome 6, *CTLA-4* on chromosome 2, *PTPN22*, and *NALP1*, but may or may not be related to *AIRE* mutations.

Although the exact mechanisms remain relatively poorly understood, a pathway has been postulated. First, a patient must have a predisposed genetic susceptibility and then be exposed to some autoimmune trigger. This trigger could be an environmental one or even an intrinsic factor. Next, this trigger imitates the structure of a body's self-antigen. At this point, the self-antigen reproduces in an organ, and organ-specific antibodies are replicated. Autoimmune activity increases in that organ to the extent that there is notable glandular destruction. This infection, if left untreated, can continue to spread until excessive organ damage has occurred because of autoimmune activity and the organ is filled with chronic inflammatory infiltrate, which is composed primarily of lymphocytes.

SYMPTOMS

For a diagnosis of APS-1 to be given, at least two out of the following three symptoms must be present: chronic mucocutaneous candidiasis (CMC), autoimmune adrenal gland insufficiency, or chronic hypoparathyroidism. Other diseases observed when APS-1 is present are vitiligo, alopecia, hypogonadism, chronic hepatitis, malabsorption, keratoconjunctivitis, autoimmune Addison's disease (AAD), and chronic atrophic gastritis. CMC is the first symptom to become visible and usually attacks the skin. Still, it can spread to the mouth, esophagus, vagina, nails, and intestines. The second overall symptom to appear is the endocrine disease hypoparathyreosis.

SCREENING AND DIAGNOSIS

Most of the symptoms for APS-1 become evident in the first twenty years of life, APS-2 in adulthood (though earlier or later onset is possible). Most cases of APS-2 involve the combination of Addison's disease with Hashimoto's thyroiditis (an autoimmune thyroid disease). In contrast, the fewest diagnosed APS-2 cases are a combination of Addison's disease, diabetes mellitus type 1, and Graves' disease (a type of autoimmune hyperthyroidism). To classify a patient with APS-2, both AAD in combination with diabetes mellitus type 1 and/or thyroid autoimmune diseases must occur. Other diseases that occur along with those three are celiac disease, pernicious anemia, and myasthenia gravis.

MYASTHENIA GRAVIS

There is also an APS type 3, which occurs when autoimmune thyroiditis is present without autoimmune adrenalitis. The other diseases that can symptomatically mimic APS 3 are alopecia, Sjögren's syndrome, pernicious anemia, and diabetes mellitus type 1.

TREATMENT AND THERAPY

Treatment options vary depending on the type, but there is no cure since all cases are chronic, lifelong diseases. APS-1 requires hormone replacement therapy with ketoconazole (an antifungal medication) to combat the CMC. Ketoconazole inhibits the production of testosterone and cortisol, which can significantly impact the function of the adrenal gland of patients who already exhibit a lower-than-average pituitary-adrenal reserve. Other treatments of Addison's disease include oral glucocorticoids (hydrocortisone) and fludrocortisone to replace aldosterone. Chronic hepatitis can be treated with immunosuppressive therapy by using medications such as prednisone or azathioprine. Other treatment options are available, but all depend on the combination of ailments and their symptoms.

PREVENTION AND OUTCOMES

Although APS cannot be cured, patients can continue to live an everyday life if the infections caused by APS are controlled. This control can best be achieved if the hormone deficiencies are corrected or by treating the yeast infections or treating diabetes through the use of insulin.

—*Jeanne L. Kuhler, PhD and Steven Matthew Atchison*

Further Information

"Autoimmune Polyglandular Syndrome." *Genetics & Inherited Conditions*. Salem Press. 2010.

Barker, Jennifer M. "Polyglandular Deficiency Syndromes." *Merck Manual for Health Care Professionals*. Merck & Co., Jan. 2014. Accessed 22 Jul. 2014.

Gibson, Toby, Chenna Ramu, Christina Gemund, and Rein Aasland. "The APECED Polyglandular Autoimmune Syndrome Protein, AIRE-1, Contains the SAND Domain and Is Probably a Transcription Factor." *Trends in Biochemical Sciences*, vol. 23, no. 7, 1988, pp. 242-44.

Husebye, E. S., J. Perheentupa, R. Rautemaa, and O. Kämpe. "Clinical Manifestations and Management of Patients with Autoimmune Polyendocrine Syndrome Type I." *Journal of Internal Medicine*, vol. 265, 2009, pp. 514-29.

Peterson, Pärt, and Eystein S. Husebye. "Polyendocrine Syndromes." *The Autoimmune Diseases*, edited by Noel R. Rose and Ian R. Mackay, Elsevier, 2014, pp. 605-18.

Wass, John A. H., and Paul M. Stewart, editors. *Oxford Textbook of Endocrinology and Diabetes*. Oxford UP, 2011.

Zlotogora, J., and M. S. Shapiro. "Polyglandular Autoimmune Syndrome Type I among Iranian Jews." *Journal of Medical Genetics*, vol. 29, 1992, pp. 824-26.

Congenital hypothyroidism

Category: Diseases/Disorders
Also known as: Infantile hypothyroidism, cretinism
Anatomy or system affected: Endocrine system, musculoskeletal system, neck, nervous system
Specialties and related fields: Endocrinology, internal medicine, perinatology, preventive medicine
Definition: Retardation of mental and physical growth arising from prenatal or neonatal hypothyroidism.

KEY TERMS

goiter: the gross enlargement of the thyroid gland to produce hormones when insufficient iodine is available

L-thyroxine (T4): a less potent thyroid hormone than the T3 form that cells convert to T3

L-triiodothyronine (T3): the most potent of the thyroid hormones

thyroid gland: the endocrine gland in humans that produces the hormones that control metabolism

CAUSES AND SYMPTOMS

In humans, the thyroid gland consists of two connected lobes in the front of the neck, on either side of the thyroid cartilage or Adam's apple. It produces the thyroid hormones, the most important of which are L-triiodothyronine (T3) and L-tetraiodothyronine or L-thyroxine (T4). These compounds circulate in the blood serum to the body's cells and regulate virtually all metabolism: the production and consumption of proteins, carbohydrates, fats, and vitamins and the generation of energy that makes body heat. In these activities, the T3 molecule (which is made in cells from T4) has two to four times the effectiveness of T4. Because of the high iodine content of both T3 and T4, sufficient dietary iodine must be supplied to maintain normal thyroid function.

Abnormal levels of T3 and T4 have a profound effect on all bodily functions. In adults, the low production of T3 and T4, known as hypothyroidism, leads to reduced mental and physical activity, weight gain, general weakness, and other symptoms. Elevated thyroid activity, or hyperthyroidism, produces restlessness and irritability, weight loss, and symptoms generally the opposite of those seen with hypothyroidism. When either of these conditions develops in adults, surgery or drug regimens are available to control them and produce normal metabolism in the patient. When these conditions occur in utero, however, there is almost no way to counteract their effects.

A child born with congenital hypothyroidism (CH) has developmental disabilities with little or no chance of improvement. The typical infant with CH can show a variety of symptoms: low body temperature, poor appetite, decreased activity, flabbiness, low pulse rate, delayed union of bones of the skull, feeding difficulties even to the point of choking and cyanosis (turning blue from lack of oxygen), and thickened, off-color skin. They may also be physically disabled or dwarfed unless immediately treated with thyroid hormones, with the bone ends not growing or maturing normally.

TREATMENT AND THERAPY

For the child born with CH, no treatment is available for the brain damage that has taken place. Thyroid replacement therapy from birth, using either

---

INFORMATION ON CONGENITAL HYPOTHYROIDISM

Causes: Thyroid disorder

Symptoms: Mental retardation, low body temperature, poor appetite, decreased activity, flabbiness, low pulse rate, a delayed union of skull bones, feeding difficulties, off-color skin

Duration: Lifelong

Treatments: Thyroid replacement therapy from birth

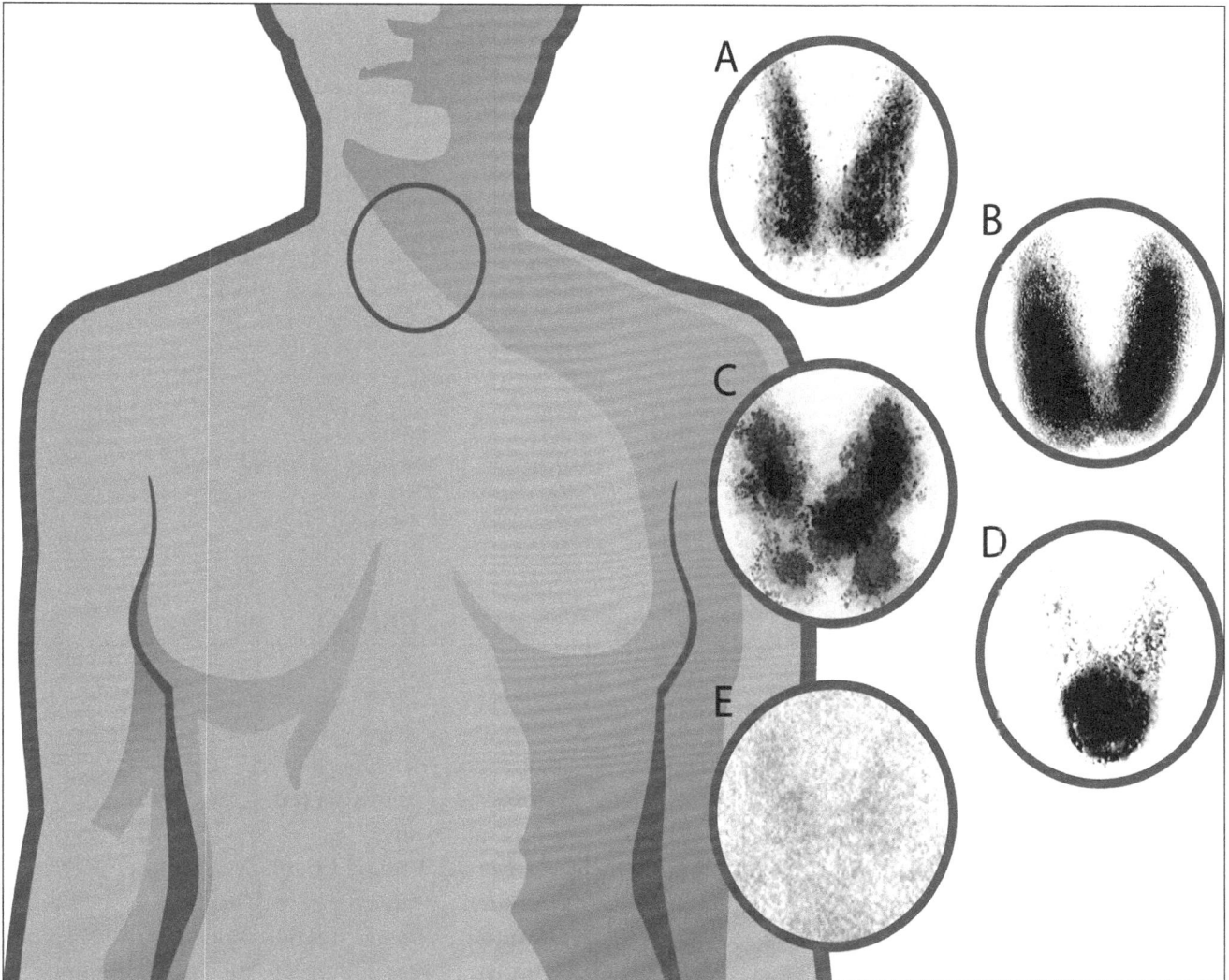

Five scintigrams taken from thyroids with different syndromes: A) normal thyroid; B) Graves disease, diffuse increased uptake in both thyroid lobes; C) Plummer's disease; D) Toxic adenoma; E) Thyroiditis. By Petros Perros, PLoS Medicine, via Wikimedia. [CC 3.0.]

natural or synthetic hormones, will avert most physical effects, but the intellectual disability is irreversible.

The most effective way to avoid this problem is to ensure that a pregnant woman consumes enough iodine to be made into her fetus's T3 and T4 molecules. The thyroid hormones do not transfer readily from the placental blood supply to the fetus, but the iodide ion does. When made available before the end of the second trimester of pregnancy, the material iodide supply is enough to allow the fetal thyroid gland to develop normally and the unborn fetus to have a proper neurological and musculoskeletal function. Iodized salt is one of the easiest ways to supply iodide ions. Still, they can also be given as an injection of iodized oil or by the oral administration of some iodine-containing medicines, such as Lugol's iodine solution.

When hypothyroidism develops in the older child or adolescent—often appearing as a goiter, in addition to the other symptoms described above—odine therapy is sometimes sufficient to return thyroid function to normal levels. Oddly, such therapy can also be counterproductive. The complex mechanisms that maintain proper hormone levels in blood serum are artificially high iodine concentrations and may close down hormone production because it appears high. For this condition, only thyroid hormone administration is effective.

PERSPECTIVE AND PROSPECTS

Hypothyroidism, goiter, and CH are worldwide health problems because of the body's dependence on dietary iodine. Many places in the world have low soil levels of iodine, leading to low iodine levels in crops and thus inadequate iodine intake from food. Such areas include high mountain countries, such as the Himalayas, where glacial meltwater leaches iodine from the soil with no replacement from higher geologic formations. The Ganges River basin, where the sheer volume of water is used, removes iodine from croplands. Some mountainous areas of the United States—such as the hill country of West Virginia, Kentucky, and Tennessee—have been centers of endemic goiter formation. Supplying iodine to inhabitants of these areas is a medical necessity but, like so many such problems, is complicated by logistic and political considerations.

—*Robert M. Hawthorne Jr., PhD*

Further Information

"Another Reason for Iodine Prophylaxis." *The Lancet*, vol. 335, no. 8703, 16 Jun. 1990, pp. 1433-34.

Buyukgebiz, Atilla. "Newborn Screening for Congenital Hypothyroidism." *Journal of Clinical Research in Pediatric Endocrinology*, vol. 5, Mar. 2013, pp. 8-12.

Cao, Xue-Yi, et al. "Timing of Vulnerability of the Brain to Iodine Deficiency in Endemic Cretinism." *New England Journal of Medicine*, vol. 331, no. 26, 29 Dec. 1994.

Gomez, Joan. *Thyroid Problems in Women and Children*. Hunter House, 2003.

Hetzel, Basil S. "Iodine and Neuropsychological Development." *Journal of Nutrition*, vol. 130, no. 2, 1999, pp. 493S-495S.

"Key Findings: Congenital Hypothyroidism." *Centers for Disease Control and Prevention*, 7 Sept. 2011.

Kronenberg, Henry M., et al., editors. *Williams Textbook of Endocrinology*. 11th ed., Saunders/Elsevier, 2008.

Maberly, Glen F. "Iodine Deficiency Disorders: Contemporary Scientific Issues." *Journal of Nutrition*, vol. 124, no. 8, Aug. 1994, pp. 1473-78S.

"Neonatal Hypothyroidism." *Medline Plus*, 28 Jun. 2011.

Rosenthal, M. Sara. *The Thyroid Sourcebook*. 5th ed., McGraw-Hill, 2009.

Woeber, K. A. "Iodine and Thyroid Disease." *Medical Clinics of North America: Thyroid Diseases*, vol. 75, no. 1, Jan. 1991, pp. 169-78.

CROHN'S DISEASE

Category: Diseases/Conditions
Also known as: Crohn disease, ileitis, ileocolitis, regional enteritis, enteritis
Anatomy or system affected: Gastrointestinal (GI) system, intestines
Specialties and related fields: Gastroenterology, immunology, nutrition, pediatrics
Definition: A chronic inflammatory condition of the GI tract, from the mouth to the anus, but most commonly at the end of the small intestine called the "ileum" and in the adjoining large bowel (colon).

KEY TERMS

abscess: a localized collection of pus (dead cells and a mixture of live and dead bacteria)
antigen: a foreign substance in the body causing an immunological response that produces antibodies
fissure: a break in the surface tissue of the anal canal or the wall of the gastrointestinal (GI) tract

fistula: an abnormal connection between two hollow structures or between a tubular organ and the skin surface

ETIOLOGY AND THE DISEASE PROCESS

Crohn's disease (CD) belongs to the group of diseases known as inflammatory bowel disease (IBD), a generic term for disorders characterized by inflammation in the small and large bowels. Other IBDs are ulcerative colitis (UC) and indeterminate colitis (lymphocytic colitis and collagenous colitis).

Crohn's disease affecting the colon is associated with a higher risk of developing colorectal cancer.

There are many theories about the etiology of Crohn's disease, but the exact cause is unknown. Crohn's disease is known to run in families and be more common in certain ethnicities, suggesting a genetic predisposition. First-degree relatives have a 13 to 18 percent increase in incidence, and there are concordance rates of 50 percent in identical twins. However, no specific reason or factor consistently explains the origin of the disease. All available evidence links Crohn's disease to abnormally regulated inflammatory processes. The human immune system protects people from harmful foreign substances (antigens) in the environment, such as bacteria, viruses, and parasites. This protection is provided by cells and various proteins (such as antibodies) through an inflammatory reaction that responds to antigens or cell injuries. In Crohn's disease, the immune system reacts abnormally against the affected part of the gastrointestinal (GI) tract and damages it. This inappropriate inflammation leads to the clinical manifestations of Crohn's disease.

Studies have shown that the inflammation related to Crohn's disease is multifactorial and may depend on genetic factors, immune reactions, and environmental cues. Mutations in one gene found on chromosome 16, *NOD2/CARD15*, are more common in Crohn's disease patients than in the general population. The NOD2 protein binds to intracellular bacterial cell wall components and activates the transcription factor NF-?B (nuclear factor-kappaB). NF-?B activates the expression of a host of inflammation-associated genes. The GI cells of patients with Crohn's disease show increased NF-?B activation. NOD might prevent excessive immune activation and combat microbes in the Gi tract. Mutations in

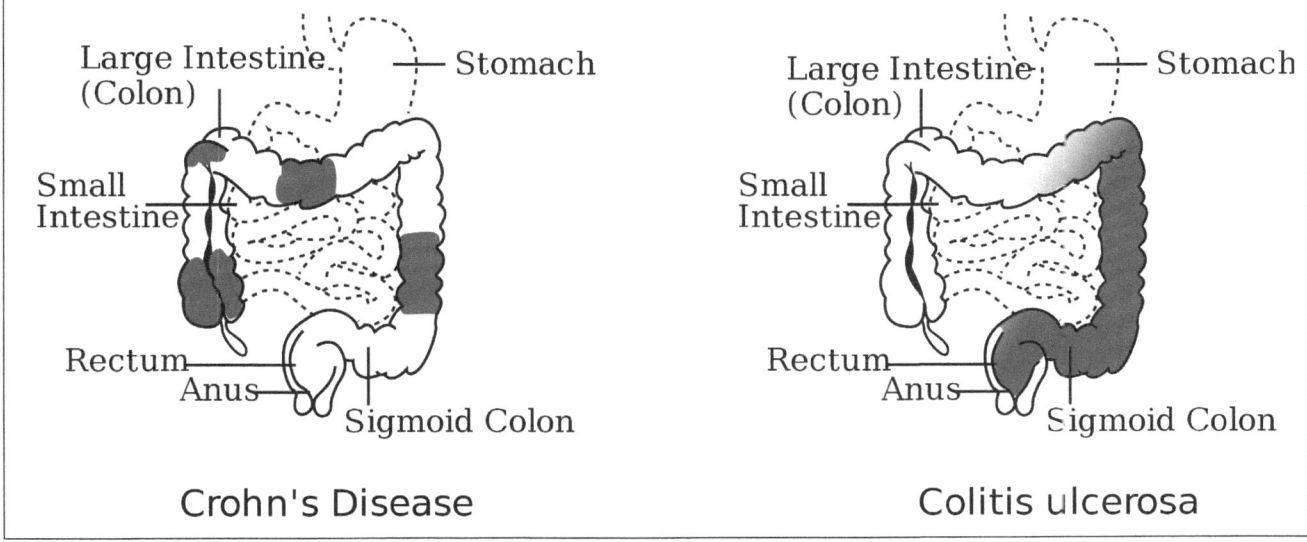

Comparison of Crohn's Disease and colitis ulcerosa. Image via Wikimedia Commons. [Public domain.]

the NOD gene cause the synthesis of a NOD protein that seems to have trouble responding modestly against GI tract bacteria. This defect somehow causes the immune system to turn against its GI microbes and vigorously attack them, injuring the GI tissues in the process. Other genes associated with susceptibility to Crohn's disease are *ATG16L1* (autophagy-related 16-like), *IRGM* (immunity-related GTPase M), and *IL23R* (interleukin-23 receptor). Both *ATG16L1* and *IRGM* are involved in autophagy, a process by which the cell recycles its internal components. Autophagy might also affect the clearance of intracellular bacteria. *IL23R* encodes a regulatory cytokine receptor that helps initiate the innate and adaptive immune activation in the intestines.

Tumor necrosis factor-alpha (TNF-alpha) is a protein produced by specific white blood cells called "macrophages." TNF is involved in various biological processes. It enhances the ability of white blood cells to defend against infections and other foreign substances. TNF is implicated in many diseases, including autoimmune diseases such as Crohn's disease. TNF may cause the inflammation associated with Crohn's disease. Crohn's disease patients have abnormally elevated TNF levels, causing excessive inflammation with its related adverse effects.

IBDs (Crohn's disease and ulcerative colitis) have similar symptoms, but they also differ significantly. Crohn's disease can affect any part of the GI tract, cause inflammation deeply penetrating through the tract linings (full thickness), and show radiographic results suggestive of Crohn's disease. Ulcerative colitis affects the colon and rectum; it can also cause a "backwash" ileitis in the junction of the small and large intestines. Ulcerative colitis inflammation is mainly in the superficial linings of the affected colon, confined to a part of or all the colon. The last part of the colon (the rectum) is usually the most affected. Tissue sampling can identify the difference between Crohn's disease and ulcerative colitis.

RISK FACTORS

Those with a family history of Crohn's disease, a genetic predisposition, or a smoking history are at the highest risk for this disease. Appendectomies, which decrease susceptibility to ulcerative colitis, do not affect susceptibility to Crohn's disease.

INCIDENCE

Crohn's disease affects approximately one in 300 adults in Europe and North America. In North America, the incidence of Crohn's disease is 3.1 to 20.2 cases per 100,000 person-years. Based on health insurance claims for 9 million Americans in 2007, the prevalence of Crohn's disease in children younger than 20 years was 43 per 100,000 and in adults was 201 per 100,000. About 20 percent of Crohn's disease cases run in families. Men and women are affected equally, but with slight female predominance in late adolescence and early adulthood. Crohn's disease is more common in people of European and Jewish heritage than those of other ethnicities. The onset of Crohn's disease has two peaks: between the ages of fifteen and thirty and sixty and eighty. However, most patients are diagnosed before the age of thirty.

SYMPTOMS

There are many manifestations of Crohn's disease, including symptoms within the GI tract and outside of it (extraintestinal). Constitutional symptoms of Crohn's disease are fatigue, fever, loss of appetite, and weight loss. The most common GI tract symptoms are prolonged diarrhea, with or without rectal bleeding, and abdominal pain (tenderness), typically in the lower right area. Sometimes the abdominal pain caused by Crohn's disease can mimic the pain of appendicitis. Malabsorption in the GI tract can lead to malnutrition and weight loss, related to delayed development and poor growth in children. Mouth ulcers may manifest along with pain in the mouth and gums. Problems of the throat, such as pain or difficulty with swallowing, can occur if the esophagus is involved.

Patients with Crohn's disease may develop perianal conditions such as "fissure-in-ano" or anal fissures (fissures or tears in the lining of the anus) and "fistula-in-ano" (an abnormal connection between the anal intestinal lining and another part of the body, such as the skin, bladder, vagina, or another part of the GI tract). Fistulas are most common in the anal region; abscesses (pockets of pus) may be present as a complication. Blockage (obstruction) and perforation of the GI tract may occur. Extraintestinal symptoms include eye disorders, skin problems, arthritis, and liver and gallbladder diseases.

SCREENING AND DIAGNOSIS

Screening begins with comprehensive patient history and physical examination. Blood tests include a complete blood count for anemia and assessing markers of inflammation such as erythrocyte sedimentation rate (ESR) and C-reactive protein (CRP) for inflammation. A stool test will assess GI tract bleeding, infection, or inflammation (Calprotectin fecal test). Special tests for antibodies, such as antineutrophil cytoplasmic antibodies and anti-Saccharomyces cerevisiae antibodies, may be used in the diagnosis of Crohn's disease is uncertain. Radiographic studies can include the upper and lower GI series (barium enema). Upper or lower GI endoscopy can identify the affected site, allow tissue sampling (biopsy), and confirm the diagnosis of Crohn's disease. Examples of GI endoscopies that use flexible tubes with light and camera at the ends for visualization include upper GI endoscopy (for the mouth, esophagus, stomach, and upper part of the small bowel), enteroscopy (for the small bowel), Ileocolonoscopy (for the lower small bowel and large bowel), colonoscopy (for the large bowel) and capsule endoscopy (which uses a pill-like camera for the whole intestine but mainly for the small bowel visualization). The severity of Crohn's disease is diverse, and its activity is described as mild-moderate, moderate-severe, severe-fulminant, and in remission.

TREATMENT AND THERAPY

Crohn's disease has no cure; however, various medications can alleviate its symptoms. Management of Crohn's disease and its complications may include medications for treating symptoms such as antidiarrheal agents (loperamide and diphenoxylate), nutritional support, surgery, or a combination of these modalities.

Medications for Crohn's disease include antibiotics such as ciprofloxacin and metronidazole; anti-inflammatory drugs such as corticosteroids, sulfasalazine, and 5-ASA or 5-aminosalicylate (which, though effective in ulcerative colitis, have uncertain benefits in Crohn's disease), immunomodulators that inhibit the immune response such as azathioprine, 6-mercaptopurine, and methotrexate; and biologic therapies such as infliximab (Remicade), adalimumab (Humira) certolizumab pegol (Cimzia), and golimumab (Simponi), which are monoclonal antibodies that block tumor necrosis factor (TNF)-alpha activity.

A class of biologic therapies called "anti-integrin antibodies," such as natalizumab (Tysabri) and vedolizumab (Entyvio), are also effective. Gastroenterologists prescribe these medications when all others are poorly tolerated or fail to provide a satisfactory response. Natalizumab and vedolizumab are "a4 integrin" inhibitors. Integrins are prominent cell adhesion molecules, and all leukocytes, except neutrophils, express a4ß1 integrins on their surfaces. Leukocytes use the a4ß1 integrin to bind to blood vessels and squeeze through them to enter the central nervous system or GI tract. Natalizumab also used to treat multiple sclerosis, inhibits white blood cell migration across the bloodstream into the GI tract, thereby staunching inflammation in the GI tract. Vedolizumab binds to a different integrin, a4ß7, which blocks leukocyte migration into the GI tract but not the central nervous system.

Another biologic therapy that effectively treats Crohn's disease is ustekinumab (Stelara). This monoclonal antibody specifically targets the p40 subunit of interleukin-12 and -23, effectively inhibiting IL-12 and -23. IL-12 and IL-23 support inflammation and immune responses. Ustekinumab is Food and Drug Administration (FDA)-approved for patients with moderately to severely active Crohn's disease after failure with other medications. A recent study using an early treatment of combined immunosuppression (immunomodulator + antibody to TNF) showed improved clinical outcomes (decreased need for surgery or hospital admissions and decreased Crohn's disease-related complications). These medications may have side effects ranging from nausea, vomiting, and headaches to infection susceptibility and other more serious potential outcomes. The risks and benefits of medicines are assessed, and modifications are implemented on an individual basis.

If the patient has an inflammatory flare-up, corticosteroids, including ileal-released budesonide, induce remission. However, corticosteroids are not recommended for the maintenance of remission. Azathioprine or mercaptopurine effectively maintains remission in most moderate to severe disease cases, and methotrexate is an alternative treatment. If these treatments prove ineffective, then a TNF inhibitor, such as infliximab, adalimumab, golimumab, or certolizumab pegol alone or in combination with azathioprine or mercaptopurine usually induce and maintain remission. If these treatment regimens produce satisfactory results, then ustekinumab or vedolizumab may effectively induce and maintain remission when other drugs are ineffective or intolerable.

Regular nutritional assessments are necessary to prevent malnutrition, which can result from malabsorption in the inflamed small and large bowels. In some cases, surgical intervention is needed, such as failure of medical treatment and complications such as obstruction, perforation, nonstop bleeding, abscess, and fistula.

PROGNOSIS, PREVENTION, AND OUTCOMES
Crohn's disease is a chronic medical condition. It can manifest in recurrent episodes of the active disease (flares) or remain in remission for variable periods. Patients with Crohn's disease are monitored closely for related conditions such as associated cancers. Regular cancer screening using colonoscopy is recommended for patients with colonic Crohn's disease ten years after its diagnosis because of its association with colorectal cancer. Patients on biological treatments must undergo regular screening for tuberculosis and cancer, as biologics can increase the patient's susceptibility to both diseases.

Stem cell therapies may revolutionize the treatment of fistulas. Adipose-derived mesenchymal stem cells (ADSCs) quell inflammation in the fistulas and facilitate tissue healing, often with minimal scarring. While such treatments are not yet part of standard care protocols, they do show remarkable efficacy in animal and clinical trials.

—Miriam E. Schwartz, MD, MA, PhD,
Colm A. Ó'Moráin, MA, MD, MSc, DSc,
and Michael A. Buratovich, PhD

Further Information
Cao, Y., Q Su, B. Zhang, et al. "Efficacy of Stem Cells Therapy for Crohn's Fistula: A Meta-Analysis and Systematic Review." *Stem Cell Research Therapies*, vol. 12, no. 32, 2021, doi.org/10.1186/s13287-020-02095-7. A review and summary of the clinical trials testing the efficacy of fat-derived stem cells to heal fistulas in Crohn's disease patients.

Kappelman, Michael D., et al. "The Prevalence and Geographic Distribution of Crohn's Disease and

Ulcerative Colitis in the United States." *Clinical Gastroenterology and Hepatology*, vol. 5, no. 12, 2007, pp. 1424-29. An article that reported an estimation of the prevalence of Inflammatory Bowel Diseases (Crohn's Disease and Ulcerative Colitis) in the United States; the study intended to quantify the overall burden of disease and assist the planning for appropriate clinical services.

Khanna, Reena, et al. "Early Combined Immunosuppression for the Management of Crohn's Disease (REACT): A Cluster Randomised Controlled Trial." *The Lancet*, vol. 386, no. 10006, 2015, pp. 1825-34. The REACT study evaluated using an early treatment of Crohn's Disease with combined immunosuppression (immunomodulator + antibody to TNF); the results showed improved clinical outcomes (decreased need for surgery or hospital admissions and decreased Crohn's disease-related complications).

Lichtenstein, Gary R., et al. "Management of Crohn Disease in Adults." *American Journal of Gastroenterology*, vol. 104, no. 2, pp. 465-83. This is the practice guideline developed by the American College of Gastroenterology for managing Crohn's Disease in adults. This article is available to the public and can be accessed at www.nature.com/ajg/journal/v104/n2/full/ajg2008168a.html.

McGovern, Dermot, P. B. "Crohn Disease and NOD2/CARD15." *Medscape*, 11 Dec. 2020. emedicine.medscape.com/article/1790325-overview#showall. Accessed 20 Aug. 2021. A review of the evidence that supports the role of NOD2 in the etiology of Crohn's disease.

Sandborn, William J. "Crohn Disease Evaluation and Treatment: Clinical Decision Tool." *Gastroenterology*, vol. 147, no. 3, 2014, pp. 702-5. This article conveys that the treatment of Crohn's Disease is in evolution. This clinical decision tool is designed to assist clinical providers in identifying, assessing, and treating patients with Crohn's Disease. This article is available to the public and can be accessed free at www.gastrojournal.org/article/S0016-5085%2814%2900918-4/fulltext.

Singh, Siddharth, and Edward V. Loftus, Jr. "Crohn Disease: REACT to Save the Gut." *The Lancet*, vol. 386, no. 10006, 2015, pp. 1800-1802. This article is a commentary on the most recent findings of the REACT Study that showed high-quality evidence supporting the early treatment of Crohn's Disease in community gastroenterology practices using combined immunosuppression with an immunomodulator and antibody to TNF.

U.S. Department of Health and Human Services, National Institutes of Health (NIH). National Institute of Diabetes and Digestive and Kidney Diseases (NIDDK). *Crohn Disease*. NIH Publication No. 14-3410. The National Digestive Diseases Information Clearinghouse (NDDIC), Sept. 2014, www.niddk.nih.gov/health-information/health-topics/digestive-diseases/crohns-disease/Pages/facts.aspx. This is a government publication that provides basic information for patients regarding the identification, assessment, diagnosis, and treatment of Crohn's Disease.

CUSHING'S SYNDROME

Category: Diseases/Disorders
Anatomy or system affected: Abdomen, back, blood, bones, endocrine system, glands, hair, muscles, skin
Specialties and related fields: Endocrinology, family medicine, immunology, internal medicine, nutrition, radiology, urology
Definition: A hormonal disorder caused primarily by chronic exposure of body tissues to excessive levels of cortisol.

KEY TERMS

adrenal cortex: the outer layer of the adrenal glands that synthesize and secrete two main types of steroid hormones, glucocorticoids, and mineralocorticoids

adrenal glands: paired glands above the kidneys that secrete steroid and catecholamine hormones

adrenocorticotropic hormone (ACTH): a peptide hormone secreted by the corticotropes anterior lobe of the pituitary gland that signals to the adrenal cortex to secrete glucocorticoid hormones

corticotropin-releasing hormone (CRH): a peptide hormone secreted by the paraventricular nuclei of the

hypothalamus that stimulates corticotropes in the anterior lobe of the pituitary to secrete ACTH.
cortisol: also known as hydrocortisone, is the main glucocorticoid secreted by the adrenal cortex
glucocorticoids: steroid hormones secreted by the adrenal cortex that regulates glucose metabolism

CAUSES AND SYMPTOMS

The adrenal or suprarenal glands are triangular-shaped glands situated on top of the kidneys. Adrenal glands have an outer layer called the "adrenal cortex" and an "inner adrenal medulla." The adrenal cortex contains three concentric zones of densely layered cells. The adrenal cortex synthesizes steroid hormones, specifically glucocorticoids and mineralocorticoids. The inner adrenal medulla contains loose clusters of chromaffin cells surrounding medullar veins, interspersed with sympathetic ganglion cells. The adrenal medulla makes catecholamine hormones like epinephrine and norepinephrine.

Glucocorticoid hormones regulate glucose metabolism. Specifically, they stimulate the synthesis of glucose (gluconeogenesis) in the liver between meals, raising the blood glucose level. Second, glucocorticoids mobilize amino acids from tissues to use as substrates for gluconeogenesis. Third, they prevent glucose uptake in muscle and fat tissues. Fourth, glucocorticoids stimulate fat breakdown in fat storage tissues. Fat degradation produces small organic acids called "ketone bodies" that provide energy for muscles and other tissues. Glucocorticoids, therefore, maintain normal blood glucose levels during periods of starvation. This ensures that the brain, which has a relatively absolute requirement for glucose, has adequate glucose supplied to it.

The anterior lobe of the pituitary gland and the hypothalamus secrete trophic and releasing hormones, respectively, to control glucocorticoid synthesis. The hypothalamus secretes a small peptide hormone called "corticotropin-releasing hormone" (CRH) that signals to specific cells in the pituitary called "corticotropes" to secrete a second peptide hormone called "adrenocorticotropic hormone" or ACTH. ACTH travels through the blood to the adrenal cortex and stimulates the synthesis and secretion of glucocorticoids. The increase in blood glucose levels caused by glucocorticoids downregulates ACTH and CRH secretion by the anterior pituitary and hypothalamus, respectively.

Cushing's syndrome is a group of abnormalities resulting from excessively high glucocorticoids produced by the adrenal cortex or taking steroid hormones. The primary source of the disorder is the main glucocorticoid hormone, cortisol. This condition is typically triggered by an excess production of ACTH from the pituitary gland. Excessive ACTH production may result from a pituitary gland tumor or cancer in another organ (e.g., carcinoid or small cell tumors of the lung, medullary carcinomas of the thyroid), or as a side effect from taking steroid hormones used to treat asthma, rheumatoid arthritis, and other serious diseases. Adrenal gland tumors also produce excess amounts of cortisol. A rare inherited tendency to develop endocrine gland tumors is another cause of Cushing's syndrome.

Since the hormones produced by the adrenal glands regulate glucose metabolism, excess production can cause widespread disorders. Because Cushing's syndrome causes the metabolism to slow, hydrolyzed fat is not metabolized, and the body redistributes fat around the middle. Some of the more common symptoms of Cushing's syndrome are a rounded face, an obese trunk with thin arms and legs, fat pads over the neck and shoulders, purple stretch marks on the skin, easy bruising, muscle weakness, poor wound healing, fractures in weakened bones, high blood pressure, diabetes mellitus, emotional instability, and severe fatigue. Men can experience diminished desire for sex, while women may experience increased hairiness, acne, and de-

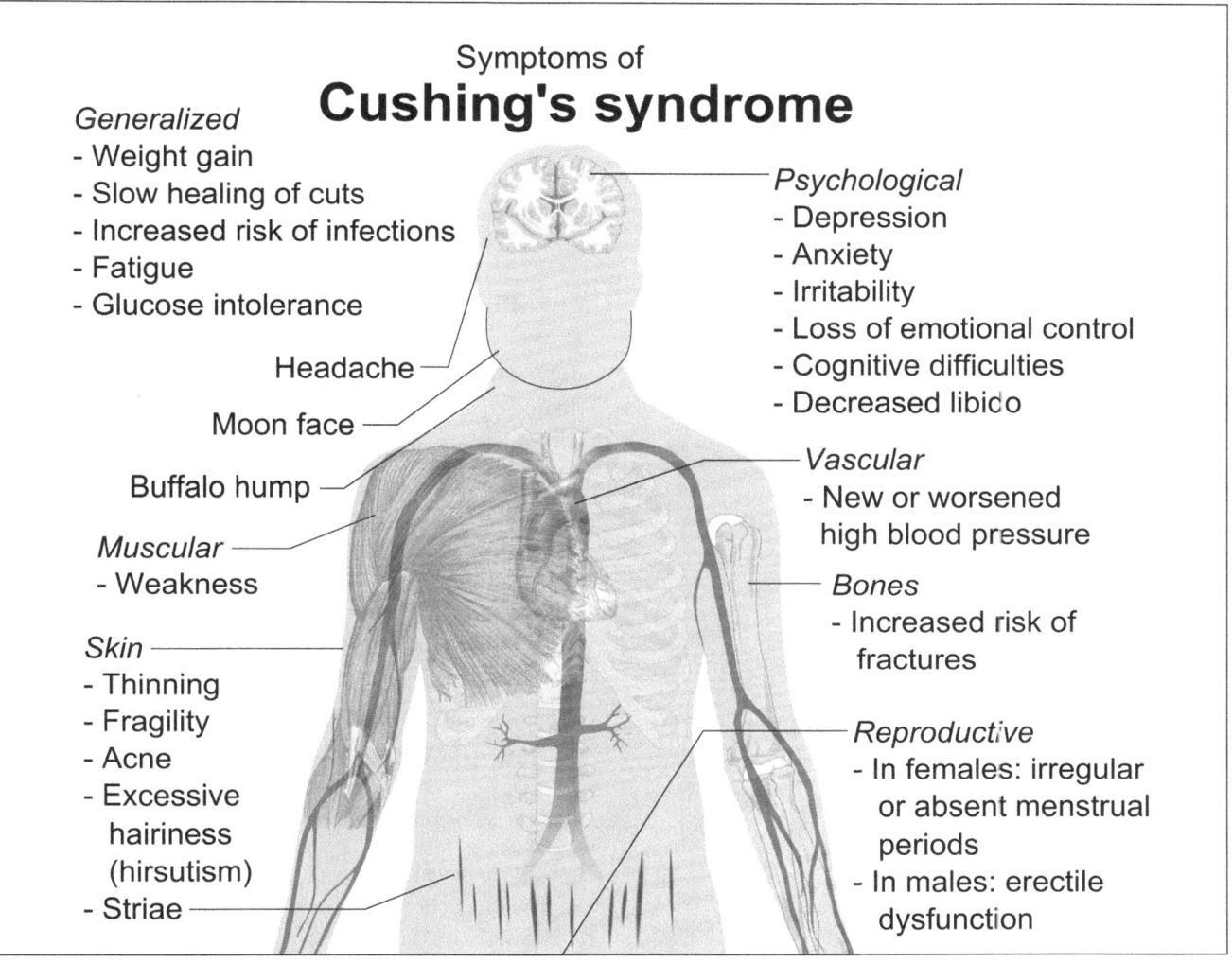

Symptoms of Cushing's Syndrome. Image by Mikael Häggström, via Wikimedia Commons. [Public domain.]

creased or absent menstrual periods. Children are usually obese, and their growth rate is slow.

TREATMENT AND THERAPY

Cushing's syndrome is treated by restoring the hormonal balance within the body, which may take several months. If Cushing's syndrome is left untreated, it can lead to death. The disease is diagnosed through blood and urine tests to detect excessive amounts of cortisol. Pituitary tumors and tumors at other locations in the body that produce ACTH are surgically removed, when possible, or are treated with radiation or chemotherapy. Transsphenoidal surgical resection of the pituitary adenomas, usually combined with radiotherapy, is the treatment of choice for pituitary tumors.

Oral drug therapy, sometimes combined with surgery or on its own, can restore the hormonal balance in the body. Steroidogenesis inhibitors impede glucocorticoid synthesis and include the antifungal drug ketoconazole, metyrapone (Metopirone), mitotane (*Lysodren*), and the newer medication,

> **INFORMATION ON CUSHING'S SYNDROME**
>
> **Causes**: Chronic exposure of body tissues to excess cortisol from overproduction by adrenal glands (tumor) or steroid use
>
> **Symptoms**: Rounded face, fat trunk with thin arms and legs, fat pads over neck and shoulders, purple stretch marks, easy bruising, muscle weakness, poor wound healing, fractures, high blood pressure, diabetes mellitus, emotional instability
>
> **Duration**: Chronic until treated
>
> **Treatments**: Restoration of hormonal balance, surgical removal of the tumor, discontinuance of steroid use

osilodrostat (*Isturisa*). Ketoconazole is inexpensive and inhibits multiple steps in cortisol synthesis. However, it has numerous adverse effects and must be avoided during pregnancy. Metyrapone is an 11-beta-hydroxylase inhibitor Food and Drug Administration (FDA)-approved for diagnostic use to test ACTH function and is safe during pregnancy. Mitotane is FDA-approved for adrenal carcinomas, but this medicine destroys the adrenal cortex and may permanently reduce adrenal function. Mitotane is also not safe during pregnancy. Osilodrostat is another 11-beta-hydroxylase inhibitor that effectively treats. Off-label treatments for Cushing's syndrome include the pituitary-targeting drugs cabergoline and pasireotide, and the glucocorticoid receptor antagonist mifepristone. These drugs can severely suppress the adrenal cortex and cause disruptions in salt concentrations, decreased energy levels, abnormal blood pressure, fatigue, nausea, headache, and swelling.

Cortisol replacement therapy is provided after surgery until cortisol production resumes. Lifelong cortisol replacement therapy may be necessary. If steroids are not being used to control a life-threatening illness, then their use should be discontinued.

Adrenal and pituitary tumors are always surgically removed. The remaining adrenal gland, which has usually diminished in size due to inactivity, will return to its normal size and function. As it is doing so, steroid hormones are administered to supply the needed cortisol and then tapered off over time. Some tumors may recur after surgical excision.

PERSPECTIVE AND PROSPECTS

Harvey Cushing made the first diagnosis of Cushing's syndrome in 1912. In 1932, he linked the syndrome to an abnormality in the pituitary gland that stimulated an overproduction of cortisol from the adrenal glands; this condition is Cushing's disease. Pituitary tumors cause approximately 70 percent of cases of Cushing's syndrome. The syndrome is more common in women than in men, with most cases occurring between twenty-five and forty-five. The disease can be severe, possibly even fatal, unless diagnosed and treated early.

—Alvin K. Benson, PhD, Sharon W. Stark, RN, APRN, DNSc, and Michael A. Buratovich, PhD

Further Information

A.D.A.M. Medical Encyclopedia. "Cushing Syndrome." *MedlinePlus*, 11 Dec. 2011.

Badash, Michelle. "Cushing's Syndrome." *HealthLibrary*, 1 May 2013.

Fox, Stuart Ira. *Human Physiology*. 16th ed., McGraw-Hill, 2021.

Kronenberg, Henry M., et al., editors. *Williams Textbook of Endocrinology*. 11th ed., Saunders/Elsevier, 2008.

National Endocrine and Metabolic Diseases Information Service. "Cushing's Syndrome." *National Institutes of Health*, 6 Apr. 2012.

"Osilodrostat (*Isturisa*) for Cushing's Disease." *Medical Letter on Drugs and Therapy*, vol. 63, no. 1617, 8 Feb. 2021, pp. 21-23.

Diabetes mellitus

Category: Diseases/Disorders
Anatomy or system affected: Abdomen, blood vessels, circulatory system, endocrine system, eyes, gastrointestinal system, glands, heart, kidneys, nervous system, pancreas
Specialties and related fields: Endocrinology, family medicine, genetics, internal medicine, nephrology, neurology, pediatrics, vascular medicine
Definition: A hormonal disorder in which proper blood sugar levels are not maintained; due either to insufficient production of insulin by the pancreas or to an inability of the body's cells to use insulin efficiently. If left untreated, diabetes mellitus leads to blindness, cardiovascular disease, dementia, kidney disease, and, eventually, death.

KEY TERMS

beta cells: the insulin-producing cells located at the core of the islets of Langerhans in the pancreas; the alpha, or glucagon-producing, cells form an outer coat

cross-linking: a chemical reaction triggered by the binding of glucose to tissue proteins that results in the attachment of one protein to another and the loss of elasticity in aging tissues

glucosuria: a condition in which the concentration of blood glucose exceeds the ability of the kidney to reabsorb it; as a result, glucose spills into the urine, taking with it body water and electrolytes

hyperglycemia: excessive levels of glucose in the circulating blood

insulin-dependent diabetes mellitus (IDDM): type 1 diabetes, a state of absolute insulin deficiency in which the body does not produce sufficient insulin to move glucose into the cells

insulin resistance: a lack of insulin action; a reduction in the effectiveness of insulin to lower blood glucose concentrations; characteristic of type 2 diabetes

insulitis: the selective destruction of the insulin-producing beta cells in type 1 diabetes

islets of Langerhans: clusters of cells scattered throughout the pancreas; they produce three hormones involved in sugar metabolism: insulin, glucagon, and somatostatin

ketoacidosis: high levels of ketones in the blood that result from a lack of circulating insulin

non-insulin-dependent diabetes mellitus (NIDDM): type 2 diabetes, which is the state of a relative insulin deficiency; although insulin is released, its target cells do not adequately respond to it by taking up blood glucose

CAUSES AND SYMPTOMS

Diabetes mellitus is by far the most common of all endocrine (hormonal) disorders. The disorder's name is derived from the Greek word *diabetes*, meaning "siphon" or "running through," referring to the potentially large urine volume that can accompany the condition. The Latin word *mellitus*, meaning "honey," was added to the name when physicians began to diagnose diabetes mellitus based on the sweet taste of the patient's urine. The disease has been depicted as a state of starvation amid plenty. Although there is plenty of sugar in the blood, the sugar does not reach the cells that need it for energy without proper insulin action. Glucose, the simplest form of sugar, is the primary source of energy for many vital functions. When cells are deprived of glucose, they starve, and tissues begin to degenerate. The unused glucose builds up in the bloodstream, which leads to a series of secondary complications.

The most common symptoms of diabetes mellitus are related to hyperglycemia, glycosuria, and ketoacidosis. The acute symptoms of diabetes mellitus are all attributable to inadequate insulin action. The immediate consequence of insulin insufficiency is a marked decrease in the ability of muscle, liver, and adipose (fat) tissue to remove glucose from the blood. In the presence of inadequate insulin action, a second problem manifests itself. People with diabetes continue to make the hormone glucagon. Glucagon, which raises the level of blood sugar, can be considered insulin's biological opposite. Like insulin, glucagon is released from the pancreatic islets. The release of glucagon is usually inhibited by insulin; therefore, in the absence of insulin, glucagon action elevates glucose concentrations.

For this reason, diabetes may be considered a two-hormone disease. With a reduction in the conversion of glucose into its storage forms of glycogen in liver and muscle tissue and lipids in adipose cells, glucose concentrations in the blood steadily increase (hyperglycemia). When the amount of glucose in the blood exceeds the capacity of the kidney to reabsorb this nutrient, glucose begins to spill into the urine (glucosuria). Glucose in the urine then drags additional body water along with it so that the volume of urine dramatically increases. In the absence of adequate fluid intake, the loss of body water and accompanying electrolytes (sodium) leads to dehydration and, ultimately, death caused by the failure of the peripheral circulatory system.

Insulin deficiency also results in a decrease in the synthesis of triglycerides (storage forms of fatty acids). It stimulates the breakdown of fats in adipose tissue. Although glucose cannot enter the cells and be used as an energy source, the body can use its supply of lipids from the fat cells as an alternate source of energy. Fatty acids increase in the blood, causing hyperlipidemia. With large amounts of circulating free fatty acids available for processing by the liver, the production and release of ketone bodies (breakdown products of fatty acids) into the circulation are accelerated, causing both ketonemia and an increase in the acidity of the blood. Since the ketone levels soon also exceed the capacity of the kidney to reabsorb them, ketone bodies soon appear in the urine (ketonuria).

Insulin deficiency and glucagon excess also cause pronounced effects on protein metabolism and result in an overall increase in the breakdown of proteins and a reduction in the uptake of amino acid precursors into muscle protein. A lack of insulin leads to the wasting and weakening of skeletal muscles. Diabetic children show a reduction in overall growth. The increased level of amino acids in the blood provides an additional source of material for glucose production (gluconeogenesis) by the liver. All these acute metabolic changes in carbohydrates, lipids, and protein metabolism can be prevented or reversed by administering insulin.

There are three distinct types of diabetes mellitus. Type 1, or insulin-dependent diabetes mellitus (IDDM), is an absolute deficiency of insulin that accounts for approximately 5 to 10 percent of all cases of diabetes. Until the discovery of insulin, people with type 1 diabetes faced certain death within about a year of diagnosis. In type 2, or non-insulin-dependent diabetes mellitus (NIDDM), the most common form of the disorder, insulin secretion may be normal or even increased. However, the target cells for insulin are less responsive than usual (insulin resistance); therefore, insulin is not as effective in lowering blood glucose concentrations. Although diabetes mellitus can manifest at any age, type 1 diabetes has a greater prevalence in children.

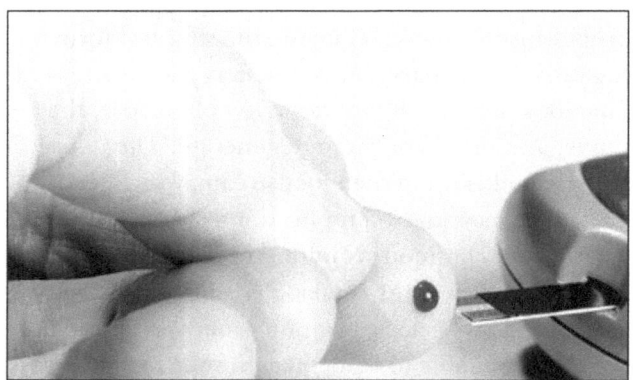

A person with diabetes performs a glucose level check using a finger blood test. Photo via Istock.com/Eugene Bochkarev. [Used under license.]

In contrast, the incidence of type 2 diabetes increases markedly after the age of forty. Genetic and environmental factors are essential in the expression of both of these types of diabetes mellitus. The third type is gestational diabetes, characterized by high blood glucose during pregnancy in a person who did not previously have diabetes.

Type 1 diabetes is an autoimmune process that involves the selective destruction of the insulin-producing beta cells in the islets of Langerhans (insulitis). The triggering event that initiates this process in genetically susceptible persons is linked to environmental factors resulting from an infection, a virus, or, more likely, toxins in the diet. The body's T lymphocytes progressively attack the beta cells but leave the other hormone-producing cell types intact. T lymphocytes are white blood cells that usually attack virus-invaded cells and cancer cells. For up to ten years, there remain enough insulin-producing cells to respond effectively to a glucose load. Still, when approximately 80 percent of the beta cells are destroyed, there is insufficient insulin release in response to a meal, and the death spiral of the consequences of diabetes mellitus is triggered. Insulin injection can halt this lethal process and prevent it from recurring. Still, it cannot mimic the regular pattern of insulin release from the pancreas. Interestingly, not everyone who has insulitis progresses to experience overt symptoms of the disease.

Type 2 diabetes is usually associated with obesity and lack of exercise. Recently, with the reported increased rates of obesity and inactivity in children, there has also been an increase in type 2 diabetes at younger and younger ages. Genetic factors also play a vital role in the development of the disorder. Research has shown that individuals who have a sibling or parent with type 2 diabetes are about three times as likely to develop diabetes themselves.

Because there is a reduction in the sensitivity of the target cells to insulin, people with type 2 diabetes

> **INFORMATION ON DIABETES MELLITUS**
>
> **Causes**: Genetic and environmental factors
>
> **Symptoms**: Large urine output, excessive thirst, dehydration, low blood pressure, weight loss despite increased appetite, fatigue, nausea, vomiting, blurred vision
>
> **Duration**: Chronic
>
> **Treatments**: Insulin or oral hypoglycemic drugs, lifestyle changes (diet modification and exercise)

must secrete more insulin to maintain blood glucose at normal levels. Because insulin is a storage, or anabolic, hormone, this increased secretion further contributes to obesity. In response to the elevated insulin concentrations, the number of insulin receptors on the target cell gradually decreases, triggering an even greater insulin secretion. In this way, the excess glucose is stored despite the reduced availability of insulin binding sites on the cell. Over time, the demands for insulin eventually exceed even the reserve capacity of the "genetically weakened" beta cells, and symptoms of insulin deficiency develop as the plasma glucose concentrations remain high for increasingly longer periods. This phenomenon is known as beta-cell burnout. Because the symptoms of type 2 diabetes are usually less severe than those of type 1 diabetes, many persons have the disease but remain unaware of it. By the time the diagnosis of diabetes is made in these individuals, they also exhibit symptoms of long-term complications that include atherosclerosis and nerve damage. Hence, type 2 diabetes has been called the "silent killer."

Gestational diabetes develops during pregnancy in a person who did not have diabetes before becoming pregnant. It occurs in 3 to 8 percent of all pregnancies. Women with gestational diabetes have an increased risk of developing diabetes after pregnancy. Children of women with gestational diabetes have a higher risk of obesity, glucose intolerance, and diabetes in adolescence.

Prediabetes is a condition in which individuals have high blood glucose levels but not high enough for them to be diagnosed with type 2 diabetes. Persons with prediabetes are at higher risk of developing diabetes in the future.

In the News: Increase in Type 2 Diabetes in Adults and Children

There is no doubt that the United States and many other countries around the world are affected by an "obesity epidemic." Poor eating habits and sedentary lifestyles are causing higher rates of obesity across all age groups and ethnic backgrounds. Approximately 30 percent of adults in the United States are obese. The rate of obesity in children ages two to five and ages twelve to nineteen has tripled since the mid-1970s. In children ages six to eleven, this rate has quadrupled from 4 to an alarming 19 percent.

Type 2 diabetes is occurring with increasing frequency in children, adolescents, and adults. The number of people with diabetes has more than doubled in the United States, from 15 percent in 1980 to 34 percent in 2006. Type 2 diabetes accounts for 90 to 95 percent of these cases. In 2005–2006, 72 percent of adults ages twenty to seventy-four were overweight or obese.

The Centers for Disease Control and Prevention estimates that 8 to 43 percent of new cases of diabetes in children are type 2 diabetes. These young people are usually overweight or obese, have a family history of diabetes, have signs of insulin resistance such as acanthosis nigricans, are members of an ethnic group with a high risk of type 2 diabetes, and are more often girls than boys.

This increase has many causes. The serving sizes of foods sold in stores and restaurants have increased. In many neighborhoods, there are more fast-food restaurants than grocery stores. Approximately 30 percent of all calories consumed by Americans are in the form of sodas and fruit-flavored drinks. Teenagers drink more soda than milk, and about half of the children ages six to eleven drink soda daily. Less than 25 percent of Americans eat five or more servings of fruit and vegetables daily. To compound the problem, more than 30 percent of high school students do not exercise regularly, and more than half of adults do not get enough physical activity.

There are several ways to stop this epidemic. Healthier eating habits and regular physical activity can decrease obesity, diabetes, and many other chronic diseases. Breastfeeding is associated with lower rates of obesity in children. Parents can advocate for regular physical activity in schools and healthy snacks and drinks in vending machines. Limiting television viewing and computer time, encouraging physical activity at home, and providing nutritious meals and smaller portions can all contribute to controlling the "obesity epidemic" in children.

—*Julie M. Slocum, RN, MS, CDE*

TREATMENT AND THERAPY

Insulin is the only treatment available for type 1 diabetes. In many cases, it is used to treat individuals with type 2 diabetes. Insulin is available in many formulations, which differ in the time of onset of action, activity, and duration of action. Insulin preparations are classified as rapid-acting, fast-acting, intermediate-acting, and long-acting.

The native insulin protein typically clumps together to form groups of six (hexamers). Subcutaneously injected insulin must dissociate from the hexamers before blood vessels absorb it. Rapid-acting insulins (aspart, lispro, insulin glulisine) are genetically engineered not to form hexamers. Consequently, they experience accelerated absorption. The effects of rapid-acting insulin peak at about thirty minutes and lasts for five hours. Fast-acting, or regular, insulin forms hexamers that must dissociate before it is absorbed. Fast-acting insulin (regular U-100) peaks at two hours and lasts until eight hours. Intermediate insulin contains regular insulin complexed with protamine sulfate salts. The insulin hexamers must dissociate from the salts and then from each other before absorption. This two-step process delays insulin absorption and activity. Intermediate insulin (neutral protamine Hagedorn [NPH]) peaks about four-five hours and lasts until approximately sixteen hours. Long-lasting insulins (insulin glargine, insulin degludec, insulin detemir) tend not to peak (peakless). Instead, these insulins provide constant, low-level activity for twenty-four to forty-two hours. Insulin glargine (Lantus) precipitates in the tissue, delaying absorption and prolonging the duration of action. Insulin detemir

(Levemir) has an attached fatty acid side chain that allows reversible binding to blood proteins, extending its action. Insulin degludec (Tresiba) has two changes (threonine at position B30 and an attached fatty acid) facilitating self-association and blood protein binding. Degludec has a long duration of action (40 hours) and stable blood concentration. *Afrezza* is a rapid-acting, inhaled, dry powder Food and Drug Administration (FDA)-approved for use in adults with diabetes mellitus. Factors that affect the rate of insulin absorption include the site of injection, the patient's age and health status, and their level of physical activity. For a person with diabetes, however, insulin is a reprieve, not a cure.

For type 2 diabetes mellitus patients who are highly insulin resistant, a more concentrated formulation of regular insulin, U-500, contains 500 units per mL of regular insulin. U-500 works better for treating severely insulin-resistant patients. Its high concentration of insulin delays absorption and U-500 activity most closely resembles that of NPH, peaking at about three hours and lasting for about twenty-two hours.

Newer insulins include *Admelog*, a slightly cheaper version of insulin lispro, *Semglee* and *Basaglar*, a less expensive version of insulin glargine, *Fiasp*, a new rapid-acting insulin, and *Lyumjev*, another type of insulin lispro.

Because of the complications that arise from chronic exposure to glucose, the patient should maintain their glucose concentrations as close to physiologically normal levels as possible. For this reason, it is preferable to administer multiple doses of insulin during the day. By monitoring plasma glucose concentrations, the diabetic person can adjust the dosage of insulin administered and thus closely mimic normal glucose concentrations. Electromechanical insulin delivery systems, also known as insulin pumps, maintain basal plasma insulin concentrations throughout the day. Such insulin pumps can be programmed to deliver a constant infusion of insulin at a rate designed to meet minimum requirements, whether internal or external. A bolus injection can then supplement the infusion before a meal. Increasingly sophisticated systems automatically monitor blood glucose concentrations and adjust the delivery rate of insulin accordingly. These alternative delivery systems are intended to prevent the development of long-term tissue complications.

In 2016, the FDA approved the first hybrid closed loop (HCL) insulin delivery system, the Medtronic MiniMed 670G System. HCL insulin delivery systems automatically monitor blood sugar with a subcutaneously implanted constant glucose monitor (CGM). The HCL delivers these continuous blood glucose readings to an insulin pump that delivers precisely calculated quantities of insulin to the patient. HCL insulin delivery systems can provide tight blood glucose control that reduces the risk of dangerously low blood glucose levels (<60 mg/dL) and high blood glucose levels (≥250 mg/dL).

Several chronic complications account for the shorter life expectancy of diabetic persons. These include atherosclerotic changes throughout the entire vascular system. The thickening of basement membranes surrounding the capillaries can affect their ability to exchange nutrients (diabetic vasculitis). Cardiovascular lesions are the most common cause of premature death in diabetic persons (diabetic cardiopathy). Kidney disease, commonly found in longtime diabetics, can ultimately lead to kidney failure (diabetic nephropathy). For these persons, expensive medical care, including dialysis and the possibility of a kidney transplant, overshadows their lives. Diabetes is the leading cause of new blindness in the United States (diabetic retinopathy). Delayed gastric emptying (gastroparesis) occurs when the stomach takes too long to empty its contents; it damages the vagus nerve from long-term exposure to high glucose levels. In addition, diabetes leads to a gradual decline in the ability of nerves to conduct sensory information to the brain (diabetic neuropathy). For example, the feet of some people with diabetes feel more like stumps of wood than living tissue.

Consequently, weight is not distributed properly; in concert with the reduction in blood flow, this problem can lead to pressure ulcers. If not carefully cared for, areas of the foot can develop gangrene, which may lead to amputation of the foot. Finally, in male patients, there are problems with the reproductive function that generally result in impotence. However, large clinical trials in the United States and the United Kingdom have shown that tight control over blood sugar levels can significantly delay the onset of these complications.

The mechanism responsible for the development of these long-term complications of diabetes is genetic in origin and dependent on the amount of time the tissues are exposed to the elevated plasma glucose concentrations. What, then, is the link between glucose concentrations and diabetic complications?

As an animal ages, most of its cells become less efficient in replacing damaged material. At the same time, tissues lose elasticity and gradually stiffen. For example, the lungs and heart muscle expand less successfully, blood vessels become increasingly rigid, and ligaments tighten. These various age-related changes are accelerated in diabetes, and the causative agent is glucose. Glucose becomes chemically attached to proteins and deoxyribonucleic acid (DNA) in the body without enzymes to speed the reaction along. What is important is the duration of exposure to the elevated glucose concentrations. Once glucose is bound to tissue proteins, a series of chemical reactions is triggered that, over the passage of months and years, can result in the formation and eventual accumulation of cross-links between adjacent proteins. The higher glucose concentrations in people with diabetes accelerate this process, and the

> **IN THE NEWS: ACCORD TRIAL**
>
> The Action to Control Cardiovascular Risk in Diabetes (Accord) trial, sponsored by the National Heart, Lung, and Blood Institute, was a large-scale clinical study of adults with type 2 diabetes who were at high risk for cardiovascular disease. More than ten thousand adults across the United States and Canada were enrolled in the study; participants were between the ages of forty and seventy, had diabetes for an average of ten years, and were at high risk for cardiovascular disease owing to a minimum two risk factors in addition to type 2 diabetes.
>
> The Accord trial examined cardiovascular disease events in three treatment strategies compared to standard treatments: intensive lowering of blood glucose levels, treating cholesterol and triglycerides with a fibrate plus a statin, and intensive blood pressure reduction.
>
> In 2008, researchers stopped the intensive glucose control arm of the trial nearly eighteen months early because of safety concerns. The traditional treatment group included 5,123 participants and aimed to lower blood sugar levels to a hemoglobin A1C (HbA1C) of 7 to 7.9 percent. The intensive therapy group included 5,128 participants and aimed to reduce HbA1C to less than 6 percent. After an average of 3.5 years of treatment, the intensive control group exhibited a 22 percent increased risk of death compared to the standard treatment group.
>
> The causes of death were similar in both groups, and approximately half of the deaths were caused by cardiovascular events, including heart attack, stroke, heart failure, or sudden cardiac death. The intensive treatment group had a 35 percent higher cardiovascular death rate than the standard treatment group. The death rates were consistent between the groups, regardless of baseline characteristics such as gender, age, race, or existing cardiovascular disease. The participants in the intensive treatment group were moved to the standard treatment arm of the study and followed to the study's planned conclusion.
>
> Researchers have been unable to identify the exact cause of the increased risk of death. Still, they believe it is due to a combination of factors and not a specific medication or treatment. The results underscore the importance of individualized therapy for type 2 diabetes. No changes to standard treatment guidelines are recommended. The results of the trial do not apply to people with type 1 diabetes.
>
> The Accord trial began in 2003 and followed patients through 2009. The researchers published the final results of the study in 2010.
>
> —*Jennifer L. Gibson, PharmD*

In the News:
Benefits and Risks of Diabetes Drugs

The benefits and risks of diabetes drugs have caused concern among patients and health-care providers and challenged traditional treatment options as safety concerns of new medications mount. The effectiveness of older medications is confirmed.

Metformin is the most used oral medication to treat type 2 diabetes. Metformin reduces triglycerides and low-density lipoprotein (LDL) cholesterol and increases high-density lipoprotein (HDL) cholesterol. According to the United Kingdom Prospective Diabetes Study, metformin reduces the risk of myocardial infarction and stroke, making it a first-choice treatment option for most patients with diabetes.

Sulfonylureas interact with the beta cells in the pancreas to increase insulin secretion. Three drugs, glimepiride (Amaryl and generics), glipizide (Glucotrol, and others), and glyburide (Glynase, Prestab, and others), reduce blood sugar and reduce long-term complications of diabetes mellitus. However, the effects of sulfonylureas are not as durable as those with metformin. Sulfonylureas cause hypoglycemia and weight gain, but combining them with metformin mitigates weight gain.

Thiazolidinediones can cause significant weight gain and fluid retention, leading to an increased risk of heart failure. Several studies suggest but do not prove that one agent, rosiglitazone, may increase the risk of heart attack and cardiovascular death. Conversely, another agent, pioglitazone, may reduce the risk of heart attack and stroke. Both thiazolidinediones have shown an increased risk of fractures in women. More research is needed to verify these findings. Pioglitazone may increase the risk of bladder cancer.

Glucagon-like peptide-1 (GLP-1) receptor agonists are incretin hormone-based therapies. Exenatide (Byetta), a GLP-1 agonist, causes substantial gastrointestinal side effects, but these typically resolve after a few weeks of treatment. Of benefit in diabetes, exenatide leads to significant weight loss. Several cases of pancreatitis have been reported using exenatide; most of the issues are resolved with the discontinuation of the drug. Also, several cases of kidney dysfunction have been reported with exenatide. The U.S. Food and Drug Administration (FDA) advises caution when using exenatide in patients with existing kidney or pancreatic disease. Other GLP-1 agonists include dulaglutide (Trulicity), liraglutide (Victoza), lixisenatide (Adlyxin), and semaglutide (Ozempic–injected; Rybelsus–oral). Exenatide is injected twice a day, liraglutide and lixisenatide are injected once a day, and dulaglutide and semaglutide are injected once per week. Exenatide, however, comes in an extended-release formulation called "Bydueron" that is administered once a week.

GLP-1 receptor agonists potentiate glucose-dependent secretion of insulin by pancreatic beta cells. These drugs also suppress glucagon secretion, slow gastric emptying, and promote satiety. Consequently, these medications facilitate weight loss in diabetic patients. Semaglutide is FDA-approved as a weight loss agent. GLP-1 receptor agonists can reduce the incidence of major adverse cardiovascular events and may benefit the kidneys.

Dipeptidyl peptidase-4 (DPP4) inhibitors are also incretin-based drugs. DPP-4 degrades GLP-1 and GIP (Glucose insulinotropic peptide), and DPP-4 inhibitors increase the half-life and activity of incretins. Rare cases of severe allergic reactions, including angioedema and Stevens-Johnson syndrome, have occurred using DPP4 inhibitors. Sitagliptin, a DPP4 inhibitor, is also associated with several cases of severe pancreatitis; most of the issues are resolved with the discontinuation of the drug. In late 2009, the FDA ordered the manufacturer of sitagliptin to change the prescribing information to warn of the increased risk of pancreatitis with sitagliptin. Other DPP-4 inhibitors include alogliptin (Nesina), linagliptin (Tradjenta), saxagliptin (Onglyza), and sitagliptin (Januvia). These drugs are weight neutral and reduce blood glucose levels. Unfortunately, they do not protect against heart attacks and strokes.

Newer drugs for type 2 diabetes mellitus include the SGLT2 (sodium-glucose co-transporter 2) inhibitors that work in the kidney. SGLT2 inhibitors prevent glucose reabsorption by the kidney and increase urinary glucose excretion. These drugs effectively reduce blood glucose levels. However, they significantly reduce heart attacks and strokes and preserve kidney function. SGLT-2 inhibitors also facilitate weight loss. The side effects of these drugs include urinary tract infections, dehydration, low blood pressure, and increases in blood lipid levels. More severe adverse effects include an increased risk of lower limb amputation, fractures, and ketoacidosis. SGLT2 inhibitors include canagliflozin (Invokana), dapagliflozin (Farxiga), empagliflozin (Jardiance), and ertugliflozin (Steglatro).

Many experts have questioned the urgency with which new diabetes medications have emerged. Clinicians now advocate weighing the benefits of blood glucose control with the undesirable risks associated with many diabetes drugs.

—*Jennifer L. Gibson, PharmD*

effects become evident in specific tissues throughout the body.

Understanding the chemical basis of protein cross-linking in diabetes has permitted the development and study of compounds that can intervene in this process. When added to the diet, certain compounds can limit the glucose-induced cross-linking of proteins by preventing their formation. One of the best-studied compounds, aminoguanidine, can help prevent the cross-linking of collagen; this fact is shown in a decrease in the accumulation of trapped lipoproteins on artery walls. Aminoguanidine also prevents the thickening of the capillary basement membrane in the kidney. Aminoguanidine acts by blocking glucose's ability to react with neighboring proteins. Vitamins C and B6 are also effective in reducing cross-linking. Aminoguanidine and vitamins C and B6 are thought to have antiaging properties. They may also improve the complications resulting from the high blood glucose levels seen in diabetes mellitus.

Alternatively, transplantation of the entire pancreas effectively achieves an insulin-independent state in persons with type 1 diabetes mellitus. However, the technical problems of pancreas transplantation and the possible rejection of the foreign tissue have limited this procedure as a treatment for diabetes. Diabetes is usually manageable; therefore, a pancreas transplant is not necessarily lifesaving. Success in treating diabetes has been achieved by transplanting only the insulin-producing islet cells from the pancreas or grafts from fetal pancreas tissue. One day, it may be possible to use genetic engineering to permit liver cells to self-regulate glucose concentrations by synthesizing and releasing their insulin into the blood.

Oral hypoglycemic agents that reduce blood glucose can control some of the less severe forms of type 2 diabetes mellitus. Sulfonylureas are oral medications that drive the beta cells to release even more insulin than usual. These drugs also increase the ability of insulin to act on the target cells, which ultimately reduces the insulin requirement. The use of these agents remains controversial because they overwork the already strained beta cells. Suppose a diabetic person relies on these drugs for extended periods. In that case, the insulin cells could "burn out" and completely lose their ability to synthesize insulin. In this situation, the previously non-insulin-dependent person would have to be placed on insulin therapy for life. Other hypoglycemic agents lower blood glucose by decreasing hepatic glucose output, reducing insulin resistance, and delaying glucose absorption from the gastrointestinal tract.

Suppose obesity is a factor in the expression of type 2 diabetes. In that case, as it is in most cases, the best therapy is a combination of a reduction of calorie intake and an increase in activity. More than any other disease, type 2 diabetes is related to lifestyle. It is often the case that people prefer having an injection or taking a pill to improve their quality of life by changing their diet and level of activity. Extensive research has shown that increased attention to diet and exercise results in a dramatic decrease in the need for drug therapy in most diabetics.

In some cases, the loss of only a small percentage of body weight results in an increased sensitivity to insulin. Exercise is beneficial in managing both types of diabetes because working muscle does not require insulin to metabolize glucose. Thus, exercising muscles take up and use some of the excess glucose in the blood, which reduces the overall need for insulin. Permanent weight reduction and exercise also help to prevent long-term complications and permit a healthier and more active lifestyle.

PERSPECTIVE AND PROSPECTS
Diabetes mellitus is a disease of ancient origin. The tomb of Thebes in Egypt (1500 BCE) contains the first known written reference to diabetes. This refer-

ence described an illness associated with the passage of vast quantities of sweet urine and excessive thirst.

The study of diabetes owes much to the Franco-Prussian War. In 1870, during the siege of Paris, it was noted by French physicians that the widespread famine in the besieged city had a curative influence on diabetic patients. Their glycosuria decreased or disappeared. These observations supported the view of clinicians at the time who had previously prescribed periods of fasting and increased muscular work for the treatment of the overweight, diabetic individual.

It was Oscar Minkowski of Germany who, in 1889, accidentally traced the origin of diabetes to the pancreas. Minkowski's technician noted the animal's subsequent copious urine production after the complete removal of the pancreas from a dog. Acting based on a hunch, Minkowski tested the urine and determined that its sugar content was greater than 10 percent.

The clinical application of a discovery usually takes a long time. In 1921, Frederick Banting and Charles Best, at the University of Toronto in Canada, successfully extracted the antidiabetic substance insulin using a cold alcohol-hydrochloric acid mixture to inactivate the harsh digestive enzymes of the pancreas. Using this substance, Banting and Best first controlled the disease in a depancreatized dog and then, a few months later, successfully treated the first human diabetic patient. Still, in this case, a mere twenty weeks had passed between the first injection of insulin into the diabetic dog and the first trial with a diabetic human. In 1923, Banting and Best won the Nobel Prize in physiology or medicine for their remarkable achievement.

Although insulin, when combined with an appropriate diet and exercise, alleviates the symptoms of diabetes to such an extent that a person with diabetes can lead an essentially normal life, insulin therapy is not a cure. The complications that arise in people with diabetes are typical of those found in the general population, except that they happen much earlier in people with diabetes. In 1908, chemists first hypothesized that sugars could react with proteins. In 1912, Louis Camille Maillard further characterized this reaction at the Sorbonne and realized that the consequences of this reaction were relevant to diabetics. Maillard suggested that sugars were destroying the body's amino acids, leading to increased excretion in diabetics. However, it was not until the mid-1970s that Anthony Cerami in New York introduced the concept of the nonenzymatic attachment of glucose to protein and recognized its potential role in diabetic complications. A decade later, this development led to the discovery of aminoguanidine, the first compound to limit the cross-linking of tissue proteins and thus delay certain diabetic complications.

In 1974, Josiah Brown published the first report showing that transplanting fetal pancreatic tissue could reverse diabetes. By the mid-1980s, procedures had been devised to isolate massive numbers of human islets that could then be transplanted into people with diabetes. For persons with diabetes, both approaches represent more than a treatment; they may offer a cure for the disease.

By the turn of the twenty-first century, there was a noticeable rise in the prevalence of type 2 diabetes in both developing and developed countries. According to the World Health Organization (WHO), an estimated 347 million people worldwide have diabetes, a number expected to rise. Although the incidence of type 2 diabetes typically increases with age, the first decades of the twenty-first century have seen a dramatic rise in the number of cases in younger people.

Obesity is linked to the increase of type 2 diabetes. The WHO reported that worldwide obesity nearly doubled between 1980 and 2013. By 2008, about 35 percent of adults were overweight, and 11 percent were obese. The growing sedentary lifestyle and increase in energy-dense food intake are significant risk factors. Due in large part to these factors, the WHO has predicted that diabetes will become the seventh leading cause of death by 2030.

—*Hillar Klandorf, PhD, Sharon W. Stark, RN, APRN, DNSc and Michael Buratovich, PhD*

Further Information

American Diabetes Association, www.diabetes.org.
American Diabetes Association. "Gestational Diabetes." *Diabetes Care*, vol. 26, 2003, pp. S103-5.
American Diabetes Association. *Managing Type 2 Diabetes for Dummies*. For Dummies, 2018.
American Diabetes Association Complete Guide to Diabetes. 5th rev. ed., American Diabetes Association, 2011.
Becker, Gretchen. *The First Year-Type 2 Diabetes: An Essential Guide for the Newly Diagnosed*. 3rd ed., Marlowe, 2015.
Campbell, Jacqueline E. *A Patient's Guide to the Treatment of Diabetes Mellitus.* ? Jacqueline Elaine Campbell, 2009.
"Diabetes." *MedlinePlus*, 2 Aug. 2021, medlineplus.gov/diabetes.html. Accessed 26 Aug. 2021.
Jovanovic-Peterson, Lois, Charles M. Peterson, and Morton B. Stori. *A Touch of Diabetes*. 3rd ed., Chronimed, 1998.
Kronenberg, Henry M., et al., editors. *Williams Textbook of Endocrinology*. 14th ed., Saunders/Elsevier, 2019.
Magee, Elaine. *Tell Me What to Eat If I Have Diabetes: Nutrition You Can Live With*. 4th ed., Career Press, 2014.
McCulloch, David. *The Diabetes Answer Book: Practical Answers to More than Three Hundred Top Questions*. Sourcebooks, 2008.
Shaw, Michael. *Diabetes Mellitus: An Incredibly Easy! Miniguide*. Springhouse Pub. Co., 2000.

Eczema

Category: Diseases/Disorders
Also known as: Dermatitis
Anatomy or system affected: Skin
Specialties and related fields: Dermatology, pediatrics
Definition: An inflammation of the skin.

KEY TERMS

dyshidrotic eczema: a type of dermatitis in which blisters form on the hands and feet
nummular eczema: a kind of dermatitis in which itchy, coin-shaped spots or patches appear on the skin
seborrheic eczema: A skin condition that causes scaly patches and red skin, mainly on the scalp

CAUSES AND SYMPTOMS

The term *eczema* refers to a noncontagious inflammation of the skin. Several types of eczema exist, resulting in a range of symptoms that vary in appearance, duration, and severity. The common characteristic, however, is red, dry, and itchy skin. Other symptoms may include scaling, thickening, or cracking of the skin, leading to infections and severe discomfort.

Atopic dermatitis, the most common form of eczema, is characterized by itchy and cracked cheeks, arms, and legs. The onset of this chronic type of eczema occurs most often during infancy or childhood, although symptoms may continue into adulthood. The cause of atopic dermatitis is a hereditary predisposition to skin sensitivities to various environmental factors. These factors include irritants

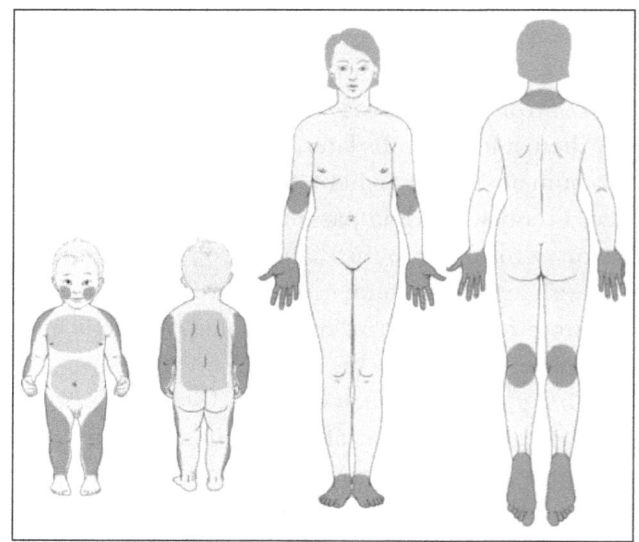

Eczema in children and adults: Skin areas typically affected.Image via National Center for Biotechnology Information (ncbi.nlm.nih.gov).

such as soaps, detergents, rough clothes; allergens such as certain foods, pollen, or animal dander; and changes in climate or temperature. Other forms of eczema, such as contact dermatitis, have similar environmental causes. Seborrheic eczema, nummular eczema, and dyshidrotic eczema may result from a combination of several possible causes. Emotional factors, such as stress or frustration, may aggravate the symptoms.

The diagnosis of eczema requires careful and detailed observation of symptoms. Family and personal medical histories are often helpful to determine the presence of allergies or exposure to allergens or irritants. Dermatologists may also use skin biopsies or blood tests to determine a tendency toward elevated allergic or immune response.

TREATMENT AND THERAPY

The treatment of eczema involves minimizing exposure to possible causes while at the same time managing symptoms to maintain a high quality of life. Identifying known allergens and irritants specific to the individual is an essential first step. Lifestyle changes aimed at avoiding exposure to these possible causes can dramatically lower the frequency and duration of symptoms. Proper skincare to prevent excessive drying of the skin, including moisturizers or creams and minimizing exposure to water, may also help reduce skin irritation. Avoiding scratching existing irritations and eliminating sources of emotional stress are other ways that patients can lessen the severity of their symptoms. Dermatologists may prescribe additional treatments, such as corticosteroid creams and ointments, antihistamines, or antibiotics. In more severe cases, systemic corticosteroid treatments or phototherapy, the use of ultraviolet (UV) light, may be tried.

The approval of a new type of treatment for eczema called "topical immunomodulators" has changed how eczema is treated in recent years. This new class of drugs counteracts the inflammation of

> **INFORMATION ON ECZEMA**
>
> **Causes**: Genetic sensitivity to irritants (soaps, detergents, rough clothes), allergens (certain foods, pollen, animal dander), and climate or temperature changes
>
> **Symptoms**: Red, dry, and itchy skin; scaling, thickening, or cracking of the skin
>
> **Duration**: Often chronic
>
> **Treatments**: Minimal exposure to irritants, drugs (corticosteroid creams and ointments, antihistamines, antibiotics); in severe cases, oral corticosteroids or phototherapy

the skin without interfering with the body's normal immune response. This treatment has been successful in preventing and even eliminating symptoms of eczema.

—*Paul J. Frisch*

Further Information

"Atopic Dermatitis." *MedlinePlus*, 5 Aug. 2021, medlineplus.gov/ency/article/000853.htm. Accessed 24 Aug. 2021.

Fry, Lionel. *An Atlas of Atopic Eczema* Parthenon, 2004.

Hellwig, Jennifer. "Eczema." *Health Library*, 11 Mar. 2013.

National Eczema Society, eczema.org/. Accessed 24 Aug. 2021.

Rakel, Robert E., and Edward T. Bcpe, editors. *Conn's Current Therapy*. Saunders, 2007.

Ring, J., B. Przybilla, and T. Ruzicka, editors. *Handbook of Atopic Eczema*. 2nd ed., Springer, 2006.

Turkington, Carol A., and Jeffrey S. Dover. *Skin Deep: An A-Z of Skin Disorders, Treatments, and Health*. 3rd ed., Checkmark, 2007.

Westcott, Patsy. *Eczema: Recipes and Advice to Provide Relief*. Welcome, 2000.

Graft-versus-host disease (GVHD)

Category: Diseases/Conditions

Anatomy or system affected: Blood, bones, gastrointestinal system, immune system, liver, musculoskeletal system, skin, tissue

Specialties and related fields: Dermatology, epidemiology, gastroenterology, hematology, immunology, internal medicine, oncology, pathology

Definition: A multiorgan inflammatory condition associated with bone marrow and stem cell transplants.

KEY TERMS

bone marrow transplant: a procedure whereby a recipient receives multipotent hematopoietic stem cells derived from the bone marrow of a donor

immunosuppression: the partial or complete suppression of someone's immune response to help the survival of an organ after a transplant operation

stem cell transplant: a procedure in which a patient receives healthy blood-forming cells (*stem cells*) from a donor to replace their stem cells that have been destroyed by disease, chemicals, or radiation

T-cytotoxic cells: a subtype of T lymphocytes that can kill specific cells, including foreign cells, cancer cells, and virally infected cells

T lymphocytes: a type of lymphocyte that differentiates in the thymus, possesses specific cell-surface antigen receptors, and controls the initiation or suppression of cell-mediated and humoral immunity or destroys antigen-bearing cells.

umbilical cord blood transplant: a procedure in which hematopoietic stem cells collected from the blood left in the umbilical cord after a baby's birth are used to replace someone's damaged bone marrow

THE BASICS

Graft-versus-host disease (GVHD) occurs as a complication of a bone marrow transplant or stem cell transplant when new cells are transplanted from a donor to a recipient. The tissue sample that is taken from the donor and inserted into the recipient is called a "graft." In the graft, the donor lymphocytes, T and B cells begin to attack foreign cells and synthesize and secrete antibodies (proteins the immune system produces to fight infection). These foreign antibodies attack the recipient's healthy cells in the digestive system, skin, and liver. The foreign T-cytotoxic cells destroy cells in the recipient's body.

Acute GVHD can occur soon after the transplantation, usually within the first one hundred days. Chronic GVHD can occur after the first one hundred days and can flare up at different times for several years after the transplantation. A person can experience both acute and chronic GVHD or just one of the syndromes.

GVHD differs from transplant rejection, in which the recipient's immune system rejects the donor's tissue. GVHD consists of immune cells from the donor's tissue attacking the recipient's cells. Blood transfusions can also cause GVHD if the blood or blood products were not irradiated or treated with an approved pathogen reduction system.

CAUSES

GVHD is an immune response generated from the newly transplanted cells from an allogeneic donor. A donor is a person who is related or unrelated to the patient. Each person's chemical makeup is unique, and for transplantation to succeed, physicians must find donors similar to the recipient in chemical makeup.

Physicians look for specific proteins on blood cells called "histocompatibility antigens" (also known as human leukocyte antigen [HLA] markers). These proteins are responsible for recognizing foreign invaders and activating the immune system to eliminate any potential infections. The HLA markers will be similar but never identical to the recipient's healthy cells unless the donor and recipient are identical twins.

As the graft of cells begins to grow and integrate into the patient's body, the new cells recognize these slight differences and react by attacking other

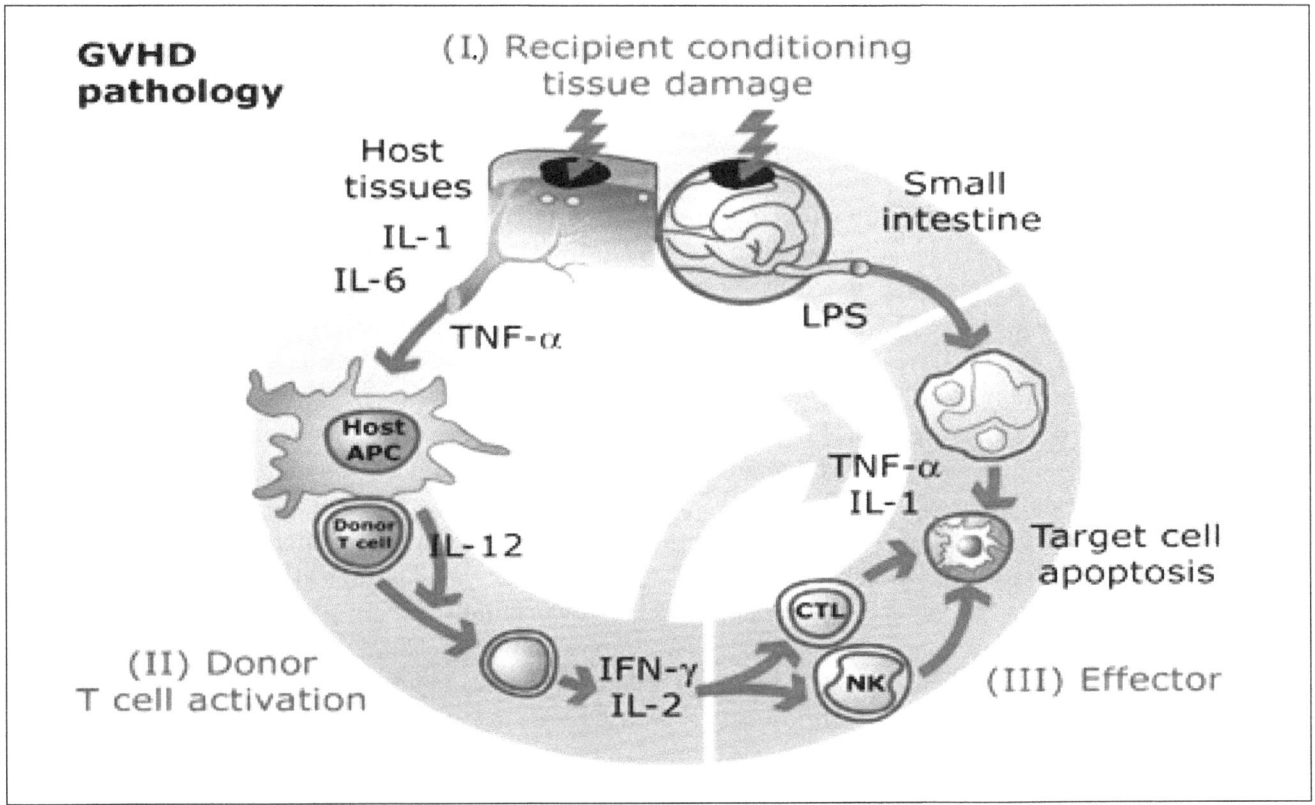
Three phases of GVHD. Image by P. Reddy and J.L.M. Ferrara, via Wikimedia Commons. [CC 3.0.]

healthy cells within the patient's body. The donor immune cells mainly attack cells in the digestive tract, skin, and liver, just as a healthy immune system attacks bacteria or viruses. This process causes damage to these areas and complications for the patient.

RISK FACTORS

GVHD occurs only in persons who receive allogeneic grafts of peripherally collected stem cells, bone marrow, or umbilical cord blood to treat various diseases, including certain cancers and sickle cell anemia. Umbilical cord blood grafts have less of a risk for GVHD than the other grafts, and grafts from unrelated donors have greater potential for causing GVHD than grafts from biological family members. Other risk factors include receiving a graft from a person of the opposite gender, older age of either the donor or the recipient, receiving a poorly matched graft, and having a cytomegalovirus (herpes) infection. Transplant recipients who have had their spleen removed are also at risk for GVHD. Men experience GVHD more often than do women.

People who have acute GVHD are at risk for developing chronic GVHD. Acute GVHD occurs in as many as 90 percent of allogeneic transplant recipients, with about 50 percent of occurrences considered clinically significant (that is, requiring medical intervention). Chronic GVHD affects as many as 80 percent of bone marrow transplant recipients.

SYMPTOMS

Symptoms depend upon the area of the body that is affected. The skin is usually affected first, and the patient will usually experience burning, itching, and a rash. The skin will darken and have a reddish tone. The hands, feet, upper back, cheeks, neck, and ears are the most commonly affected. GVHD can progress to other body areas and include more severe skin complications, including blisters filled with a clear liquid. GVHD can resemble a severe burn. The most severe form can cause tissue necrosis (progressive skin-cell death).

When GVHD affects the liver, typical symptoms of liver disease occur, including jaundice (a yellowish tone to the skin and whites of the eyes), abdominal pain and cramping, weight gain, and ascites an increase of fluid in the abdomen.

When GVHD includes the digestive tract, it affects the outer lining of the system (known as the mucosal lining). The most common symptom is diarrhea, which can be severe. The patient may also experience nausea and appetite loss.

The symptoms for each system can occur independently or at the same time. All three organ systems may be affected or only one or two. Symptoms can range from mild to life-threatening.

SCREENING AND DIAGNOSIS
To determine if a person has GVHD, physicians must rule out other diseases with similar symptoms, which often occur in people who have bone marrow or stem cell transplants. These conditions include drug toxicity, reactions to radiation therapy or chemotherapy, bacterial or viral infections, or complications from total parental nutrition (tube feeding).

Diagnostic studies will depend on the part of the body that is affected. Because the risk is so high for GVHD in patients who receive an allogeneic stem cell or bone marrow transplant, they are often monitored for early signs of the disease through blood tests. Imaging scans and tissue biopsies of the affected system are usually performed to rule out GVHD in persons experiencing symptoms. Endoscopy can be performed on persons who are experiencing digestive tract symptoms.

TREATMENT AND THERAPY
GVHD treatment depends on the severity of the condition and whether the disease is acute or chronic. GVHD is "graded" according to the percentage of the skin involved and the degree of liver and gastrointestinal dysfunction observed. Standard treatment for GVHD consists in suppressing the immune system.

Treatment of acute, cutaneous GVHD includes applying mid- to high-potency topical steroids twice daily to moist skin and covered with warm wet towels. Cutaneous GVHD that does not respond to steroids may respond to topical tacrolimus, a calcineurin inhibitor, or oral ruxolitinib, a JAK kinase inhibitor. There is little clinical agreement on the ideal treatment for steroid-resistant GVHD.

For severe, acute GVHD, high-dose, intravenous or oral steroids, such as methylprednisolone, are the standard treatment. If the patient has substantial gastrointestinal involvement, the oral beclomethasone, a nonabsorbable glucocorticoid, improves outcomes. If the condition resists steroid treatment, then oral ruxolitinib seems the best option.

The addition of antithymocyte globulin (ATG) or the monoclonal antibody alemtuzumab to preparative regimens reduces the rate of chronic GVHD. The administration of high-dose cyclophosphamide on days three and four after the transplant procedure further reduces the risk of chronic GVHD. Should chronic GVHD develop, the standard treatment also includes high-dose steroids, particularly prednisone. Adding cyclosporine or tacrolimus while tapering prednisone dosages decreases the risk of GVHD recurrence. While many other immunosuppressive agents are available, the evidence for their efficacy remains equivocal.

PREVENTION AND OUTCOMES

Suppressing the immune system is also used as an approach to GVHD prevention. In addition, finding the proper donor match is crucial to preventing GVHD. Taking steps to prevent acute GVHD will also help to prevent chronic GVHD.

—Laura J. Pinchot, BA
and Michael A. Buratovich, PhD

Further Information

Chao, Nelson J., and Robert Zeiser. "Pathogenesis of Graft-Versus-Host Disease (GVHD)." *UpToDate*, 8 Apr. 2021, www-uptodate-com.arbor.idm.oclc.org/contents/pathogenesis-of-graft-versus-host-disease-gvhd?search=GvHD&source=search_result&selectedTitle=3~150&usage_type=default&display_rank=3. Accessed 25 Aug. 2021.

Eggert, Julie, editor. *Cancer Basics*. Oncology Nursing Society, 2010.

"Graft-Versus-Host Disease." *Memorial Sloan Kettering Cancer Center*, n.d., www.mskcc.org/cancer-care/types/graft-versus-host-disease-gvhd. Accessed 25 Aug. 2021.

Latchford, Teresa. "Cutaneous Effects of Blood and Marrow Transplantation." *Principles of Skin Care and the Oncology Patient*. Oncology Nursing Society, 2010.

MacDonald, Kelli Pa, et al. "Cytokine Mediators of Chronic Graft-Versus-Host Disease." *The Journal of Clinical Investigation*, vol. 127, no. 7, 2017, pp. 2452-63, doi:10.1172/JCI90593.

Penack, Olaf, et al. "Prophylaxis and Management of Graft Versus Host Disease After Stem-Cell Transplantation for Haematological Malignancies: Updated Consensus Recommendations of the European Society for Blood and Marrow Transplantation." *The Lancet (Haematology)*, vol. 7, no. 2, 2020, pp. e157-e167, doi:10.1016/S2352-3026(19)30256-X.

Guillain-Barré Syndrome

Category: Diseases/Disorders
Also known as: Acute inflammatory demyelinating polyneuropathy
Anatomy or system affected: Immune system, muscles, musculoskeletal system, nerves, nervous system
Specialties and related fields: Internal medicine, neurology
Definition: An acute degeneration of peripheral motor and sensory nerves, known to physicians as acute inflammatory demyelinating polyneuropathy, a common cause of acute generalized paralysis.

KEY TERMS

antibody: a substance produced by plasma cells that usually binds to a foreign particle; in Guillain-Barré syndrome, antibodies bind to myelin protein

antigen: any substance that stimulates white blood cells to mount an immune response

areflexia: loss of reflex

autoimmune disorder: a condition in which the immune system attacks the body's tissue instead of foreign tissue

B cell: a type of white blood cell that produces antibodies

CSF protein: a protein in the cerebrospinal fluid which is usually very low

demyelination: a loss of the myelin coating of nerves

electromyogram: the external recording of electrical impulses from muscles

macrophage: a white blood cell that engulfs foreign protein; in Guillain-Barré syndrome, it also attacks myelin

motor weakness: muscle weakness resulting from the failure of motor nerves

nerve conduction velocity: the speed at which a nerve impulse travels along a nerve

neurogenic atrophy: shrinkage of muscle caused by a loss of nervous stimulation

neuropathy: a condition in which nerves are diseased, are inflamed, or show abnormal degeneration

phagocytosis: the process of engulfing particles

polyneuropathy: neuropathy found in many areas

CAUSES AND SYMPTOMS

Guillain-Barré syndrome (GBS) is an acute disease of the peripheral nerves, especially those that connect to muscles. It causes weakness, areflexia (loss of reflex), ataxia (difficulty in maintaining balance), and sometimes ophthalmoplegia (eye muscle paralysis). GBS demonstrates a variable, multifocal pattern of inflammation and demyelination of the spinal roots and the cranial nerves. However, the brain itself is not affected. By the 1990s and early 2000s, it was the most common cause of generalized paralysis in the United States, averaging one to two cases per 100,000 people per year. The disease was first described in the early twentieth century by Georges Guillain and Jean-Alexander Barré, two French neurologists. However, little was known of the cause of GBS or the mechanism for its symptoms until the 1970s. Since then, symposia sponsored by the National Institute of Neurological and Communicative Disorders and Stroke have shed more light on this condition.

Most individuals with GBS have a rapidly progressing muscular weakness in more than one limb and experience paresthesia (tingling) and numbness in the hands and feet. These sensations have the effect of reducing fine muscle control, balance, and one's awareness of limb location. The prevailing scientific opinion regarding GBS is that it is an autoimmune disorder involving white blood cells, which for some unknown reason, attack nerves and produce antibodies against myelin, the insulating covering of nerves. The weakness is usually ascending, beginning with numbness in the toes and fingers and progressing to total limb weakness. The demyelination is more prominent in the nerves of the trunk. It occurs to a lesser extent in the more distal nerves. The brain and spinal cord are protected from GBS by the blood-brain barrier. However, antibodies to myelin have been found in the cerebrospinal fluid of some patients.

There is often a precipitating event with GBS such as surgery, pregnancy, upper respiratory infection, viral infection (such as cytomegalovirus), or vaccination. The increased risk with such surgery may be attributable to the stress associated with the procedure. Preexisting debilitating illnesses such as systemic lupus erythematosus (SLE) or Hodgkin's disease also seem to predispose a person to GBS. GBS has been diagnosed in patients having heart transplants even though they are receiving immunosuppressive drugs. Most patients who come down with GBS have had some prior condition that prioritized the immune system before the appearance of GBS.

The patient with GBS is frequently incapable of communicating as a result of paralysis of the vocal

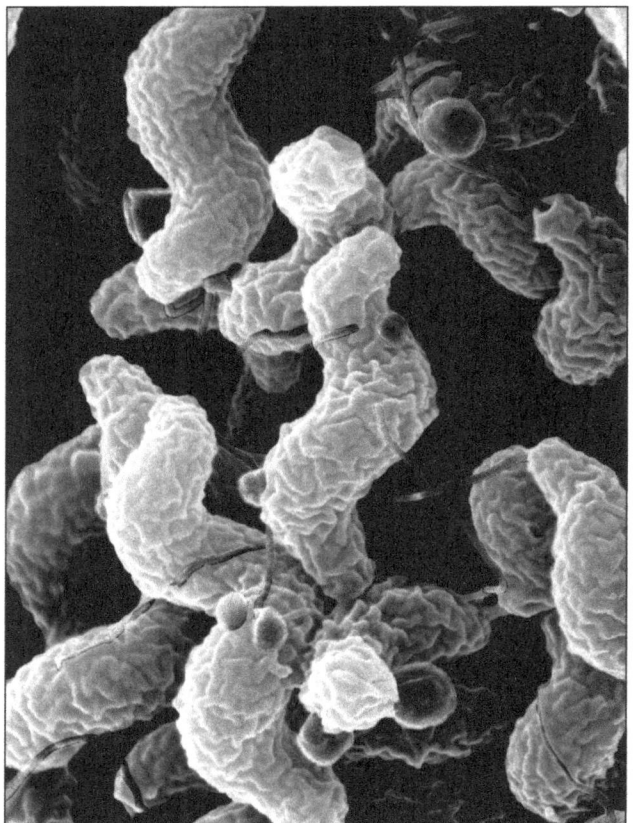

A scanning electron microscope-derived image of Campylobacter jejuni, which triggers about 30% of cases of Guillain–Barré syndrome. Photo via Wikimedia Commons. [Public domain.]

cords. Typically, motor paralysis worsens rapidly and then plateau after four weeks, with the patient bedridden and often needing respiratory support. Autonomic nerves can also be affected, causing gastrointestinal disturbances, adynamic ileus (loss of function in the ileum of the small intestine), and indigestion. Other, less common symptoms include pupillary disturbances, pooling of blood in limbs, heart rhythm disturbances, and a decrease in the heart muscle's strength. These patients are usually hypermetabolic because considerable caloric energy goes into a self-destructive immune response and mechanisms to repair the damage.

In addition to the loss of myelin, nerve damage may result in permanent deficits. If the nerve cell itself is not severely damaged, regrowth and remyelination can occur. Antibodies to myelin proteins and acidic glycolipids are seen in a majority of patients. Blood serum taken from patients with GBS has been shown to block calcium channels in muscle, and experiments in Germany have found that cerebrospinal fluid from GBS patients blocks sodium channels.

Like most autoimmune conditions, GBS is cyclic; the patient will have good days and bad days because the immune system is sensitive to steroid hormones in the body, which are known to fluctuate. In addition to paralysis, there is significant pain with GBS. Many nerve fibers that register the pain response (nociceptors) are nonmyelinated (C fibers) and, therefore, not interrupted in GBS. Pain management can be complex, requiring the use of such drugs as fentanyl, codeine, morphine, and other narcotics. The course of the disease is variable and is a function of the level of reactivity of the patient's immune system. The autoimmune attack is augmented in those patients experiencing activation of serum complement protein induced by antibodies. Recovery usually takes months, and frequently the patient requires home health care. Complications can lead to death, but most patients recover fully, though some have a residual weakness.

The physician must be careful to distinguish GBS from lead poisoning, chemical or toxin exposure, polio, botulism, and hysterical paralysis. Diagnosis can be confirmed using cerebrospinal fluid (CSF) analysis. GBS patients have protein levels greater than 0.55 grams per deciliter of CSF. Macrophages are frequently found in the CSF, as well as some B cells. Nerve conduction velocity will be decreased in these patients to a value that is 50 percent of normal in those nerves that are still functioning. These changes can take several weeks to develop.

With GBS, macrophages and T cells are in contact with nerves, as evidenced in electron micrographs. T-cell and macrophage activation in these individuals point to an immune response gone awry, possibly precipitated by a virus or exposure to an antigen that is foreign but similar in appearance to one of the proteins in myelin. When T cells encounter an unrecognizable antigen, they produce interleukin-2, initiate an attack, and recruit macrophages. Using an anti-T-cell drug theoretically should improve nerve function. However, researchers at the University of Western Ontario failed to benefit from an anti-T-cell monoclonal antibody infusion. Unexpectedly, GBS occurs in asymptomatic patients who test positive for the human immunodeficiency virus (HIV) even though their T-cell levels are below normal. Although myelin proteins are thought to be the immunogens, other candidates include gangliosides in the myelin. Antiganglioside antibodies have been seen in a majority of GBS patients. This trait may distinguish GBS from amyotrophic lateral sclerosis (Lou Gehrig's disease) and multiple sclerosis, which seem to involve different myelin proteins as antigens.

In GBS, the white blood cells attack peripheral motor nerves more often than other types of nerves, implying a biochemical difference between motor and sensory nerves that has yet to be discovered.

> **INFORMATION ON GUILLAIN-BARRÉ SYNDROME**
>
> **Causes**: Autoimmune disorder; often with precipitating events such as surgery, pregnancy, upper respiratory infection, viral infection (such as cytomegalovirus), vaccination
>
> **Symptoms**: Weakness; loss of reflex; difficulty maintaining balance; eye muscle paralysis; tingling and numbness in hands and feet; reduced fine motor control, balance, and awareness of limb location; paralysis of vocal cords
>
> **Duration**: Chronic with acute episodes
>
> **Treatments**: Plasmapheresis, administration of cyclosporine or corticosteroids

One possible cause of this disease is a similarity between a protein or glycolipid that is present normally in myelin and coincidentally on an infectious agent, such as a virus. The immune system responds to the agent, resulting in a sensitization of the macrophages and T cells to that component of myelin. B cells are then stimulated to produce antibodies against this antigen. Unfortunately, they cross-react with parts of the myelin protein. The severity of the disease will depend on the number of macrophages and lymphocytes activated and whether serum complement-binding antibodies are being produced. Serum complement proteins are activated by a particular class of antibodies, resulting in proteins that cause tissue destruction and neurogenic atrophy. A serum complement fixation test can determine serum complement levels.

In severe cases of GBS, intercostal muscles are more severely compromised, and respiratory function needs to be monitored closely. The immune response will subside when T-suppressor cells have reached their peak levels. Halting the autoimmune response will not reverse the symptoms immediately since it takes time for antibody levels to decrease and for the nerves to regrow and remyelinate, which occurs at the rate of 1 to 2 millimeters per day. Some nerves will undergo retrograde degeneration and be lost from the neuronal pool. Other nerves will have more closely spaced nodes and conduct impulses at a lower velocity. Nerve sprouting will also occur, which will result in one nerve's being responsible for more muscle fibers or serving a larger sensory area and in decreased fine motor control.

An electromyogram effectively assesses the amount of muscle and nerve involvement in people with Guillain-Barré syndrome. This technique determines the degree of motor nerve interruption and the conduction velocity of the nerves that continue to function.

TREATMENT AND THERAPY

Since clinicians treated Guillain-Barré syndrome as an autoimmune response, treatments typically involved suppressing the immune system. Therefore, physicians administered corticosteroids such as prednisolone and methylprednisolone in high doses. However, these drugs have a deleterious effect on the disease and are no longer used.

More recently, a procedure known as plasmapheresis has shown better results, especially when performed in the first two weeks. This procedure involves removing 250 milliliters (a little more than a pint) of plasma from the blood every other day and replacing this volume with a solution containing albumin, glucose, and suitable salts. Six treatments are typical and usually result in a faster recovery of muscle control than for those not receiving plasmapheresis. Because relapses may occur if the patient produces new antibodies to myelin, immunosuppressants are given to the patient after plasmapheresis. Another procedure, intravenous immunoglobulin therapy, is based on blocking the binding of antibodies to nerves, which lessens the severity of the immune attack.

Cyclosporine, a T-cell inhibitor, is also used, with some promising results. However, some researchers note that transplant patients, who routinely take cyclosporine, have a higher-than-normal risk of developing GBS. Others emphasize that no one knows what their risk for GBS would be without the administration of cyclosporine. Because of the variability of the body's immune response, the benefits of this drug will depend on whether, in a given individual, it is an antibody response or T-cell response. Cyclosporine will benefit those who have a robust T-cell response. T-cell reactivity can be tested with the mixed lymphocyte assay, and T-cell counts can be done.

Cerebrospinal fluid filtration is also being tried to remove antibodies. Filtered serum loses its nerve-inhibiting effect, as evidenced by its application to in vitro nerve and muscle cells. GBS has been mimicked in animal models, which show antibody and T-cell reactivity to myelin protein. Guillain-Barré syndrome has many of the characteristics of autoimmune disease. It could serve as a model for an acquired autoimmune condition.

Not related to the neurology of this sudden-onset disease, but equally devastating, is the protracted psychological impact of simultaneously being able to think and have emotions while not being able to move limbs, fingers, toes, and facial and eye muscles. Even though most patients recover, progress is always torturously slow, as the myelin sheath gradually regenerates. Ongoing psychological support is an essential element in treating these patients.

PERSPECTIVE AND PROSPECTS

Guillain-Barré syndrome is an example of a delicate physiological balance gone awry. The immune system has the difficult task of distinguishing between self and enemy. If it detects the latter, it must either inactivate or eliminate the intruder. Mistakes in recognition or communication between immune cells can cause either an unintended attack or the failure to attack when appropriate. GBS probably represents an unnecessary self-attack on tissue, in this case, myelin, and may be considered a form of hyperimmunity. Many diseases fall into this category. They include rheumatoid arthritis, juvenile diabetes, Crohn's disease, ulcerative colitis, Graves' disease, multiple sclerosis, amyotrophic lateral sclerosis, ankylosing spondylitis (inflammation of the joints between the vertebrae), and systemic lupus erythematosus. The other type of response, hypoimmune, is seen in cancer and immunodeficiency diseases such as acquired immunodeficiency syndrome (AIDS).

Questions that arise with GBS are the same ones that occur in many other diseases. It must be determined why the immune system chose this time to initiate an attack against a self-antigen. The answer could be a mistake in recognition, an error in translating the deoxyribonucleic acid (DNA) code in the bone marrow cells, an alteration of the antigen by some environmental factor, or an alteration of an antigen-detector protein on a white blood cell. Researchers also try to discover if there is a genetic predisposition for GBS. Seeking answers about GBS may shed light on other conditions, and treatments beneficial to GBS patients have a high probability of benefiting patients with other immune disorders. GBS is a reminder that physiological stress can translate to immunological stress, and under pressure, the immune system can make mistakes.

—*William D. Niemi, PhD*

Further Information

Abbas, Abul K., Andrew H. Lichtman, and Shiv Pillai. *Basic Immunology: Functions and Disorders of the Immune System.* 6th ed., Saunders/Elsevier, 2019.

Adelman, Daniel C., et al., editors. *Manual of Allergy and Immunology.* 5th ed., Lippincott Williams & Wilkins, 2012.

Baron-Faust, Rita, and Jill P. Buyon. *The Autoimmune Connection.* Contemporary Books, 2003.

"Guillain-Barré Syndrome." *MedlinePlus*, 25 Oct. 2019, medlineplus.gov/guillainbarresyndrome.html. Accessed 25 Aug. 2021.

"Guillain-Barré Syndrome Fact Sheet." *National Institute of Neurological Disorders and Stroke*, 16 Mar. 2021, www.ninds.nih.gov/Disorders/Patient-Caregiver-Educati

on/Fact-Sheets/Guillain-Barr%C3%A9-Syndrome-Fact-Sheet. Accessed 25 Aug. 2021.

Kierman, John A., and Nagalingam Rajakumar. *Barr's The Human Nervous System: An Anatomical Viewpoint*. 10th ed., Wolters Kluwer/Lippincott Williams & Wilkins, 2013.

Nicholls, John G., et al. *From Neuron to Brain*. 5th ed., Sinauer, 2011.

Noback, Charles R., et al. *The Human Nervous System: Structure and Function*. 6th ed., Humana Press, 2005.

Parker, James N., and Philip M. Parker, editors. *The Official Patient's Sourcebook on Guillain-Barré Syndrome*. Icon Health, 2002.

Sticherling, Michael, and Enno Christophers, editors. *Treatment of Autoimmune Disorders*. Springer, 2003.

Hashimoto's thyroiditis

Category: Diseases/Disorders
Also known as: Struma lymphomatosa, lymphadenoid goiter, chronic lymphocytic thyroiditis, autoimmune thyroiditis
Anatomy or system affected: Endocrine system, glands, immune system, neck
Specialties and related fields: Endocrinology
Definition: An autoimmune disease that results in inflammation of the thyroid gland caused when abnormal blood antibodies and white blood cells infiltrate and attack thyroidal cells.

KEY TERMS

goiter: enlargement of the thyroid gland
thyroid gland: a small, butterfly-shaped gland in the front of the neck that controls how your body uses energy
thyroiditis: inflammation of the thyroid gland

CAUSES AND SYMPTOMS

Hashimoto's thyroiditis is a common type of hypothyroidism. The cause and etiology of this disorder are not fully understood; however, it is thought to have an autoimmune origin, in which ab-

> **INFORMATION ON HASHIMOTO'S THYROIDITIS**
>
> **Causes**: Unknown; possibly autoimmune in origin
>
> **Symptoms**: Mild pressure on the thyroid gland, goiter, fatigue, weight gain, cold intolerance, constipation, hair loss
>
> **Duration**: Chronic
>
> **Treatments**: Hormonal therapy with thyroxine, surgery if required

normal blood antibodies and white blood cells, called "lymphocytes," infiltrate and attack thyroid cells. The combative interplay between the lymphocytes and the thyroid may lead to a complete absence of thyroid cells. A family history of thyroid disease is commonly traced.

The highest incidence of the disease is observed in young or middle-aged women, but it may occur at any age. The onset is prolonged, and the disease may progress for many months or years before it is fully detected. The symptoms may vary, but the condition is usually characterized by mild pressure on the thyroid gland. In some cases, a firm, slightly irregular, and sometimes tender goiter (enlarged thyroid gland) may develop in the neck region. In more severe cases, the disease may cause symptoms related to low thyroid function (hypothyroidism), such as fatigue, weight gain, intolerance to cold, constipation, and hair loss.

The symptomatology of Hashimoto's thyroiditis may resemble other medical conditions. Therefore, in addition to a complete medical examination, the diagnostic procedure must also include blood tests to determine thyroid hormone levels and thyroid antibodies. Suppose a patient has developed the classic symptoms accompanying Hashimoto's thyroiditis but has normal blood test results. In that case, a biopsy in which a needle is inserted into the thyroid and some cells are removed may be performed to confirm the diagnosis.

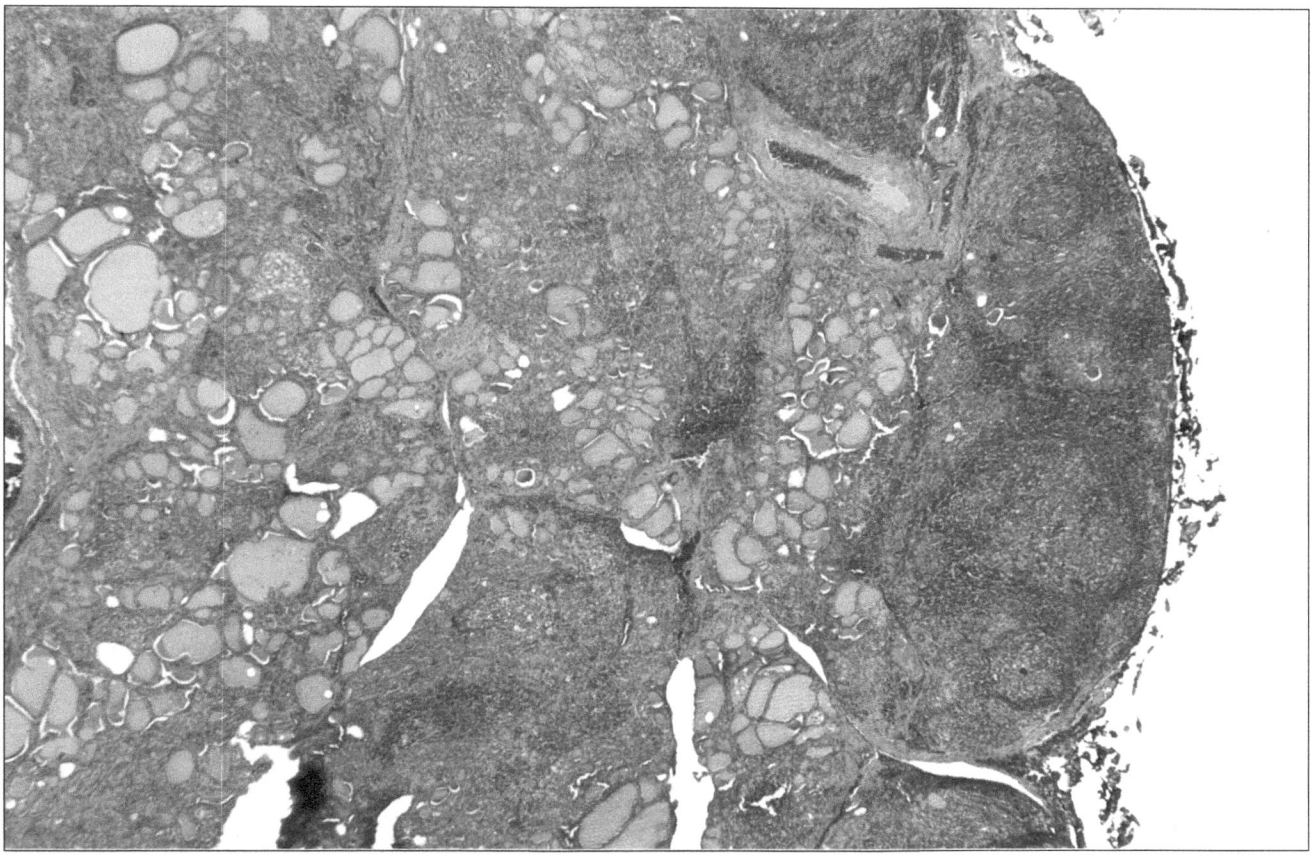
Micrograph showing a thyroid gland with Hashimoto's thyroiditis. H&E stain. Photo by Librepath, via Wikimedia Commons. [CC 3.0.]

TREATMENT AND THERAPY

Oral thyroid hormones can treat the hypothyroidism that results from Hashimoto's thyroiditis. Nevertheless, specific treatments for this condition are not yet available. Medical practitioners opt to commence hormone therapy in the form of thyroxine as soon as a diagnosis is made, even if thyroid function is normal at the time. The hormone therapy is expected to shrink any goiter that has developed. If hormone treatment does not sufficiently shrink the thyroid, the patient may require surgery. The prognosis for a full recovery is usually good because the disease remains dormant or stable for many years.

*—Nicholas Lanzieri and
Sharon W. Stark, RN, APRN, DNSc*

Further Information

Bayliss, R. I. S., and W. M. Tunbridge. *Thyroid Disease: The Facts*. 4th ed., Oxford UP, 2008.

Braverman, Lewis E. *Werner & Ingbar's The Thyroid*. 11th ed., Lippincott Williams & Wilkins, 2020.

Burman, Kenneth D., and Derek LeRoith, editors. *Thyroid Function and Disease*. Saunders/Elsevier, 2007.

"Chronic Thyroiditis (Hashimoto's Disease). *Medline Plus*, 5 Aug. 2021, medlineplus.gov/ency/article/000371.htm. Accessed 26 Aug. 2021.

"Hashimoto's Disease." *National Institute of Diabetes and Digestive and Kidney Diseases*, July 2020, www.niddk.nih.gov/health-information/endocrine-diseases/hashimotos-disease. Accessed 26 Aug. 2021

"Hashimoto's Disease." *Office of Women's Health*, 18 Oct. 2018, www.womenshealth.gov/a-z-topics/hashimotos-disease. Accessed 26 Aug. 2021.

Melmed, Shlomo, Ronald Koenig, et al. *Williams Textbook of Endocrinology*. 14th ed., Saunders/Elsevier, 2019.

Mincer, D. L., and I. Jialal. *Hashimoto Thyroiditis*. StatPearls Publishing, 10 Aug. 2020, pubmed.ncbi.nlm.nih.gov/29083758/. Accessed 26 Aug. 2021.

Shannon, Joyce Brennfleck, editor. *Thyroid Disorders Sourcebook: Basic Consumer Health Information About Disorders of the Thyroid and Parathyroid Glands*. Omnigraphics, 2005.

Wood, Lawrence C., David S. Cooper, and E. Chester Ridgway. *Your Thyroid: A Home Reference*. 4th rev. ed., Ballantine Books, 2005.

HISTIOCYTOSIS

Category: Diseases/Disorders

Also known as: Langerhans cell histiocytosis (LCH), histiocytosis X, eosinophilic granuloma, Hand-Schüller-Christian disease, Letterer-Siwe disease

Anatomy or system affected: Blood, bones, ears, gastrointestinal system, immune system, liver, lungs, nervous system, skin, throat

Specialties and related fields: Hematology, immunology

Definition: A group of relatively rare blood disorders characterized by the abnormal accumulation of white blood cells called "histiocytes," leading to a wide range of adverse bodily responses.

KEY TERMS

histiocyte: large white blood cells resident in tissues, including Langerhans cells, monocytes/macrophages, and dermal/interstitial dendritic cells

Langerhans cell histiocytosis (LCH): a disorder characterized by a buildup of excess immune system cells called "Langerhans cells" that damage tissues or cause lesions in multiple locations in the body

monocytes: large, phagocytic white blood cell with a simple oval nucleus and clear, grayish cytoplasm that regulates and participated in the immune response

---

INFORMATION ON HISTIOCYTOSIS

Causes: Response to underlying immunodeficiency or secondary effect from viral infection

Symptoms: Depends on severity; may include bone lesions (especially skull), rashes, respiratory problems (cough, shortness of breath), gastrointestinal problems (bleeding, elevated liver enzymes)

Duration: Short term or long term

Treatments: Depends on the severity; may include chemotherapy

---

CAUSES AND SYMPTOMS

There is no clear understanding of the exact etiology of histiocytoses, blood disorders characterized by an accumulation of white blood cells called "histiocytes," including monocytes and macrophages. Langerhans cell histiocytosis (LCH) is the most common type. At least four or five people per million are affected, with more males affected than females. The disorder affects both children and adults.

LCH may develop in response to underlying immunodeficiency or as a secondary effect from a viral infection. Symptoms vary based on the severity of the disease, and patients may be relatively symptom-free. LCH may be localized to one area or organ or more diffuse, involving multiple organs. It can cause lesions on bone, especially skull bones, or manifest itself as a skin rash. Respiratory symptoms such as cough or shortness of breath may signify that LCH has affected the lungs. Gastrointestinal manifestations of the disease include bleeding within the gastrointestinal tract or elevated liver enzymes. LCH can also affect the lymph nodes or the central nervous system and may contribute to the development of diabetes insipidus, growth hormone deficiency, and hypopituitarism (underactive pituitary gland).

Definitive diagnosis requires a biopsy, and the differential diagnosis (other diseases similar to it) is broad. Making the diagnosis requires a high index of suspicion because it is rare and easily missed. Helpful radiologic tests might include a chest X-ray or a skeletal survey.

TREATMENT AND THERAPY
Treatment options vary widely based on the severity of the disease. On the one hand, minimal treatment may be needed for symptom-free, single-system involvement, especially as LCH affecting only one system often remits completely. On the other hand, a more severe disease affecting many systems may warrant chemotherapy, with characteristic remissions and relapses.

PERSPECTIVE AND PROSPECTS
The histiocytoses are classified into three types: LCH, hemophagocytic lymphohistiocytosis (HLH), and malignant histiocytosis. The impacts of LCH can be many, some with short-term and others with long-term consequences: stunted growth, dental problems, hearing loss, and hepatic fibrosis, to name a few. Though caregivers from various medical specialties are often involved in caring for LCH patients, and tremendous strides in diagnosis and treatment have been made, many patients still suffer from complex, recurrent diseases.

—*Leonard Berkowitz, DO and Paul Moglia, PhD*

Further Information
Arceci, Robert J., B. Jack Longley, and Peter D. Emanuel. "Atypical Cellular Disorders." *Hematology*, 2002, pp. 297-314.
Egeler, R. Maarten, and Giulio J. D'Angio, editors. *Langerhans Cell Histiocytosis*. W. B. Saunders, 1998.
Gersten, Todd. "Histiocytosis." *MedlinePlus*, 30 Apr. 2012, Histiocytosis Association, www.histio.org.
Irvine, Alan, Peter Hoeger, and Albert C. Yan. *Harper's Textbook of Pediatric Dermatology*. Wiley-Blackwell, 2011.
Jaffe, Elaine Sarkin. *Hematopathology*. Saunders/Elsevier, 2011.
James, William D., and Dirk M. Elston. *Andrews' Diseases of the Skin: Clinical Dermatology*. Saunders Elsevier, 2011.
Lichtman, Marshall A. *Williams Manual of Hematology*. McGraw-Hill, 2011.
Osband, Michael E., and Carl Pochedly, editors. *Histiocytosis-X*. W. B. Saunders, 1987.

Hyperthyroidism

Category: Diseases/Disorders
 Related terms: Graves' disease, subacute thyroiditis, thyroid hormone, excess, thyrotoxicosis
Anatomy or system affected: Blood, brain, eyes, gastrointestinal system, immune system, intestines, liver, lungs, lymphatic system, mouth, psychic-emotional system, reproductive system, respiratory system, skin, throat
Specialties and related fields: Dermatology, endocrinology, gastroenterology, gynecology, hematology, immunology, internal medicine, nuclear medicine, oncology, ophthalmology, otorhinolaryngology, pathology, pharmacology, Principal proposed natural treatments: None
 Other proposed natural treatments: Bugleweed, L-carnitine, glucomannan, motherwort, royal jelly
 Herbs and supplements to avoid: Ashwagandha, bladderwrack, kelp
Definition: Treatment for excessive amounts of thyroid hormone released by the thyroid gland.

KEY TERMS
goiter: abnormal enlargement of the thyroid gland
Graves' hyperthyroidism: an immune system disorder that results in the overproduction of *thyroid* hormones
thyroid eye disease: an autoimmune disorder characterized by ocular inflammation and protrusion
thyroid-stimulating hormone: a peptide hormone secreted by the anterior lobe of the pituitary gland that stimulates the thyroid to produce thyroid hormone

INTRODUCTION

Disorders of the thyroid gland will affect a person's "3 Ms": movement, mentation, and metabolism. Hyperthyroidism is a condition in which the thyroid gland releases excessive amounts of thyroid hormone. (In contrast, the thyroid gland does not secrete adequate amounts of thyroid hormone in hypothyroidism, discussed separately.) Symptoms of hyperthyroidism include weight loss, fatigue, headache, insomnia, fast heart rate, heart palpitations, shortness of breath with exertion, intolerance to heat, insomnia, anxiety, tremor, frequent bowel movements, scant and/or irregular menstruation, bone thinning, hair loss, nail pitting and breakages, and goiter (visible enlargement of the neck caused by a swollen thyroid gland). This condition is more common in women than men.

The most common form of hyperthyroidism is Graves' disease. In this condition, the body manufactures antibodies that have the unintended effect of stimulating the thyroid gland. In addition to the classic symptoms of hyperthyroidism, specific features of Graves' disease include bulging eyes, swelling around the eyes, eyelid retraction, double vision or blurred vision, reduced color perception, swelling of the shin areas of the lower extremities, and clubbing of fingers and toes accompanied by swelling of the hands and feet. In another condition, Hashimoto's thyroiditis, the body produces antibodies that attack and destroy thyroid cells, causing a transient hyperthyroid phase due to the release of preformed thyroid hormones, followed by a lasting hypothyroid condition. In addition, benign thyroid tumors can secrete excessive thyroid hormone on their own (cancerous tumors seldom do). Viral infection of the thyroid (subacute thyroiditis) causes short-lived hyperthyroidism occasionally followed by a more prolonged period of hypothyroidism. Thyroid hormone levels in patients with subacute thyroiditis tend to return to baseline over time. Other causes of hyperthyroidism include toxicity of iodine-containing compounds (e.g., the heart medication, amiodarone), induction via other medications (e.g., lithium used in bipolar disorder, cancer medications such as interferon-alpha and tyrosine kinase inhibitors, highly active antiretroviral therapy used for human immunodeficiency virus/acquired immunodeficiency syndrome [HIV/AIDS]), metastatic thyroid cancer, postpartum thyroiditis, and a condition called "hyperemesis gravidarum," which involves excessive vomiting during pregnancy due to the high levels of alpha-hCG (the hormone present in positive urine pregnancy tests) that stimulates the thyroid. Lastly, an interesting and infrequent condition called "Struma Ovarii" can occur when thyroid tissue abnormally grows in an ovarian tumor, producing thyroid hormones, causing hyperthyroidism irrespective of the normal thyroid gland.

Measurement of a hormone called "thyroid-stimulating hormone" (TSH) is the preferred laboratory test to screen for thyroid abnormalities. The pituitary gland releases TSH to control the function of the thyroid gland. The pituitary gland constantly measures the thyroid hormone level in the blood and adjusts TSH levels as necessary. When thyroid hormone levels are low, the pituitary raises TSH levels to stimulate the thyroid to produce more thyroid

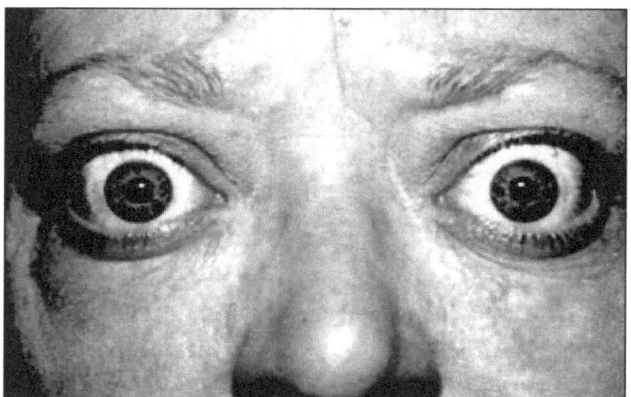

Example of a person with Graves disease, an autoimmune disease that strikes the thyroid. Photo by Jonathan Trobe, M.D. - University of Michigan Kellogg Eye Center, via Wikimedia Commons. [CC 3.0.]

hormone. If the thyroid gland is overactive and secretes excess thyroid hormones, the pituitary responds by suppressing TSH secretion. This, in turn, should allow the thyroid to take a break from creating too much hormone. When the TSH is below normal levels, it represents a state where the thyroid produces too much thyroid hormone. In other words, the person has entered a hyperthyroid state or is about to enter such a state.

STANDARD TREATMENTS

Hyperthyroidism causes increased blood pressure and high heart rate (tachycardia). To treat hyperthyroidism symptoms, patients should take a cardioselective beta-blocker. The best choice is probably atenolol or metoprolol. These drugs relieve anxiety, heart palpitations, heat intolerance, tremors, and hypertension associated with hyperthyroidism. Tiredness and shortness of breath are the two main side effects of beta-blockers.

Successful treatment of hyperthyroidism must decrease thyroid hormone synthesis. Three different approaches accomplish this, but all three have significant side effects. The first employs drugs called "thionamides." These medications can induce permanent remission of hypothyroidism. They also avoid permanent hypothyroidism and have low costs. They commonly cause rash, hives, achiness in the joints, transient low white blood cell counts, and upset stomach. In some people, thionamides cause long-term low white blood cell counts, liver damage, and lupus-like syndrome. They can cause fetal goiter, hypothyroidism, and congenital disabilities if taken during pregnancy. These drugs also require frequent monitoring. Methimazole is the preferred treatment for Graves' hyperthyroidism, but propylthiouracil is a safer drug during pregnancy.

Radioiodine is the second approach, and this treatment can produce a permanent resolution of hyperthyroidism. The downsides of this approach are the permanent hypothyroidism that results from it. Second, patients on radioiodine must take any necessary precautions for several days after treatment to ensure that their children and pregnant women are not exposed to radiation. Some patients experience a worsening of ophthalmopathy with radioiodine treatments, and others rarely have radiation thyroiditis. Finally, patients sometimes have concerns about the long-term effects of radiation.

The third approach is surgery, which provides a rapid, permanent cure of hyperthyroidism but causes permanent hypothyroidism. Surgery also carries risks of hypoparathyroidism and recurrent laryngeal nerve damage. Surgery also has a high cost.

A newer drug called "teprotumumab" (*Tepezza*), an insulin-like growth factor-1 receptor (IGF-1R) inhibitor, is Food and Drug Administration (FDA)-approved for IV treatment of thyroid eye disease. Fibroblasts overexpress IGF-1R in the eyes of thyroid eye disease patients. Teprotumumab is a monoclonal antibody that blocks IGF-1R activation and signaling. It prevents the pathologic immune responses inactive thyroid eye disease.

PROPOSED NATURAL TREATMENTS

Physician supervision is necessary to determine why the thyroid is overactive to design a specific treatment plan. None of the treatments discussed in this section get to the root of the problem, nor have they been proven effective. Self-treatment of hyperthyroidism is not recommended.

Traditional Chinese herbal medicines such as Jiakangxin Koufuye, Longdanxiegan Wan, Chenxiangshuqi Wan, or Zhibaidihuang Wan combined with other routine treatments (e.g., methimazole) may show some benefit by improving patient's symptoms and thyroid function as opposed to using the herbal medication alone. However, the studies do not provide strong evidence of their use in hyperthyroidism.

Test-tube and animal studies suggest that the herb bugleweed may reduce thyroid hormone by decreasing levels of TSH (the hormone that stimulates the thyroid gland) and impairing thyroid hormone synthesis. In addition, bugleweed may block the action of thyroid-stimulating antibodies found in Graves' disease.

The supplement L-carnitine was shown to be effective in reversing and preventing symptoms of hyperthyroidism and has a beneficial effect on bone mineralization. It has shown promise for treating a unique form of hyperthyroidism that may occur during the treatment of benign goiter. People with benign goiter often take thyroid hormone pills as treatment. Sometimes, successful treatment of this condition requires taking slightly more thyroid hormone than the body needs, resulting in symptoms of mild hyperthyroidism. A double-blind, placebo-controlled trial found evidence that the use of the supplement L-carnitine could alleviate many of these symptoms. This six-month study evaluated the effects of L-carnitine in fifty women who were taking thyroid hormone for benign goiter. The results showed that a dose of 2 grams (g) or 4 g of carnitine daily protected participants' bones and reduced other symptoms of hyperthyroidism. Carnitine is thought to affect the thyroid hormone by blocking its action in cells. A preliminary trial found evidence that normal thyroid hormone levels are restored more rapidly when the supplement glucomannan is added to standard treatment.

For many people, the most problematic symptom of hyperthyroidism is a rapid or irregular heartbeat. In cases of temporary high thyroid hormone levels (as in a viral infection), conventional treatment may involve simply protecting the heart. Germany's Commission E (the herbal regulating body in that country) has authorized the use of the herb motherwort as part of an overall treatment plan for an overactive thyroid (hyperthyroidism). Motherwort is said to calm the heart; however, there is no meaningful evidence to indicate that it is effective for the heart-related symptoms of hyperthyroidism (or any other heart-related symptoms). Royal jelly has been proposed for use in Graves' disease, but there is no meaningful evidence that it is effective.

HERBS AND SUPPLEMENTS TO AVOID
According to one study in animals, the herb ashwagandha may raise thyroid hormone levels. For this reason, it should not be used by people with hyperthyroidism. Excessive kelp, bladderwrack, or other forms of seaweed can cause hyperthyroidism by overloading the body with iodine.

—*Michael Raghunath, MD*

Further Information
Azezli, A. D., T. Bayraktaroglu, and Y. Orhan. "The Use of Konjac Glucomannan to Lower Serum Thyroid Hormones in Hyperthyroidism." *Journal of the American College of Nutrition*, vol. 26, 2007, pp. 663-68.
Benvenga, S., et al. "Usefulness of L-carnitine, a Naturally Occurring Peripheral Antagonist of Thyroid Hormone Action, in Iatrogenic Hyperthyroidism." *Journal of Clinical Endocrinology and Metabolism*, vol. 86, 2001, pp. 3579-94.
Benvenga, S., M. Lakshmanan, and F. Trimarchi. "Carnitine Is a Naturally Occurring Inhibitor of Thyroid Hormone Nuclear Uptake." *Thyroid*, vol. 10, 2000, pp. 1043-50.
Erem, C., et al. "The Effects of Royal Jelly on Autoimmunity in Graves' Disease." *Endocrine*, vol. 30, 2006, pp. 175-83.
Gardner, David, and Dolores Shoback. *Greenspan's Basic and Clinical Endocrinology*. 10th ed., McGraw-Hill Educational, 2017.
Glatstein, M., et al. "Pharmacologic Treatment of Hyperthyroidism During Lactation." *Canadian Family Physician*, vol. 55, 2009, pp. 797-98.
Kravets, I. "Hyperthyroidism: Diagnosis and Treatment." *American Family Physician*, vol. 93, 2016, pp. 363-70.
Malek, N. Z. H., et al. "Association of Transient Hyperthyroidism and Severity of Hyperemesis Gravidarum." *Hormone Molecular Biology and Clinical Investigation*, vol. 3, 2017, doi:10.1515/hmbci-2016-0050.

Zen, X. X., et al. "Chinese Herbal Medicines for Hyperthyroidism." *The Cochrane Database of Systematic Reviews,* vol. 2007, no. 2, CD005450, doi:10.1002/14651858.CD005450.pub2.

Idiopathic thrombocytopenic purpura

Also known as: Immune thrombocytopenic purpura
Category: Diseases/Conditions
Anatomy or system affected: Blood, immune system, spleen
Specialties and related fields: Hematology, immunology, internal medicine, pharmacology, proctology
Definition: An autoimmune disease in which the immune system attacks and destroys platelets.

KEY TERMS

platelet: cells in the blood that initiate the clotting cascade
spleen: an abdominal organ that forms part of the immune system and produces and removes blood cells
thrombocytopenia: a deficiency of platelets

INTRODUCTION

Idiopathic thrombocytopenic purpura (ITP) is a treatable blood disorder. Antibodies produced in the spleen attack and destroy the body's blood-clotting cells (platelets), which help stop bleeding. Normally, platelets move to damaged areas of the body and stick together, forming a sort of barrier against germs. If there are not enough platelets in the body, bleeding injuries are difficult to stop. Although people with ITP have a lower than normal number of platelets in their blood, all other blood cell counts are normal.

There are two types of ITP. Acute ITP, which lasts less than six months and usually occurs in children, is the most common. Chronic ITP lasts more than six months and usually occurs in adults.

CAUSES

The cause of most cases of ITP is unknown. In children, the disorder has been linked to viral infections. It is believed that in these cases, the immune system becomes confused and begins attacking healthy platelet cells. When too many platelets are destroyed, ITP can result. The disorder in adults has not been linked to viral infections. Some cases of ITP are thought to be caused by drugs, infections, or other immune disorders. Pregnant women, too, sometimes develop the disease.

RISK FACTORS

Persons with an increased chance of developing ITP include children who have had a recent viral infection or have had a live-virus vaccination (which may sometimes put a child at higher risk); women, usually younger than age forty years; and women in general, who are two to three times more likely to get ITP than are men.

SYMPTOMS

Both adults and children may notice the following symptoms of ITP: easy bruising, dark urine or stools, bleeding for longer than usual following an injury, unexplained nosebleeds, bleeding from the gums, heavier-than-normal menstrual periods (in adult women), red dots called "petechiae" on the skin (petechiae may occur in groups and resemble a rash), and, in rare cases, bleeding within the intestinal tract or brain.

SCREENING AND DIAGNOSIS

A doctor will ask about symptoms and medical history and will perform a physical exam. Tests may include a complete blood count (CBC), in which a blood sample is tested to see if the numbers of different blood cells are normal; and a bone marrow

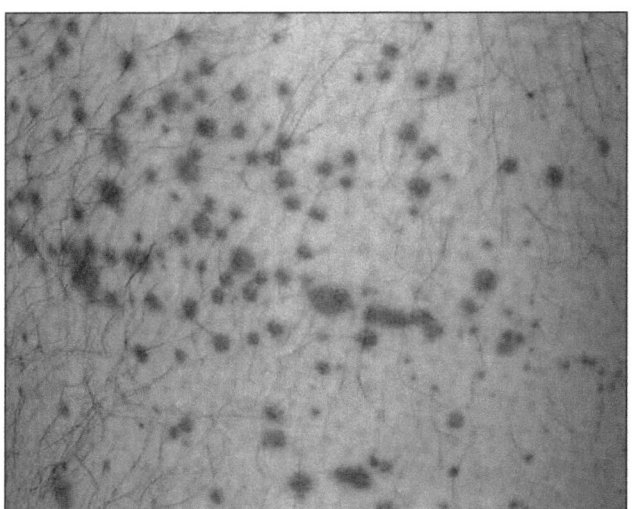
Petechiae, or small bruise-like markings, may occur in ITP. Photo by Hektor, via Wikimedia Commons. [CC 3.0.]

test, in which a needle is inserted through the skin and the bone and a small amount of bone marrow is removed. The sample is tested to ensure the marrow contains normal numbers of platelet-producing cells. This test is done to rule out other disorders. Another test is a computed tomography (CT) scan (in rare cases). The CT scan is done if there is a concern about bleeding in the brain.

TREATMENT AND THERAPY
Treatment for ITP is different for children and adults. Most children recover from ITP without any treatment. However, a doctor may recommend the following: medications to increase platelet counts in the blood, such as steroids (e.g., prednisone), which lowers the activity of the immune system and keeps it from destroying platelets; and gamma globulin infusions (an antibody-containing protein that slows down platelet destruction). An infusion means that the injection is given by IV (intravenously) or through a shot. It usually works more quickly than steroids. Both of these treatments work, but both can have side effects. Eighty-five percent of children who have ITP recover within a year and do not experience the problem again.

Two newer drugs stimulate platelet production: eltrombopag (Promacta) and romiplostim (Nplate). Using these drugs and the targeted monoclonal antibody rituximab (Rituxan) may prevent the need for splenectomy. A splenectomy is the surgical removal of the spleen. This procedure stops the destruction of platelets because the antibodies are made in the spleen. If drug intervention does not do enough to raise platelet counts in adults, the doctor may recommend a splenectomy.

A splenectomy leaves the body more vulnerable to infection from other sources. This surgery is usually not performed until medications have proven ineffective. Doctors also sometimes recommend lifestyle changes when platelet counts are low, including avoiding contact sports; patients also are advised to wear a helmet during sports activities.

PREVENTION AND OUTCOMES
Because the cause of ITP is unknown, there are no specific ways to prevent the disease. However, because bleeding and injury can be severe for people with ITP, one should take precautions to avoid injury, such as using padding on an infant's crib or around a play area and ensuring that older children wear helmets and protective gear when playing sports (to help reduce bruising injuries). Persons with low platelet counts should stop playing contact sports.

People who have ITP should also avoid medications that contain aspirin or ibuprofen. These medicines can reduce platelet function. To help stay healthy, one should eat a healthful diet, low in saturated fat and rich in whole grains, fruits, and vegetables; get regular exercise; lose weight if overweight; stop smoking; and drink alcohol, if desired, only in moderation (two drinks per day for men and one drink per day for women).

—*Amanda Dameron*

Further Reading

Bick, Roger L. *Disorders of Thrombosis and Hemostasis: Clinical and Laboratory Practice*. 3rd ed., Lippincott Williams & Wilkins, 2002.

Bussel, J. B., et al. "Eltrombopag for the Treatment of Chronic Idiopathic Thrombocytopenic Purpura." *New England Journal of Medicine*, vol. 357, no. 22, 2007, pp. 2237-47.

George, J. N. "Platelets." *The Lancet*, vol. 355, 2000, pp. 1531-39.

George, J. N., et al. "Update on Idiopathic Thrombocytopenic Purpura." www.hematology.org/publications/hematologist/2010/4965.aspx.

Ishida, Yoji, and Yoshiaki Tomiyama, editors. *Autoimmune Thrombocytopenia*. Springer, 2017.

Karpatkin, S. "Autoimmune (Idiopathic) Thrombocytopenic Purpura." *The Lancet*, vol. 349, 1997, pp. 1531-36.

Kaushansky, Kenneth, Marshall Lichtman, and Josef Prchal. *Williams Hematology*. 10th ed., McGraw-Hill, 2021.

McCrae, Keith R., editor. *Thrombocytopenia*. Taylor & Francis, 2006.

Newland, A., et al. "An Open-Label, Unit Dose-Finding Study of AMG 531, a Novel Thrombopoiesis-Stimulating Peptibody, in Patients with Immune Thrombocytopenic Purpura." *British Journal of Haematology*, vol. 135, no. 4, 2006, pp. 547-53.

JUVENILE IDIOPATHIC ARTHRITIS

Category: Diseases/Disorders

Anatomy or system affected: Back, circulatory system, eyes, heart, immune system, joints, musculoskeletal system

Specialties and related fields: Exercise physiology, family medicine, immunology, ophthalmology, orthopedics, pediatrics, psychology, rheumatology

Definition: A usually chronic autoimmune disease of unknown cause, characterized by joint swelling, pain, and sometimes the destruction of joints.

KEY TERMS

articular: of or relating to a joint or joints

autoimmune disease: a disease in which the body's immune system attacks itself

cytokines: small proteins, such as interferon, interleukin, and growth factors, secreted by specific cells that affect other cells.

interleukins: a type of small glycoproteins, secreted by leukocytes that regulate immune response

manifestation: an outward or visible expression

systemic: relating to the body as a whole, not limited to a particular part

CAUSES AND SYMPTOMS

Juvenile idiopathic arthritis (JIA, formerly called "Still's disease" or "systemic-onset juvenile rheumatoid arthritis") is an autoimmune disease of children that attacks the joints. It appears in three different subgroups that vary according to severity and type of extraarticular manifestation. Other significant variations within these subgroups include age at disease onset, the sex of affected children, genetic predisposition, and prognosis.

The first major clinical pattern is a systemic disease, including about 10 percent of children with JIA. This type has the most dramatic onset and is the least common form of the illness. It affects boys more than girls and can begin at any age. The most characteristic manifestations are high, intermittent fevers and a temporary red rash that occurs during periods of fever. Occasionally, more severe complications are involved. In some cases, systemic-onset is marked by polyarthritis, which affects large and small multiple joints, and moves subsequently to disease of the knee or hip with no further involvement of other joints. The systemic complaints, which are often sudden and explosive, may recur months or years later. Some children with systemic-onset, however, never develop lasting arthritis.

Polyarticular JIA, the second subgroup, includes children in whom five or more joints have been involved in the first six months of illness. It affects more girls than boys and can begin at any age. This subgroup includes about 40 percent of children with JIA and is frequently mild. Within this subgroup exists a smaller subgroup, which includes about 5 percent of children with JIA is and rarely begins before the eighth birthday. The arthritis is often severe, with joint destruction occurring within the first year. Polyarthritis may involve swelling of the joints over time, in which pain is not a prominent feature, or a sudden articular swelling, which can be severe. Weight-bearing joints, usually knees and ankles, are often involved initially.

The third major subgroup is pauciarticular disease, which involves about 50 percent of all children with JIA. In the initial episode of this type, only one joint is involved. More joints usually become involved within a few weeks or months, although occasionally, involvement is restricted to one joint. The knee is often the primary area, with the ankles and hips being the sites of minimal involvement.

TREATMENT AND THERAPY
The first step in treating JIA is identifying the child's problems and potential problems, which include active joint disease, disabilities, ocular disease, growth retardation, and psychosocial disability. Because the cause of chronic arthritis is not known, treatment suppresses the symptoms and does not cure the disease itself.

Drug therapy relieves inflammatory pain and immobility. The primary medication used is the standard nonsteroidal anti-inflammatory drugs (NSAIDs), such as aspirin, ibuprofen, and naproxen. If NSAIDs are ineffective, another pharmacological intervention is disease-modifying antirheumatic drugs (DMARDs), of which the most common is methotrexate. DMARDs slow the progression of arthritis but take a long time to act. Another powerful drug treatment is corticosteroids, administered either by mouth or injected directly into the joint; these are used sparingly, however, because of their serious side effects for children.

> **INFORMATION ON SYSTEMIC JUVENILE IDIOPATHIC ARTHRITIS**
>
> **Causes**: Unknown
>
> **Symptoms**: High, intermittent fevers; temporary red rash occurring during periods of fever; joint pain; occasionally polyarthritis
>
> **Duration**: Acute and recurrent
>
> **Treatments**: Alleviation of symptoms through medication (anti-inflammatory drugs), physical and occupational therapy, orthopedic treatment (e.g., splinting)

Pediatric rheumatologists prefer prescribing a biologic DMARD over glucocorticoids in patients from whom NSAIDs fail to provide satisfactory treatment. Children with systemic JIA consistently display increased circulating levels of multiple cytokines. Several lines of evidence show that monoclonal antibodies or soluble receptors that inhibit inflammatory cytokines in systemic JIA patients improve patient symptoms and decrease disease progression. Based on data from clinical trials, the cytokines that play the most significant role in JIA pathology are interleukin (IL) 1 and IL-6. Three different biologic DMARDs block IL-1 activity: anakinra (recombinant IL-1 receptor antagonist), rilonacept (IL-1 trap), and canakinumab (anti-IL-1-beta monoclonal antibody). The anti-IL-6 medicine that effectively treats JIA is tocilizumab (anti-Il-6 monoclonal antibody).

Anti-tumor necrosis factor-alpha (TNF-alpha) biologic DMARDS generally benefit children with nonsystemic types of JIA and systemic JIA. Etanercept, a soluble TNF-alpha receptor fusion protein that binds TNF-alpha, has been widely tested in systemic JIA patients. There is less data for infliximab or adalimumab, but both agents seem to provide relief if etanercept treatment fails.

Physical and occupational therapy attempts to maintain strength and stamina and preserve and increase the range of motion in the joints and supporting muscles. In addition to exercise, the program consists of moist heat, adequate rest, and a proper diet aimed at maintaining strength. All children with significant joint involvement should have a daily home program of activities and exercises directed toward preventing and correcting disabilities that their parents can supervise. Children with severe disabilities may need hospitalization for intensive therapy.

Beyond physical therapy, orthopedic treatment for the joints may include splinting to preserve or repair joint motion. In rehabilitating older children who have suffered severe damage, the replacement of affected joints may provide good results.

JIA offers significant challenges for families. The family pediatrician or physician must act as a teacher and adviser both to the patient and family members. Other health-care professionals who may be necessary to the care of a child with JIA are ophthalmologists, pediatric nurses, social workers, psychiatrists, and the child's schoolteachers.

PERSPECTIVE AND PROSPECTS
George R. Still's finding in 1896 that JIA includes at least three distinct joint afflictions first brought the subgroups to the medical profession's attention and has fostered a greater understanding of the disease; in fact, systemic arthritis was initially known as Still's disease.

For most children with JIA, early diagnosis and appropriate therapy point to a good prognosis. Of the children with systemic-onset, at least 75 percent will enjoy a good outcome. In contrast, the rest may suffer severe arthritis, possibly resulting in disability. Between 80 and 90 percent of children with polyarthritis escape without permanent joint damage, although the disease may be chronic. The overall prospects for children with pauciarticular disease are not known.

Although most children suffering from JIA eventually outgrow it, it is difficult for most parents to accept that accurate prediction for the outcome for their child is impossible. Nevertheless, a positive attitude, careful medical management, physical therapy, and psychological support can improve the quality of life for all children with JIA.

—*Mary Hurd and Michael A. Buratovich, PhD*

Further Information
Arthritis Foundation, www.arthritis.org.
Brewer, Earl J., Jr., and Kathy Cochran Angel. *The Arthritis Sourcebook*. 3rd ed., Lowell House, 2000.
Brewer, Earl J., Jr., Edward H. Giannini, and Donald A. Person. *Juvenile Rheumatoid Arthritis*. 2nd ed., W. B. Saunders, 1982.
"Childhood Arthritis." *Centers for Disease Control and Prevention*, 27 Jul. 2020, www.cdc.gov/arthritis/basics/childhood.htm. 31 Aug. 2021.
Judd, Sandra J. *Childhood Diseases and Disorders Sourcebook: Basic Consumer Health Information About the Physical, Mental, and Developmental Health of Pre-Adolescent Children*. 2nd ed., Omnigraphics, 2009.
"Juvenile Idiopathic Arthritis." National Institute of Arthritis and Musculoskeletal and Skin Diseases, Mar. 2021, www.niams.nih.gov/health-topics/juvenile-arthritis. Accessed 31 Aug. 2021
"Juvenile Rheumatoid Arthritis." *Johns Hopkins Medicine*, www.hopkinsmedicine.org/health/conditions-and-diseases/arthritis/juvenile-idiopathic-arthritis. Accessed 31 Aug. 2021.
Kliegman, Robert M., et al., editors. *Nelson Textbook of Pediatrics*. 21st ed., Elsevier, 2019.
Melvin, Jeanne L., and Virginia Wright, editors. *Pediatric Rheumatic Diseases*. Vol. 3. American Occupational Therapy Association, 2000.
Merenstein, Gerald B., David W. Kaplan, and Adam A. Rosenberg. *Handbook of Pediatrics*. 18th ed., Appleton & Lange, 1999.
Parker, James N., and Philip M. Parker, editors. *Juvenile Rheumatoid Arthritis: The Official Patient's Sourcebook*. Icon Health, 2002.
Tarp, S., et al. "Efficacy and Safety of Biological Agents for Systemic Juvenile Idiopathic Arthritis: A Systematic Review and Meta-Analysis of Randomized Trials." *Rheumatology*, vol. 55, no. 4, 2016, p. 669.

Multiple sclerosis

Category: Diseases/Disorders
Anatomy or system affected: Muscles, musculoskeletal system, nerves, nervous system, spine
Specialties and related fields: Immunology, internal medicine, neurology, pediatrics
Definition: A debilitating chronic inflammatory disease affecting the central nervous system.

KEY TERMS

autoimmunity: a condition in which the immune system fails to recognize its tissues as "self" and mounts an immune response against its cells
demyelination: the destruction of myelin
disseminated sclerosis: another name for multiple sclerosis (MS)
myelin: a fatty substance wrapping nerves as a sheath that accelerates electric impulse propagation
primary progressive multiple sclerosis (PPMS): the most aggressive form of MS, characterized by the absence of remissions and continual decline
relapsing-remitting multiple sclerosis (RRMS): the most common form of MS, characterized by unpredictable attacks (relapses) followed by periods free of symptoms (remission)
remyelination: the repair of myelin
sclerosis: a process of hardening of tissues
secondary progressive multiple sclerosis (SPMS): a form that occurs in patients who initially had RRMS and transition to a more aggressive MS

CAUSES AND SYMPTOMS

Multiple sclerosis (MS) is a chronic and disabling disease of the nervous system. Symptoms can be mild, such as limb numbness, or severe, such as paralysis and loss of vision. How the disease will progress, and its severity in specific individuals are difficult to predict because it progresses differently in each of its victims.

Multiple sclerosis is caused by degeneration of the nervous system. A fatty substance called "myelin" surrounds and protects many nerve fibers of the brain and spinal cord. Myelin is important because it speeds up signals that move along the nerve fibers. In MS, the body attacks its tissues, termed an "autoimmune reaction." A breakdown in the myelin layer along the nerves occurs. Destruction of any part of the myelin sheath slows, distorts, or interrupts nerve impulses to and from the brain. The disease is called "multiple" because it affects many areas of the brain. Scleroids are hardened, scarred patches that form over the damaged areas of myelin.

The initial symptoms of MS may include tingling, numbness, slurred speech, blurred or double vision, loss of coordination, and muscle weakness. Later manifestations include unusual fatigue, muscle tightness, bowel and bladder control difficulties, sexual dysfunction, and paralysis. The most common cognitive functions influenced are short-term memory, abstract reasoning, verbal fluency, and information processing speed. All the mental and physical symptoms listed may come or go in any combination. The symptoms may also vary from mild to severe in intensity throughout the disease.

The symptoms of MS vary from person to person and may periodically vary within the same person. The nature of MS makes its prognosis challenging to foresee. Although the general course of the disease may be anticipated, the symptoms and their severity seem to be quite unpredictable in most individuals. In the "classic" course of MS, as time progresses, chronic problems gradually accumulate over many years, slowly worsening the sufferer's quality of life. The total level of disability will vary from patient to patient.

There are four main types of MS and a pre-MS condition. Each type of MS displays a distinct clinical progression. A radiologically isolated syndrome or RIS is a neurological abnormality consistent with MS on a brain magnetic resonance imaging (MRI). RIS patients have no MS symptoms and usually have a brain MRI for other reasons. Just over half of people with RIS go on to develop MS within ten years. There are no protocols for people with RIS since there is no way to predict if they will develop MS. Clinically isolated syndrome (CIS) results from the first episode of MS symptoms lasting at least 24 hours. If lesions on a brain MRI accompany this episode, the likelihood of developing MS is high. Relapsing-remitting MS (RRMS) is the most common type of MS. It is characterized by flares with new or increasing neurologic symptoms followed by remittance periods. Secondary progressive MS (SPMS) begins with an initial relapsing-remitting course that transitions to progressively worsening neurologic function (accumulation of disability) over time. Finally, primary progressive MS (PPMS) worsens neurologic function and disability at the start, without early relapses or remissions.

The typical pattern of MS is marked by active periods of the disease during which the immune system is ravaging the nerves. These periods are called "attacks," "relapses," or "exacerbations." The active periods of the disease are followed by calm periods called "remissions." The cycle of attack and remission will differ from sufferer to sufferer. Some people have few attacks, and their MS disabilities slowly accumulate over time; it takes decades to become genuinely debilitated in these sufferers. Most people with MS have what is known as the relapsing-remitting form of the disease. They suffer many attacks over time. These attacks occur unpredictably; the attacks are then followed by complete remission, which may last months or years. Again, the injuries may take many years to accumulate to complete disability.

The most aggressive form of the disease is PPMS. In this type of MS, the disease follows a rapid course that steadily worsens from its first onset. Although there are still attacks and partial remission, the attacks are severe and occur more regularly in time. Complete paralysis may develop in PPMS in three to five years. SPMS occurs in patients who initially have the relapsing-remitting type and later develop the more aggressive form.

Both genetic and environmental factors have been implicated in inducing the onset of MS. Viral infection has been suggested as a cause. Still, no single virus has ever been shown to be associated with MS. Although infections such as the common cold, flu, and gastroenteritis increase the risk of relapse, flu vaccination is safe in patients with MS. Risk may be conferred by exposure to a specific environment during adolescence. However, that environment and the genetic risk factors have not yet been characterized. The support for the genetic component comes from examining identical twins. The likelihood of MS in the second identical twin, when the first twin has MS, is 30 percent.

Researchers Sharon Lynch and John Rose suggested that specific racial and geographic populations are less susceptible to the disease. MS is uncommon in Japanese people as well as among American Indians. The disease is more common among Northern European Caucasians as well as among North Americans of higher latitudes. There is an additional sexual dimorphism in the epidemi-

---

INFORMATION ON MULTIPLE SCLEROSIS

Causes: Genetic and environmental factors; possibly a viral infection

Symptoms: Tingling, numbness, slurring of speech, blurred or double vision, loss of coordination, muscle weakness and tightness, fatigue, bowel and bladder control difficulties, sexual dysfunction, paralysis, impaired cognitive functions

Duration: Chronic with recurrent episodes

Treatments: Steroids, human interferons, regular exercise

ology of MS; the disease is found more frequently in women by a ratio of 2:1.

The disease usually begins its first manifestations in late adolescence (around age eighteen) to early middle age (around age thirty-five). It is not clear how the interaction between the genetics of the sufferer and the environment may trigger onset. The progressive type of MS is more common over the age of forty, so those with late-onset MS often have the quickest deterioration of motor function. The reason that an older age predisposes someone to primary chronic progressive MS is still not apparent.

Studies by Swiss researcher Avinoam Safran have shown that occasionally MS manifests after the age of fifty. This condition has been named late-onset multiple sclerosis. Late-onset MS is not rare. Nearly 10 percent of MS patients demonstrate their first symptom after the age of fifty. Physicians, who do not expect it in the aged, often do not recognize this type of MS.

TREATMENT AND THERAPY

Scientists have been encouraged by advancements in MS diagnosis using the MRI brain scan. In 2002 they announced that these scans appear to detect damage around nerve fibers in patients with possible early signs of MS. This detection helps doctors predict those who will eventually develop MS and how severe one's experience with the disease might be. In turn, this allows a drug regimen to begin earlier. In the past, doctors did not officially diagnose MS or start treatment until patients had two episodes of nerve problems in different areas of the body. During this time, reoccurrences that could come years apart while damage nonetheless continued silently. New research has found that putting patients on MS drugs at the first sign of nerve inflammation drastically slows the chances of developing MS within a few years. However, most will eventually still develop the disease.

While there is no cure for MS, there are many effective treatments. In most cases, steroidal drugs treat relapses or attacks of the disease. Corticotropin was the first steroidal immunosuppressant to be used widely in MS treatment. The primary effect

Multiple sclerosis. Image by Mikael Häggström, via Wikimedia Commons. [Public domain].

of the drug is to shorten the duration of an attack. However, it does not appear to reduce the severity of the attack. Although it is still used by patients who respond well to it, other drugs have supplanted corticotropin. Methylprednisolone is an immunosuppressant and steroid that has replaced corticotropin. It controls the inflammation that accompanies demyelination. These steroids seem to work by sealing leaking blood vessels in the brain and reducing the responsiveness of the white blood cells of the immune system so that they cannot attack the myelin as easily.

Several federally approved drugs can slow the rate of attacks: Avonex, Rebif, and Betaseron are interferon preparations (proteins regulating the immune system), and Copaxone is a mixture of small peptides that protects myelin. Although these drugs do not stop MS entirely, they limit the level of myelin destruction, as observed in MRI scans of the brain. Avonex slows down the rate of progression to disability, and all four slow down the natural course of MS. University of Western Ontario researcher George Ebers was the first to perform experimental treatments on MS patients with interferons. The myelin sheath is produced by a particular nerve cell called an "oligodendrocyte"; presumably, interferons stimulate the oligodendrocytes to protect themselves. Patients treated with human interferons demonstrated a 34 percent reduction in the frequency of attacks; that reduction was sustained over five years of treatment. More impressive was the 80 percent reduction of MS activity detected in their brains. These patients rarely required steroid treatments.

Eighty-five percent of MS patients have the relapsing-remitting form of MS. Treatment in these patients includes a disease-modifying drug, corticosteroids for acute exacerbations, and medicines to manage fatigue, depression, and pain. Interferon-beta (INF-ß) was the first Food and Drug Administration (FDA)-approved disease-modifying drug for MS. INF-ß reduces clinical relapse rates by

> **IN THE NEWS: NEW DRUG TREATMENTS FOR MULTIPLE SCLEROSIS**
>
> The neurodegeneration that characterizes multiple sclerosis (MS) results from the destruction of myelin that surrounds and protects nerves by the immune system. Myelin-specific T cells are required for this attack. Corticosteroids have been used as therapy because of their known immunosuppressive properties. They have proved to be effective against the symptoms of MS episodes, but they have serious side effects and can be taken only for short times. Because they suppress the immune system in a general, nonspecific way, they inhibit the destruction of myelin and the body's ability to fight infection. This problem has led to the deaths of some MS patients. In addition, corticosteroids do not delay the long-term progression of MS. More recently, interferon-ß has been used to treat MS. Although interferon-ß therapy can be given for long periods and has been shown to reduce the frequency of relapses and slow the disease's progression. Interferon's mechanism remains unknown. One theory is that it reduces inflammation.
>
> New drugs on the horizon aim to stop the progression of MS and eliminate all relapses. The theory behind them is that a drug should be targeted to inhibit only the components of the immune system that destroy myelin. Unlike the drugs currently available, such drugs would be attacking the underlying cause of MS rather than its symptoms. They would be expected to cause few or no side effects.
>
> Two of these new drugs, Tovaxin from Opexa Therapeutics and a not-yet-named candidate, now called "RTL1000," from Artielle Immuno-Therapeutics, act by specifically inactivating the patient's own myelin-specific T cells without interacting with other immune system cells. Myelin-specific T cells are required for the destruction of myelin. Inactivation of many of them slows down myelin destruction.
>
> Immune Response is developing another approach. Their drug NeuroVax acts by specifically stimulating patients' cells that down-regulate myelin-specific T cells. Clinical trials of NeuroVax are underway.

30 to 35 percent. It also decreases the appearance of new brain lesions on MRI. Interferons cause a flu-like syndrome and injection-site reactions. Pegylated INF-ß1 *(Plegridy)* is injected subcutaneously or intra-

muscularly every two weeks. INF-ß is safe for pregnant and breastfeeding women.

Glatiramer acetate (Copaxone) is a mixture of small polypeptides that suppressed T-cell activation. It is about as effective as INF-ß and is the safest of all disease-modifying MS medications. This drug is also safe for pregnant and breastfeeding women. Unfortunately, Glatiramer acetate must be injected subcutaneously daily or three times a week.

The most effective medication for RRMS is the monoclonal antibody natalizumab (Tysabri). This anti-a4 integrin antibody inhibits white blood cell migration across the blood-brain barrier. It is given as an intravenous (IV) infusion for one hour every four weeks. It reduces relapse rates by 68 percent, new brain lesions by 82 percent, and disease progression rates by 42 percent. This wonder drug, however, comes with a significant drawback. The immune system suppression provided by natalizumab increases the risk of the John Cunningham (JC) virus infection. JC virus causes progressive multifocal leukoencephalopathy (PML), a potentially fatal infection. The PML risk is low during the first two to three years of treatment (0.02 percent). Still, it increases with each additional year of natalizumab use. Natalizumab is safe for breastfeeding but not during pregnancy.

Alemtuzumab (Lemtrada) is an anti-CD52 monoclonal antibody that depletes the body of B and T lymphocytes that express this protein. It is more effective than interferon and is infused IV for five consecutive days and then twelve months later for three consecutive days. However, alemtuzumab causes severe autoimmune reactions, infusion reactions, and tumors. It is restricted to those patients who did not achieve satisfactory relapse with other medications. Alemtuzumab is safe for breastfeeding but not during pregnancy.

At least three MS disease-modifying medications bind to the B lymphocyte surface protein CD20. Ocrelizumab (Ocrevus) and ofatumumab (Kesimpta) decrease flares and the appearance of new brain lesions. Ocrelizumab also treats PPMS, and it is the only drug approved to treat this form of MS. Ocrelizumab and ofatumumab cause PML and cancers. Rituximab (Rituxan) is not FDA-approved for MS, but it is used off-label as a cheaper alternative. Though probably safe for breastfeeding women, the anti-CD20 drugs are not safe during pregnancy.

Mitoxantrone is an anticancer drug that can reduce relapses in RRMS patients. Unfortunately, this drug is poisonous to the heart and significantly increases the cancer risk. Therefore, clinicians use this drug infrequently.

Oral medications are far more convenient to take than injected ones, and several oral disease-modifying medications for MS are available. The first group is the sphingosine-1-phosphate (S1P) receptor modulators, fingolimod (Gilenya), siponimod (Mayzent), ozanimod (Zeposia), and ponesimod (*Ponvory*). T cells use the S1P receptor to enter the central nervous system. Blocking this receptor keeps autoreactive T-cells from accessing the brain and its myelin, decreasing relapses and the appearance of new lesions. These drugs are more effective than INF-ß. As a group, they decrease the effectiveness of live vaccines and can cause heart arrhythmias. The S1P receptor modulators have multiple drug-drug interactions and are safe for neither pregnancy nor breastfeeding.

A second oral disease-modifying MS medication is cladribine (*Mavenclad*). However, this medication is a second-line drug for patients who failed other medicines because of its toxicity. Cladribine prevents the synthesis of the building blocks of deoxyribonucleic acid (DNA). Therefore, it selectively depletes B lymphocytes and prevents relapses. Cladribine can cause lymphopenia and severe infections, and it is not safe during pregnancy or breastfeeding.

The fumarates include dimethyl fumarate (*Tecfidera* and generics) and diroximel fumarate

(Vumerity). The body metabolizes both drugs to monomethyl fumarate (MMF), which reduces inflammation. These drugs significantly reduce relapse rates and the development of new or enlarging brain lesions. The fumarates are well tolerated but can cause an upset stomach. PML was reported with dimethyl fumarate, but it is not common. The fumarates are not recommended during pregnancy or when breastfeeding.

Teriflunomide (Aubagio) also prevents the synthesis of DNA and ribonucleic acid (RNA) building blocks and reduces T- and B-cell levels. It reduces relapses but is less effective than the fumarates. Teriflunomide is not safe during pregnancy or when breastfeeding.

Early use of disease-modifying therapy significantly improves clinical outcomes.

During the 1990s, in a study supported by the National Institutes of Health and conducted at the Mayo Clinic, plasma exchange, also called "plasmapheresis," was proven to be an effective treatment for certain patients suffering from severe symptoms of multiple sclerosis who were not responsive to conventional methods of treatment. Plasma exchange involves removing the patient's blood; the elimination of the plasma-containing antibodies that target myelin, which is then replaced by a fluid with similar properties, usually containing albumin; and its subsequent return to the patient. This procedure has been used to treat other autoimmune diseases such as myasthenia gravis and Guillain-Barré syndrome in the past.

Investigators concluded that plasma exchange might contribute to recovery from an acute attack in people with MS who have not responded to standard steroid treatment. Therefore, they recommended that this treatment only be considered for individuals experiencing a severe, acute attack that is not responding to high-dose steroids. Since the vast majority (90 percent) of people experiencing acute attacks respond well to the standard steroid treatment, plasma exchange would be considered a treatment alternative only for the approximately 10 percent who do not. For those 10 percent, however, plasma exchange may offer an essential and beneficial treatment option. Because the exact reasons for the effectiveness of plasmapheresis are unknown, researchers feel that further studies are warranted based on the idea that some people may have antibodies in their plasma that are instrumental in certain disease activities that allow disabilities to occur.

As additional therapy, patients with MS should participate in a regular exercise program. Exercise is vital to the maintenance of functional ability in MS sufferers. It strengthens muscles, benefits gait, and generally improves coordination. The best type of exercise is aquatic. Sufferers are often heat-intolerant, and participation in a regular aerobic program would be unpleasant. Also, aquatic exercise is a low-impact activity that puts less stress on chronically sore muscles. Exercise programs also encourage the socialization of patients and engender peer support.

PERSPECTIVE AND PROSPECTS
The first written report of MS was published in 1400 when the famed Dutch skater Lydwina of Schieden was diagnosed. It was recognized initially as a wasting disease of unknown origin. The disease was described clinically by Jean-Martin Charcot in 1877. Charcot initially characterized the clinical signs and symptoms of MS. He recognized that the disease affects the nervous system and tried many remedies without success. In 1890, the cause of MS was thought to be suppression of sweat; the treatment was electrical stimulation and bed rest. At the time, life expectancy for a sufferer was five years after diagnosis. By 1910, MS was thought to be caused by toxins in the blood, and purgatives were the best treatment. In the 1930s, poor circulation was believed to cause MS, and blood-thinning agents be-

came the treatment of choice. In the 1950s through the 1970s, MS was caused by severe allergies; treatments included antihistamines. Not until the 1980s was the basis of MS understood and effective treatment developed.

By the early twenty-first century, it was estimated that thousands of people had this disorder of the brain and spinal cord, which disrupts the smooth flow of electrical messages from the brain and nerves to the body. The progress of the disease is slow and may take decades to achieve complete nerve degeneration and paralysis. Although often considered a disease of youth, MS can become an increasing problem in aging populations. More cases of late-onset MS have come to light in individuals over forty years of age, including such celebrities as comedian Richard Pryor, entertainer Annette Funicello, and talk-show host Montel Williams.

Current clinical trials are likely to reveal treatment strategies that will further facilitate controlling the symptoms and progression of MS.

—*James J. Campanella, PhD, W. Michael Zawada, PhD, and Michael A. Buratovich, PhD*

Further Information
"About MS." *National Multiple Sclerosis Society*, 2013.
Alan, Rick, and Rimas Lukas. "Multiple Sclerosis-Adult." *Health Library*, 30 Sept. 2012.
Alan, Rick, Rebecca Stahl, and Kari Kassir. "Multiple Sclerosis-Child." *Health Library*, 6 Jun. 2012.
Blackstone, Margaret. *The First Year-Multiple Sclerosis: An Essential Guide for the Newly Diagnosed*. 2nd ed., Avalon, 2007.
"Drugs for Multiple Sclerosis." *Medical Letter on Drugs and Therapeutics*, vol. 63, no. 1620, 2021, pp. 42-48.
Halbreich, Uriel. *Multiple Sclerosis: A Neuropsychiatric Disorder*. American Psychiatric Press, 1993.
Iams, Betty. *From MS to Wellness*. Iams House, 1998.
Kalb, Rosalind, editor. *Multiple Sclerosis: The Questions You Have, the Answers You Need*. 5th ed., Demos Vermande, 2012.
Litin, Scott C., editor. "Multiple Sclerosis." *Mayo Clinic Family Health Book*. 4th ed., HarperResource, 2009.
Matthews, Bryan. *Multiple Sclerosis: The Facts*. 4th ed., Oxford UP, 2001.
"Multiple Sclerosis." *MedlinePlus*, 7 May 2013.
National Multiple Sclerosis Society. www.nationalmssociety.org/. Accessed 6 Sept. 2021.
Polman, Chris H., et al. *Multiple Sclerosis: The Guide to Treatment and Management*. 6th ed., Demos Vermande, 2006.
Rae-Grant, Alexander et al. "Practice Guideline Recommendations Summary: Disease-Modifying Therapies for Adults with Multiple Sclerosis: Report of the Guideline Development, Dissemination, and Implementation Subcommittee of the American Academy of Neurology." *Neurology*, vol. 90, no. 17, 2018, pp. 777-88, doi:10.1212/WNL.0000000000005347.
Russell, Margot. *When the Road Turns: Inspirational Stories About People with MS*. Health Communications, 2001.
Salter, Robert Bruce. *Textbook of Disorders and Injuries of the Musculoskeletal System*. 3rd ed., Williams & Wilkins, 1999.

MYASTHENIA GRAVIS

Category: Diseases/Disorders
Anatomy or system affected: Immune system, musculoskeletal system, nervous system
Specialties and related fields: Immunology, neurology
Definition: A disorder characterized by selective muscle fatigue following repeated use caused by an abnormal immune reaction to specific receptors on the muscle surface.

KEY TERMS

acetylcholine: a chemical released by motor neuron terminals; it causes muscle contraction
acetylcholine receptor: a protein on the surface of muscle cells; binding of acetylcholine to this receptor causes muscle cells to contract
acetylcholinesterase: an enzyme that degrades acetylcholine
antibody: a protein produced by the immune system to inactivate substances detected as foreign

autoimmune disease: a disorder in which the immune system targets proteins that are normal components of body tissues

paraneoplastic syndrome: a cluster of rare disorders triggered by an abnormal immune system response induced by a tumor

thymus: a gland located at the base of the neck; part of the immune system

CAUSES AND SYMPTOMS

Myasthenia gravis derives from a Latin phrase that means "grave muscle weakness." It is a neuromuscular disorder characterized by weakness of skeletal muscles following repeated use. The prevalence of the disease in the United States is approximately 14 in 100,000. It occurs in both genders of all ethnic groups, although myasthenia gravis preferentially affects young women in their 20s and 30s and older men in their 60s and 70s. The cause of this starkly bimodal distribution of age-of-onset remains unclear.

Usually, body movements result from the contraction of skeletal muscles, which are voluntary muscles attached to the bone. These muscles are stimulated to contract by motor neurons in the brain and spinal cord. Nerve impulses travel down the motor neurons to their axon terminals, where a small amount of a substance known as a "neurotransmitter" is released onto the muscle's surface. In this case, the neurotransmitter is the chemical acetylcholine. When acetylcholine binds to specific receptors called "nicotinic acetylcholine receptors" at the motor endplate, contraction results. The motor endplate is a specialized structure where the axon of the motor neuron contacts the skeletal muscle.

In myasthenia gravis, an autoimmune disease, someone's B cells inappropriately make antibodies that bind to nicotinic acetylcholine receptors on the muscle cells. Once bound to the antibodies, the nicotinic acetylcholine receptors cannot bind acetylcholine. Consequently, they don't respond to the "contract" signal from the central nervous system. These antiniconic acetylcholine receptors antibodies also activate the classical complement pathway. The complement system consists of small proteins that work in an enzymatic cascade to destroy invading bacteria. The classical complement pathway is activated by antibodies, closely packed together, tightly bound to a surface. Complement activation results in inflammation and destruction of the muscle cells. This significantly reduces the number of nicotinic acetylcholine receptors on the muscle cell surfaces. With fewer remaining receptors, the muscle's contractile response is weakened.

In very rare cases, myasthenia gravis results from a "paraneoplastic syndrome." Paraneoplastic syndromes result from underlying cancers like bronchogenic carcinomas or thymic neoplasms (thymomas) produce an immune response that produces autoantibodies.

The root cause of this aberrant immune response remains unknown. The thymus, a gland involved in immune function, is abnormal in about 75 percent of patients with the disease. Two distinct thymic anomalies may occur in myasthenia gravis: Thymic hyperplasia (an increase in the number of specific immune cells in the thymus) or thymoma (a thymic tumor). In some late—onset cases of myasthenia

> **INFORMATION ON MYASTHENIA GRAVIS**
>
> **Causes**: Autoimmune disorder in which immune system fails to recognize muscle receptors as "self"
>
> **Symptoms**: Weakness of muscles following repeated use, resulting in visual disorders, difficulty chewing and swallowing, slurred speech, limb weakness, breathing difficulties; in most cases, abnormal thymus gland
>
> **Duration**: Chronic, usually progressive
>
> **Treatments**: Alleviation of symptoms; may include medications (neostigmine, prednisone, azathioprine), surgery (removal of thymus), plasma exchange

gravis, however, the thymus appears normal or even shrunken—yet these cases are also accompanied by elevated levels of antibodies recognizing acetylcholine receptors. Such inconsistencies are part of the reason that the relationship between the thymus and myasthenia gravis is not fully understood.

Skeletal muscle weakness is a symptom common to all forms of myasthenia gravis. Because this weakness is exacerbated with muscle use, it is not surprising that the first muscles to be affected are those used most often. Thus, the earliest signs of the disease often involve the eye's muscles, including drooping of the eyelids and double vision. As other muscle groups become affected, advancing symptoms may include difficulty chewing and swallowing, slurred speech, limb weakness, and breathing difficulties. Although symptoms vary from patient to patient, they often fluctuate in severity with a similar daily pattern: Weakness is usually more pronounced in the evening than in the morning. Factors other than exertion that can provoke symptoms include viral illness, excitement, elevated temperature, menses, and pregnancy.

Although the long-term course of the disease can vary, it is usually progressive. In a minority of patients, weakness affects only the eye muscles. In other cases, progression is often most rapid within the first three years and may be punctuated with spontaneous temporary remissions. Treatment can help keep the symptoms under control.

Myasthenic crises result when the disease affects the muscles that control breathing. This life-threatening condition is a consequence of the disease spreading beyond the muscles that control the appendages.

Early symptoms are not always recognized as being linked to myasthenia gravis. A definitive diagnosis includes testing for the presence of antibodies that bind acetylcholine receptors. In addition, impaired nerve-muscle communication should be demonstrated in the form of specific muscle weakness elicited by repetitive nerve stimulation. Finally, it should be shown that muscle weakness is briefly relieved following the administration of edrophonium. This drug blocks the breakdown of acetylcholine, temporarily increasing the amount of the neurotransmitter available to act on muscle receptors.

TREATMENT AND THERAPY
Several treatment options have been developed with the goal of symptomatic control of myasthenia gravis. Treatment must be individually tailored depending on disease history and severity. Therapies include medications, surgery, and plasma exchange.

Acetylcholinesterase is a naturally occurring enzyme that degrades acetylcholine and regulates its activity. Acetylcholinesterase inhibition prolongs the availability of acetylcholine, enhancing its contractile effect. Drugs that inhibit the action of acetylcholinesterase can improve neuromuscular transmission: such drugs include neostigmine and pyridostigmine. Another pharmacological approach is to suppress the immune system with drugs such as prednisone and azathioprine, reducing the production of abnormal antibodies.

Thymectomy, the surgical removal of the thymus, is commonly recommended as a treatment for myasthenia gravis. In general, this procedure is considered the most effective approach for obtaining sustained relief or remission. Maximum postsurgical improvement may take several years to occur, and results are usually best in younger patients early in their disease.

Plasma exchange is an immediate intervention to combat the sudden onset of severe symptoms such as respiratory failure or in cases where the patient has not responded to other treatments. This procedure removes abnormal antibodies from the blood plasma.

PERSPECTIVE AND PROSPECTS
The British physician Thomas Willis first described myasthenia gravis in 1685. Although relatively rare,

it was the first neurological disease to be identified as having an autoimmune basis. The understanding of the disease was aided by converging research among neurophysiologists, neurologists, and immunologists; these combined approaches have helped to elucidate other autoimmune diseases.

Although patients undergoing treatment for myasthenia gravis can expect an average life span marked by significant improvement of their symptoms, as of 2013, there was no cure for the disease. Present research aims to understand better the factors triggering the autoimmune response in myasthenia gravis, elucidate the relationship between the thymus and the disease, and fully understand the molecular basis of normal and aberrant nerve-muscle transmission. This research should guide developments in treatment strategy, with a key goal being to cure the immune abnormality that underlies the disease.

—*Sharon W. Stark, RN, APRN, DNSc
and Michael A. Buratovich, PhD*

Further Information

Carson-DeWitt, Rosalyn. "Myasthenia Gravis (MG)." *Health Library*, 10 Sept. 2012.

Farmakidis, Constantine, et al. "Treatment of Myasthenia Gravis." *Neurologic Clinics*, vol. 36, no. 2, 2018, pp. 311-37, doi:10.1016/j.ncl.2018.01.011.

Kaminski, Henry J., editor. *Myasthenia Gravis and Related Disorders*. 2nd ed., Humana Press, 2010.

Kasper, Dennis L., et al., editors. *Harrison's Principles of Internal Medicine*. 16th ed., McGraw-Hill, 2005.

MedlinePlus. "Myasthenia Gravis." *MedlinePlus*, 19 Apr. 2013.

National Institute of Neurological Disorders and Stroke. "NINDS Myasthenia Gravis Information Page." *NINDS*, 4 Dec. 2012.

Parker, James N., and Philip M. Parker. *Myasthenia Gravis: A Medical Dictionary, Bibliography, and Annotated Research Guide to Internet References*. ICON Health Publications, 2004.

Sanders, Donald B., et al. "International Consensus Guidance for Management of Myasthenia Gravis: Executive Summary." *Neurology*, vol. 87, no. 4, 2016, pp. 419-25, doi:10.1212/WNL.0000000000002790.

Vincent, Angela. "Unravelling the Pathogenesis of Myasthenia Gravis." *Nature Reviews Immunology*, vol. 2, Oct. 2002, pp. 797-804.

Myositis

Category: Diseases/Conditions
Also known as: Idiopathic inflammatory myopathy, inflammatory myopathy
Anatomy or system affected: Muscles, musculoskeletal system
Specialties and related fields: Cardiology, dermatology, hematology, immunology, internal medicine, neurology, ophthalmology, otorhinolaryngology, pathology, rheumatology
Definition: A group of rare chronic conditions characterized by inflammation of the skeletal muscles.

KEY TERMS

dermatomyositis: inflammation of the skin and underlying muscle tissue due to collagen destruction, leading to discoloration, and swelling, typically results from an autoimmune condition or associated with cancer.

Electromyogram (EMG): a technique that measures the electrical activity produced by skeletal muscles

erythrocyte sedimentation rate: a laboratory test that measures the rate at which red blood cells in anticoagulated whole blood descend in a standardized tube over one hour. It is a nonspecific measure of inflammation

polymyositis: a muscle disease characterized by chronic muscle inflammation and muscle weakness

INTRODUCTION

"Myositis" is a general term for rare chronic conditions characterized by inflammation of the skeletal muscles. This inflammation can cause muscle weakness. Myositis refers to the inflammatory myopathies, including polymyositis, dermatomyositis, inclusion-body myositis, and juvenile myositis. All these disorders are autoimmune diseases. Inflammatory myopathies can also be caused by certain medications or by exposure to a toxic substance; these myopathies are usually not chronic and resolve once the harmful substance is removed.

CAUSES
It is not known what causes myositis. It is believed that an environmental factor, such as a viral infection, triggers myositis in people who might be genetically predisposed to the condition. The damage in myositis is caused by the body's immune system, as white blood cells and antibodies attack the muscle and, in some cases, the skin.

RISK FACTORS
Generally, women are more affected than men, although inclusion-body myositis affects twice as many men as women. Polymyositis occurs in persons between twenty and sixty years of age. In contrast, inclusion-body myositis is more common after age fifty years. Children can develop dermatomyositis. African Americans are at higher risk for myositis. In contrast, the lowest rates of myositis occur in persons of Japanese origin.

SYMPTOMS
Common symptoms of the inflammatory myopathies include muscle weakness, sometimes with muscle pain that lasts for more than a few weeks; general tiredness and fatigue; difficulty climbing stairs, standing up from a seated position, or reaching up; and difficulty swallowing. Additional symptoms for the various myopathies include various skin symptoms (such as a rash or scaly, dry, and rough skin) in dermatomyositis; and hardened lumps of calcium (calcinosis) under the skin in juvenile dermatomyositis. Unlike other inflammatory myopathies, the muscle weakness in inclusion-body myositis is often asymmetrical.

SCREENING AND DIAGNOSIS
Myositis varies from person to person and can often resemble other diseases, such as scleroderma or systemic lupus erythematosus (SLE, or lupus). Tests used to help confirm a diagnosis include a physical exam; tests of muscle strength; magnetic resonance imaging (MRI) scan; an electromyogram (EMG); blood tests, including erythrocyte sedimentation rate, creatinine kinase, and antinuclear antibodies; and muscle and skin biopsies.

TREATMENT AND THERAPY
Treatment for myositis generally includes rest, physical therapy, and the use of anti-inflammatories (corticosteroids as first-line therapy and methotrexate, hydroxychloroquine, and azathioprine), and intravenous immunoglobulin. If left untreated, inflammatory myopathy can cause permanent damage.

PREVENTION AND OUTCOMES
Because the cause of myositis is unknown, there is no known way to prevent the condition. To lessen the severity of dermatomyositis, however, persons with the condition should avoid excessive exposure to the sun, which can worsen any dermatomyositis-associated skin rashes.

—*Anita P. Kuan, PhD*

Further Information
Isenberg, D. A., et al. "International Consensus Outcome Measures for Patients with Idiopathic Inflammatory Myopathies: Development and Initial Validation of Myositis Activity and Damage Indices in Patients with Adult-Onset Disease." *Rheumatology*, vol. 43, no. 1, 2004, pp. 49-54.

Kagen, Lawrence J., editor. *The Inflammatory Myopathies*. Humana Press, 2009.

Marieb, Elaine N., and Katja Hoehn. *Human Anatomy and Physiology*. 11th ed., Pearson/Benjamin Cummings, 2018.

Murphy, Kenneth, Paul Travers, and Mark Walport. *Janeway's Immunobiology*. 7th ed., Garland Science, 2008.

Parker, James N., and Philip M. Parker, editors. *Myositis: A Medical Dictionary, Bibliography, and Annotated Research Guide to Internet References*. ICON Health, 2004.

Psoriasis and psoriatic arthritis

Category: Diseases/Disorders
Anatomy or system affected: Skin, eyes, joints, nails
Specialties and related fields: Dermatology, internal medicine, ophthalmology, orthopedics, rheumatology
Definition: A chronic skin disease in which red, scaly patches develop, overlaid with thick, silvery-gray scales, causing physical discomfort as well as damage to self-esteem.

KEY TERMS

dermatologist: a physician who treats the skin and its structures, functions, and diseases

dermis: the layer of skin directly beneath the epidermis, consisting of dense connective tissue and numerous blood vessels

enthesitis: inflammation of the insertion sites of tendons and ligaments to the bone surface

epidermis: the outermost part of the skin, composed of four or five different layers called "strata"

methotrexate: a powerful drug originally developed to treat cancer that treats patients with severe cases of psoriasis

onchonylysis: pitting and destruction of the fingernails or toenails

psoralens: chemicals found in plants that make the skin more sensitive to light

psoriatic arthritis: a subtype of psoriasis characterized by the extension of the inflammation that involves the skin to the joints and nails

PUVA: a treatment for psoriasis that exposes the patient to ultraviolet A (UVA) light after receiving one of the psoralens

stratum corneum: the outermost layer of the epidermis; its cells are generally dead, hard, and removed by regular bathing

ultraviolet light (UV): invisible light composed of waves that are shorter than the ordinary light waves able to be seen by humans

CAUSES AND SYMPTOMS

Psoriasis is a common skin problem afflicting approximately two of every hundred people, affecting males and females with relatively equal frequency. Although it affects all races, it is most prevalent among northern Europeans. This stubborn, chronic, and incurable disease most commonly appears in one's teens or twenties. However, it can appear in early childhood. Seventy percent of psoriasis patients develop it by the age of twenty. However, another typical danger period occurs in the fifties and sixties, with many patients developing their first symptoms at that time.

There are several different types of psoriasis, making diagnosis difficult. The most widespread is the "plaque type"; because it accounts for 95 percent of all cases, this type is also called "common psoriasis." Plaque-type psoriasis gets its name from the appearance of the patches of affected skin. Each patch resembles a plaque or small disk stuck to the body's surface. These dull, wine-colored patches of abnormal skin are often rounded or oval; they may be very irregular when several nearby patches join together. The surface of each thickened patch is rough and scaly, with the scales ranging in color from red to white to the most typical silvery gray. These psoriatic plaques can be small (the size of coins) or become palm-sized and larger. Whatever their final size, they generally begin as purple or reddened areas the size of a pinhead. The original areas expand in size, usually for a few weeks, until they reach a stable phase and stop expanding. The average size of a plaque in the stable phase is between two and three inches. A patch of stable psoriasis may eventually grow pale, become less scaly, and disappear completely, or it may begin to enlarge for no apparent reason. Even those plaques that have disappeared may be reactivated and later reappear in the same place.

Certain body parts seem most prone to psoriatic lesions, namely the elbows, the knees, the scalp, and the lower back. The patches may appear elsewhere, including the genitals and the buttocks, but the face, hands, and feet are rarely affected. Severe cases may cover the entire chest or back. In a few cases, psoriasis is symmetrical, appearing in the same area on the left and right sides of the body simultaneously. The patches are, however, more likely to develop in a random, scattered manner.

Almost 50 percent of patients with psoriasis have lesions on their scalps. When these plaques are extensive and widespread, they are challenging to treat and very difficult to hide. Although very uncomfortable, scalp psoriasis does not affect the growth of hair or cause baldness. It can cause a temporary thinning of the hair. Still, hair usually grows again once the disease is controlled by medication. About one-third of psoriasis patients have affected finger-

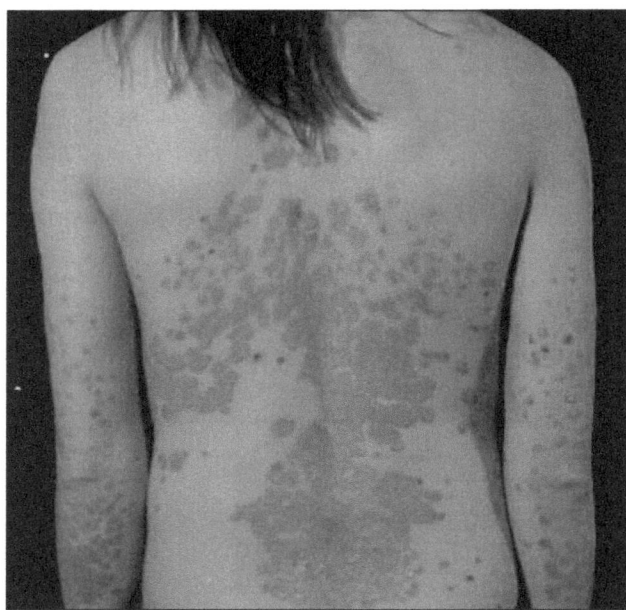

Back and arms of a person with psoriasis. Photo by James Heilman, MD, via Wikimedia Commons. [CC 4.0.]

nails and toenails. The diseased nails show pits or pinpoint indentations, loosening, thickening, and yellowish discoloration. Surprisingly, in some people, the condition remains on the nails alone, never developing elsewhere.

In addition to psoriasis of the nails, several rare and unusual types of psoriasis are different from the common or plaque type. These include flexural or inverse, guttate, pustular, and erythrodermic psoriasis. Flexural psoriasis appears in folds and creases on the body. It usually occurs in people who are particularly overweight and who are in their mid-forties or older. The patches tend to be very moist rather than scaly and are particularly sore and uncomfortable. Guttable psoriasis consists of an enormous number of highly scattered but minute plaques. It is rare and occurs between the ages of eight and sixteen. Although the spots usually clear up in a few weeks, they sometimes recur or change into large lesions of common psoriasis. Pustular psoriasis is the only form of the disease that occurs on the palms of the hands or the soles

---

INFORMATION ON PSORIASIS

Causes: Failure in the mechanism by which normal skin renews itself; often hereditary

Symptoms: Red, scaly patches; thick, silvery-gray scales; physical discomfort; loose, thick, and yellowish fingernails and toenails; thinning hair

Duration: Chronic with acute episodes

Treatments: Corticosteroids, tar-containing agents, sun exposure, methotrexate, disease-modifying antirheumatic drugs (DMARDs), and biologic agents

of the feet. It was named for the yellow or white pus-filled spots that form on the skin and eventually drop off. These spots form when hordes of white blood cells invade the skin even though no infection is present. Erythrodermic psoriasis means "red skin." This rare condition receives its name because flaming red patches that do not turn scaly cover the entire body. Since the extensive nature of this condition makes internal temperature control very difficult and dehydration inevitable, it can be perilous and may require hospitalization.

Common psoriasis, by comparison, is not dangerous or life-threatening. It is usually not painful and does not even cause itching in most patients. It is, however, very annoying because of its unsightly appearance and its tendency to flare up repeatedly. Once the disease has appeared, it stays with the person for life, improving or worsening periodically. After periods of relative quiet, during which the skin may appear quite normal, patients with psoriasis experience new eruptions and scaling for no apparent reason. Plaques continue to form for an unpredictable amount of time until the condition spontaneously quiets down again.

The source of the plaques is a failure in the mechanism by which normal skin renews itself. Ordinarily, the cells at the base of the epidermis reproduce themselves at a slow and steady rate. They then move upward in about twenty-eight days, changing chemically, dying, and detaching from the surface, the stratum corneum. However, there is a considerable increase in the number of basal cells in the epidermis in psoriatic skin. These basal cells reproduce so rapidly that they push upward to the surface in only four days, forming thick disks of sticky, abnormal cells. Below the epidermis, the dermis of a patient with psoriasis is also abnormal. Its normally fine blood vessels are wide and highly twisted, causing the red appearance of the plaques. Consequently, the skin readily bleeds if bumped or scratched. An unusually high number of white blood cells called "neutrophils" and T lymphocytes are also present. They move up into the epidermis, creating inflammation and swelling within the plaques.

Dermatologists noted that psoriasis runs in families long before they discovered the facts about the structure and the functioning of psoriatic skin. If one parent has the problem, there is a one-in-three chance that a child will eventually be afflicted; if both parents have the disease, the risk for their offspring is one in two. If one non-identical twin has psoriasis, there is a 70 percent chance that the other will have psoriasis. With identical twins, the chances of having psoriasis can be as high as 90 percent, according to some studies. Geneticists suspect that people do not inherit psoriasis in a simple Mendelian manner. It seems more likely that the condition results from several genetic factors from each parent, much like how height and intelligence are inherited.

PSORIATIC ARTHRITIS

Psoriatic arthritis (PsA) is a widely variable type of psoriasis in which skin inflammation extends to the joints. PsA affects not only the joints but also structures associated with the joint. For example, involvement of the tendon area that inserts onto bone (entheses) results in enthesitis. Inflammation of the tendons and joints of the fingers causes dactylitis. PsA can also afflict the nails, causing nail pitting, also known as onchonylysis. Fingernail, toenail, and tendon insertion involvement distinguish psoriatic arthritis from rheumatoid arthritis, localizing to the joints.

The most significant risk factor for psoriatic arthritis is having psoriasis. The prevalence of PsA is between 6 to 42 percent in people with patients with psoriasis. PsA prevalence ranges from 0.3 to 1 percent of the general population. Psoriatic arthritis most commonly occurs in 30 to 50 years old and is nearly equal in both sexes. There is a higher incidence in people of Northern European descent and a lower incidence in Japanese descent.

Genetic factors have a significant role in the cause of PsA. PsA shows strong familial association and links with several major histocompatibility complex (MHC) class I alleles. As many as 40 percent of all PsA patients have a family history of arthritis or psoriasis. Most PsA patients experience skin manifestations of psoriasis before suffering any joint involvement. However, ten percent of PsA patients experience joint pain before any skin lesions. Psoriasis patients who suffer from scalp lesions, nail dystrophy, uveitis, and intergluteal/perianal skin lesions are at higher risk of PsA.

The clinical presentation of PsA differs from patient to patient. The severity and the course of the disease show extensive ranges. Some PsA patients have mild joint stiffness and soreness, while others have severe irreversible inflammatory joint destruction. Most PsA cases begin with pain in one to four joints (oligoarthritis). This condition may lead to the involvement of five or more joints (polyarthritis). PsA patients with polyarthritis, extensive skin involvement early in life (before age 20), and a strong family history of psoriasis are at higher risk for aggressive disease.

Why does psoriasis spread to the joints in some people but not others? The answer to this burning question remains unknown. However, an ensemble of genetic, environmental, and immunologic factors probably plays a role in the onset, severity, and presentation of PsA. Activated T cells are present in psoriatic skin lesions and joints. Therefore, a breakdown in the regulation of the immune response may lead to uncontrolled inflammation in the skin and joints. Consequently, PsA treatment usually involves inhibiting cytokines that stimulate inflammation, including tumor necrosis factor-alpha (TNF-a) and other proinflammatory cytokines (e.g., interleukin-6, interleukin-17, interleukin-12, interleukin-23).

PsA symptoms vary, but a common thread is stiffness, pain, swelling, and tenderness of one or more joints. This pain tends to limit motion. PsA commonly affects the spine, hips, and shoulders. PsA subtypes include: (1) distal interphalangeal joint-predominant arthritis (10 percent of cases), (2) symmetrical polyarthritis-predominant arthritis (5 to 20 percent of cases), (3) asymmetric oligoarthritis or monoarthritis (70 to 80 percent of cases), (4) axial disease (5 to 20 percent of cases), and (5) arthritis mutilans (rare).

The most critical factors when diagnosing PsA are the patient's medical history and clinical presentation. Distinguishing PsA from other types of arthritis requires blood tests to rule out rheumatoid arthritis (i.e., the absence of rheumatoid factor and anticyclic citrullinated peptide antibody). Other blood tests have varying usefulness for diagnostic purposes. Imaging affected joints with X-rays, computer-aided tomography (CAT) scans, or magnetic resonance imaging (MRI) shows joint destruction in a pattern known as a "pencil in cup" deformity.

TREATMENT AND THERAPY

More than 90 percent of psoriasis patients have their lesions cleared significantly or even made lesion-free by contemporary medicines and methods. For minor outbreaks, limited to a small body area,

---

INFORMATION ON PSORIATIC ARTHRITIS

Causes: Inflammation in the skin that spreads to the joints and structures associated with joints; often hereditary, but environmental factors are also involved in the onset and manifestation of the disease

Symptoms: Pain, stiffness, swelling, and tenderness of one or several joints that limits motion. It can also affect tendon insertion sites (entheses), particularly in the hand and some forms of psoriatic arthritis affect the spine, hips, and shoulders.

Duration: Chronic with acute episodes

Treatments: Nonsteroidal anti-inflammatory drugs (NSAIDs), interarticular and systemic corticosteroids, disease-modifying antirheumatoid drugs (DMARDs), apremilast, and biologic agents

the first choice for treatment is corticosteroid cream or ointments applied directly to the plaques. Corticosteroids are derivatives of glucocorticoid hormones produced by the adrenal glands that reduce glucose metabolism and suppress inflammation. Corticosteroids reduce inflammation and decrease blood flow to psoriatic lesions. Dermatologists have a large variety of such preparations ranging from mild to superpotent. Superpotent topical corticosteroids include 0.5 percent betamethasone dipropionate ointment and 0.05 percent halobetasol propionate cream. Potent topical steroids include amcinonide 0.1 percent ointment and halcinonide 0.1 percent cream. Moderate topical corticosteroids include upper-, mid-, and lower-mid strength preparations. Upper-mid strength includes triamcinolone acetonide 0.5 percent cream and mometasone furoate 0.1 percent ointment, and lower-mid strength consists of desoximetasone 0.05 percent cream and flurandrenolide 0.05 percent. Mild topical corticosteroids include alclometasone dipropionate 0.05 percent cream or ointment and desonide 0.05 percent cream. Finally, the least potent topical corticosteroids contain hydrocortisone, flumethasone, dexamethasone, prednisolone, or methylprednisolone. Dermatologists and rheumatologists must find a topical corticosteroid strong enough to suppress the inflammation but not cause unwanted side effects.

Topical steroids cause thinning of the skin and stretch marks if the patient uses it for a prolonged period, too much, or apply it to the face or intertriginous areas. Rarely, superpotent topical corticosteroids can suppress adrenal gland function if applied to large skin areas. Additionally, psoriatic skin absorbs substances more quickly than normal skin. Excess steroids enter the bloodstream and can change the output of hormones by the pituitary and adrenal glands, dangerously altering the body's chemical balance. The other danger is the skin itself, which becomes abnormally thin, easily damaged, and prone to infections. Another drawback to using corticosteroids is the tendency for the psoriatic plaques to reappear soon after discontinuation of the creams or ointments.

To decrease corticosteroid use, some patients opt for topical vitamin D analogs that decrease psoriatic skin lesions. Two synthetic vitamin D analogs, calcipotriene (*Dovonex*) and calcitriol (*Vectical*), are about as effective as medium-potency corticosteroids for topical treatment of plaque psoriasis. Both agents are well-tolerated, but calcipotriene causes burning and itching when applied to the skin, calcitriol less so. Ultraviolet (UV) light exposure inactivates calcipotriene. Another topical agent, tazarotene (Tazorac), is a retinoid (vitamin A derivative) that effectively treats plaque psoriasis. Tazarotene increases the sunburn risk and causes itching, burning, peeling, and itching. The combination of these topical agents with corticosteroids augments their efficacy.

Another group of topical agents, the calcineurin inhibitors, effectively treat psoriasis but are not Food and Drug Administration (FDA)-approved and used off-label. Tacrolimus (Protopic) and pimecrolimus (Elidel) work well for psoriatic lesions on the face and provide alternatives to corticosteroids. Tacrolimus and pimecrolimus cause burning, redness, and itching, but pimecrolimus is the better tolerated of the two. Long-term use seems to increase the risk of lymphomas.

Many patients find relief from an entirely different class of medications that contain tar. This thick, black, oily liquid, made from coal, contains thousands of chemical substances, and biochemists do not know which helps heal the skin. Tar-containing ointments, creams, gels, shampoos, and bath additives help remove the scales without problematic side effects. However, a significant drawback is their tendency to stain clothing, bedding, bathroom tiles, and bathtubs. Covering the treated skin area with bandages, cotton underwear, or a shower cap avoids some of this staining. In addition to the staining, many patients find the tar odor quite unpleasant; pharmaceutical companies are constantly trying to improve this aspect of these quite effective products.

The third type of preparation is particularly effective for removing very thick scales. These medications contain a compound called "salicylic acid." Like corticosteroids, salicylic acid ointments and gels are most effective when they contact the plaques for an extended period. After treatment, patients should cover their lesions with plastic gloves, plastic bags (for the feet), or taped-down plastic wrap for four to eight hours.

Patients with psoriasis have noted for years that exposure to the sun is beneficial in clearing their lesions. Daily sunlight exposure is effective for as many as 80 percent of patients. This treatment is relatively accessible for at least part of the year and inexpensive compared to the various medications available. Patients should have repeated but brief sun exposure and use sunblock creams and lotions to avoid sunburn, given the increased risk of skin cancer. Although sun exposure is helpful to most patients with common psoriasis, it rarely helps and can even worsen the pustulate and erythrodermic types. Since too much exposure to sunlight will damage rather than help any skin, even plaque-type patients should stop their sun exposure once psoriasis has improved.

For patients in many climates, sunbathing is possible for only a few months of the year. The development of sunlamps for use at home or in a dermatologist's office, hospital, psoriasis care center, or tanning parlor has made this therapy possible all year round. Because of the danger of severe sunburns, sunlamp treatments remain controversial. To reduce their danger, a dermatologist must carefully determine the amount of time of each treatment, the precise distance from the lamp, and the appropriate frequency of treatments for each patient to achieve maximal and safe results.

The curative effect of sunlight depends on the very short wavelength part of the light, called "ultraviolet." Ultraviolet B (UVB) waves help heal psoriasis, possibly by slowing down the high growth rate of cells in the epidermis. Both natural sunlight and sunlamps contain UVB and, therefore, have the potential to help psoriasis. They also have the potential, however, to burn the skin. Narrow-band UVB is safer and more effective than broad-band UVB. UVB phototherapy is the preferred treatment for breastfeeding women.

Patients with severe psoriasis may require ultraviolet A (UVA) waves from a special kind of sunlamp. The patient takes a dose of a psoralen. This substance makes the skin more light-sensitive. Then the patient exposes their skin to UVA inside a full-body light cabinet. Narrowband UVB is safer and more effective than broad-band UVB. Patients may require up to thirty treatments to clear their skin completely. The psoralen is often given in tablet form. However, some patients suffer fewer side effects if they paint it onto the skin or bathe in it. The early side effects of PUVA (psoralen plus UVA) treatment include nausea, itching, colored blotches on the skin, and occasional worsening of psoriasis. More worrisome are the possible later side effects: skin cancer and cataracts in the eyes. The danger of developing cataracts also exists from natural sunlight and UVB sunlamps; patients using any light therapy must use dark sunglasses that block out all rays harmful to the eyes. Excimer laser therapy is safe and effective for localized psoriasis and is FDA-approved for it. Narrow-band UVB and the excimer laser are safe during pregnancy. Breastfeeding women should not breastfeed for at least twenty-four hours after PUVA.

For patients with pustular and erythrodermic psoriasis, the retinoid acitretin can be very useful if its side effects are carefully monitored. Some dermatologists have been especially successful in combining PUVA or UVB and acitretin therapies; the improvement in the psoriasis is greater than with either alone, while the lower dosage of each minimizes risk and side effects. Acitretin should never be used with alcohol and is not safe during pregnancy.

A newer medication for psoriasis and psoriatic arthritis is apremilast (Otzela). This drug prevents the breakdown of a cell-signaling molecule called "cyclic AMP" (cAMP). Increasing intracellular levels of cAMP in immune cells slow them down. Apremilast improves symptoms in people with moderate to severe plaque psoriasis. In people with psoriatic arthritis, it improves symptoms but does not decrease disease progression. Apremilast causes diarrhea, nausea, upper respiratory infection, and headache. It can also increase the risk of depression. Another downside to this drug is its costliness.

For patients with widespread psoriasis who do not respond to corticosteroids, tar preparations, or the various light therapies, methotrexate is effective in more than 80 percent of patients. Patients with mild to moderate psoriatic arthritis also benefit from methotrexate. Methotrexate was initially developed to treat various kinds of cancer because it slows down cell multiplication. Thus, the psoriatic epidermal cells are prevented from reproducing and forming the scaly plaques. Often methotrexate must be taken for six months or a year, in pill form or by injection, to impact an extensive case significantly. Such a dosage poses a risk of severe and numerous side effects, including persistent feelings of sickness, indigestion, and diarrhea. Frequent tests are necessary to monitor the blood condition since methotrexate can interfere with the bone marrow's normal blood cells and liver and kidney function. Periodic liver biopsies, removing sample liver cells using a special needle are necessary because methotrexate can cause irreversible damage to this crucial organ. It is imperative that a pregnant woman never takes methotrexate or that a woman never become pregnant while taking it. The drug's ability to interfere with cell growth can cause many abnormalities in a developing embryo or fetus. Drugs called "retinoids" cause similar fetal abnormalities.

Patients with mild psoriatic arthritis that have few joints involved can manage their pain with nonsteroidal anti-inflammatory drugs (NSAIDs). NSAIDs include over-the-counter drugs like aspirin, ibuprofen, naproxen sodium, and stronger prescription NSAIDs like meloxicam, piroxicam, celecoxib, indomethacin, ketorolac, and diclofenac. Long-term NSAID use can cause stomach ulcers, kidney failure, and increased risk of heart attacks and strokes. If only a few joints show signs of arthritis, intra-articular injections of corticosteroids or low-dose systemic corticosteroids provide short-term relief. High-dose injections of corticosteroids into joints accelerate cartilage destruction and should be avoided.

Conventional disease-modifying antirheumatoid drugs (DMARDs) are first-line treatments for mild to moderate psoriatic arthritis. These DMARDS, besides methotrexate, include leflunomide (*Arava* and generics) and sulfasalazine (*Azulfidine* and generics). DMARDS are not effective in patients with axial disease.

Another medication effective in treating severe psoriasis and psoriatic arthritis is cyclosporine. It has brought dramatic improvement to patients with lifelong disabling symptoms. Many people, however, can tolerate the drug only for short periods. Because of its potential to cause high blood pressure and kidney damage, multiple drug-drug interactions, as well as an increased risk of cancer, this medicine is prescribed only with extreme caution.

Should the medicines mentioned above fail to provide relief, biologic therapies usually bring satisfactory improvement of symptoms. The first group of biologic therapies includes tumor necrosis factor-alpha (TNF-a) inhibitors. Five TNF-a inhibitors, adalimumab (*Humira* and biosimilars), certolizumab pegol (*Cimzia*), etanercept (*Enbrel*, and biosimilars), golimumab (*Simponi*), and infliximab (*Remicade* and biosimilars), are FDA-approved to treat severe plaque psoriasis and active psoriatic arthritis. TNF-a inhibitors are first-line treatments for severe plaque psoriasis and moderate to severe psoriatic arthritis, especially those who did not respond satisfactorily to DMARDS. Suppose a patient does not find relief with one specific TNF-a inhibitor. In that case, a different one may provide a better response.

If TNF-a inhibitors do not provide adequate relief, then ustekinumab (Stelara) may halt disease progression. Typically, patients who fail treatment with TNF-a inhibitors find relief with ustekinumab. This monoclonal antibody binds to and inhibits a common subunit used by the proinflammatory cytokines IL-12 and IL-23. Should ustekinumab fail, the following medications are two different drugs that inhibit IL-17A, secukinumab (Cosentyx) and ixekizumab (Taltz). IL-12, IL-23, and IL-17A are upregulated in the skin of psoriasis patients, particularly during psoriatic flares. Inhibition of these proinflammatory cytokines tamps down inflammation of disease progression. Rheumatologists typically prescribe IL-17A inhibitors to patients who did not respond to one or more TNF-a inhibitors. If these drugs fail, an alternative treatment is abatacept, an inhibitor of T-cell costimulation.

Suppose the patient cannot find relief with any of these medications or prefer oral medications. In that case, the Janus kinase (JAK) inhibitor, tofacitinib (Xeljanz), can help. JAK receives stimulatory signals inside immune cells and activates them. JAK inhibitors shut down the stimulatory signals in immune cells.

IL-23 antagonists can treat severe plaque psoriasis, but not psoriatic arthritis. Guselkumab *(Tremfya)*, tildrakizumab *(Ilumya)*, and risankizumab *(Skyrizi)* are FDA-approved for the treatment of moderate to severe plaque psoriasis in adults. They bind to IL-23 and prevent it from binding to the IL-23 receptor. IL-23 inhibition prevents the downstream release of proinflammatory cytokines (such as IL-17A) and chemokines.

All biologic therapies increase the risk of infection and tumors. Still, they can relieve the symptoms of severe psoriasis and psoriatic arthritis and arrest joint deterioration.

All these therapies described can bring partial or total clearing of lesions and even bring remission of the disease for a time. Until the cause of psoriasis is completely understood, no research group will find a permanent cure.

PERSPECTIVE AND PROSPECTS

Descriptions of psoriasis appear in the records of the earliest known civilizations. The term *psora* comes from the ancient Greek language. Psoriasis was considered a form of leprosy in biblical times. Despite this ancient history and extensive modern research, however, the exact cause of psoriasis is still unknown. Unlike many human diseases, psoriasis does not afflict animals; therefore, no adequate animal model systems exist to study it in a controlled laboratory environment.

Early work on psoriasis by dermatologists centered on differential diagnosis—the ability to distinguish psoriasis from various rashes caused by fungi, such as ringworm, and from the many forms of eczema or dermatitis caused by allergies. Skin biopsies developed by oncologists can now determine that the condition is not cancer; the portion of skin removed, when placed under a microscope, will clearly show the dermal and epidermal appearance characteristic of psoriatic skin.

While skin scientists have proven that psoriasis is not contagious, it has been known since the 1930s that many cases develop soon after strep throat and other upper respiratory infections. However, the bacteria involved are not the cause of psoriasis but rather a trigger for developing a condition for which the patient is genetically predisposed. Another trigger, excessive scratching or rubbing of the skin, can precipitate outbreaks in susceptible people; this is named the Koebner phenomenon for its discoverer. Neurologists and psychologists have proved that the disease is not caused by "nerves," even though stress of all kinds can make its symptoms worse. Health-care providers must help patients lower their stress levels if they are to keep the disease under control.

Nutritionists have searched for ways to use diet to help psoriatics, but to no avail. Although no particular foods either help or hinder the course of the disease, most dermatologists now recognize that drinking alcohol can precipitate and aggravate the disfiguring plaques.

Immunologists have been very involved in the study of psoriasis, even though it is not an allergic reaction to any substance in one's environment. In the late twentieth century, they pursued many possible connections between the streptococci bacteria that cause strep throat, the white blood cells called "T lymphocytes" that seek to destroy them, and the development of psoriasis. They believe that, in predisposed people, chemicals from the bacteria cause the T lymphocytes to give off substances that trigger the skin's uncontrolled and excessive production of epidermal cells.

Geneticists have been searching diligently for the source of the predisposition to psoriasis. Among the genes children receive from their parents are those that build particular proteins on their white blood cells called "human leukocyte antigens" (HLAs). Out of the hundreds of different HLAs that one can inherit, those who develop psoriasis always seem to possess similar combinations. Identifying the genes responsible for HLAs and the role of those genes in precipitating psoriasis may bring about significant improvements in the treatment and possibly a cure for this disease afflicting millions of people throughout the world.

—*Grace D. Matzen and Michael A. Buratovich, PhD*

Further Information

"About Psoriasis." *National Psoriasis Foundation*, 2013.

Camisa, Charles. *Handbook of Psoriasis*. 2nd ed., John Wiley & Sons, 2004.

Carvalho Ana L., and Hedrich Christian M. "The Molecular Pathophysiology of Psoriatic Arthritis—The Complex Interplay Between Genetic Predisposition, Epigenetics Factors, and the Microbiome." *Frontiers in Molecular Biosciences*, vol. 8, 2021, p. 190, www.frontiersin.org/article/10.3389/fmolb.2021.662047. DOI=10.3389/fmolb.2021.662047.

Cram, David L. *Coping with Psoriasis: A Patient's Guide to Treatment*. Addicus Books, 2000.

"Drugs for Psoriasis." *Medical Letters on Drugs and Therapeutics*, vol. 61, no. 1574, 2019, pp. 89-96.

"Drugs for Psoriatic Arthritis." *Medical Letters on Drugs and Therapeutics*, vol. 61, no. 1588, 2019, pp. 203-10.

Freinkel, Ruth K., and David T. Woodley. *Biology of the Skin*. Parthenon, 2001.

Husni, Elaine M. "Psoriatic Arthritis." *Cleveland Clinical Center for Continuing Education*, Oct. 2016, www.clevelandclinicmeded.com/medicalpubs/diseasemanagement/rheumatology/psoriatic-arthritis/. Accessed 5 Sept. 2021.

Mackie, Rona M. *Clinical Dermatology*. 5th ed., Oxford UP, 2003.

Marks, Ronald. *Psoriasis*. 2nd rev. ed., Sheldon Press, 1994.

"An Overview of Psoriasis and Psoriatic Arthritis." *National Psoriasis Foundation*, Feb. 2011.

Parker, James N., and Philip M. Parker, editors. *The Official Patient's Sourcebook on Psoriasis*. Icon Health, 2004.

"Psoriasis." *MedlinePlus*, 6 May 2013.

Shuman, Jill, and Purvee S. Shah. "Psoriasis." *Health Library*, 25 Feb. 2013.

Singh, Jasvinder A., et al. "Special Article: 2018 American College of Rheumatology/National Psoriasis Foundation Guideline for the Treatment of Psoriatic Arthritis." *Arthritis & Rheumatology*, vol. 71, no. 1, 2019, pp. 5-32, doi:10.1002/art.40726.

Turkington, Carol, and Jeffrey S. Dover. *The Encyclopedia of Skin and Skin Disorders*. 3rd ed., Facts On File, 2007.

Weedon, David. *Skin Pathology*. 3rd ed., Churchill Livingstone/Elsevier, 2010.

"What Is Psoriasis?" *National Institute of Arthritis and Musculoskeletal and Skin Diseases*, Sept. 2009.

Rheumatoid arthritis

Category: Diseases/Disorders
Also known as: Rheumatism
Anatomy or system affected: Heart, immune system, musculoskeletal system, respiratory system
Specialties and related fields: Geriatrics and gerontology, immunology, orthopedics, rheumatology
Definition: A chronic, systemic, and inflammatory autoimmune disease that affects the synovial membranes of joints and other organs in the body.

KEY TERMS

autoimmune: relating to an immune response by the body against itself

erythrocyte sedimentation rate: a screening test for active inflammation in the body

metacarpophalangeal: referring to the joints of the fingers closest to the body or knuckles

proximal interphalangeal: referring to the middle joints of the fingers

rheumatoid factor: an antibody found in the blood that identifies an inflammatory process

rheumatoid nodule: a small hard growth under the skin of the hands and elbows that may be present in those with rheumatoid arthritis

Sjögren's syndrome: dry eyes and mouth-related to rheumatoid arthritis

symmetric: occurring on both sides of the body at the same time

synovial membrane: a sac in a joint space filled with synovial fluid that reduces friction during movement of the joint

white blood cell: a component of the blood that indicates an infective or inflammatory process occurring in the body

CAUSES AND SYMPTOMS

Most experts believe that rheumatoid arthritis (RA) results from stress on the body that triggers an autoimmune response characterized by chronic inflammation, swelling, and pain in joint spaces as cartilage erodes and bony cysts cause deformities in the joints, and joint motion is lost. Specific genes associated with the immune system increase the possibility of developing RA.

Initially, persons with RA may have general, vague complaints such as fatigue, weakness, weight loss, anorexia, low-grade fever, and tingling in the hands and feet during the weeks or months after some traumatic physical event in their life. Joint stiffness lessens as the day progresses but may recur after inactivity and is worse after strenuous activity. Although all joints may be affected, the proximal interphalangeal or metacarpophalangeal joints and joints of the wrists, knees, ankles, and toes are most often affected. Rheumatoid nodules may appear on the hands and elbows. Sjögren's syndrome may also be present. There is also potential for renal, cardiovascular, pulmonary, neurological, and ophthalmological involvement. RA is a disease of remissions and exacerbations and therefore should be monitored regularly.

Diagnosis of RA involves identifying at least one painful or swollen joint that has been that way for at least six weeks, as well as a variety of blood tests intended to identify autoimmune disease. These tests may measure rheumatoid factor, anticitrullinated protein antibodies, erythrocyte sedimentation rate, and C-reactive protein. X-rays to identify erosions, bony calcifications, and narrowing in affected joints may also be undertaken.

TREATMENT AND THERAPY

The goals of rheumatoid arthritis treatment are to reduce inflammation and pain, slow disease progression, improve function, and maintain quality of life. RA medications have analgesic, anti-inflammatory, cytotoxic, and immunosuppressive effects. The three main categories of medication used in treating RA are nonsteroidal anti-inflammatory drugs (NSAIDs), disease-modifying antirheumatic drugs (DMARDs), glucocorticoids, biologic agents, and JAK inhibitors.

NSAIDs such as aspirin, ibuprofen, naproxen, and more powerful prescription NSAIDs, like meloxicam, nabumetone, celecoxib, piroxicam, and indomethacin, reduce joint pain and swelling but do nothing to slow the progression of RA. These drugs staunch inflammation by preventing the synthesis of prostaglandins, small molecules that promote inflammation. Additionally, NSAIDs relieve pain. Unfortunately, NSAIDs cause stomach ulcers, diminished kidney function, and increased heart attack risk with routine use. Therefore, NSAIDs are not long-term solutions for rheumatoid arthritis.

DMARDS, which include methotrexate, hydroxychloroquine, sulfasalazine, gold salts, azathioprine, cyclosporine, and leflunomide, slow the progression of RA. Methotrexate, even at low doses, decreases symptoms, limits joint damage, and improves outcomes. This drug interferes with single-carbon transfer reactions involved in making the building blocks for deoxyribonucleic acid (DNA) and ribonucleic acid (RNA). Unfortunately, methotrexate can cause substantial gastrointestinal distress, liver and kidney damage. Some patients tolerate it well, but others do not, and it is contraindicated during pregnancy. Hydroxychloroquine is an antimalaria medication that suppressed inflammation by unknown mechanisms. It is moderately effective for patients with mild RA and is usually well tolerated. Hydroxychloroquine causes nausea and retinopathy and is not safe during pregnancy. Patients on this drug should see their eye doctor routinely.

Sulfasalazine prevents joint erosions in RNA patients. It takes two to three months before it starts to work. This drug is commonly combined with methotrexate or hydroxychloroquine. Sulfasalazine

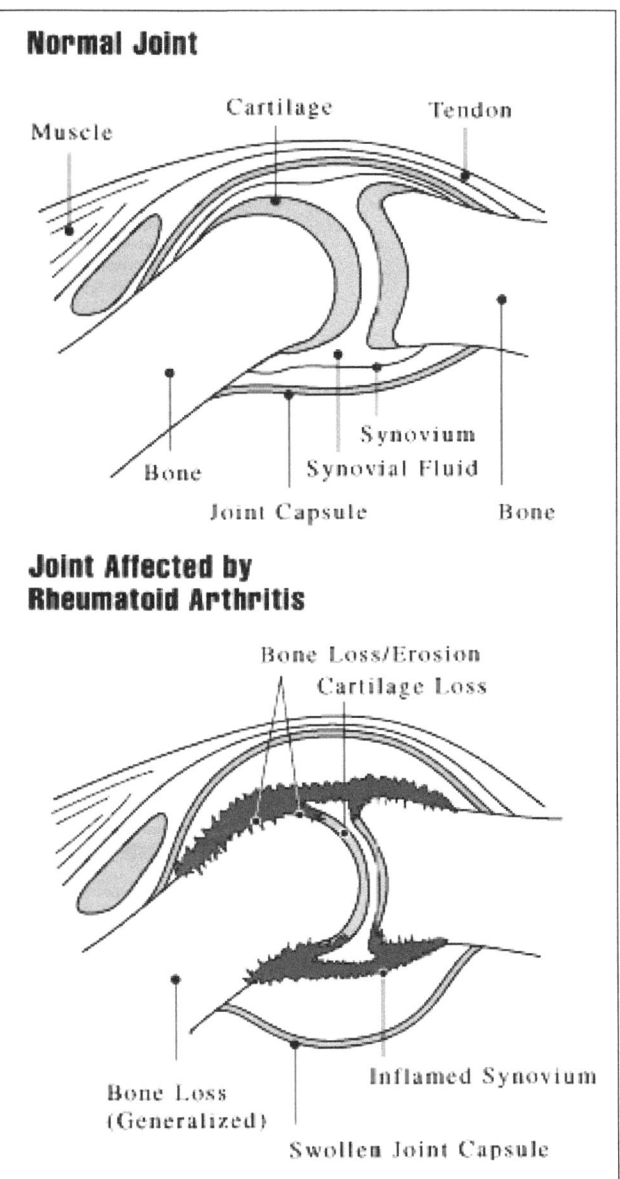

A diagram showing how rheumatoid arthritis affects a joint. Image via Wikimedia Commons. [Public domain.]

causes nausea, appetite loss, and rash, but it is safe to take during pregnancy. Gold salts include Myochrysine, Solganal, and others, and these drugs decrease inflammation in joints by unknown means. These medications cause pulmonary fibrosis and sensitivity to light. The availability of better-toler-

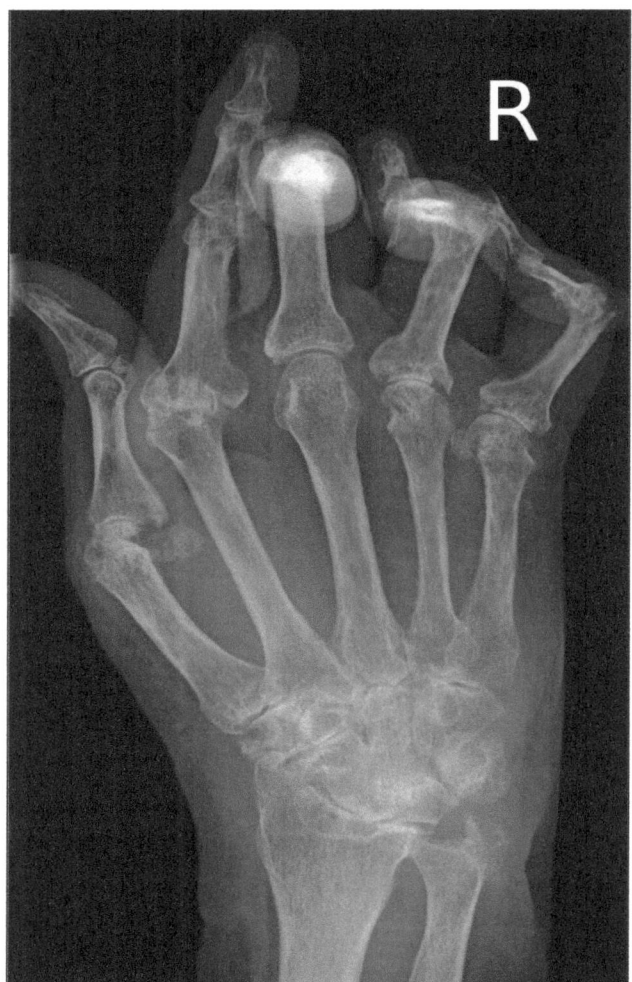

Hand X-ray of a person suffering rheumatoid arthritis. Photo by Dr. Martin Steinhoff, via Wikimedia Commons. [CC 3.0.]

ated options limits the utility of gold salts. Azathioprine is effective for RA patients whose disease extends beyond their joints. This drug is another DNA/RNA building block inhibitor, and it is safe for pregnant women. Azathioprine causes upset stomach, liver damage, and bone marrow suppression. It also increases the risk of developing lymphoma. Cyclosporine inhibits T-cell activation and diminishes joint erosion in RA patients. Cyclosporine is not safe for pregnant women and causes high blood pressure and kidney damage.

Leflunomide also inhibits the synthesis of DNA and RNA building blocks, effectively limiting RA symptoms and joint damage. Diarrhea commonly afflicts those who take leflunomide, as does hair loss, liver damage, rash, bone marrow suppression, and neuropathy. Leflunomide is also poisonous to an unborn baby, and future mothers and fathers should avoid this drug altogether.

Glucocorticoids are effective for rapidly reducing joint inflammation. Short-term courses of oral corticosteroids provide effective bridge therapy before the effects of a DMARD appear. Prednisone reduces joint and bone erosion. However, most clinicians do not prescribe them for long periods due to the extensive number of side effects corticosteroids cause. Injections of corticosteroids into the joints or interarticular injections relieve inflamed rheumatoid joint. Unfortunately, high-dose corticosteroid injections accelerate cartilage destruction. Therefore, low-dose triamcinolone or methylprednisolone remain better options for RA patients.

Biologic disease response modifiers are a newer class of drugs targeting areas of the immune system that cause joint and tissue damage. The two main biologic agents include tumor necrosis factor-alpha (TNF-a) inhibitors and interleukin-6 (IL-6) inhibitors. TNF-a is a cytokine that promotes inflammation, and inhibiting TNF-a activity effectively quells inflammation. Five TNF inhibitors are Food and Drug Administration (FDA)-approved for RA treatment and include adalimumab, certolizumab pegol, etanercept, golimumab, and infliximab. These drugs are monoclonal antibodies that bind to TNF-a and render it innocuous. All these drugs relieve RA symptoms and limit joint destruction more effectively than methotrexate alone. TNF inhibitors work faster than conventional DMARDs. Some patients report substantial improvement after the first dose. Combining a TNF-a inhibitor with methotrexate has synergistic beneficial effects. TNF-a inhibitors increase the risk of infections, particularly tuberculosis and lymphomas. Because they come in injector pens for subcutaneous injections, health-care providers can easily teach patients to administer their medication at home, increasing the convenience of these drugs.

IL-6 is another proinflammatory cytokine, and preventing IL-6 from binding to its receptor diminishes joint inflammation and RA progression. Two IL-6 inhibitors, tocilizumab, and sarilumab, effectively treat RA in patients who failed to achieve satisfaction with other treatments. The adverse effects of IL-6 inhibitors include infusion reactions, high blood pressure, low white blood cell counts, liver damage, and high blood lipid levels. Severe infections and hypersensitivity reactions can occur.

Other biologics that treat RA include the T-cell costimulation blocker abatacept and the anti-CD20 B-cell depleting monoclonal antibody rituximab. Both these agents treat RA patients who failed with other anti-RA drugs. Rituximab steeply increases the risk of various infections. Abatacept increases blood pressure, causes headaches, dizziness, and, rarely, allergic reactions. It also increases the risk of serious infections.

JAK inhibitors inhibit an intracellular enzyme called "Janus kinase" that transduces activating signals within immune cells. JAK inhibitors constrain cytokine and growth factor signaling. These drugs are available in the United States for use in RA and include tofacitinib, baricitinib, upadacitinib. These oral medications cause diarrhea, upper respiratory tract infections, headaches, and high blood pressure. Liver damage may occur with high blood lipids, low white blood cell numbers, and an increased risk of infections and cancers.

Research has shown that fish oils containing omega-3 fatty acids may also decrease inflammation in joints.

Fish oils containing omega-3 fatty acids may also decrease inflammation in joints.

> **INFORMATION ON RHEUMATOID ARTHRITIS**
>
> **Causes**: Autoimmune response, possibly resulting from stress on the body, genetic factors
>
> **Symptoms**: Chronic inflammation, swelling, and pain in joint spaces; morning stiffness; fatigue; weakness; weight loss; anorexia, low-grade fever; tingling in hands and feet
>
> **Duration**: Chronic
>
> **Treatments**: NSAIDs (aspirin, ibuprofen, naproxen), DMARDs (methotrexate, hydroxychloroquine, sulfasalazine, gold salts, minocycline, azathioprine, cyclosporine, leflunomide), glucocorticoids, surgical repair

Education for the management of RA includes isometric exercise, stress control, methods to protect joint integrity, and support groups that assist individuals and their families in maintaining independence and planning for care during exacerbations of RA. Surgical interventions to repair damaged joints and joint replacement are also part of RA therapy.

PERSPECTIVE AND PROSPECTS

More than two million Americans have rheumatoid arthritis, the majority of them women. The peak onset for RA is among people in their sixties. Juvenile rheumatoid arthritis occurs in children younger than sixteen years of age. Research has indicated a possible link between infections and the development of rheumatoid arthritis.

—*Sharon W. Stark, RN, APRN, DNSc*
and Michael A. Buratovich, PhD

Further Information

Arthritis Foundation. *Raising a Child with Arthritis: A Parent's Guide*. National Book Network, 1998.

"Drugs for Rheumatoid Arthritis." Medical Letter on Drugs and Therapeutics, vol. 60, no. 1552, 2018, pp. 123-28.

Firestein, Gary S., Gabriel S. Panayi, and Frank A. Wollheim, editors. *Rheumatoid Arthritis*. 2nd ed., Oxford UP, 2006.

Foltz-Gray, Dorothy. *The Arthritis Foundation's Guide to Good Living with Rheumatoid Arthritis*. 3rd ed., Arthritis Foundation, 2006.

Krause, Megan L, and Ashima Makol. "Management of Rheumatoid Arthritis during Pregnancy: Challenges and Solutions." *Open Access Rheumatology: Research and Reviews*. vol. 8, 2016, pp. 23-36, doi:10.2147/OARRR.S85340.

Paget, Stephen A., Michael D. Lockshin, and Suzanne Loebl. *The Hospital for Special Surgery Rheumatoid Arthritis Handbook*. John Wiley & Sons, 2002.

Poehlmann, Katherine M. *Rheumatoid Arthritis: The Infection Connection*. Satori Press, 2002.

"Rheumatoid Arthritis." *Centers for Disease Control and Prevention*, 19 Nov. 2012.

"Rheumatoid Arthritis." *Health Library*, 30 Sept. 2012.

"What Is Rheumatoid Arthritis?" *National Institute of Arthritis and Musculoskeletal and Skin Diseases*, Dec. 2009.

Sjögren's syndrome

Category: Diseases/Disorders
Also known as: Dry eye/dry mouth or sicca syndrome
Anatomy or system affected: Eyes, immune system, mouth
Specialties and related fields: Dentistry, family medicine, rheumatology
Definition: An autoimmune disorder resulting in the loss of tears and saliva.

KEY TERMS

Sicca syndrome: a condition characterized by dryness of the mouth and eyes
xerophthalmia: dry eyes
xerostomia: dry mouth

CAUSES AND SYMPTOMS

Sjögren's (pronounced SHOW-grins) syndrome is a chronic autoimmune disease in which the body's immune cells attack and eliminate the glands that produce tears and saliva. This results in dryness of the eyes and mouth and is referred to as sicca syndrome.

> **INFORMATION ON SJÖGREN'S SYNDROME**
>
> **Causes**: Unknown; possibly viral infection, heredity, hormones
>
> **Symptoms**: Dry eyes, dry mouth, blurred vision, eye discomfort, recurrent mouth infections, swollen salivary glands, hoarseness, difficulty swallowing and eating, extreme fatigue
>
> **Duration**: Chronic
>
> **Treatments**: Moisture replacement (eyedrops, saliva-stimulating drugs, salivary packets); immunosuppressive drugs or nonsteroidal anti-inflammatory drugs (NSAIDs)

The causes of Sjögren's syndrome are unknown, although evidence suggests that viral infection, heredity, and hormones may be involved. Sjögren's syndrome is one of the more prevalent autoimmune disorders, affecting as many as four million Americans. Nine of ten patients with Sjögren's syndrome are female.

Sjögren's syndrome can be challenging to diagnose because the symptoms are similar to those caused by other diseases. The symptoms can also mimic the side effects of several medications and may vary from individual to individual. Even when the symptoms are reported to a physician, dentist, or eye specialist, the proper diagnosis can be overlooked.

The classic symptoms are dry eyes (xerophthalmia) and dry mouth (xerostomia). Individuals with Sjögren's syndrome often have blurred vision, constant eye discomfort, recurrent mouth infections, swollen parotid (salivary) glands, hoarseness, and difficulty swallowing and eating. Dryness of other mucous membranes of the body, such as the intestines, lungs, and reproductive system, may also occur. Extreme fatigue can also seriously alter the quality of life.

Sjögren's syndrome is most commonly diagnosed in people in their mid-forties. In some individuals,

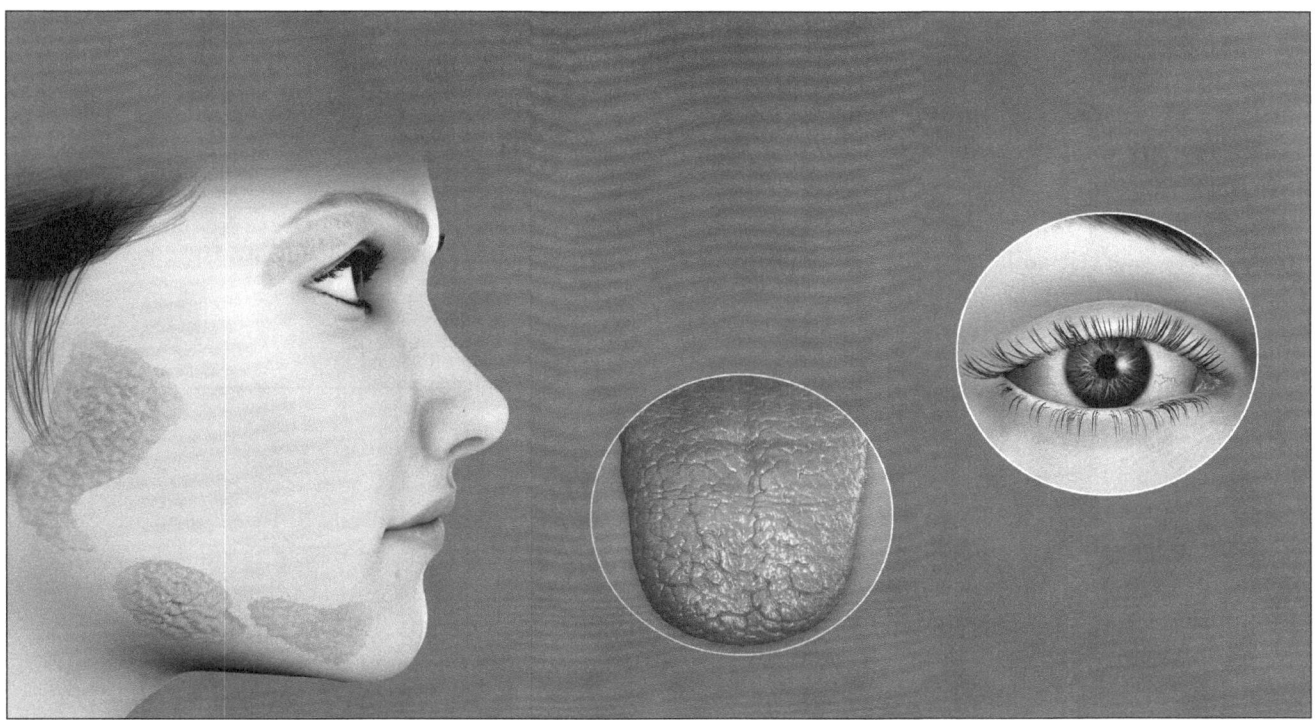

Characteristic dryness appears at multiple locations, such as the tongue, face, and eyes. Image by Scientific Animations, via Wikimedia Commons. [CC 4.0.]

primary Sjögren's syndrome affects only the tear ducts and salivary glands. In other patients, it is present in conjunction with other diseases such as rheumatoid arthritis, systemic lupus erythematosus, systemic sclerosis (scleroderma), or polymyositis/dermatomyositis (secondary Sjögren's syndrome).

Sjögren's syndrome also adversely affects dental hygiene. Saliva contains many different compounds that discourage cavity formation in the teeth. Also, the constant washing of the teeth keeps them clean. The xerostomia experience by Sjögren's syndrome patients increases tooth sensitivity and the risk of dental caries and periodontal disease.

TREATMENT AND THERAPY

Once Sjögren's syndrome is suspected, a doctor will order blood tests for autoantibodies against nuclear or cytoplasmic proteins. Other tests for Sjögren's syndrome include the Schirmer's test, which measures tear production, and salivary scintigraphy, which determines salivary gland function, may also be performed. A lower lip biopsy to determine the extent of inflammation may also be needed.

Moisture replacement therapies are designed to ease the symptoms of dryness. Routine use of over-the-counter artificial tears effectively wets the eyes and temporarily relieves the pain of dry eyes. Many artificial tears preparations are available. They usually contain some form of cellulose as a lubricant and polyethylene glycol or polyvinyl alcohol to prevent evaporation. Some artificial tear formulations contain preservatives that may irritate the eyes, but other preparations are preservative-free. Lacrisert, a daily insert, gradually releases hydroxypropylcellulose, a lubricant, after placement.

Other ocular medications diminish eye inflammation. These include ocular cyclosporine preparations: 0.05 percent (Restasis) and 0.09 percent (*Cequa*) formulations. These drugs help tear formation and reduce inflammation at the eye surface. Another ocular anti-inflammatory is the 5 percent ophthalmic solution of lifitegrast (*Xiidra*).

The everyday use of eyedrops controls dryness of the eyes, and saliva-stimulating drugs and salivary packets help with difficulties in chewing and swallowing food. For individuals with more severe complications, their doctors may prescribe immunosuppressive or nonsteroidal anti-inflammatory drugs (NSAIDs).

Dentists and dental hygienists treat Sjögren's syndrome patients with local anesthetics to mitigate tooth sensitivity during dental cleanings. Additionally, dentists treat Sjögren's syndrome patients' teeth with fluoride applications to strengthen the tooth enamel and discourage tooth decay. Sjögren's syndrome patients have difficulty wearing dentures due to dry and sensitive gums. Consequently, tooth implants seem to be a better choice for these patients rather than dentures.

PERSPECTIVE AND PROSPECTS
Sjögren's syndrome is named after the Swedish eye doctor Henrik Sjögren, who first identified the syndrome in 1933. There is no known cure for Sjögren's syndrome or a current treatment to restore gland secretion. The outlook for individuals with this condition is usually good because Sjögren's syndrome is generally not life-threatening.

—*Thomas L. Brown, PhD and Michael A. Buratovich, PhD*

Further Information
Masterson, Susan. *You Mean It Isn't in My Head?: What Sjogren's Syndrome Is and What You Can Do About It*. Independently published, 2021.
Ng, Wan-Fai, editor. *Sjögren's Syndrome*. Oxford UP, 2016.
Parker, James N., and Philip M. Parker, editors. *The Official Patient's Sourcebook on Sjögren's Syndrome*. Icon Health, 2002.
Rose, Noel R., and Ian R. Mackay, editors. *The Autoimmune Diseases*. 4th ed., Academic Press/Elsevier, 2006.
"Sjögren Disease." *Oral Health Topics, American Dental Association*, 16 May 2019, www.ada.org/en/member-center/oral-health-topics/sjogren-disease. Accessed 28 Aug. 2021.
Wallace, Daniel J., et al., editors. *The New Sjogren's Syndrome Handbook*. 3rd ed., Oxford UP, 2005.

Spondylitis

Category: Diseases/Disorders
Also known as: Ankylosing spondylitis
Anatomy or system affected: Eyes, joints, spine
Specialties and related fields: Cardiology, immunology, rheumatology, ophthalmology, orthopedics
Definition: A form of arthritis that affects the spine.

KEY TERMS
arthritis: inflammation of joints leading to painful stiffness
spondyloarthropathies: a family of long-term (chronic) diseases of joints that occur in children and adults

CAUSES AND SYMPTOMS
Spondylitis, also known as ankylosing spondylitis, is a form of arthritis that is chronic and affects the spine. It is a specific disease within a family of diseases called "spondyloarthropathies." Examples include psoriatic arthritis, Reiter's syndrome, and arthritis associated with inflammatory bowel disease (IBD). Spondylitis has unique features differentiating it from the other spondyloarthropathies and its prognosis. The cause of spondylitis is unknown, but the condition may be genetic. Most people with this condition or other spondyloarthropathies are born with a particular allele of class I major histocompatibility complex genes, *HLA-B27*. However, having this allele gene does not mean that a person will definitely develop spondylitis.

Symptoms include mild to severe back and buttock pain that is often worse in the early morning hours. This pain usually decreases with activity. The condition may begin in the teens or twenties and appears gradually over time. Continued inflammation of the ligaments and joints of the spine can cause the spine to fuse, leading to deformity and disability. The inflammation of ankylosing spondylitis can affect other parts of the body, most commonly other joints, and the eyes, but sometimes the lungs and heart valves. Other complications include arthritis of the hip joints and the joints between the ribs and sternum, bone spurs and inflammation in the feet, inflammation of the eyes, scarring of the lungs, inflammation of the prostate, and the aorta and aortic valve. Severe disease may lead to poor posture and deformities.

> **INFORMATION ON SPONDYLITIS**
>
> **Causes**: Unknown; possibly genetic
>
> **Symptoms**: Pain in lower back, buttocks, and hips in the morning or after inactivity; difficulty bending spine; bent posture; difficulty walking; pain in heels and soles; fever; appetite loss and weight loss; fatigue and decreased energy; eye swelling, redness, and pain; sensitivity to light; difficulty with chest expansion for deep breathing; heart failure; heart block
>
> **Duration**: Chronic
>
> **Treatments**: Exercise and physical therapy; medications (pain relievers, nonsteroidal anti-inflammatory drugs [NSAIDs]); assistive devices (canes, walkers)

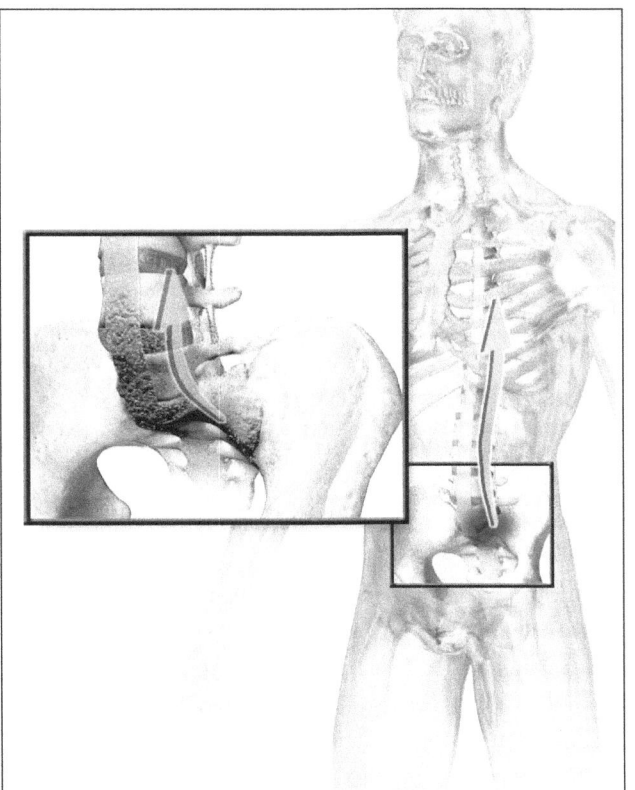

A diagram showcasing spondylitis. Image by Bruce Blaus, via Wikimedia Commons. [CC 3.0.]

Men are more likely than women to develop spondylitis; however, females may develop milder cases that sometimes go undiagnosed. Most spondylitis symptoms appear in early adulthood, before age forty. However, young males may have symptoms in early adolescence or even in childhood.

The hallmark signs and symptoms are stiffness and pain in the lower back, buttocks, and hips upon waking in the morning or after a period of inactivity; back pain relieved by movement and exercise; difficulty bending the spine; pain in the hips and difficulty walking; pain in the heels and soles of the feet; bent posture; straightening of the normal curvature of the spine; fever; loss of appetite and weight loss; fatigue and decreased energy; eye swelling, redness, and pain; sensitivity to light; difficulty with chest expansion for deep breathing; Heart failure; and heart block.

No definitive test can diagnose ankylosing spondylitis. Most doctors expect to see X-ray evidence of inflammation of the joint between the sacrum and the ilium, as well as any one of the following: inflammatory back pain, reduced mobility of the spine, and reduced ability to expand the chest. Blood tests results that can suggest spondylitis include an elevated erythrocyte sedimentation rate and anemia. The aspiration of synovial fluid from the joint will confirm inflammation.

TREATMENT AND THERAPY
Treatment includes exercise and physical therapy to help reduce stiffness and to maintain good posture and mobility. To treat pain and inflammation, physicians prescribe medications known as nonsteroidal anti-inflammatory drugs (NSAIDs). Celecoxib (Celebrex) provides effective pain relief and is well tolerated. Treatment of iritis involves regular eye examinations. Steroid eye drops reduce inflammation of the eye and dilating eyedrops reduce iritis pain. Dilating eye drops also protect from developing complications that interfere with pupil function.

If NSAIDs fail to treat the patient's condition adequately, biologic medications may provide relief. Clinical trials support using two classes of biologic agents, tumor necrosis factor-alpha (TNF-a) inhibitors and anti-interleukin-17 drugs. Anti-TNF-a drugs include etanercept (Enbrel), infliximab (Remicade), adalimumab (Humira), golimumab (Simponi), and certolizumab (Cimzia). Interleukin-17 inhibitors include ixekizumab (Taltz) and secukinumab (Cosentyx). There is no evidence that one anti-TNF-a is any better than the other, and patients who fail on one drug may find satisfactory relief with another. Patients who fail to find adequate relief with anti-TNF-a drugs should try anti-interleukin-17 drugs.

Assistive devices, such as a cane or walker, help reduce joint stress and inflammation. Surgery is rarely performed. Patients should choose chairs that help them avoid slumped or stooped postures. Other treatments include hip replacement surgery, treatment for iritis with steroid and dilating drops, and a pacemaker for severe heart block.

—*Jane C. Norman, PhD, RN, CNE*

Further Information
Klippel, John H., Paul A. Dieppe, and Fred F. Ferri. *Primary Care Rheumatology*. W. B. Saunders, 2002.
Koopman, William J., and Larry W. Moreland, editors. *Arthritis and Allied Conditions: A Textbook of Rheumatology*. 15th ed., Lippincott Williams & Wilkins, 2005.
McCormack, Paul L. "Celecoxib: A Review of Its Use for Symptomatic Relief in the Treatment of Osteoarthritis, Rheumatoid Arthritis and Ankylosing Spondylitis." *Drugs*, vol. 71, no. 18, 2011, pp. 2457-89, doi:10.2165/11208240-000000000-00000.
Royen, Barend J. van, and Ben A. C. Dijkmans, editors. *Ankylosing Spondylitis: Diagnosis and Management*. Taylor & Francis, 2006.
Schulze-Koops H., and A. Skapenko, "Biosimilars in Rheumatology: A Review of the Evidence and Their Place in the Treatment Algorithm." *Rheumatology*, vol. 56, no. suppl 4, 2017, pp. iv-30.
Van der Linden, S., and D. van der Heijde. "Ankylosing Spondylitis: Clinical Features." *Rheumatic Disease Clinics of North America*, vol. 24, no. 4, 1998, pp. 663-76.
Ward, M. M., et al. "2019 Update of the American College of Rheumatology/Spondylitis Association of America/Spondyloarthritis Research and Treatment Network Recommendations for the Treatment of Ankylosing Spondylitis and Nonradiographic Axial Spondyloarthritis." *Arthritis and Rheumatology*, vol. 71, no. 10, 2019, p. 1599.
Weisman, Michael H., Désirée van der Heijde, and John D. Reveille, editors. *Ankylosing Spondylitis and the Spondyloarthropathies*. Mosby/Elsevier, 2006.

Systemic lupus erythematosus (SLE)

Category: Diseases/Disorders
Also known as: Lupus
Anatomy or system affected: All
Specialties and related fields: Cardiology, dermatology, endocrinology, family medicine, gastroenterology, histology, immunology, internal medicine, nephrology, nutrition, orthopedics, pharmacology, physical therapy, psychiatry, psy-

chology, pulmonary medicine, rheumatology, vascular medicine

Definition: A chronic, inflammatory autoimmune disease in which the immune system attacks the body's structures. SLE can affect any organ or body system, especially the skin, joints, blood vessels, and kidneys. It is distinguished from two other forms of lupus: drug-induced lupus, which is caused by certain prescription medications, and discoid lupus, which primarily affects the skin.

KEY TERMS

antibodies: proteins manufactured by the body to attack and neutralize foreign substances, such as bacteria

antinuclear antibody (ANA): an unusual antibody that is directed against structures within the nucleus of cells

autoantibodies: antibodies that attack the body's cells and tissues

autoimmune: a term describing a disease in which the body produces antibodies against its cells

connective tissue: the substance holding the body and organs together

cytotoxic: having a damaging effect on cells

discoid rash: raised red patches

erythematosus: characterized by redness of the skin

hyperlipidemia: an excess of lipids (for example, cholesterol and triglycerides) in the blood

malar rash: a redness or rash on the face covering the cheeks and the bridge of the nose; also called "butterfly rash"

photosensitivity: sensitivity to light or sunlight

Raynaud's phenomenon: discoloration and pain in the fingertips induced by cold

serositis: inflammation of the lining of the lung or heart

CAUSES AND SYMPTOMS

The cause of lupus is unknown, but scientists believe that both genetic and environmental factors are involved. Although there is a genetic predisposition to lupus, and researchers have identified an associated gene in some cases, only 10 percent of lupus patients have a familial connection. Only 5 percent of children born to individuals with lupus will develop the disease. People of African, American Indian, Asian, and Hispanic origin seem to develop the disease more frequently than non-Hispanic Caucasians. Lupus affects both men and women, but the incidence is ten to fifteen times higher in women. Between 85 and 90 percent of patients are women. The majority of lupus diagnoses occur in young women in their late teens to thirties. Hormonal factors may play a role in this disparity because it is known that symptoms in women increase before menstrual cycles and during pregnancy. Environmental triggers include infections, exposure to ultraviolet light, extreme stress, and antibiotic usage (particularly penicillin and those in the sulfa group). Certain other drugs, particularly hydralazine, procainamide, and isoniazid, can also cause lupus. Still, this type of drug-induced lupus usually disappears after discontinuation of the offending drug.

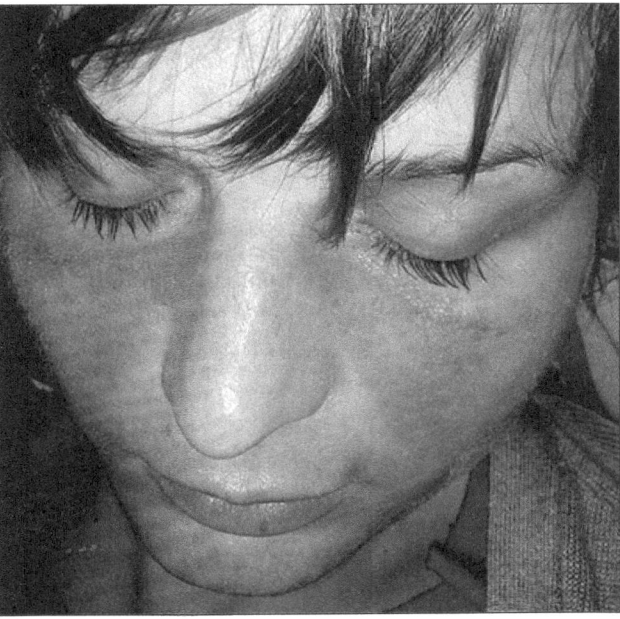

Young woman with the typical butterfly rash found in lupus. Photo by Doktorinternet, via Wikimedia Commons. [CC 4.0.]

> **INFORMATION ON
> SYSTEMIC LUPUS ERYTHEMATOSUS (SLE)**
>
> **Causes**: Unclear; possibly related to paramyxoviral infection
>
> **Symptoms**: Red or purple facial lesions, joint pain and swelling, fatigue, low-grade fever
>
> **Duration**: Chronic
>
> **Treatments**: None; alleviation of symptoms

Symptoms may begin suddenly with fever or may develop gradually over months or years. The clinical course is usually marked by remissions, periods when symptoms are minimal or absent, and relapses (called "flare-ups") when the patient experiences an aggravation of symptoms and general malaise.

SLE can affect all organ systems of the body. The production of autoantibodies is the underlying physiologic problem in lupus. These autoantibodies can appear in a significant number and variety, differing from patient to patient, thus causing their varying symptoms. General symptoms include fatigue, fever, anemia, weight loss, Raynaud's phenomenon, and headaches. Joint inflammation and pain (arthritis) occur in about 90 percent of patients and are often the disease's earliest manifestation. It usually occurs intermittently and generally does not cause permanent joint damage or deformity. Skin manifestations in most patients include malar (butterfly) and/or discoid skin rashes; redness on the hands, fingertips, and nails; mucous membrane ulcers in the mouth and nose; and photosensitivity. Inflammation of the sac around the lungs (pleurisy) or heart (pericarditis) is frequent, resulting in pain upon deep breathing or chest pain. There may be severe complications on rare occasions, such as bleeding into the lungs, which is life-threatening, or cardiac failure. Neurologic complications may also occur, including headaches, thinking impairment, personality changes, seizures, strokes, depression, dementia, and psychosis. Kidney involvement may be either minor or progressive, leading to severe nephritis that can be fatal. Ocular changes sometimes occur, causing conjunctivitis or blurred vision. In rare cases, retinitis, inflammation of the blood vessels at the back of the eye, can occur, leading to blindness if not treated quickly.

SLE is difficult to diagnose due to its variety of symptoms and similarity to many other diseases. The constellation of symptoms appears and progresses differently for each patient and initially may seem vague and unrelated. Usually, patients will first see their family doctors. Upon diagnosis or discovering particular body system involvement, the family doctor may refer the patient to one or more specialists. There is no single test for lupus. A physician will perform several laboratory tests as part of the differential diagnostic process, including blood and urine tests and biopsies of the skin and kidney. For a positive diagnosis of SLE, a patient must have at least four of the eleven criteria established by the American College of Rheumatology: malar rash, discoid rash, photosensitivity, oral ulcers, arthritis, serositis, renal disorder, neurologic disorder, hematologic disorder, immunologic disorder, and the presence of antinuclear antibodies (ANA).

TREATMENT AND THERAPY

There is no cure for lupus. Treatment is aimed at minimizing symptoms, reducing inflammation, and maintaining normal bodily functions. The treatment approach will vary according to the specific symptoms and organ involvement of the individual patient.

Preventive therapy involves lifestyle strategies aimed at reducing the risk of flare-up episodes. Patients are advised to follow a healthy diet, get adequate rest, and participate in moderate weight-bearing exercise to combat fatigue and muscle weakness. Counseling, support groups, and patient education help reduce stress and protect emotional well-being.

Other recommendations include smoking cessation, limited alcohol intake, and adequate intake of vitamin D and calcium. Avoidance of excessive sun exposure through protective clothing and sunscreens can reduce the occurrence of skin rashes and possibly systemic disease flares. Patients can learn to recognize the warning signs of an impending flare-up, such as increased fatigue, headaches, dizziness, stomach upset, fever, or the appearance of a rash. Regular laboratory tests can also detect an imminent flare-up. Early treatment of flare-ups can make them easier to control, prevent tissue damage, and reduce the length of time that the patient is given high doses of drugs.

Medications are an integral part of treating lupus and fall into four main categories: nonsteroidal anti-inflammatory drugs (NSAIDs), corticosteroids, antimalarial drugs, and cytotoxic and immunosuppressive agents.

NSAIDs are used to control symptoms and reduce muscle and joint pain and inflammation. Commonly used NSAIDs include acetylsalicylic acid (aspirin), ibuprofen, naproxen, indomethacin, sulindac, nabumetone, tolmetin, and ketoprofen. Since these drugs can cause stomach upset, patients are usually advised to take them with meals or take antacids or prostaglandins. Some NSAIDs have a prostaglandin added to the capsule. Patients taking NSAIDs must be monitored because of the potential adverse effects on the liver, kidney, and central nervous system.

Corticosteroids are synthetic hormones that have excellent anti-inflammatory and immunoregulatory effects and reduce symptoms promptly. They are used to treat a spectrum of lupus manifestations, especially in cases when organs are threatened. Prednisone is the most commonly used, followed by hydrocortisone, methylprednisolone, and others. Topical formulations are used for skin rashes, and oral doses are given for systemic involvement. Dosages are monitored carefully and tapered after initial inflammation reduction is achieved to reduce possible side effects. Corticosteroids may also be administered by injection into the skin or joint. For severe cases, intravenous (IV) administration of large doses of methylprednisolone (called "pulse steroids") for three days is given. Unfortunately, high doses of corticosteroids over long periods can produce unpleasant side effects, such as weight gain, rounded face, acne, emotional lability, hypertension, hyperlipidemia, increased risk of infection, diabetes, and osteoporosis.

Antimalarial drugs effectively manage skin rashes, joint inflammation, and serositis. However, it may take months before their beneficial effects become apparent. They also help protect against the damaging effects of ultraviolet light. The most common agents are hydroxychloroquine (Plaquenil), chloroquine (Aralen), and quinacrine (Atabrine). SLE patients can take antimalarial medications in combination with NSAIDs and other drugs to increase their effectiveness. They are beneficial when used with corticosteroids to decrease the dose of steroids needed. Damage to the retina is a potential side effect and is dose-related. Patients must be evaluated by an ophthalmologist twice a year.

Cytotoxic and immunosuppressive agents are potent drugs utilized in cases requiring aggressive therapy to protect major organs. They are used with, or in place of, corticosteroids to diminish the side effects of the corticosteroids. Cytotoxics are not approved by the Food and Drug Administration (FDA) for use in treating SLE; however, they are considered part of standard practice. These drugs target autoantibodies, thus suppressing the overactive immune response of lupus patients.
Cyclophosphamide (Cytoxin) and azathioprine (Imuran) are both used in the treatment of lupus nephritis. They are also effective in combating blood cell deficiencies, pulmonary bleeding, vasculitis, and central nervous system disease. Imuran is less potent but causes fewer side effects than does Cytoxin.

Methotrexate, mycophenolate mofetil (CellCept), cyclosporine, chlorambucil, and nitrogen mustard are other cytotoxic agents that have been used in the management of lupus. Intravenous immunoglobulin injections are given to some patients to increase the production of blood platelets. Side effects of cytotoxic drugs include nausea, hair loss, increased risk of certain cancers, increased risk of infection, sterility, and bone marrow suppression.

The FDA-approved belimumab *(Benlysta)* in 2011 for adults with active SLE. Belimumab is a human monoclonal antibody that blocks the binding of "soluble B-lymphocyte stimulator" (BLyS) to its receptors on B cells. BLyS is a small polypeptide that regulates B cell differentiation and stability. BLyS levels are elevated in SLE. The levels of BLyS correlate with disease activity. Inhibiting BLyS function diminishes the number of SLE flares and symptoms.

About 50 to 60 percent of patients with systemic lupus erythematosus (SLE) develop a kidney disease called "lupus nephritis." Lupus nephritis occurs during the first ten years, and up to 10 percent of these patients develop end-stage renal disease. Black and Hispanic/Latino patients have a significantly higher prevalence of lupus nephritis and generally have more severe disease. Standard treatment for lupus nephritis includes corticosteroids plus oral or IV cyclophosphamide *(Cytoxan* and generics) or mycophenolate mofetil. Upon resolution of nephritis, maintenance treatment to prevent it from recurring consists of continuing mycophenolate mofetil (preferred) or azathioprine (Imuran and others). A new FDA-approved therapy for lupus nephritis is voclosporin *(Lupkynis)*, an oral calcineurin inhibitor. Voclosporin should be used with mycophenolate mofetil *(CellCept* and generics) and a corticosteroid.

Pregnancy in a lupus patient requires special care. Even though more than 50 percent of lupus pregnancies follow an ordinary course, all lupus pregnancies are considered high risk. Doctors recommend planning pregnancy during times of remission. Recent studies contradict the traditional belief that pregnancy increases the chance of flare-ups and also suggest that most flare-ups during pregnancy are mild, consisting only of rashes, fatigue, and arthritis. Frequent doctor visits are a necessity to detect and treat any problems early. The obstetrician will regularly check the baby's growth and heartbeat to detect any abnormalities that might signal problems. Some lupus medications, such as prednisone, are safe to take during pregnancy because they do not cross the placenta. Others, such as cyclophosphamide, need to be used with caution or discontinued during the pregnancy.

Preeclampsia is a severe condition during pregnancy in which there is a sudden increase in blood pressure and protein in the urine. It requires immediate treatment of the patient and delivery of the baby. Preeclampsia affects approximately 20 percent of women with SLE during their pregnancy.

About one-third of women with lupus have antiphospholipid antibodies. These antibodies cause blood clots, which puts the patient at risk of developing them in the placenta, interfering with the baby's nourishment. Since these blood clots usually form in the placenta in the second trimester, often, the baby has developed enough to be delivered prematurely. Treating the mother with heparin reduces the chance of clots and miscarriage.

About 50 percent of lupus pregnancies result in birth before full term. The majority of babies born between thirty and thirty-six weeks will grow normally with no problems. Those born before thirty-six weeks are considered premature. Approximately 3 percent of women with lupus will have a baby with a syndrome called "neonatal lupus." This syndrome consists of a transient rash and blood count abnormalities and disappears by three to six months. Sometimes, a permanent heartbeat abnormality also occurs, but it is treatable, and the baby can grow normally.

The drugs of choice in pregnant women with SLE are hydroxychloroquine and low-dose aspirin. Other safe medications during pregnancy with caveats include glucocorticoids (lower dose), azathioprine (do not exceed 2 mg/kg/day), and tacrolimus. Safe blood pressure medicines for pregnancy include methyldopa, labetalol, nifedipine, and hydralazine.

PERSPECTIVE AND PROSPECTS
The identification of lupus as a distinct medical entity dates back to the twelfth century when the term *lupus* (Latin for "wolf") was used to describe ulcerative facial lesions because they looked similar to either a wolf's bite or a wolf's facial markings. Physicians noted other descriptions of the various dermatologic manifestations of lupus over several centuries; the first medical textbook illustration occurred in 1856. The Viennese physician Moriz Kaposi, in 1872, was the first physician to recognize and describe the systemic manifestations of lupus, as well as the fact that there seemed to be two distinct forms of lupus, discoid and systemic. In 1909, Canadian physician Sir William Osler described, in detail, the major organ manifestations of SLE. In the late nineteenth century, the usefulness of quinine and salicylates in treating lupus was reported. In the mid-twentieth century, the identification of antinuclear antibodies initiated the immunologic aspects of lupus. Around this same time, the first animal models were used to study lupus. Studies of animal models revealed a genetic component of lupus. A significant advance was the discovery of the effectiveness of cortisone in the treatment of systemic lupus. Corticosteroids remain the primary treatment modality, complemented by antimalarials (for skin and joint involvement) and cytotoxic agents (for severe kidney manifestations and other life-threatening complications).

The prognosis for lupus patients has improved dramatically as a result of earlier diagnosis and better treatment. However, the long-term prognosis for a given patient is still variable. It is often related to the severity and controllability of the initial inflammation. Also, the morbidity patterns of lupus patients have changed because of the increased usage of corticosteroids and cytotoxic drugs. Infections, accelerated atherosclerosis, and osteoporosis have become significant risk factors. Overall, however, the outlook for survival and quality of life has dramatically improved. As of 2005, more than 90 percent of lupus patients lived more than ten years postdiagnosis. Those with the organ-threatening disease had a lower rate, with only 60 percent surviving fifteen to twenty years.

A proliferation of research into the treatment of lupus that began in the 1950s continues and brings much promise for additional insight into the pathogenesis of lupus and new treatment modalities and agents. Some focus areas of current research include investigations into patterns of gene activity, the role of the protein interferon-alpha in the progression of lupus, environmental factors, immune ablation, stem cell transplantation, and the targeting of destructive white blood cells. An intensified effort by the federal government, private industry, and nonprofit organizations, such as the Alliance for Lupus Research and the Lupus Foundation of America, fuels the hope that better treatments, prevention, and ultimately a cure for lupus will be found.

—*Barbara C. Beattie and Michael A. Buratovich, PhD*

Further Information
"Belimumab (Benlysta) for Systemic Lupus Erythematosus." *Medical Letter on Drugs and Therapeutics*, vol. 53, no. 1366, 2011, pp. 45-46. An introduction to belimumab for SLE.
Hanger, Nancy C. *Lupus-The First Year: An Essential Guide for the Newly Diagnosed*. Marlowe, 2003. A "patient-expert" guides the reader step-by-step through the first year after diagnosis.
Kasitanon, Nuntana, Laurence S. Magder, and Michelle Petri. "Predictors of Survival in Systemic Lupus

Erythematosus." *Medicine*, vol. 85, no. 3, 2006, pp. 147-56. This large study correlates various factors to overall survival rates, such as demographics, clinical manifestations, and disease activity.

Lahita, Robert G., and Robert H. Phillips. *Lupus Q & A: Everything You Need to Know.* Rev. ed., Avery, 2004. Written jointly by an expert on lupus and a psychologist, this book provides straightforward information about all aspects of lupus in an easy-to-read, question-and-answer format.

Lupus Foundation of America, www.lupus.org. An organization dedicated to improving the diagnosis and treatment of lupus, supporting individuals and families affected by the disease, increasing awareness of lupus among health professionals and the public and finding a cure.

Meadows, Michelle. "Battling Lupus." *FDA Consumer*, vol. 39, no. 4, 2005, pp. 28-34. A complete overview of lupus written for the patient. Includes symptoms, diagnosis, treatment, and prospects.

Phillips, Robert H. *Coping with Lupus: A Practical Guide to Alleviating the Challenges of Systemic Lupus Erythematosus.* 3rd ed., Avery, 2001. Written by an eminent psychologist, this book provides valuable assistance to patients and families coping with the medical and psychological problems caused by lupus.

Scofield, R. Hal, and James Oates. "The Place of William Osler in the Description of Systemic Lupus Erythematosus." *The American Journal of the Medical Sciences*, vol. 338, no. 5, 2009, pp. 409-12, doi:10.1097/MAJ.0b013e3181acbd71. A description of the historic contribution of Sir William Osler in our understand of SLE.

Seppa, N. "Self-Help: Stem Cells Rescue Lupus Patients." *Science News*, vol. 169, no. 5, 4 Feb. 2006, pp. 67-68. A description of a promising new therapy procedure for patients with severe forms of lupus.

"Voclosporin (Lupkynis) for Lupus Nephritis." *Medical Letter on Drugs and Therapeutics*, vol. 63, no. 1631, 2021, pp. 134-36. An introduction to voclosporin for lupus nephritis.

Wallace, Daniel J. *The Lupus Book: A Guide for Patients and Their Families.* 3rd ed., Oxford UP, 2005. A complete compendium of information from a leading authority, this book provides thorough coverage of the pathogenesis and management of lupus and a discussion of standard, alternative, and promising new therapies. Includes references and sources of additional information.

Zonali, M. "Taming Lupus." *Scientific American*, vol. 292, no. 3, 2005, pp. 70-77. Authoritative coverage on the complexities of managing the various manifestations and complications of lupus.

THYROID DISORDERS

Category: Diseases/Disorders
Anatomy or system affected: Endocrine system, glands, neck
Specialties and related fields: Endocrinology
Definition: Underactivity (hypothyroidism) or overactivity (hyperthyroidism) of the thyroid gland.

KEY TERMS

cretinism: congenital hypothyroidism
Graves' disease: an autoimmune disease of the thyroid that causes overproduction of thyroid hormone
Hashimoto's thyroiditis: an autoimmune disease resulting in chronic inflammation of the thyroid; the most common cause of hypothyroidism in the United States
hyperthyroidism: a condition characterized by overactivity of the thyroid gland
hypothyroidism: a condition characterized by underactivity of the thyroid gland
thyroxine: the primary hormone released by the thyroid gland

CAUSES AND SYMPTOMS

The thyroid gland weighs about twenty to thirty-five grams and is located in the neck just below the larynx, or voice box. The gland is named for the shield-shaped "thyroid" cartilage that forms the front of the larynx. The thyroid has two lateral lobes connected by an isthmus that crosses in front of the trachea. Placing a finger on the trachea below the larynx makes it possible to feel the ridge-like isthmus pass under the finger after swallowing. The bilobed (two-lobed) shape of the rest of the gland is under the skin of the neck on either side of the midline. However, its boundaries are generally indistinct except to a trained examiner.

The thyroid produces two major hormones. Thyroxine, a product of the follicular cells, is the primary hormone produced by the thyroid that helps regulate metabolism. Within the thyroid are also parafollicular cells that produce calcitonin, an essential hormone involved in calcium metabolism. In the tissue of the thyroid are also embedded two pairs of parathyroid glands. The parathyroid glands produce parathyroid hormone, which is required to maintain normal levels of blood calcium. In the case of thyroid surgery, the parathyroid glands mustn't be damaged or removed; otherwise, there may be life-threatening tetanus—the sustained contraction of muscles, including those needed for breathing.

The normal functioning of the thyroid results from an elaborate physiological control system involving the brain's hypothalamus, the anterior lobe of the pituitary gland, and the thyroid gland. The hypothalamus produces thyrotropic-releasing hormone (TRH), which is passed by special blood vessels to the anterior lobe of the pituitary, the adenohypophysis. The TRH-stimulated cells in the adenohypophysis produce thyroid-stimulating hormone (TSH) released into the general circulation. When it reaches the thyroid gland, it stimulates the gland to produce thyroxine. Usually, thyroxine has a negative feedback effect on its production; that is, thyroxine can inhibit the activity of the hypothalamus and the pituitary to maintain its concentration in the blood. Various thyroid disorders, which are more common in women than in men, can develop from tumors that increase or decrease the hormones produced in these three interdependent structures.

The normal thyroid (or euthyroid state) produces mainly thyroxine, which is converted into triiodothyronine in the body's tissues before it has its

> **INFORMATION ON THYROID DISORDERS**
>
> **Causes**: Tumors, iodine deficiency, autoimmune disorders
>
> **Symptoms**: In hypothyroidism, intolerance of cold, low body temperature, tendency to sleep longer, lack of energy, infrequent bowel movements, constipation, possible weight gain, puffy face and hands; in hyperthyroidism, bulging eyes, intolerance of heat, weight loss, nervousness, increased or decreased skin pigmentation, more frequent bowel movements, hair loss, rapid heart rate
>
> **Duration**: Several months to chronic
>
> **Treatments**: Thyroxine, antithyroid drugs (propylthiouracil, methimazole), radioactive iodine, surgery

effects, which are generally to increase the body's metabolic rate. The thyroid directly produces some triiodothyronine. The thyroxine molecule contains iodide, the negative ion of iodine; iodine is, therefore, an essential component of one's diet. Suppose iodine is not available in the diet, as in vegetables grown in geographical areas glaciated in the past, such as mountainous terrain and the American Midwest. In that case, the body cannot produce thyroxine. Industrialized countries have iodine added to table salt to ensure an adequate supply of this element in the diet. A lack of iodine, and therefore a lack of thyroxine, prevents the functioning of the negative feedback effect of thyroxine on the hypothalamus and pituitary, resulting in deficient thyroxine levels and high TSH levels in the blood. High levels of TSH cause substantial thyroid growth, which will bulge from the neck as a goiter. A person with such a condition would be hypothyroid (that is, have lower-than-normal thyroxine levels in the blood) and may be affected by cretinism (mental impairment and stunted physical growth) if this condition occurs early in childhood.

Hypothyroidism can arise in other ways as well. Hashimoto's thyroiditis is a common type of hypothyroidism caused by an autoimmune reaction whereby white blood cells known as lymphocytes infiltrate the thyroid and gradually destroy its tissue. Individuals with this condition have detectable antibodies against normal thyroid proteins in their blood. The usual signs of hypothyroidism are intolerance of cold, a low body temperature, a lower rate of metabolism, a tendency to sleep longer, a general lack of energy, infrequent bowel movements, constipation, possible weight gain, a puffy face and hands, a slow heart rate, cold and scaly skin, a lack of perspiration, and potential emotional withdrawal and depression.

Graves' disease, the most common type of hyperthyroidism, is an autoimmune disorder in which antibodies mimic the action of TSH and therefore stimulate the thyroid to produce excessive thyroxine. Sometimes, nodules develop in the thyroid that make excessive thyroxine. Although a nodule in the thyroid may cause someone to suspect cancer, the nodules are usually benign. Hyperthyroidism may be associated with bulging eyes, but this orbitopathy does not always occur. Generally, there is an intolerance of heat, bodyweight loss, a high degree of nervousness, increased or decreased skin pigmentation, more frequent bowel movements, loss of hair, and a very rapid heart rate.

TREATMENT AND THERAPY
Patients suspected of having hypothyroidism or hyperthyroidism will have their blood tested for levels of TSH and thyroxine. Ultrasonography can detect tumors and serve as an anatomical guide for potential surgery. Hypothyroidism patients have prescribed a small oral dose (less than 1 milligram per day) of synthetic thyroxine (levothyroxine), which is adjusted until a euthyroid state is obtained within a few months. The usual replacement dose is about 1.6 to 1.8 microgram/kilogram body weight/day. Healthy patients under the age of 50 usually start with 50 to 100 micrograms/day. Older patients, especially those with heart conditions, begin at lower doses. Patients are maintained on thyroxine, with perhaps yearly checkups by a physician. Patients should also take levothyroxine on an empty stomach with a full glass of water, about one hour before breakfast. Other drugs, such as iron or calcium, and foods (soy, fiber, coffee) can interfere with thyroxine absorption or metabolism. Levothyroxine is safe during pregnancy and while breastfeeding.

For hyperthyroidism patients, several modes of treatment are possible. Antithyroid drugs, such as propylthiouracil (PTU) or methimazole, inhibit thyroxine synthesis. Radioactive iodine is commonly given to destroy part of the thyroid gland and thus reduce its thyroxine output. Second or even third doses of radioactive iodine may be given if the blood thyroxine levels remain high. Radioactive iodine is not used during pregnancy because damage to the fetal thyroid is likely. Additionally, surgery can be performed to remove enough thyroid tissue to restore normal thyroxine levels. Following any of the treatments, hypothyroidism may be induced, requiring that the patient receive thyroxine supplements.

Finally, surgery can reduce the bulging of the eyes caused by hyperthyroidism. However, the Food and Drug Administration (FDA) approved a new drug called "teprotumumab" (*Tepezza*) for IV treatment of thyroid eye disease. Teprotumumab is a monoclonal antibody that binds to the insulin-like growth factor-1 receptor (IGF-1R), inhibiting it. IGF-1R is overexpressed by cells called "fibroblasts" in the eyes of patients with thyroid eye disease. By blocking the activation of IGF-1R, teprotumumab decreases the progression of active thyroid eye disease. Adverse effects of teprotumumab include muscle spasms, nausea, hair loss, diarrhea, high blood sugar, and pain at the injection site.

—*John T. Burns, PhD and Matthew Berria, PhD*

Further Information

Bar, Robert S. *Early Diagnosis and Treatment of Endocrine Disorders*. Humana Press, 2003.

Braverman, Lewis E., editor. *Diseases of the Thyroid*. 2nd ed., Humana Press, 2003.

Hershman, Jerome M., editor. *Endocrine Pathophysiology: A Patient-Oriented Approach*. 3rd ed., Lea & Febiger, 1988.

Holland, Kimberly, "What's Hypothyroidism?" *HealthLine*, 19 Dec. 2020, www.healthline.com/health/hypothyroidism/symptoms-treatments-more. Accessed 27 Aug. 2021.

"Hyperthyroidism." *MedlinePlus*, 24 Aug. 2021, medlineplus.gov/hyperthyroidism.html. Accessed 27 Aug. 2021.

"Hypothyroidism." *MedlinePlus*, 17 Aug. 2021, medlineplus.gov/hypothyroidism.html. Accessed 27 Aug. 2021.

Kovacs, William J.., and Sergio R. Ojeda, editors. *Textbook of Endocrine Physiology*. 6th ed., Oxford UP, 2012.

Lights, Verneda. "Hyperthyroidism." *HealthLine*, 22 Mar. 2019, www.healthline.com/health/hyperthyroidism. Accessed 27 Aug. 2021.

Melmed, Shlomo, et al. editors. *Williams Textbook of Endocrinology*. 13th ed. Elsevier/Saunders, 2019.

Rubin, Alan L. *Thyroid for Dummies*. For Dummies, 2006.

Ruggieri, Paul, and Scott Isaacs. *A Simple Guide to Thyroid Disorders: From Diagnosis to Treatment*. Addicus Books, 2003.

ULCERATIVE COLITIS

Category: Diseases/Disorders
Anatomy or system affected: Abdomen, anus, gastrointestinal system, immune system, intestines
Specialties and related fields: Gastroenterology, general surgery
Definition: An inflammatory bowel disease that causes open sores in the colon.

KEY TERMS

antibodies: specialized proteins that bind to those foreign substances in the body that triggered their production, and neutralize them

B lymphocytes: special white blood cells that make and secrete antibodies in response to stimulation by foreign substances known as antigens

monoclonal antibodies: antibodies made by a single B-lymphocyte clone that are homogeneous and recognize only one antigen

mucosae: the innermost, mucus-secreting layer that lines the gastrointestinal tract

T lymphocytes: a group of closely related white blood cells that develop in the thymus and regulate the immune system's response to infections and tumors

CAUSES AND SYMPTOMS

Crohn's disease and ulcerative colitis (UC) are the two types of inflammatory bowel diseases (IBDs). UC only affects the large intestine (colon) and its upper mucosal layer, but Crohn's disease can cause lesions anywhere in the gastrointestinal tract and affects all layers of it. The incidence of UC varies widely and ranges from 0.2 to 24.5/100,000 persons.

The exact cause of UC remains unknown, but studies with identical twins and families with a history of UC have established a strong genetic component. However, environmental and behavioral factors contribute to the severity of the disease. Psychological stress, diet, smoking, the use of nonsteroidal anti-inflammatory drugs, breastfeeding, and isotretinoin (Accutane) have all been implicated as factors that influence the course and onset of UC.

UC presents as an autoimmune disease of the colon, since white blood cells called "T lymphocytes" accumulate at the bottom of the mucosal epithelium, attack it, and damage it. Yet another type of white blood cell, "B lymphocytes," which produce and secrete antibodies, release antibodies that bind to the colonic tissues and damage them. The continuous damage to the colon causes ulcers, which are replaced by granulation tissue (a mass of new connective tissue and capillaries that form on the surface of a healing wound). Accumulation of granulation tissue leads to the formation of pseudopolyps.

UC is graded as mild (rectal bleeding and fewer than four bowel movements a day), moderate (rectal bleeding and more than four bowel movements a day), severe (bleeding from the rectum, more than four bowel movements a day and the symptoms of systemic illness, e.g., fever, elevated heart rate, and low blood cell counts), or fulminant (more than ten bowel movements a day, continuous bleeding and a vastly enlarged colon or megacolon).

Another classification scheme for UC depends on the parts of the colon affected by the disease. Proctitis is limited to the rectum; proctosigmoiditis extends from the rectum to the sigmoid colon; left-sided colitis involves the rectum, sigmoid colon, ascending colon, and the beginning of the transverse colon; and pancolitis involves the entire colon.

UC patients typically complain of rectal bleeding, frequent bowel movements with mucous discharge, lower abdominal pain, and a constant feeling of needing to pass a stool even though the colon is empty (tenesmus). In severe disease, the patient also shows fever, severe diarrhea, cramps, and abdominal distension. Complete blood counts reveal an elevated white blood cell count (leukocytosis).

Some UC patients show symptoms outside the colon. These include inflammation of the iris of the eye (uveitis), arthritis, skin lesions (erythema nodosum), clubbing at the ends of the fingers, in-

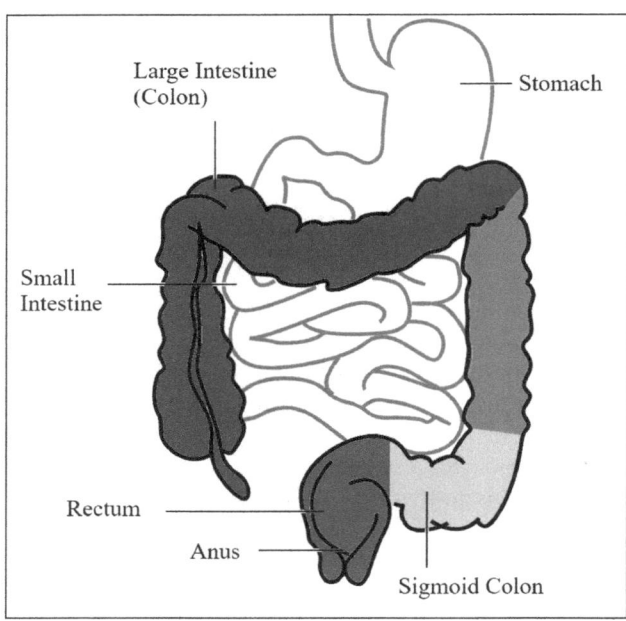

Representation of staging system for colitis, based on the Montreal classification, which is used to define the extent of involvement of ulcerative colitis. Proctitis (blue), proctosigmoiditis (yellow), left sided colitis (orange) and pancolitis (red). Image by Connormah, via Wikimedia Commons. [CC 4.0.]

flammation of the bile ducts (cholangitis), ulcers in the mouth, and blood clots (deep vein thrombosis).

Diagnosis of UC requires a colonoscopy or flexible sigmoidoscopy to rule out Crohn's disease, intestinal cancer, or diverticulitis. The gastroenterologist inserts a colonoscope through the anus and into the colon to view the colon. A colon from a UC patient contains continuous ulcers without the scarring normally observed in Crohn's disease. Biopsies of the colon reveal the involvement of the mucosae and not the lower layers.

TREATMENT AND THERAPY

Patients with active UC may require hospitalization and treatment with high-dose corticosteroids (e.g., prednisone). These drugs can relieve symptoms and induce remission. Because corticosteroids have significant side effects, they are typically not used long term.

INFORMATION ON ULCERATIVE COLITIS

Causes: Autoimmune response against the colon

Symptoms: Abdominal pain, bloody diarrhea with mucus for an extended period, fever, nausea

Duration: A chronic disease that lasts for the remainder of the patient's life, unless the colon is removed

Treatments: Aminosalicylates, corticosteroids, immunomodulators, surgery

The first-line treatments for managing UC include anti-inflammatory drugs that quell inflammation in the colon. Sulfasalazine (Azulfidine and generic), mesalamine (Asacol HD, Canasa, Delzicol, Rowasa, and others), balsalazide (Colazal and generic), and olsalazine (Dipentum) come in oral forms specially formulated so that they release their medicine primarily in the colon, and liquid forms for enemas. Anti-inflammatory drugs have few side effects, but if they do not control the patient's disease, then immunomodulators are added. These drugs include azathioprine (Azasan, Imuran), 6-mercaptopurine (Purinethol), and cyclosporine (Gengraf, Neoral, and Sandimmune). Because they suppress the immune response, immunomodulators cause severe side effects.

Biological immunomodulators, monoclonal antibodies that bind to and inactivate the pro-inflammatory protein tumor necrosis factor-alpha (TNF-a), include infliximab (Remicade), adalimumab (Humira), and golimumab (Simponi). Because of their potentially severe side effects and high cost, these drugs are a last resort. A newer biological immunomodulator, vedolizumab (Entyvio), is Food and Drug Administration (FDA)-approved for UC patients when other medications, such as corticosteroids, immunosuppressants, or TNF-a inhibitors fail to provide satisfactory relief. Vedolizumab is a monoclonal antibody that binds to and inhibits a specific "integrin," a type of cell adhesion protein. White blood cells use the integrin targeted by vedolizumab (a4ß7 integrin) to migrate from the bloodstream into the gastrointestinal (GI) tract. By blocking this integrin, vedolizumab quells inflammation in the GI tract.

If medications do not properly manage UC, then surgical options remain. Surgical removal of the colon (colectomy) or colon and rectum (proctocolectomy) can cure UC. A surgical procedure called "ileoanal anastomosis" reattaches the severed end of the small intestine to the anus and eliminates the need for a colostomy bag. Because UC increases the risk of colon cancer, some long-term UC patients have their colons removed as a preventative measure or when routine colon biopsies show signs of colon cancer.

PERSPECTIVE AND PROSPECTS

Although historical accounts contain several probable descriptions of UC, Sir Samuel Wilks first referred to UC by name in 1859. Some years after Wilk's discovery, the Surgeon General of the Union Army directly referred to UC and showed microscopic pictures of tissue sections from the colon of a UC patient. In the decades that followed, detailed clinical and pathological descriptions of UC sealed its place as a recognized condition.

Alicaforsen is a first-generation antisense oligonucleotide that binds to the messenger ribonucleic acid (mRNA) for the *ICAM-1* gene and inhibits the synthesis of ICAM-1 protein. Increased ICAM-1 expression in the colon correlates with the severity of the disease and inhibition of ICAM-1 decreases inflammation. In the future, antisense oligonucleotide treatments that specifically bind to and inactivate the messenger RNAs expressed by particular pro-inflammatory genes might be used to successfully treat UC. The FDA originally granted alicaforsen orphan drug designation as a treatment of pouchitis and left-sided UC. On the strength of a positive open-label trial and a case series in patients with chronic refractory pouchitis, the FDA granted alicaforsen (Camligo) a rolling submission for a license application for the treatment of pouchitis.

—*Michael A. Buratovich, PhD*

Further Information

Ali, Tauseef. *Crohn's and Colitis for Dummies*. For Dummies, 2013.

"Drugs for Inflammatory Bowel Disease." *Medical Letter on Drugs and Therapy*, vol. 60, no. 1550, 2018, pp. 107-14.

Sabil, Fred. *Crohn's Disease and Ulcerative Colitis: Everything You Need to Know*. 3rd ed., Firefly Books, 2011.

Zinser, Stephanie. *The Good Gut Guide: Help for IBS, Ulcerative Colitis, Crohn's Disease, Diverticulitis, Food Allergies, and Other Gut Problems.* Thorsons, 2012.

UVEITIS

Category: Condition
Related terms: Acute anterior uveitis, anterior uveitis, iridocyclitis, iritis
Anatomy or system affected: Eyes
Specialties and related fields: Immunology, ophthalmology, rheumatology
Definition: Treatment of the inflammation of the uvea, the middle layer of the tissues surrounding the eyeball.

KEY TERMS

anterior chamber: the from part of the eye between the cornea and the iris

choroid body: a structure within the eye that connects the iris to the choroid and consists of the ciliary muscles, radial ciliary processes to which the lens is attached by ligaments, and the ciliary ring that merges with the choroid

ciliary muscles: muscles that attach to the lens from the choroid body and alter the curvature of the lens to accommodate differing focal distances

cornea: the transparent part of the eye that covers the iris and transmits light to the eye's interior

iris: a flat, colored, ring-shaped membrane behind the cornea of the eye that has an adjustable circular opening or pupil in its center

Principal proposed natural treatments: None
Other proposed natural treatments: Turmeric, curcumin, vitamin E with vitamin C

INTRODUCTION

Uveitis is a condition marked by inflammation of the uvea. The uvea is the middle layer of the tissues surrounding the eyeball, stretching from the iris at the front of the eye to a lining beneath the retina at the back of the eye. The three main types of uveitis are named based on where the inflammation occurs: iritis (or "anterior uveitis"), which affects the front of the eye; cyclitis (or "intermediate uveitis"), for inflammation along the body of the eye; and choroiditis (or "posterior uveitis"), which affects the rear of the eye. Uveitis can also be called "acute" or "chronic," depending on whether it is short or long in duration.

Uveitis usually occurs in only one eye. In the most common forms of uveitis, the eye reddens, and the redness reaches into the area just next to the iris. The affected pupil may be smaller than the other, and its shape may be irregular. Vision is often blurred or misty, and blinking will not clear it. Deep, aching pain generally accompanies uveitis.

Uveitis can begin after injury to the eye or after eye surgery. Still, it can also start with no apparent trigger. While the underlying cause of uveitis is unknown, autoimmune processes probably play a role, given its association with autoimmune diseases, such as juvenile idiopathic arthritis, Behçet syndrome, ulcerative colitis, and ankylosing spondylitis. If left untreated,

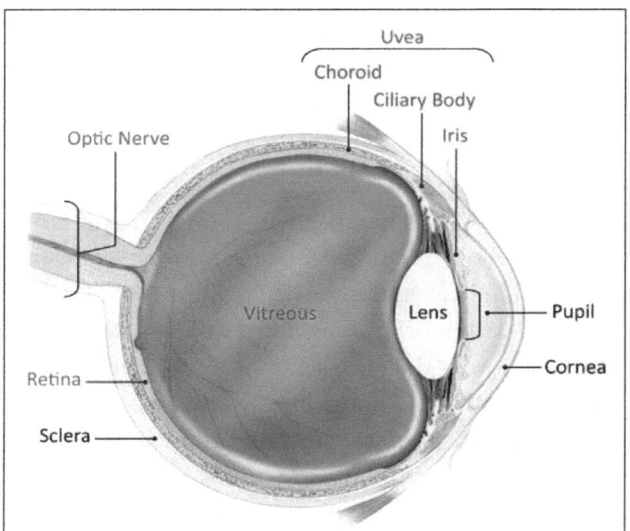

Diagram of the uvea; parts of the eye most affected by uveitis. Image via the National Eye Institute (nei.nih.gov).

uveitis can cause permanent damage to vision, including blindness. For this reason, one should seek medical examination and treatment. Uveitis is diagnosed with a special medical tool called a "slit lamp." Treatment involves medications to reduce inflammation and to control pressure in the eye.

STANDARD TREATMENTS

Initial treatment of noninfectious uveitis includes topical glucocorticoids such as prednisone acetate (1 percent). Dilating drops such as cyclopentolate (one percent) relieve pain due to the spasm of the muscles controlling the pupil and help prevent posterior adhesions (synechiae) can interfere with pupil function. Generally, uveitis posterior to the lens does not respond to topical medications. Still, a drug called "difluprenate" (Durezol) penetrates the vitreous humor better than other topical corticosteroids. Unfortunately, it also has a greater tendency to raise intraocular pressure and cause cataracts. Triamcinolone Injections into the eye with triamcinolone or slow-release polymers that release steroids are riskier but provide more sustained benefits. Some patients, however, may decline a periocular or intraocular injection.

Uveitis that resists treatment requires systemic remedies. Likewise, patients with glaucoma also require system treatments since topical or interocular steroids raise eye pressures. Systemic treatments vary but include immunosuppressive agents, such as azathioprine, mycophenolate mofetil, methotrexate, calcineurin inhibitors, such as cyclosporine and tacrolimus, and, rarely, alkylating agents, such as cyclophosphamide and oral corticosteroids. Alternative treatments include the tumor necrosis factor-alpha (THF-a) inhibitors infliximab and adalimumab. Because of their costliness, TNF-a inhibitors are not first-line treatments. However, some causes of non-infectious uveitis, such as Behçet syndrome, juvenile idiopathic arthritis, or ankylosing spondylitis, respond well to TNF-a inhibitors.

PROPOSED NATURAL TREATMENTS

No natural treatment can substitute for standard medical care for uveitis. However, two natural substances, vitamin C and vitamin E have shown promise when combined with standard treatment.

In a double-blind trial of 145 people undergoing treatment for acute anterior uveitis, participants received either a placebo or combined treatment with vitamin C (500 milligrams [mg] twice daily) and vitamin E (100 mg twice daily). People receiving the actual treatment had better visual acuity at the end of the eight-week study period. Researchers hypothesized that free radicals (a class of dangerous, naturally occurring chemicals) play a role in the eye injury caused by uveitis. Vitamin C and vitamin E are antioxidants, and they tend to neutralize free radicals. While further study is necessary to corroborate these results, it appears plausible that the use of these antioxidants may help keep the eye healthy while it recovers from the condition.

Other antioxidants have also been recommended for acute uveitis, but there is no objective evidence that they are helpful. These include flavonoids such

---

ANTIOXIDANTS FOR TREATING UVEITIS

Antioxidants are substances that may prevent potentially disease-producing cell damage that can result from natural bodily processes or exposure to certain chemicals. Several different antioxidants occur in foods and dietary supplements, including vitamins C and E.

Oxidation—one of the body's natural chemical processes—can produce reactive oxygen species (ROS), highly unstable molecules that damage cells. For example, when the body breaks down foods for energy or storage, it produces ROSs. The body also makes ROSs when it encounters tobacco smoke, radiation, and environmental contaminants. ROSs cause damage, known as oxidative stress, which plays a role in the onset of many diseases, including eye disease, Alzheimer's disease, cancer, heart disease, Parkinson's disease, and rheumatoid arthritis. In laboratory experiments, antioxidant molecules counter oxidative stress and its associated damage.

as curcumin, carotenoids, plant sterols, selenium, and zinc.

Antioxidants are also often recommended for chronic uveitis (combined with conventional care). One study examined the potential benefits of an antioxidant extract made from the herb turmeric and appeared to find benefit. However, this study lacked a placebo group and, therefore, cannot be taken as reliable.

Vitamin D may also play a role in uveitis activity. In a retrospective case-control study with 765 patients, patients with low vitamin D levels were more likely to have active uveitis than patients with normal vitamin D levels. A prospective case-control study with 151 participants compared serum vitamin D levels of those with active uveitis and those with inactive uveitis; low serum levels of vitamin D were associated with active uveitis, and vitamin D supplementation, as well as sun exposure, were associated with decreased uveitis activity.

Manufacturers of natural treatments for uveitis make numerous other recommendations based on speculation only. These treatments include fish oil, flax oil, manganese, vitamin B complex (a mixture of vitamins B_1, B_2, B_3, B_6, and B_{12}; pantothenic acid; biotin; and folate), olive leaf extract, red clover, and zinc.

—Ekta Patel, MD

Further Information

Chiu, Zelia K., et al. "Patterns of Vitamin D Levels and Exposures in Active and Inactive Noninfectious Uveitis Patients." *Ophthalmology*, vol. 127, no. 2, 2020, pp. 230-37.

Dawczynski, J., et al. "Selenium and Zinc in Patients with Acute and Chronic Uveitis." *Biological Trace Element Research*, vol. 113, no. 2, 2006, pp. 131-37.

Gaby, A. R. "Nutritional Therapies for Ocular Disorders." *Alternative Medicine Review*, vol. 13, 2008, pp. 191-204.

Jaffe, Glenn, J., et al. "Adalimumab in Patients with Active Noninfectious Uveitis." *The New England Journal of Medicine*, vol. 375, no. 10, 2016, pp. 932-43, doi:10.1056/NEJMoa1509852.

Lal, B., et al. "Efficacy of Curcumin in the Management of Chronic Anterior Uveitis." *Phytotherapy Research*, vol. 13, 1999, pp. 318-322.

Liu, Xiu-Fen, et al. "Curcumin, a Potential Therapeutic Candidate for Anterior Segment Eye Diseases: A Review." *Frontiers in Pharmacology*, vol. 8, no. 66, 14 Feb. 2017.

Llop, Stephanie, M., et al. "Association of Low Vitamin D Levels with Noninfectious Uveitis and Scleritis." *Ocular Immunology and Inflammation*, vol. 27, no. 4, 2019, pp. 602-9.

Van Rooij, J., et al. "Oral Vitamins C and E as Additional Treatment in Patients with Acute Anterior Uveitis." *British Journal of Ophthalmology*, vol. 83, 1999, pp. 1277-82.

Yadav, U. C. S., et al. "Emerging Role of Antioxidants in the Protection of Uveitis Complications." *Current Medicinal Chemistry*, vol. 18, no. 6, 2011, pp. 931-42.

VASCULITIS

Category: Diseases/Disorders

Anatomy or system affected: Abdomen, blood vessels, chest, circulatory system, ears, eyes, gastrointestinal system, hands, immune system, intestines, kidneys, legs, lungs, nerves, nose, respiratory system, skin

Specialties and related fields: Cardiology, dermatology, gastroenterology, nephrology, neurology, ophthalmology, otolaryngology, pulmonary medicine, rheumatology

Definition: Several conditions characterized by inflammation of blood vessels, both arteries, and veins, that leads to decreased circulation in the affected tissue or organ, which can damage the tissue or organ. Inflammation may be continuous or spotty and can damage the blood vessel walls, leading to the destruction of the blood vessel or the formation of an aneurysm.

KEY TERMS

blood vessels: tubular structures that carry blood throughout the body, into tissues and organs, consisting of veins, arteries, or capillaries

corticosteroids: a group of synthetic or natural steroid hormones produced by the adrenal cortex that regulate metabolic functions, salt balances, and treat inflammation.

endothelium: a thin, cellular membrane that lines the insides of the heart and blood vessels

inflammation: a protective reaction to injury, disease, or irritation of tissues, characterized by pain, redness, heat, and swelling

CAUSES AND SYMPTOMS

There is no definite cause of vasculitis. Some types may be autoimmune, in which the body attacks its tissues. Some types of vasculitis may result from allergic reactions to a medication, exposure to a toxic chemical, or viruses, such as hepatitis B and hepatitis C viruses. Vasculitis may occur with connective tissue diseases such as rheumatoid arthritis, Sjögren's syndrome, and lupus, or with a blood cell cancer such as leukemia or lymphoma.

These conditions are often classified by the size of the blood vessels involved or the type of cells involved in the blood vessel inflammation. Large vessel vasculitis includes Takayasu arteritis, Behçet's syndrome, polymyalgia rheumatica, and giant cell arteritis. Medium vessel vasculitis includes Buerger's disease, polyarteritis nodosa, Kawasaki disease, cutaneous vasculitis, and primary central nervous system vasculitis. Small vessel vasculitis includes Wegener's granulomatosis, Churg-Strauss arteritis, microscopic polyarteritis/angiitis, hyperallergic vasculitis, Henoch-Schonlein purpura, essential cryoglobulinemic vasculitis, hypersensitivity vasculitis, and vasculitis secondary to connective tissue disorders. The cells observed in the various vasculitis types are neutrophils, lymphocytes, leukocytes, eosinophils, or granulomatous cells. The two classification systems tend to overlap, and the cell type can change in a type of vasculitis as the condition progresses.

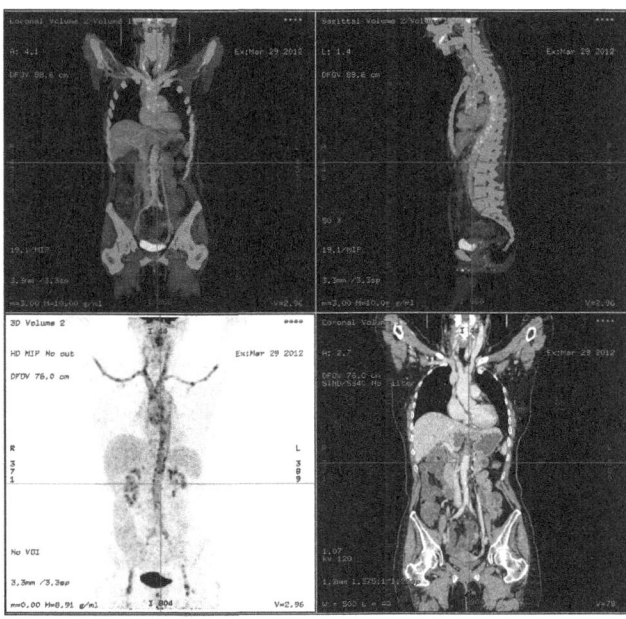

Severe vasculitis of the major vessels, displayed on FDG-PET/CT. Photo by Hg6996, via Wikimedia Commons. [CC 3.0.]

The first symptoms reported are usually systemic. They include fatigue, fever, night sweats, weakness, weight loss, anorexia, muscle, and joint pain, and numbness. More specific symptoms depend on the type of vasculitis. Some of the types demonstrate only skin lesions, which can be purple spots (purpura), areas of necrosis, or skin ulcers. They include hypersensitivity vasculitis, Buerger's disease, and cutaneous vasculitis. Each type of vasculitis then has symptoms based on the part of the body that is affected. Symptoms can include a skin rash, joint or extremity pain, neuropathy, ulcerations of the skin, headache, visual problems, abdominal pain, vomiting, diarrhea, anemia, coughing up blood, muscle pain, conjunctivitis, weakness, heart failure, palpitations, sinus problems, bleeding into the lungs, and abnormal kidney function. Some types of vasculitis are self-limiting, but most are chronic conditions. The damage that vasculitis can cause can be life-threatening.

> **INFORMATION ON VASCULITIS**
>
> **Causes**: Body attacking its blood vessels as a result of autoimmunity, certain viral infections, some cancers, some connective tissue diseases (rheumatoid arthritis), allergies to some medications
>
> **Symptoms**: Depends on type; fatigue, fever, night sweats, weakness, weight loss, anorexia, muscle, and joint pain, numbness, skin rash, skin ulcers, headache, visual problems, abdominal pain, vomiting, diarrhea, anemia, coughing up blood, muscle pain, heart failure, sinus problems, kidney problems
>
> **Duration**: Some self-limiting, others chronic
>
> **Treatments**: Drugs suppressing inflammation or immune system, particularly corticosteroids (prednisone, Cytoxan)

Vasculitis is diagnosed by blood tests, including a complete blood count (CBC), general chemistry, liver function tests, and kidney function tests. These tests demonstrate what body organs are affected by vasculitis. Some tests that are commonly abnormal with vasculitis are erythrocyte sedimentation rate (ESR), C-reactive protein (CRP), antinuclear antibody (ANA), and antineutrophil cytoplasmic antibody (ANCA). These tests indicate the presence of inflammation in the body, which is a sign of vasculitis. The most specific test for vasculitis is a biopsy of an affected body area, such as the skin or a kidney. The biopsy demonstrates the presence of vasculitis. Sometimes, angiograms (X-rays of the blood vessels) detect vasculitis. If kidney problems are suspected, then urine is tested for the presence of microscopic blood and protein.

TREATMENT AND THERAPY

The treatment for vasculitis depends on the type of disease. The most common treatment is the administration of corticosteroid drugs, such as prednisone or methylprednisolone. Patients can take these medicines orally or intravenously. Corticosteroids control the inflammation in the blood vessels. Often, other immune system suppressant drugs are administered with corticosteroids. They include cyclophosphamide, azathioprine, and methotrexate. Like corticosteroids, patients can receive these three immunosuppressant medications orally or intravenously. Both of these groups of medications have many side effects. Corticosteroids can cause weight gain, diabetes, osteoporosis, insomnia, hypertension, increased risk of infection, mood changes, stomach upset, and cataracts. The immune system suppressant drugs are cytotoxic substances that treat some types of cancer and prevent the rejection of transplanted organs. They, too, have many side effects. They can cause hair loss, fatigue, bladder cancer, hemorrhagic cystitis, increased risk of infections, nausea, vomiting, diarrhea, and liver damage.

Usually, vasculitis responds well to one or both of these medications, mainly if diagnosed early. If vasculitis does not respond well to this treatment, plasmapheresis or the medication interferon-alpha are viable alternative treatments. Plasmapheresis is a procedure that removes the plasma from blood drawn from the body. Centrifuging the blood separates it into plasma with other immune cells and the red blood cells, and the patient receives their enriched red blood cells. Eliminating many of the white blood cells can interfere with the immune response. Interferon-alpha is a biological drug that can affect the immune response. This drug is still under study as a potential treatment for vasculitis.

PROSPECTIVE AND PROSPECTS

Although symptoms of conditions that sound like vasculitis have appeared in ancient medical writings, vasculitis was not identified until 1866 by Adolf Kussmaul. Kussmaul noted that the affected patient had nodules under his skin. During the autopsy, he saw nodules on the patient's arteries. Kussmaul called this condition "periarteritis nodosa." He attributed the arterial nodules to inflammation of the blood vessels. He considered it a novel condition that had not been described previously.

After Kussmaul's description of periarteritis nodosa, pathologists compared other cases of apparent vasculitis to it. However, many of these conditions were different types of vasculitis. There are approximately twenty different types of vasculitis. Giant cell arteritis was described in 1890. Giant cell arteritis is inflammation of the large temporal arteries of the head. It causes localized pain and tenderness, and it can lead to blindness if untreated. A biopsy of a temporal artery diagnosed it. Polymyalgia rheumatica was first described in 1957, and it occurs in roughly 50 percent of those who develop giant cell arteritis. Polymyalgia rheumatica affects the large arteries of the shoulders and hips and causes muscle pain in the arms and legs.

Takayasu's arteritis, first described in 1908, is inflammation of the aorta and its major branches, the optical arteries. This vasculitis affects young women and can lead to heart failure. Buerger's disease was also described in 1908. It is characterized by a severe lack of blood flow to the hands and feet, causing severe pain, blue fingers and toes, and tissue death. Buerger's disease is caused by cigarette smoking. Kawasaki's disease was described in 1939. It demonstrates inflammation of the medium-sized arteries of the mucous membranes, lymph nodes, and coronary arteries. This condition occurs only in young children and causes swollen glands in the neck, conjunctivitis, inflammation around the mouth and on the palms of the hands and the bottom of the feet, a skin rash, and aneurysms of the coronary arteries.

The more severe forms of vasculitis are Wegener's granulomatosis, Churg-Strauss syndrome, and microscopic polyarteritis. These conditions can be rapidly fatal unless treated aggressively. All three are associated with the presence of antineutrophil cytoplasmic antibodies in the blood. Wegener's granulomatosis, first described in 1936, affects the small blood vessels of the skin, lungs, eyes, sinuses, and kidneys. Churg-Strauss syndrome, first described in 1951, begins with the development of asthma and then progresses to affect the nerves, skin, heart, lungs, gastrointestinal tract, and kidneys. Microscopic polyarteritis, first described in 1948, affects the smallest blood vessels of the lungs and kidneys. All three conditions can lead to bleeding by the small blood vessels in the lungs and kidney failure.

—Christine M. Carroll, RN, BSN, MBA

Further Information
Qontro Medical Guides. *Vasculitis Medical Guide*. Author, 2008.
Schwar, Sheri Lyn. *Vasculitis: Sick and Tired of Being Sick and Tired*. iUniverse, 2006.
Swart, Myrna. *There Must Be a Reason: My Daughter's Battle with Wegener's Granulomatosis*. iUniverse, 2008.
"Vasculitis." *MedlinePlus*, 16 May 2013.
"Vasculitis Syndromes of the Central and Peripheral Nervous Systems Fact Sheet." *National Institute of Neurological Disorders and Stroke*, 7 Feb. 2012.
"What Is Vasculitis?" *The Johns Hopkins Vasculitis Center*, 2013.
"What Is Vasculitis?" *National Heart, Lung, and Blood Institute*, 1 Apr. 2011.

Vitiligo

Category: Diseases/Disorders
Anatomy or system affected: Immune system, skin
Specialties and related fields: Dermatology, endocrinology
Definition: A disorder that occurs when cells that make pigment (color) in the skin are destroyed, leading to white patches on the body. It may also affect the eyes and the mucous membranes of the mouth and nose, and it may cause hair to gray.

KEY TERMS

autoimmune disorders: conditions in which the body attacks its cells and tissues

immune system: a body system in which blood cells, proteins, and organs fight infection and other cellular abnormalities such as cancer

melanin: the substance in the skin responsible for color (pigment); melanin causes tanning from sun exposure

CAUSES AND SYMPTOMS

There is no known cause for vitiligo, but it may be an autoimmune disease or a disorder in which one or more genes contribute to its development. The white patches that develop on the skin develop when skin melanocytes, cells that produce melanin, are destroyed. The amount of melanin that the body produces determines the skin color. Contributing factors to the development of vitiligo may include emotional distress, sunburn, or preexisting autoimmune diseases such as hyperthyroidism, but they are not considered causative.

Vitiligo usually develops before the age of forty and equally affects all races and sexes, with up to 2 percent of the population affected. The disorder may run in families; those with a family history of vitiligo or premature graying of the hair are at an increased risk.

The primary symptom of vitiligo is the loss of pigment in the skin, leading to widespread, irregularly shaped white patches on the body. The white patches are more evident in dark-skinned individuals and are much less noticeable in fair-skinned individuals. The patches may develop rapidly. Cycles of depigmentation followed by stable periods may occur throughout the lifetime of the affected individual. The areas commonly affected are the areas exposed to the sun, body folds such as the armpit and groin area, body openings, the area around moles, and areas of previous injury to the skin. Premature graying of the hair, including eyelashes, eyebrows, and beards, may also be symptomatic of vitiligo. The course of the disease is difficult to predict, and the spread of the white patches may spontaneously stop. Still, in most cases, the entire surface of the body is ultimately affected.

TREATMENT AND THERAPY

There is no cure for vitiligo. People should consult a doctor if they notice skin that loses color, early graying of hair, or loss of eye color. A dermatologist, a doctor who specializes in skin disease, is usually the physician of choice to treat vitiligo, but other specialists may be involved. The goal of treatment is to restore color to the skin and stop future depigmentation, if possible.

The diagnosis of vitiligo begins with a thorough patient examination and history, including any family history of vitiligo or autoimmune disease, unusual sun exposure, sunburn, or other skin condition in the period just before the white patches' onset and recent stress or physical illness. Doctors may order a blood draw to determine if there are thyroid or other blood-related dysfunctions. A referral to an ophthalmologist (a doctor who specializes in the eye) for a comprehensive eye examination for inflammation may be indicated.

Treatment depends on the site and the extent of the discolored areas. Therapeutic cosmetics may be used to camouflage white patches and are readily available in most department stores. The use of

---

INFORMATION ON VITILIGO

Causes: Unknown cause; may be an autoimmune disease

Symptoms: Irregular white patches on the skin, most commonly in areas exposed to the sun

Duration: Progressive and lifelong

Treatments: Creams, medicine plus ultraviolet light, skin grafts, tattooing

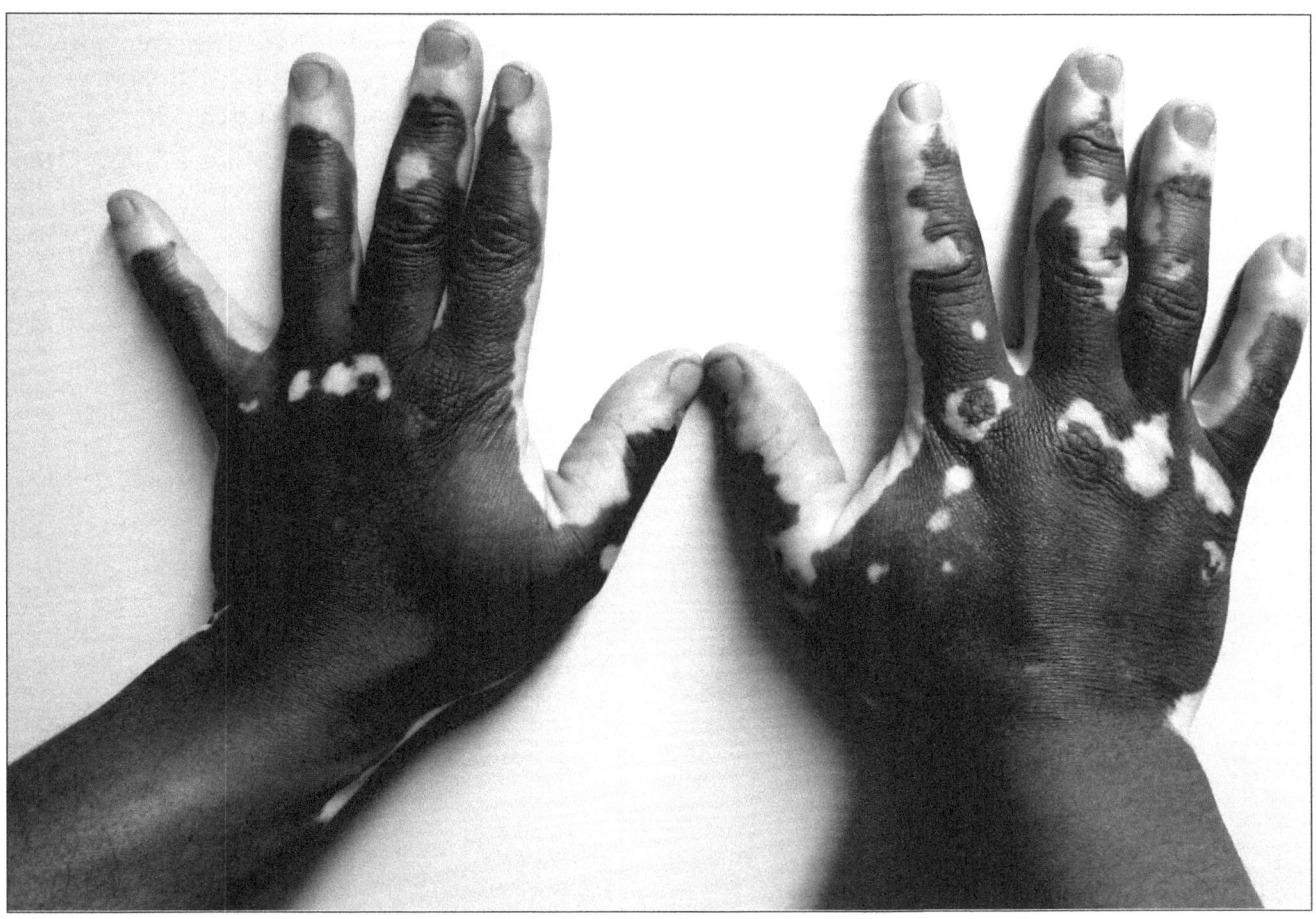
The hands of a person with vitiligo. Photo by James Heilman, MD, via Wikimedia Commons. [CC 3.0.]

sunscreen is essential to prevent normal skin from becoming increasingly darker than the vitiligo patches, especially in fair-skinned individuals. Sunless tanning preparations can also tint areas of the skin.

Topical corticosteroids may be helpful in the early stages of the disease. Vitamin D derivatives may be used in conjunction with corticosteroids or with ultraviolet (UV) light. Other topical ointments may be used in small areas of vitiligo. However, studies are small and side effects including an increased risk of lymphoma and skin cancer are possible. Topical psoralen with ultraviolet A (PUVA therapy), or photochemotherapy, may be effective, although severe sunburn, blistering, and other complications may occur. If more than 20 percent of the body is involved, oral PUVA is a possible remedy. Regardless of medical treatment, frequent visits to the doctor's office and careful monitoring are needed.

Narrowband ultraviolet B (UVB) therapy is a newer approach to treating vitiligo. No medicine is needed before the application of ultraviolet light. More research is needed, although small clinical trials have shown promise. Depigmentation therapy using monobenzyl ether of hydroquinone twice a day lightens all areas of the skin to match the areas of vitiligo in individuals with depigmentation that affects more than half the body. Autologous skin grafts and tattooing are options that may restore pigmentation or provide color to affected areas.

PERSPECTIVE AND PROSPECTS
Support for the individual experiencing vitiligo is important since the altered appearance caused by visible white patches may cause emotional distress. The extent of treatment may depend on the psychological impact of the disease on the individual. Younger and dark-skinned individuals may find the discoloration more disruptive in their daily lives and seek more aggressive therapies. Support groups are also available in many areas or online through organizations related to vitiligo therapy.

Researchers are trying to grow melanocytes in the laboratory from the patient's skin that are then transplanted into the areas of depigmentation. Other medicines are the subject of alternative lines of research: piperine, an alkaloid found in black pepper, effectively repigments skin in mice. While there are no significant clinical trials, individuals with slow-spreading vitiligo have tried alternative medicines. Patients should talk to their doctors before trying any over-the-counter treatments.

—*Christine M. Carroll, RN, BSN, MBA*

Further Information
American Academy of Dermatology. "Vitiligo."
Halder, Rebat M., and Jonathan Chappell. "Vitiligo Update." *Seminars in Cutaneous Medicine and Surgery*, vol. 28, no. 2, Jun. 2009, pp. 86-92.
Isenstein, Arin, Dean Morrell, and Craig Burkhart. "Vitiligo: Treatment Approach in Children." *Pediatric Annals*, vol. 38, no. 6, Jun. 2009, pp. 339-44.
National Library of Medicine and National Institutes of Health. "Vitiligo."
National Vitiligo Foundation.
Rosenblum, Laurie B. "Vitiligo." *Health Library*, 12 Sept. 2012.
Ta?eb, Alain, and Mauro Picardo. "Clinical Practice: Vitiligo." *New England Journal of Medicine*, vol. 360, no. 2, 8 Jan. 2009, pp. 160-69.
"Vitiligo." *Mayo Clinic*, 21 Apr. 2011.
"Vitiligo." *MedlinePlus*, 11 Jul. 2012.

DISEASES

This section discusses the complex relationship between the immune system and common medical disorders and bacterial and viral infections. Certain disorders compromise the body's ability to fight off infection, and both bacteria and viruses can have a devastating effect on an individual with a compromised immune system. The twenty essays in this section cover immune response to conditions that include anemia and other blood disorders, COVID-19, influenza, insect-borne diseases, and osteoarthritis.

Anemia	327
Blood and blood disorders	332
Coronavirus infections	338
COVID-19 disease	341
Cytomegalovirus (CMV)	345
Epstein-Barr virus	348
Goiter	352
Impetigo	354
Influenza	356
Insect-borne diseases	361
Measles	368
Nasopharyngeal disorders	371
Osteoarthritis	377
Rashes	385
Rhinitis	388
Rhinoviruses	391
Roseola	393
Shingles	396
Sinusitis	399
Skin disorders	402

Anemia

Category: Diseases/Disorders
Anatomy or system affected: Blood, heart, kidneys
Specialties and related fields: Cardiology, family medicine, geriatric medicine, hematology, internal medicine, nephrology, oncology, preventive medicine
Definition: A decrease in the oxygen-carrying capacity of blood with a reduction in the red blood cell count and/or hemoglobin.

KEY TERMS

erythrocytes: red blood cells of the circulatory system that contain hemoglobin and are responsible for delivering oxygen to the tissues

erythropoietin: the hormone protein that is produced in the kidneys and acts on the bone marrow helping in red blood cell synthesis

hematopoiesis: the process of production of red blood cells by bone marrow

hemoglobin: the pigmented protein that imparts red color to the blood and carries oxygen from the lungs to the rest of the body

hemolytic anemia: anemia attributable to increased destruction of red blood cells

macrocytic anemia: anemia with red blood cells of increased size

microcytic anemia: anemia with red blood cells of decreased size

normocytic anemia: anemia with red blood cells of normal size

CAUSES AND SYMPTOMS

Red blood cells or erythrocytes are continuously produced in the bone marrow by a process known as "hematopoiesis." This complex process requires adequate amounts of iron, vitamins such as B_{12} and folic acid, and hormones such as erythropoietin. Iron is required to form hemoglobin, which is the oxy-

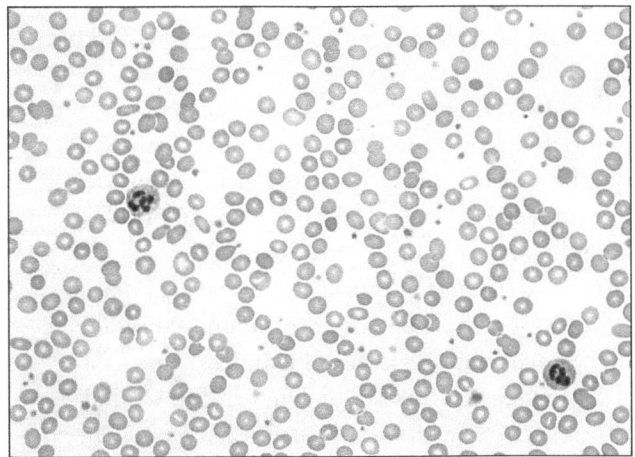

Blood smear from a person with iron-deficiency anemia. Note the red cells are small and pale. Image by Dr Graham Beards, via Wikimedia Commons. [CC 3.0.]

gen-carrying protein contained in red blood cells. Deficiency of any of the above can cause a decrease in hemoglobin or red blood cell counts, resulting clinically in anemia. Certain medications, environmental toxins, and cancers that affect the bone marrow can also cause anemia. As the kidneys produce erythropoietin, anemia is seen with chronic kidney disease as well.

The typical life span of a red blood cell, from its production in the bone marrow to its destruction in the liver and spleen, is about 120 days. If the life span is decreased in any way, either by increased destruction due to various reasons or through blood loss (during trauma, vaginal bleeding, gastrointestinal bleeding, or surgery), anemia can result. Increased destruction can also occur if the red blood cells are abnormal or the liver or spleen are enlarged. Anemia is recognized by laboratory tests when the hemoglobin falls below the normal values expected for the age and sex of the patient. The usual hemoglobin range is 13.5 to 17.5 milligrams per deciliter in males and 12 to 16 milligrams in females. Anemia is generally classified into three broad categories: microcytic, macrocytic, and normocytic, based on red blood cell size measured as the mean corpuscular volume (MCV) of red blood cells in blood tests. Microcytic anemia refers to decreased red blood cell size, usually with decreased hemoglobin as well. The most common cause of microcytic anemia is iron deficiency. Other causes include lead poisoning, thalassemia, sideroblastic anemia, and anemia of chronic disease.

Iron-deficiency anemia is a microcytic anemia with low serum iron caused by decreased intake, malabsorption, or increased iron loss. The most common cause of iron deficiency in the United States is chronic blood loss, usually seen in women of reproductive age (menstrual loss) and the elderly (gastrointestinal blood loss due to tumors, cancers, or side effects of medication that irritates the stomach). Pregnant women may have an iron deficiency due to inadequate intake that does not meet the requirements of the growing fetus; they require iron supplementation. Iron is absorbed in the small intestine. Any disease or procedure that causes problems with absorption, such as celiac sprue, inflammatory bowel disease (IBD), or intestinal surgery, can lead to iron-deficiency anemia. Iron-deficiency anemia is also prevalent in developing nations due to parasitic infestations such as hookworm. Blood tests usually diagnose iron deficiency. Still, occasionally a bone marrow biopsy may be required in which absent iron stores are noted.

Chronic lead poisoning can also cause anemia by a direct toxic effect on the bone marrow. Lead is in old house paints, pipes, bullets, batteries, and other items. Children living or playing in old houses are usually affected. They may develop learning and behavioral problems in addition to anemia. The characteristic feature of lead poisoning in anemia is the basophilic stippling of red blood cells.

Thalassemias are inherited disorders of the hemoglobin involving alpha or beta chains. These defective hemoglobin chains result in tiny, fragile red blood cells that cannot withstand passage through the spleen, causing hemolytic anemia. Patients with thalassemia may have suffered from anemia early in their childhood. Hydrops fetalis is a very severe form of thalassemia that results in fetal death. Thalassemia most commonly occurs in people of Mediterranean and Southeast Asian origin. Cooley's anemia or

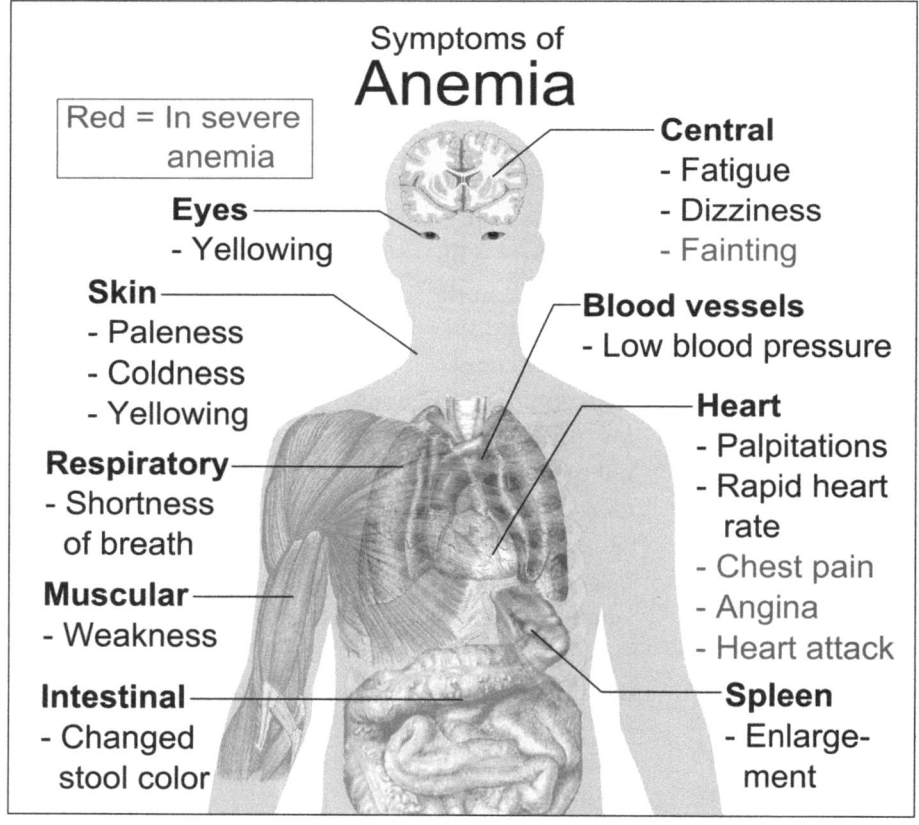

Main symptoms that may appear in anemia. Image by Mikael Häggström, via Wikimedia Commons. [Public domain.]

beta-thalassemia major occurs early in childhood and causes growth retardation. Sideroblastic anemia is also caused by defective hemoglobin in red blood cells, resulting in hemolytic anemia. Certain toxins such as lead, alcohol, drugs such as chloramphenicol, and hypothermia can cause acquired sideroblastic anemia. Occasionally, sideroblastic anemia may be normocytic. Confirmation of the diagnosis comes when blood tests reveal an excess of iron. A characteristic bone marrow study shows ringed sideroblasts.

Macrocytic anemia is characterized by an increase in red blood cell size. Common causes of macrocytic anemia are vitamin B_{12} and folic acid deficiencies, alcoholism, hypothyroidism, myelodysplastic syndromes (MDS), and hemolytic anemias. Vitamin B_{12} and folate deficiency cause megaloblastic or macrocytic anemia. Vitamin B_{12} or cobalamin is essential for deoxyribonucleic acid (DNA) synthesis. Ingested cobalamin binds to the intrinsic factor essential for its absorption in the small intestine. Most cobalamin deficiency results from a chronic dietary deficiency or pernicious anemia, a deficiency in the intrinsic factor. Folate (folic acid) is present in green leafy vegetables and fruits such as bananas. Folate deficiency is generally attributable to dietary deficiency, increased need in pregnancy, or decreased absorption in the small intestine. Dietary deficiency is prevalent in alcoholics. Pregnant women and patients on certain medications such as metformin, methotrexate, proton pump inhibitors, and sulfasalazine have increased folic acid needs and require folic acid supplements. Hemolytic anemias are characterized by increased fragility of the red blood cells and their increased destruction in the spleen and liver. The types of hemolytic anemias are sickle cell anemia, hereditary spherocytosis, thalassemia, and autoimmune hemolytic anemias.

Sickle cell anemia is common in those with African ancestry. The red blood cells assume the characteristic, abnormal "sickle" shape when exposed to

> **INFORMATION ON ANEMIA**
>
> **Causes**: A deficiency in the oxygen-carrying material of the blood and/or vitamin B_{12}
>
> **Symptoms**: Pallor, shortness of breath, heart palpitations, lethargy and fatigue, low blood pressure
>
> **Duration**: Acute or chronic
>
> **Treatment**: Replacement of deficient iron, vitamin B_{12}, or folate; blood transfusions

specific triggers. These abnormal red blood cells are unable to carry adequate oxygen to the tissues. As these fragile cells pass through the capillaries of the spleen, they rupture easily, resulting in anemia. In hereditary spherocytosis, red blood cells are spherical and rigid instead of being biconcave flexible discs. These cells are trapped in the spleen and destroyed before completing their expected life span of 120 days. In autoimmune hemolytic anemia, the immune system makes antibodies against the red blood cells, which enable them to be targets of destruction by the white blood cells of the immune system. This type of anemia is seen with unmatched blood transfusion or with the ingestion of certain drugs.

A normal red blood cell size characterizes normocytic anemia. It occurs in anemia of chronic disease, acute blood loss, and anemia of chronic kidney disease. Chronic inflammatory diseases such as rheumatoid arthritis or lupus result in the production of certain toxins that act directly on the bone marrow and decrease red blood cell production. Normocytic anemia ensues, in which there is simply an overall decrease in red blood cell production without a maturation defect. The anemia usually improves when chronic inflammation subsides. In chronic kidney disease, a decrease in erythropoietin production results in decreased red blood cell production. Aplastic anemia is another condition characterized by a marked decrease in red blood cell production because of the effect of toxins, medications, or infections such as parvovirus B19 (fifth disease). Other blood cell types may also be affected in aplastic anemia, resulting in severe infections and bleeding problems.

The symptoms of anemia are generally the same irrespective of the cause. Patients are generally pale and fatigue easily and can experience dizziness, weakness, palpitations, or rapid heartbeat. Most of the symptoms are attributable to compensatory mechanisms of the body trying to overcome decreased oxygenation. These compensatory mechanisms result in an increased circulating fluid volume that can eventually cause heart failure. Patients may have symptoms of heart failure such as foot swelling, shortness of breath, palpitations, chest pain, lightheadedness, or episodes of passing out. Patients whose anemia results from blood loss may have these symptoms if the loss is chronic and the body has adequate time to compensate. In cases of acute blood loss or when hemoglobin falls below 5 milligrams per deciliter, however, patients may experience shock, low blood pressure, heart attack, stroke, and confusion, sometimes leading to death. On the other hand, chronic mild anemia may be asymptomatic and is detected as an incidental finding on a routine laboratory test.

Other symptoms may be specific to the cause of the anemia. Iron deficiency may sometimes manifest itself as pica (a craving for materials such as clay or ice) and flattened or spoon-shaped nails. Severe thalassemia in children usually causes multiple fractures, a characteristic chipmunk face, an enlarged liver and spleen, heart failure, and gallstones. Patients with anemia caused by vitamin B_{12} deficiency may have neurological and psychiatric problems. There may be an associated thick red tongue and cracking at the angles of the mouth due to other associated vitamin deficiencies. Patients with hemolytic anemia can have jaundice, dark urine, and gallstones because of the bilirubin released from the hemolyzed red blood cells and enlarged spleen. Patients with sickle cell anemia may have acute pain crises and multiple infections. As a result of decreased oxygenation in peripheral tissues, stroke, angina, or lung clots may be the primary presentation in sickle cell disease. Patients with anemia of chronic disease usually have an obvious source of inflammation. Patients with bone marrow failure may also display symptoms of infection and bleeding.

TREATMENT AND THERAPY

The most critical step in managing anemia is evaluating the patient's condition and the cause of anemia by a physician or a nurse practitioner. A detailed history is usually elicited and should include dietary habits, occupation, associated symptoms, family history, medication history, and other medical problems. A complete physical examination looks specifically for jaundice, pallor, signs of heart failure, and enlarged liver and spleen. The most helpful tool in the diagnosis of anemia is the blood test. The physician may order further tests when the diagnosis is difficult, including invasive tests like a bone marrow biopsy. The treatment of anemia is directed toward the cause and acuteness of the problem. The use of blood transfusion is based on a person's signs and symptoms. In those without symptoms, they are not recommended unless hemoglobin levels are less than 6 to 8 milligrams per deciliter. These recommendations may also apply to some people with acute bleeding. Acute blood loss is an emergency and requires close monitoring in a hospital. It is treated with blood transfusions and fluid resuscitation. Some patients displaying signs of shock may need to be monitored in an intensive care setting. Patients with chronic anemia may be managed on an outpatient basis.

Oral iron sulfate tablets usually treat iron deficiency. Antacids and calcium supplements interfere with iron absorption and hence should not be taken simultaneously. Patients who cannot tolerate oral iron may receive iron intravenously. Lead poisoning is treated with chelating agents to remove the lead from the body. Thalassemia requires multiple blood transfusions and, if severe enough, bone marrow transplantation. Iron overload may become a problem with multiple blood transfusions, and chelating treatment with deferoxamine removes the excess iron. Oral pyridoxine treats hereditary spherocytosis. Acquired spherocytosis caused by alcohol and medications is treated with discontinuation of the offending agent.

Megaloblastic anemia due to vitamin B_{12} and folic acid deficiency is treated with oral supplements of these vitamins. Vitamin B_{12} also comes as an intramuscular injection. The neurological abnormalities are reversible if treated early. Autoimmune hemolytic anemias are treated by removal of the offending agent and with steroids. Some patients may require splenectomy (surgical removal of the spleen). Patients suffering from sickle cell crises must receive intravenous fluids, oxygen, and blood transfusions in the hospital. Supportive care is generally required, and patients may need antibiotics for infections and high doses of painkillers. Oral hydroxyurea, given as outpatient therapy, reduces the number of attacks. The treatment of anemia caused by chronic kidney disease due to low erythropoietin will require weekly subcutaneous erythropoietin and iron supplementation. Patients undergoing dialysis must maintain their hemoglobin above 10 milligrams per deciliter. Patients with aplastic anemia require multiple blood transfusions and immunosuppressive therapy and may benefit from bone marrow transplantation.

PERSPECTIVE AND PROSPECTS

The earliest mention of iron therapy is in Greek mythology in the story of Iphiclus, who was cured of impotence by drinking tea made from the rust of an iron blade. However, the use of iron for the treatment of anemia occurred much later, after the discovery of blood and blood transfusion. Jan Swammerdam first described red blood cells in 1658, and the first blood transfusion was dog-to-dog in 1665 by Oxford physician Richard Lower. The first human-to-human blood transfusion was performed successfully in 1818 by British obstetrician James Blundell to treat postpartum hemorrhage. However, death from hemolytic anemias caused by mismatched blood transfusions was a problem until Karl Landsteiner identified the ABO blood groups in 1901. He received the Nobel Prize in Medicine in 1930. He subsequently discovered Rh groups in the blood that further reduced hemolytic anemias that resulted from blood transfusions. James Herrick described the first case of sickle cell anemia in 1910. Still, it was Linus Pauling who postulated that the disease was the result of the presence of mutant hemoglobin HbS. The mortality rate of anemia has improved significantly over the past century, thanks to advances in blood transfusion and bone marrow transplantation. Current research focuses on the therapeutic potential of anemia correction in cancer, rheumatoid arthritis, human immunodeficiency virus (HIV) infection, heart failure, and kidney disease. Correction of anemia improves the quality of life significantly. Synthetic blood may become the treatment of anemia in the future.

—*Venkat Raghavan Tirumala, MD, MHA, Ophelia Empleo-Frazier, MSN, GNP-BC, WCC, DCP, and Geraldine Marrocco*

Further Information

Greer, John, et al., editors. *Wintrobe's Clinical Hematology*. 13th ed., Wolters Kluwer/Lippincott Williams & Wilkins Health, 2013.

"Iron." *National Institute of Health, Office of Dietary Supplements*. 22 Mar. 2021, ods.od.nih.gov/factsheets/Iron-Consumer/. Accessed 10 Sept. 2021.

Kasper, Dennis L., et al., editors. *Harrison's Principles of Internal Medicine*. 20th ed., McGraw-Hill, 2021.

Lights, Verneda. "What You Need to Know About Anemia." *Heathline*, 2 Aug. 2019, www.healthline.com/health/anemia. Accessed 10 Sept. 2021.

McCoy, Krisha, and Kari Kassir. "Anemia." *Health Library*, 28 Mar. 2013.

National Anemia Action Council, www.anemia.org.

"Oral Iron for Anemia: A Review of the Clinical Effectiveness, Cost-effectiveness and Guidelines Rapid Response Report: Summary with Critical Appraisal Ottawa (ON)." *Canadian Agency for Drugs and Technologies in Health*, 6 Jan. 2006.

BLOOD AND BLOOD DISORDERS

Category: Diseases/Disorders
Anatomy or system affected: Blood vessels, circulatory system, immune system, liver, lymphatic system
Specialties and related fields: Hematology, immunology, serology
Definition: The fluid that circulates in veins and arteries, carries oxygen and nutrients throughout the body, transports waste materials to excretory channels, and participates in the body's defense against infection.

KEY TERMS

blood: the fluid that circulates through the cardiovascular system; composed of a fluid and a cellular fraction that consists of erythrocytes, leukocytes, and thrombocytes

blood group system: a classification of individuals into groups based on the presence or absence of blood group antigens found on the surfaces of red blood cells

blood group antigen: glycolipid surface markers on the outer surface of red blood cell membranes that determine an individual's blood group; two main groups of blood surface antigens are called "ABO" (blood type A, B, AB, and O) and "Rh" (Rh-positive or Rh-negative)

blood typing: identification of surface blood group antigens of an individual for classification into specific blood groups

erythrocytes: red blood cells; non-nucleated, disk-shaped blood cells that contain hemoglobin

hemoglobin: oxygen-carrying red pigment present in red blood cells that is responsible for oxygen exchange in cells and tissues

leukocytes: white blood cells; any of the white or colorless nucleated cells that occur in blood

plasma: the protein-containing fluid portion of the blood in which blood cells are suspended

serum: the clear, yellowish fluid obtained from blood after it has been allowed to clot thrombocytes: platelets; small, irregularly shaped cells in the blood that participate in blood clotting

STRUCTURE AND FUNCTIONS

Blood provides a common communication channel for all organs in the body. It is responsible for the transport of oxygen, enzymes, hormones, drugs, and many other substances, as well as for the transfer of heat produced by chemical reactions in the body. The average-sized adult has about ten pints (~4.7 L) of blood. At rest, ten pints a minute (and up to forty pints during exercise) are pumped by the heart via the arteries to the lungs and other tissues and returns to the heart through veins in a continuous circuit.

THE COMPONENTS OF BLOOD

Blood consists of cells floating in a fluid called "plasma." The cells that comprise blood include red blood cells, platelets, and white blood cells, with cells comprising about half the volume of whole blood. The remainder of the blood volume is comprised of plasma, which contains dissolved proteins, sugars, fats, and minerals. Red blood cells, also known as erythrocytes, contain hemoglobin, a protein that carries oxygen. Platelets are involved in blood clotting mechanisms. White blood cells, which are di-

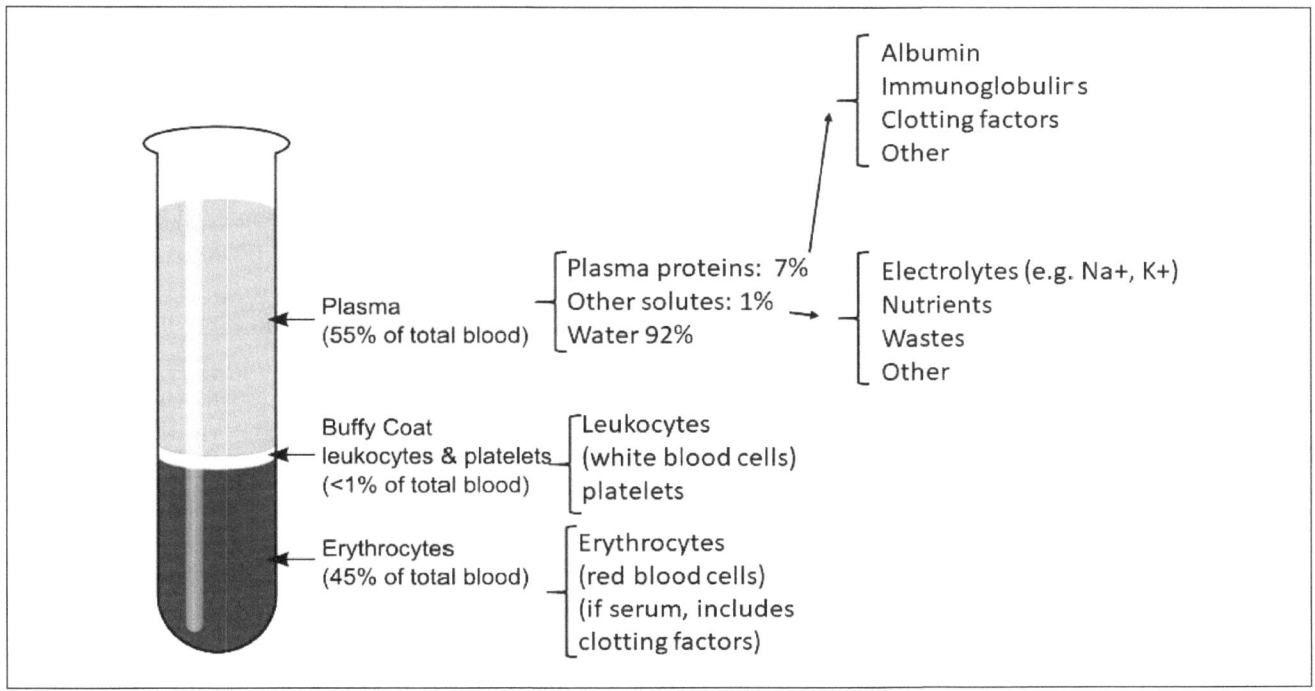

Components of blood. Image by Alan Sved, via Wikimedia Commons. [CC 4.0.]

vided into granulocytes, monocytes, and lymphocytes, are the cells primarily responsible for the immune response.

All types of blood cells are formed in the bone marrow by divisions of a single cell called a "hematopoietic stem cell." Red blood cells, or erythrocytes (from the Greek *eruthros*, "red"), are very small, have no nucleus, and require very little oxygen for survival. Red blood cells have a large surface area relative to their volume, which allows oxygen and carbon dioxide to diffuse in and out of the cell rapidly. This large surface also allows the cell to swell and shrink and to squeeze through narrow capillaries without shearing or bursting. Red blood cells cannot repair themselves, and after three or four months (roughly 120 days) in the circulation, they are eliminated by stationary phagocytic cells in the liver, spleen, and bone marrow, and replaced by the bone marrow. The main function of red blood cells is to transport oxygen employing their enriched hemoglobin content; as such, they are among the most highly specialized cells in the body.

Hemoglobin, the red, iron-containing pigment responsible for the color of blood, has a great affinity for oxygen. It will release oxygen in a situation where free oxygen is scarce, such as in working tissues. Hemoglobin gives blood an oxygen-carrying capacity eighty times greater than if the oxygen were merely dissolved in plasma. When hemoglobin releases oxygen, it becomes capable of taking up carbon dioxide, which it carries back to the lungs. Hemoglobin occupies 33 percent of the red blood cell volume and accounts for 90 percent of its dry weight.

Leukocytes, or white blood cells (from the Greek *leukos*, meaning "clear" or "white"), are larger and less plentiful than red blood cells and can also be found in tissues. The purpose of white blood cells is to remove foreign material and to defend against microorganisms. Leukocytes travel through the circulatory system and can pass through the walls of blood vessels to carry out specific effector functions in surrounding tissues. White blood cells play an important role in defense against infection by viruses, bacteria, fungi, and parasites. There are three main populations of leukocytes: granulocytes, monocytes, and lymphocytes. Granulocytes, also known as polymorphonuclear (PMN) leukocytes, contain granules and have a segmented nucleus. There are three types of granulocytes: neutrophils, basophils, and eosinophils. The most abundant are the neutrophils, which are responsible for killing invading bacteria (pus consists largely of neutrophils). They are also called "phagocytes" ("engulfing cells") because of their ability to ingest bacteria and other foreign materials. In the absence of activation, neutrophils reside in the blood for only six to nine hours, but upon activation, they can move to sites of infection, or travel to tissues where they may survive a few more days. Eosinophils are involved in allergic reactions. Monocytes are also a type of phagocyte important in the immune system.

Lymphocytes participate in the adaptive immune response, such as the production of antibodies and the rejection of tissue grafts. They play integral roles in directing the activity of other cells involved in the immune response. Lymphocytes become specialized against a specific antigen in the lymph nodes. Lymphocytes live longer, with their lifetime ranging between three months to several years. Unlike granulocytes and monocytes, lymphocytes do not engulf solid particles or phagocytose, but instead play a part in producing antibodies and important immune hormones known as cytokines. An antibody is a protein that may be soluble in blood plasma or lymph and may affix to other cells. There are many different types of lymphocytes, each of which has a different function. T lymphocytes are responsible for delayed hypersensitivity phenomena and produce substances called "lymphokines," a type of cytokine that affects the function of many cells. They also moderate the activity of other lymphocytes called "B lymphocytes," cells that produce antibodies. Antibodies help kill or specifically mark foreign material so that it is more readily detected and eliminated by scavenger cells. Most B lymphocytes are in a state of surveillance to create an early warning system to detect foreign material. If these cells encounter foreign material that binds to specific molecular pattern detection receptors (known as Toll-like Receptors or TLRs) in their membranes or if they receive such material from another cell, they move to a lymph node where they divide to produce daughter cells that manufacture antibodies specifically active against that foreign material. Natural killer, or NK cells, are also a type of lymphocyte with roles in the direct killing of virus-infected cells.

Platelets are the smallest cells in the blood; they can survive there for about nine days. They circulate in the blood in an inactive state, but under certain circumstances they begin to adhere to blood vessels and each other, producing and releasing chemicals that initiate blood clotting. Platelets are critical in hemostasis or stopping blood flow.

Plasma is the straw-colored fluid in which blood cells are suspended. It is composed mainly of water (95 percent), with a salt content similar to saltwater. Other constituents comprising plasma include nutrients, waste products, proteins, and hormones. Nutrients, such as sugars, fats, vitamins, minerals, and amino acids, are transported to tissues after absorption from the intestinal tract or following release from storage in the liver. Among the proteins in plasma are substances such as fibrinogen (involved in coagulation), immunoglobulins and complement proteins (bacteria fighters that are part of the immune system), carrier proteins known as globulins, and albumin.

The term "blood group" refers to the classification of blood according to differences in the makeup of its red blood cells. The ABO system consists of three blood group substances, the A, B, and H antigens (substances that induce the production of an antibody when injected into an animal), which are components of erythrocyte surface substances. Individuals with type-A red blood cells carry anti-B antibodies in their serum; those with type-B red blood cells carry anti-A antibodies; those with type AB red blood cells (which bear both A and B antigens) carry neither anti-A nor anti-B antibodies; and type O individuals, whose red blood cells bear neither antigen, carry both anti-A and anti-B antibodies. The transfusion of type A blood into a type B individual, for example, clumps together the transfused erythrocytes and results in an often-fatal blockage of blood vessels, which indicates the importance of blood typing before a transfusion is performed.

Another blood group system is based on the rhesus (or Rh) factor. The system involves several antigens, but the most important is called "factor D." It is found in 85 percent of the population; those individuals are called "Rh-positive." If it is not present, the person is classified as Rh-negative. Based on this system, individuals are therefore classified as O positive or AB negative, for example, based on their ABO and Rh blood groups. The main importance of the Rh group is during pregnancy. An Rh-negative woman who is pregnant with an Rh-positive baby may form antibodies against the baby's blood. Such women are given antibodies directed against factor D after delivery to prevent the development of anti-D antibodies, which would cause hemolytic disease of the newborn in successive Rh-positive infants. The transfusion of Rh-positive blood into an Rh-negative patient can cause a serious reaction if the patient has had a previous blood transfusion that contained the Rh antigen.

About four hundred other antigens have been discovered, but they are widely scattered throughout the population and rarely cause transfusion problems. Only the ABO and the Rh blood group systems have major clinical importance. Blood typing is used to categorize blood for transfusion. Knowledge of blood group substances and their inheritance has been useful for legal, historical, and medical purposes. The ABO blood groups are found in all people, but the frequency of each group varies with race and geographical distribution. This fact can aid anthropologists who are involved in investigating, for example, early population migrations. The genes inherited from someone's parents determine their blood group. Identification of a blood group can be used in a paternity case to establish that a man could not have been the father of a particular child, although blood grouping cannot positively demonstrate that a man is the father. Blood found at the scene of a crime can be typed and used to exclude suspects if the type does not match. Some blood groups are associated with particular disorders. For example, blood group A is more common in people suffering from cancer of the stomach, while group O is found more often in people suffering from peptic ulcers.

DISORDERS AND DISEASES
Blood tests can be used to ascertain the health of major organs as well as respiratory functions, hormonal balance, immune system, and metabolism. They can reveal not only blood cell abnormalities characteristic of some diseases but also healthy variations in the blood induced by the response to infections. Blood tests can be classified into three categories: hematological, biochemical, and microbiological tests. Hematological tests involve studying the components of blood itself by looking at the number, shape, size, and appearance of its cells, as well as by testing the function of clotting factors. The most important tests of this type are the blood count, blood smear, and blood-clotting tests. Biochemical tests examine chemicals in the blood such as sodium, potassium, uric acid, urea, vitamins, gases, and drugs. In microbiological tests, blood is examined for microorganisms, such as bacteria,

viruses, and viral particles, fungi, and parasites, and forms antibodies against them.

Known causes of blood disorders include genetic factors (an inherited or acquired abnormality in the production of some blood component), nutritional disorders (i.e., vitamin deficiency), infections by microorganisms, over- or underproduction of certain immune cell types or immune factors; tumors (such as bone marrow cancer), poisons (carbon monoxide, lead, snake and spider venoms), drugs (which can produce blood abnormalities as a side effect), and radiation.

Abnormalities can occur in any of the blood components. Leukemias are disorders in which the number of white blood cells is abnormally high, and can arise from multiple cell types. Leukemias can arise from lymphocytes, such as acute or chronic lymphocytic leukemias, or cells of the granulocyte lineage, such as acute or chronic myeloid leukemias. Overproduction of red blood cells can also occur and result in diseases such as polycythemia vera, an acquired blood disorder in which there is a defect in signaling that results in overproduction of red blood cells. Lymphomas are cancers of the lymph nodes or lymphatic system and include Hodgkin's and non-Hodgkin's lymphomas. These types of cancers vary in their severity, available treatment options, and prognosis. In acquired immunodeficiency syndrome (AIDS), T lymphocytes are infected by the human immunodeficiency virus (HIV), which results in immune dysfunction and increased risk for certain types of infections and cancers. Abnormal platelet numbers, or the lack of platelets, can lead to some types of bleeding disorders, such as hemophilia (inability of the blood to clot properly) or von Willebrand disease in which there is disruption of normal clotting processes. Unwanted clot formation (thrombosis) can occur from circumstances that overactivate the blood's clotting mechanisms. The most common blood disorder is anemia, which results from a hemoglobin deficiency and includes a corresponding reduction in the blood's oxygen-carrying capacity. Deficiencies of blood plasma proteins include hypoalbuminemia (albumin deficiency) and may indicate malnutrition or liver disease. Thalassemia is an inherited blood disorder characterized by less hemoglobin and fewer red blood cells than normal, resulting in anemia and fatigue and may require blood transfusions. Sickle cell anemia is an inherited condition in which there aren't enough healthy red blood cells to distribute oxygen; in this condition, red blood cells are sticky and crescent-shaped and don't flow easily through vessels.

PERSPECTIVE AND PROSPECTS

Blood is a liquid of complex structure and vital functions that has been considered the essence of life for centuries. There is no shortage of irrational or unscientific ideas about the supposed properties of human blood-one can speak of "blood brotherhood," "blood feuds," "blood relations," and of someone being "bloodthirsty."

The present medical understanding of blood has developed over the past two or three thousand years. The study of blood began in Egypt and Mesopotamia, around 500 BCE, and moved to countries around the Mediterranean that had become intellectually active. Ancient Greek thinkers noted differences between arteries and veins and that blood moved through them. According to whether the heart, the liver, or the brain was thought to be the prime organ controlling the rest of the body, various functions were tentatively ascribed to blood, such as its relation to sleep, distribution of heat, and animation of the body. The Greek school of medicine became personified in Hippocrates, who denied the widely accepted theory of the existence of spirits and proposed that the body followed natural laws. He presented the concept of body juices or "humors." There were four of them: blood, lymph or phlegm, yellow bile (or choler), and black bile (or melancholy), with blood being the most important one. The philosopher Aristotle accepted the humoral hypothesis. One of his pupils was Alexander the Great, whose military conquests spread Greek influence widely. A notable medical school developed in Alexandria, Egypt, where students learned the ideas of Hippocrates and Aristotle. There was, however, a variation regarding blood; namely, the theory of plethora, in which it was postulated that an excess of blood in the circulatory system or one organ caused illness.

Four hundred years later, Galen, a product of the Alexandria School of Medicine, denied the doctrine of plethora and returned to the humoral approach. Health and disease were thought to occur because of an upset in the equilibrium of these humors. Physicians practiced bloodletting to restore the balance of the humors by purging the body of its contaminated fluids from Hippocrates (ca. 460-ca. 370 BCE) until the nineteenth century. During Galen's time, animal dissection was widely practiced and provided a better concept of blood and its functions. It was proposed that the liver changed food to blood, which was distributed to the body along the veins. At the same time, impurities from the body were thought to be absorbed into venous blood and returned to the liver and then to the right side of the heart, where they supposedly ascended in the pulmonary artery to the lungs to be exhaled. The weakening of medieval ideas set the stage for English doctor William Harvey's discovery of blood circulation. He used the analogy of the heart as a pump and veins and arteries as pipes, where blood is moving around and is being driven in a continuous circuit. Four years after Harvey died in 1661, the Italian anatomist Marcello Malpighi observed the capillary blood vessels with the aid of the microscope. The cellular composition of blood was also recognized using a microscope, as Antoni van Leeuwenhoek, a Dutch naturalist, accurately described and measured red blood cells. The discovery of white blood cells and platelets followed after microscope lenses improved. William Hewson first observed leukocytes in the eighteenth century. He thought that these cells came from nucleated cells in the lymph that eventually emerged from the spleen as red blood cells. In the nineteenth century, interest in leukocytes intensified with studies on inflammation and microbial infection.

In 1852, Karl Vierordt published the first quantitative results of blood cell analysis after several attempts to correlate blood cell counts with various diseases. In 1865, Felix Hoppe-Seyler discovered the oxygen-carrying capacity of the red pigment (hemoglobin) in cells. The early history of protein chemistry is essentially that of hemoglobin because it was one of the first molecules to have its molecular weight accurately determined and the first to be associated with a specific physiological function, i.e., carrying oxygen.

In 1900, the German pathologist Karl Landsteiner began mixing blood taken from different people and found some mixtures were compatible and others were not. This incompatibility resulted in illness and sometimes death after transfusions. He discovered two types of marker proteins, or antigens, on the surface of red blood cells that he called "A" and "B." Landsteiner classified a person's blood according to whether it contained one or the other antigen, both, or neither. Blood with only the A antigen was type A, and blood with only the B antigen was type B. Blood with both antigens was AB blood, and blood with neither the A nor the B antigen was type O blood. He also discovered the Rh factor in 1940 during experiments with rhesus monkeys. Improved methods of blood examination in the 1920s and the growth of knowledge of blood physiology in the 1930s allowed anemias and other blood disorders to be studied. Modern hematology recognizes that alterations in the components of blood are a result of disease, and research is conducted continually for a better understanding of this relationship and of blood itself.

Currently, there are many advances in what we know about the immune system and its function. We also are continuing to learn about many blood disorders, including leukemias and lymphomas, and defects in the regulation of production of immune production and signaling. Blood continues to be an area of emerging science and vital to the maintenance and function of all life processes.

—*Catherine J. Walsh, PhD*

Further Information

American Medical Association. *American Medical Association Complete Encyclopedia of Medicine*. Random House Reference, 2003. A medical encyclopedia written by the American Medical Association and lists medical terms and definitions, explains surgical procedures and tests, includes descriptions of benefits and side effects of treatments and provides general information about blood disorders.

Bick, Roger L. *Disorders of Thrombosis and Hemostasis: Clinical and Laboratory Practice*. 3rd ed., Lippincott Williams & Wilkins, 2002. This book provides current data on antithrombotic therapy, information for diagnosis and treating bleeding and clotting disorders, and etiology, pathophysiology, clinical, laboratory diagnosis, and management of disorders of thrombosis and hemostasis.

Kaushansky, Kenneth, and Marcel Levi. *Williams Hematology Hemostasis and Thrombosis*. McGraw-Hill Education, 2017.

Lichtman, Marshall, et al., editors. *Williams Manual of Hematology*. 9th ed., McGraw-Hill, 2016. A quick-access summary of epidemiology, etiology, pathogenesis, diagnostic criteria, differential diagnosis, and therapy of blood cell and coagulation protein disorders.

Rodak, Bernadette, editor. *Hematology: Clinical Principles and Applications*. 4th ed., Elsevier Saunders, 2012. This text explores essential aspects of hematology including identification of cells, understanding hemostasis and thrombosis, normal hematopoiesis, and diseases of erythroid, myeloid, lymphoid, and megakaryocytic origins.

Saba, Hussain I., and Harold R. Roberts, editor. *Hemostasis and Thrombosis: Practical Guidelines in Clinical Management*. John Wiley & Sons, Ltd., 2014. A handbook summarizing the current understanding of hemostasis and thrombosis, with emphasis on clinical diagnosis, treatment, and daily management of thrombotic and bleeding disorders.

Zucker-Franklin, D., et al. *Atlas of Blood Cells: Function and Pathology*. 3rd ed., Lea & Febiger, 2003. Updated with biomolecular advances, including apoptosis, and advances in detect methods including immune-electron microscopy and fluorescent in situ hybridization for detecting chromosomal abnormalities.

CORONAVIRUS INFECTIONS

Category: Diseases/Conditions

Anatomy or system affected: Gastrointestinal system, lungs, respiratory system

Also known as: Common cold, severe acute respiratory syndrome (SARS), viral bronchitis, viral pneumonia

Anatomy or system affected: Blood, brain, eyes, gastrointestinal system, immune system, intestines, liver, lungs, lymphatic system, mouth, psychic-emotional system, reproductive system, respiratory system, skin, throat

Specialties and related fields: Bacteriology, dermatology, epidemiology, gastroenterology, gynecology, hematology, immunology, internal medicine, microbiology, neurology, oncology, ophthalmology, osteopathic medicine, otorhinolaryngology, pathology, pharmacology, proctology, psychiatry, public health, pulmonary medicine, virology

Definition: The largest positive-strand ribonucleic acid (RNA) virus that causes common colds and severe acute respiratory syndromes.

KEY TERMS

COVID-19: coronavirus disease discovered in 2019 caused by SARS-CoV-2

MERS: Middle East Respiratory Syndrome caused by the beta-coronavirus MERS-CoV

SARS: a severe acute respiratory syndrome caused by the beta coronavirus SARS-CoV

INTRODUCTION

The coronavirus is the largest positive-strand ribonucleic acid (RNA) virus; it is part of the Coronaviridae family. Exposure to coronaviruses results in various infections, including approximately one-third of all cases of the common cold. The virus also may be responsible for viral bronchitis, pneumonia, and SARS (severe acute respiratory syndrome), especially in persons with weakened immune systems.

CAUSES

Coronaviruses are named for the crown-like spikes on their surface. There are four main subgroupings of coronaviruses, known as alpha, beta, gamma, and delta. Human coronaviruses were first identified in the mid-1960s. The seven coronaviruses that can infect people are 229E (alpha coronavirus), NL63 (alpha coronavirus), OC43 (beta coronavirus), and HKU1 (beta coronavirus). Other human coronaviruses that cause severe disease include MERS-CoV (the beta coronavirus that causes Middle East Respiratory Syndrome, or MERS), SARS-CoV (the beta coronavirus that causes a severe acute respiratory syndrome, or SARS), and SARS-CoV-2. This novel coronavirus causes coronavirus disease 2019, also known as COVID-19.

Coronaviruses are the underlying cause of various illnesses that affect the respiratory system, the gastrointestinal system, and, in rare cases, the neurological system. Infections with the virus are often seasonal, with more occurring in winter. Contact with contaminated droplets from sneezing and coughing and direct contact by touching contaminated objects, such as surfaces and tissues, may transmit the virus from person to person.

The virus may live six to nine hours, and the live virus has been found in the stool of people diag-

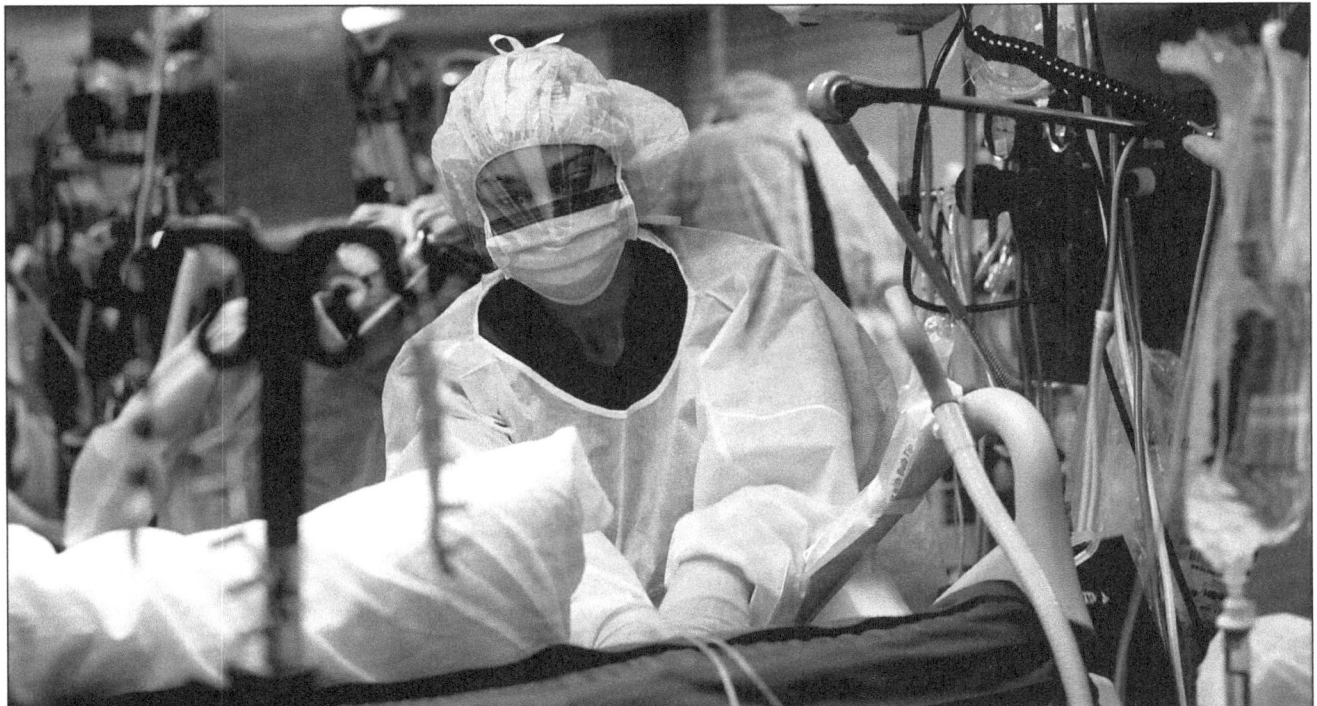

A nurse treats a COVID-19 patient in an intensive care unit aboard a US hospital ship in April 2020. Photo via Wikimedia Commons. [Public domain.]

nosed with SARS. It is highly contagious, and reinfection may occur. The virus can affect humans, cattle, pigs, rodents, cats, dogs, and birds. Still, there is no evidence of animal and bird variations infecting humans.

MERS-CoV is a zoonotic virus that is transmitted between animals and people. Infected dromedary camels transfer MERS-CoV to humans. MERS-CoV causes Middle East respiratory syndrome (MERS). MERS-CoV transmission occurs through direct or indirect contact with infected animals. MERS-CoV has been identified in camels in the Middle East, Africa, and South Asia. Twenty-seven countries have reported MER cases since 2012. MERS has caused a total of 858 known deaths due to the infection and related complications.

SARS-CoV-2 causes COVID-19. Most people who contract COVID-19 have a severe cold or flu and recover without any treatment. Others become seriously ill and require hospitalization. Older people or those with preexisting medical conditions like heart disease, diabetes mellitus, high blood pressure, or chronic respiratory diseases are more likely to suffer severe disease. However, anyone at any age can become seriously ill from COVID-19. Aerosols transmit SARS-CoV-2, and mask-wearing, though not a perfect barrier, reduces infection.

RISK FACTORS
Risk factors for coronavirus infection are exposure to an infected person through kissing and sharing living spaces and contact with droplets or contaminated surfaces containing the virus. The severity of the infection increases if a person is immunocompromised (less able to fight infections because of a weakened immune system). Risk reduction for coronavirus infections includes studious hand hygiene, distancing from other people (at least 2 meters), wearing a well-fitting, clean face mask, and ventilation of all rooms.

SYMPTOMS
Coronavirus infection that leads to the common cold comes with fatigue, a scratchy throat, sneezing, nasal congestion, and a runny nose. Fever rarely occurs with a cold, except in children. A more severe infection, such as pneumonia or SARS, may be occurring if symptoms include fever, chills, muscle aches, an acute cough, a headache, dizziness, or diarrhea.

Severe coronavirus disease symptoms include difficulty breathing, persistent pain or pressure in the chest, confusion, fatigue, discoloration of the lips, nail beds, or skin tone.

Some people who have had COVID-19, even if they had mild cases, continue to experience symptoms up to six months after the resolution of their initial symptoms. This condition is called "long COVID." The symptoms of long COVID vary but usually include fatigue, respiratory and neurological symptoms.

SCREENING AND DIAGNOSIS
A physical examination, including listening to lung sounds, reviewing symptoms, chest X-rays, and blood work, may be used to determine if a person has a cold or has developed pneumonia or SARS. Blood work may include blood chemistries and a complete blood count to determine if white blood cell counts, lymphocytes, and platelets are low. Specific tests for SARS may be ordered too.

SARS-CoV-2 is diagnosed with a PCR test from a nasal swab. This test is very sensitive and can detect the virus before patients feel any symptoms. Particles detected by PCR tests may or may not be infectious. Lateral flow tests detect whole viral particles. These tests are inexpensive and rapid.

TREATMENT AND THERAPY
If symptoms worsen or if a fever develops, one should seek medical care. In the absence of fever, symptoms may be treated with over-the-counter medications, plenty of fluids, and rest. Antibiotics,

antiviral medications, and high doses of steroids to decrease lung inflammation may be prescribed. In severe cases, the patient may need oxygen, breathing support with a respirator, and hospitalization.

PREVENTION AND OUTCOMES
The best prevention against coronavirus infection is to limit contact with infected persons. Hand hygiene, including handwashing or cleaning hands with an alcohol-based hand sanitizer, is an integral part of prevention. Infected persons should cough or sneeze into a tissue or arm to minimize droplets and airborne particles. Because coronavirus is contagious, one should not share food and drink, utensils, or personal supplies. Household areas, including doorknobs, countertops, and other surfaces, should be cleaned with disinfectant.

Infected individuals should quarantine for at least ten days and even longer if their symptoms fail to resolve. Wearing well-fitting face masks in public decreases the spread of coronaviruses. Coronavirus infections outdoors rarely occur, and masking is unnecessary unless the probability of being close to infected people is high.

—*Patricia Stanfill Edens, RN, PhD, FACHE*
and Michael A. Buratovich, PhD

Further Information
"Coronavirus Disease (COVID-19)." *World Health Organization*, 12 Oct. 2020, www.who.int/news-room/q-a-detail/coronavirus-disease-covid-19. Accessed 10 Sept. 2021.
Eccles, Ronald, and Olaf Weber, editors. *Common Cold*. Birkhäuser, 2009.
"Middle Eastern Respiratory Syndrome (MERS)." *Center for Disease Control and Prevention*, www.cdc.gov/coronavirus/mers/index.html. Accessed 10 Sept. 2021.
Peiris, M., et al., editors. *Severe Acute Respiratory Syndrome*. Blackwell, 2005.
Wagner, Edward K., and Martinez J. Hewlett. *Basic Virology*. 3rd ed., Blackwell Science, 2008.

COVID-19 DISEASE

Category: Diseases/Conditions
Also known as: Severe acute respiratory syndrome (SARS)-CoV-2, 2019-nCoV, novel betacoronavirus
Anatomy or Systems Affected: Respiratory system
Specialties and related fields: Epidemiology, hematology, immunology, internal medicine, microbiology, neurology, public health, pulmonary medicine, virology
Definition: COVID-19 is a respiratory disease caused by a novel betacoronavirus that can produce illnesses ranging from mild or even asymptomatic to severe, life-threatening pneumonia. The virus is highly contagious and has spread worldwide, causing a pandemic.

KEY TERMS
long COVID: Those who had COVID-19 recovered from it but continue to feel symptoms long after the days or weeks that represent a typical course of the disease
N95 respirators: a respiratory protective device designed to achieve a very close facial fit and very efficient filtration of airborne particles
pneumonia: an infection of the lower respiratory system that includes the bronchial tubes and alveoli of the lung

CAUSES
On December 31, 2019, China reported a cluster of pneumonia cases associated with the Huanan Seafood Market in Wuhan. One week later, the Chinese health authorities announced that the infectious agent was a novel coronavirus. The Chinese market sold various live animals, including bats; the virus is thought to have originated in bats with direct transfer to humans or indirect transfer to humans through an intermediate animal host. However, extensive surveys of local animals failed to recover the

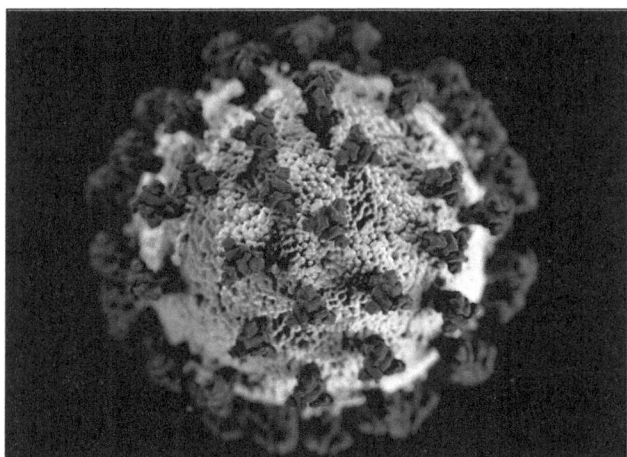
This illustration reveals ultrastructural morphology exhibited by coronaviruses. Photo via Center for Disease Control (CDC).

virus. A laboratory leak from the Wuhan Institute of Virology is a competing possibility for the origin of this pandemic. The virus is similar to another betacoronavirus—severe acute respiratory syndrome (SARS)—originating in Chinese live animal markets in 2003, causing severe respiratory distress syndrome. The first case of COVID-19 in the United States occurred on January 19, 2020, in Snohomish County, Washington state. The patient was a thirty-five-year-old man who had just returned from visiting his family in Wuhan, China.

Airborne droplets can spread the SARS-CoV-2 virus, contact contaminated surfaces, enter through mucous membranes, and possibly through fecal-oral routes. The virus is shed in the feces of infected individuals. After exposure, the incubation period is usually about five days but may be up to two weeks.

RISK FACTORS

This is a new virus, so no one is immune to infection. Older age, immunocompromised status, underlying diseases, and smoking have all been associated with more severe diseases. COVID-19 is highly transmissible, and close contact with an infected individual or contaminated surface should be avoided. Health-care workers are at an increased risk and must wear gloves, gowns, and N-95 respirators to protect themselves from infection. Infected or suspected patients should wear masks to decrease the chance of spreading infection. Wearing regular masks by uninfected individuals does not reliably protect against infection. They are not occlusive against aerosols and leave the eyes unprotected.

SYMPTOMS

Some infected persons will have few or no symptoms. Children usually have mild disease with cold-like symptoms, often with no fever. Adults will have a fever, headache, sore throat, dry cough, and shortness of breath in more severe cases. There can also be a feeling of fatigue and general malaise with accompanying myalgia. Viral pneumonia occurs with severe disease and results in impaired oxygenation manifested by shortness of breath. Such patients need immediate medical care and hospitalization.

Some patients find that even if they experienced a mild case of COVID-19, they continue to have debilitating fatigue even up to six months after recovery. This condition, known as "long COVID," is a common but poorly understood phenomenon.

SCREENING AND DIAGNOSIS

During the current pandemic, any patient with new respiratory symptoms, especially if accompanied by fever, must be considered possibly infected with COVID-19. Additionally, any patient from a highly infected country, cruise ship, or area with a high prevalence of COVID-19 infection must be considered possibly infected even if they are asymptomatic. Screening may initially be done to rule out other respiratory pathogens such as the influenza virus. Definitive testing for COVID-19 takes two swabs, one from the nose and one from the throat. These are sent to a microbiology laboratory capable of performing specific polymerase chain reaction (PCR) testing. This test can identify viral genetic material. Because this coronavirus's genome (ribonucleic acid

[RNA]) is large and capable of evolving mutations, the PCR probe has been designed to target two specific genetic areas to avoid missing cases. It is possible to have a negative PCR test very early in the COVID-19 infection when only small amounts of the virus are present.

Later flow tests for COVID-19 are rapid diagnostic tests that can quickly test for SARS-CoV-2. Lateral flow tests can deliver a positive or negative result in fifteen to thirty minutes. They work similarly to home pregnancy tests, except that the material tested comes from a patient's nose and throat. Additionally, the kit contains antibodies to specific viral proteins rather than to a pregnancy hormone. Lateral flow tests are inexpensive and easy to use and represent a powerful diagnostic tool for controlling COVID-19.

Radiological examinations are also helpful in diagnosis. Computerized tomography (CT) scanning often reveals characteristic features in COVID-19 pneumonia patients. Sometimes the findings from these exams can provide a presumptive diagnosis while awaiting PCR test results.

TREATMENT AND THERAPY

For infections in patients with mild symptoms, treatment can be initiated at home with zinc lozenges and mouth wash containing alcohol to reduce the virus in the mouth and upper respiratory tract. Fever should be treated with acetaminophen. More severe cases require hospitalization to provide intravenous fluids and respiratory therapy with oxygen and mechanical ventilation, if necessary. Antiviral agents have been used with varying success. The antimalarials, quinine, chloroquine, and hydroxychloroquine, are also being investigated for effectiveness against the virus. The antiparasitic medication ivermectin is used in third-world countries to treat COVID-19. However, double-blinded, placebo-controlled studies have yielded mixed results. The government of western countries has yet

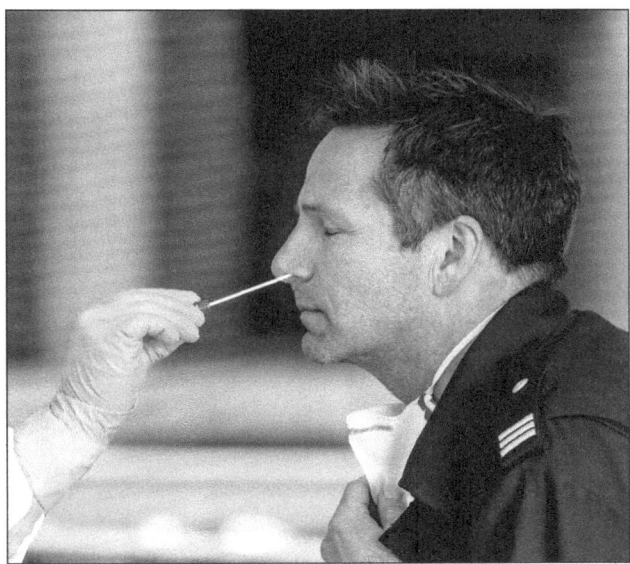

A nasopharyngeal swab being used to test for SARS-CoV-2 virus and the associated COVID-19 illness. [CC 4.0.]

to approve it as a treatment for COVID-19, even though some researchers continue to advocate for it.

Antibiotics help prevent or treat secondary bacterial infection of the damaged lung tissue of COVID-19 pneumonia patients. Some severe cases seem to show improvement from the infection and then worsen. This late-stage illness, sometimes seen in severe cases, is thought to result from continuing and overactive immune response to the infection that can lead to further damage to the lungs. Treatment with corticosteroids has been shown to benefit patients with this late-stage deterioration of pneumonia. Heparin treatment also diminishes the risk of blood clots. Intubation can increase oxygen saturation, but severely ill patients may require extracorporeal membrane oxygenation (ECMO).

Excellent vaccines exist for COVID-19. The PfizerBioNTECH (BNT162b2) and Moderna (messenger ribonucleic acid [mRNA]-1273) mRNA-vaccines confer outstanding protection against many SARS-CoV-2 strains. Adenovirus-based vaccines include the Oxford/AstraZeneca (Vaxzevria), Johnson & Johnson (JNJ-78436735), and Russian Sputnik V

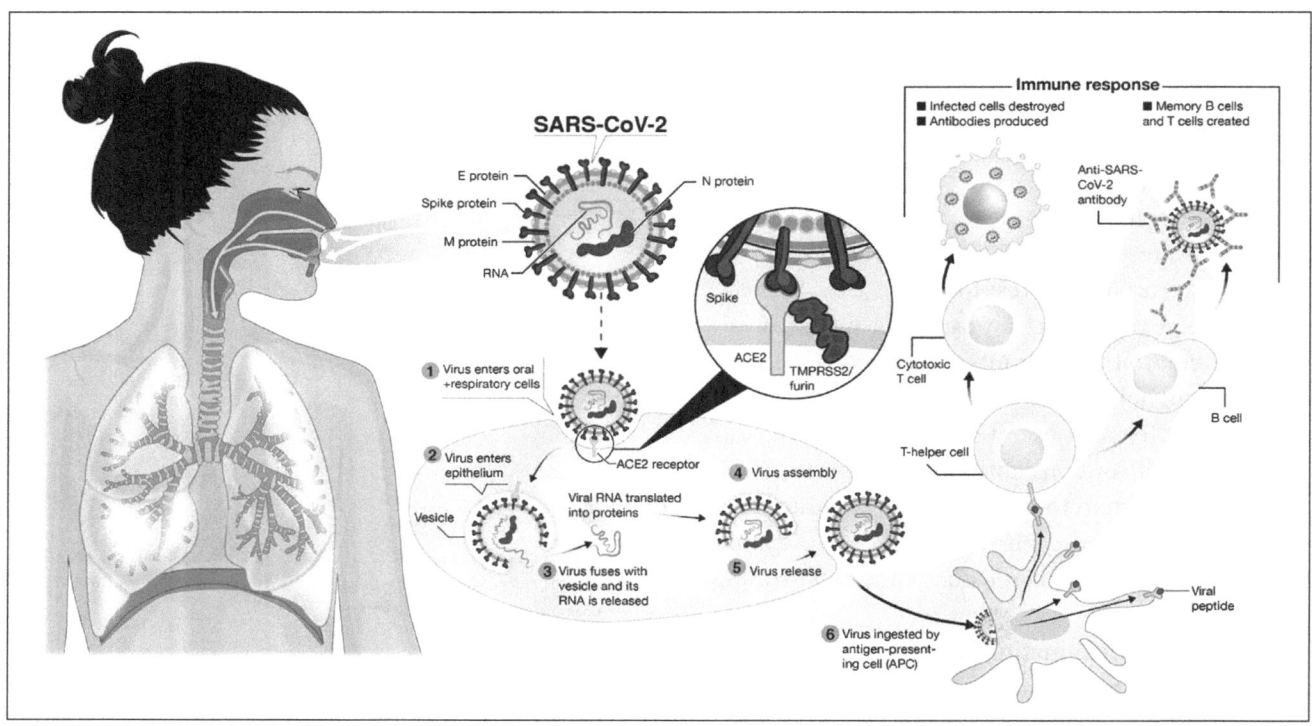

Transmission and life-cycle of SARS-CoV-2 causing COVID-19. Image by Colin D. Funk, Craig Laferrière, and Ali Ardakani, via Wikimedia Commons. [CC 4.0.]

(Gam-COVID-Vac) vaccines. These also provide reasonable protection against infection, and especially against severe disease hospitalization and death. The side effect profile of these vaccines is also excellent. The mRNA-based vaccines cause fatigue, local soreness of the arm, transient joint and muscle pain, and headaches. In younger male patients, they cause mild and temporary myocarditis at a rate of 77 cases per million vaccinations. The risk of myocarditis from COVID-19 is six times that rate. Some adenovirus-based vaccines increase the risk of blood clots, usually in younger women (7 to 11 per million). However, the risk of blood clots in COVID-19 patients is close to ten times higher. Therefore, the vaccines are much safer than COVID-19.

PREVENTION AND OUTCOMES

Prevention for the general population is being accomplished by social distancing and quarantine of infected patients or possibly infected patients. The movement of people from countries or areas of increased infection was halted entirely or restricted. A two-week period of quarantine is necessary for infected or possibly infected patients, as well as individuals exposed to an infected patient. Travelers from a country with a high incidence of COVID-19 and cruise ship passengers were required to self-quarantine for two weeks. Frequent handwashing with soap and water for at least twenty seconds or use of hand sanitizer is strongly recommended. SARS-CoV-2 is inactivated on surfaces by disinfection with 70 percent ethanol, 0.5 percent hydrogen peroxide, or 0.1 percent sodium hypochlorite for one minute. Infected or possibly infected patients should wear masks when seeking medical diagnosis or treatment to lessen the chance of spreading the disease. Health-care workers need to wear gloves, gowns, and N-95 respirators when caring for infected or possibly infected patients. This protective equipment is also necessary for healthcare workers obtaining nasal and throat swabs for diagnostic testing.

Children generally have a mild disease; the infrequent cases of severe disease in children are rarely fatal. Adults have increased risks of severe disease with older age, underlying diseases, obesity, and smoking. The overall adult mortality rate worldwide has ranged from less than 1 to 3 percent. For elderly patients, the mortality rate is much higher and may exceed 10 percent. Individuals can completely recover even from severe disease. Still, some patients recovering from severe disease may shed virus for several weeks and may require more extended quarantine. Hospitalized patients should test negative for the virus before being removed from quarantine after discharge from the hospital.

—*H. Bradford Hawley, MD
and Michael A. Buratovich, PhD*

Further Information

Baden, Lindsey R. et al. "Efficacy and Safety of the mRNA-1273 SARS-CoV-2 Vaccine." *New England Journal of Medicine,* vol. 384, no. 5, 2020, pp. 403-16, doi:10.1056/NEJMoa2035389.

Guan, W., et al. "Clinical Characteristics of Coronavirus Disease 2019 in China." *New England Journal of Medicine,* 28 Feb. 2020, doi:10.1056/NEJMoa2002032.

Holshue, M. L., et al. "First Case of 2019 Novel Coronavirus in the United States." *New England Journal of Medicine,* vol. 382, 2020, pp. 929-36, doi:10.1056/NEJMoa2001191.

Huang, Chaolin, et al. "Clinical Features of Patients Infected with 2019 Novel Coronavirus in Wuhan, China." *The Lancet,* vol. 395, no. 10223, 15 Feb. 2020, pp. 497-506, www.thelancet.com/journals/lancet/article/PIIS0140-6736(20)30183-5/fulltext.

Kampf, G., et. al. "Persistence of Coronaviruses on Inanimate Surfaces and Their Inactivation with Biocidal Agents." *Journal of Hospital Infection,* doi.org/10.1016/j.jhin.2020.01.022.

Lu, Roujian, et al. "Genomic Characterization and Epidemiology of 2019 Novel Coronavirus: Implications for Virus Origins and Receptor Binding." *The Lancet,* Jan. 2020, doi.org/10.1016/s0140-6736(20)30251-8.

Polack, Fernando P., et al. "Safety and Efficacy of the BNT162b2 mRNA Covid-19 Vaccine." *New England Journal of Medicine,* vol. 383, no. 27, 2020, pp. 2603-15, doi.org/10.1056/NEJMoa2034577.

Thevarajan, Irani, et al. "Breadth of Concomitant Immune Responses Prior to Patient Recovery: A Case of Non-Severe COVID-19." *Nature Medicine,* Mar. 2020, doi.org/10.1038/s41591-020-0819-2.

Wang, Manli, et al. "Remdesivir and Chloroquine Effectively Inhibit the Recently Emerged Coronavirus (2019-nCoV) In Vitro." *Cell Research,* vol. 30, 2020, pp. 269-71, doi.org/10.1038/s41422-020-0282-0.

Cytomegalovirus (CMV)

Category: Diseases/Disorders

Anatomy or system affected: Blood, brain, cells, ears, eyes, gastrointestinal system, immune system, liver, lungs

Specialties and related fields: Family medicine, gastroenterology, hematology, immunology, obstetrics, pediatrics, virology

Definition: A viral disease normally producing mild symptoms in healthy individuals but severe infections in the immunocompromised. Congenital infection may lead to malformations or fetal death.

KEY TERMS

hepatitis: inflammation of the liver; usually caused by viral infections, toxic substances, or immunological disturbances

hepatosplenomegaly: enlargement of the liver and spleen such that they may be felt below the rib margins

heterophil antibodies: antibodies that are detected using antigens other than the antigens that induced them

jaundice: yellow staining of the skin, eyes, and other tissues and excretions with excess bile pigments in the blood

latency: following an acute infection by a virus, a period of dormancy from which the virus may be reactivated during times of stress or immunocompromise

microcephaly: a congenital condition involving an abnormally small head associated with an incompletely developed brain

> **INFORMATION ON CYTOMEGALOVIRUS (CMV)**
>
> **Causes**: Viral infection spread during childbirth or through body fluid exchange
>
> **Symptoms**: Deafness, visual impairment, mental retardation, jaundice, microcephaly, seizures, cerebral palsy, blood disorders, infectious mononucleosis
>
> **Duration**: Varies
>
> **Treatments**: Antiviral drugs (ganciclovir, foscarnet)

CAUSES AND SYMPTOMS

Cytomegalovirus (CMV) is a member of the herpesvirus group that includes such viruses as the Epstein-Barr virus, which causes infectious mononucleosis, and the varicellazoster virus, which causes chickenpox. CMV is a ubiquitous virus that is transmitted in a number of different ways. A newly infected woman may transmit the virus across the placenta to her unborn child. Infection may also occur in the birth canal or via mother's milk. Young children commonly transmit CMV by means of saliva. Sexual transmission is common in adults. Blood transfusions and organ transplants may also transmit cytomegalovirus to recipients. As many as 80 percent of adults worldwide have antibodies indicating exposure to cytomegalovirus.

Congenital cytomegaloviral infection is universally common and especially prevalent in developing nations. According to the Centers for Disease Control and Prevention (CDC), about 0.7 percent of children are born infected. Most congenitally infected infants exhibit no symptoms. Normal development may follow, but some infants experience problems such as hearing loss, visual impairment, and developmental disabilities. Approximately 10 to 20 percent exhibit clinically obvious evidence of cytomegalic inclusion disease: hepatosplenomegaly, jaundice, microcephaly, deafness, seizures, cerebral palsy, and blood disorders such as thrombocytopenia (a decrease in platelets) and hemolytic anemia (in which red blood cells are destroyed). Giant cells having nuclei containing large inclusions are found in affected organs. Cytomegalovirus is a leading cause of developmental disabilities and has also been linked to microcephaly.

In immunocompetent adults and older children, cytomegalovirus can cause heterophil-negative mononucleosis, an infectious mononucleosis in which no heterophil antibodies are formed. Such antibodies are found in infectious mononucleosis caused by the Epstein-Barr virus. Heterophil-negative mononucleosis is characterized by fever, hepatitis, lethargy, and abnormal lymphocytes in blood.

Severe systemic cytomegalovirus infections are frequently seen in the immunocompromised. Transplant patients are intentionally immunosuppressed to reduce the likelihood of graft rejection, making them vulnerable to infection by cytomegalovirus either by reactivation or by acquisition of the virus from the donor organ. Resulting systemic infections are manifested in diseases such as pneumonia, hepatitis, and retinitis. In addition to these CMV diseases, acquired immunodeficiency syndrome (AIDS) patients may experience infections of the central nervous system and gastrointestinal tract. Their blood cells may also be affected, resulting in disorders such as thrombocytopenia. AIDS patients frequently have intestinal CMV infections leading to chronic diarrhea. Cytomegalovirus retinitis in AIDS patients is particularly serious and may lead to retinal detachment and blindness. This is the most common sight-damaging opportunistic eye infection found in AIDS patients.

TREATMENT AND THERAPY

Ganciclovir, valganciclovir, foscarnet, and cidofovir are all antiviral agents that have been found useful in treating CMV infections in immunocompromised patients. Toxic properties, however, can limit their long-term administration. Ganciclovir exhibits hematopoietic toxicity; that is, it has an adverse effect on blood cells that may result in neutropenia, a decrease in the number of neutrophils in the blood. Foscarnet has more side effects than ganciclovir. It is a nephrotoxic substance, which means that it may damage the kidneys and thus cannot be used in patients with renal failure.

Valganciclovir, the oral form of ganciclovir, has been used effectively to prevent CMV infection in transplant recipients. It is administered to CMV-seronegative transplant patients receiving organs from CMV-seropositive donors as well as in CMV-seropositive recipients who will be undergoing immunosuppression to prevent rejection of transplanted organs. Another material employed as a prophylaxis for bone marrow and renal transplant recipients is intravenous cytomegalovirus immune globulin.

Therapy for CMV retinitis involves intravenous treatment with either ganciclovir, foscarnet, or cidofovir plus oral probenecid or oral valganciclovir. Alternatively, an intraocular ganciclovir implant may be used along with one of the systemic treatments mentioned above. Therapy of retinitis as well as other types of CMV infection in AIDS patients should be accompanied by highly effective

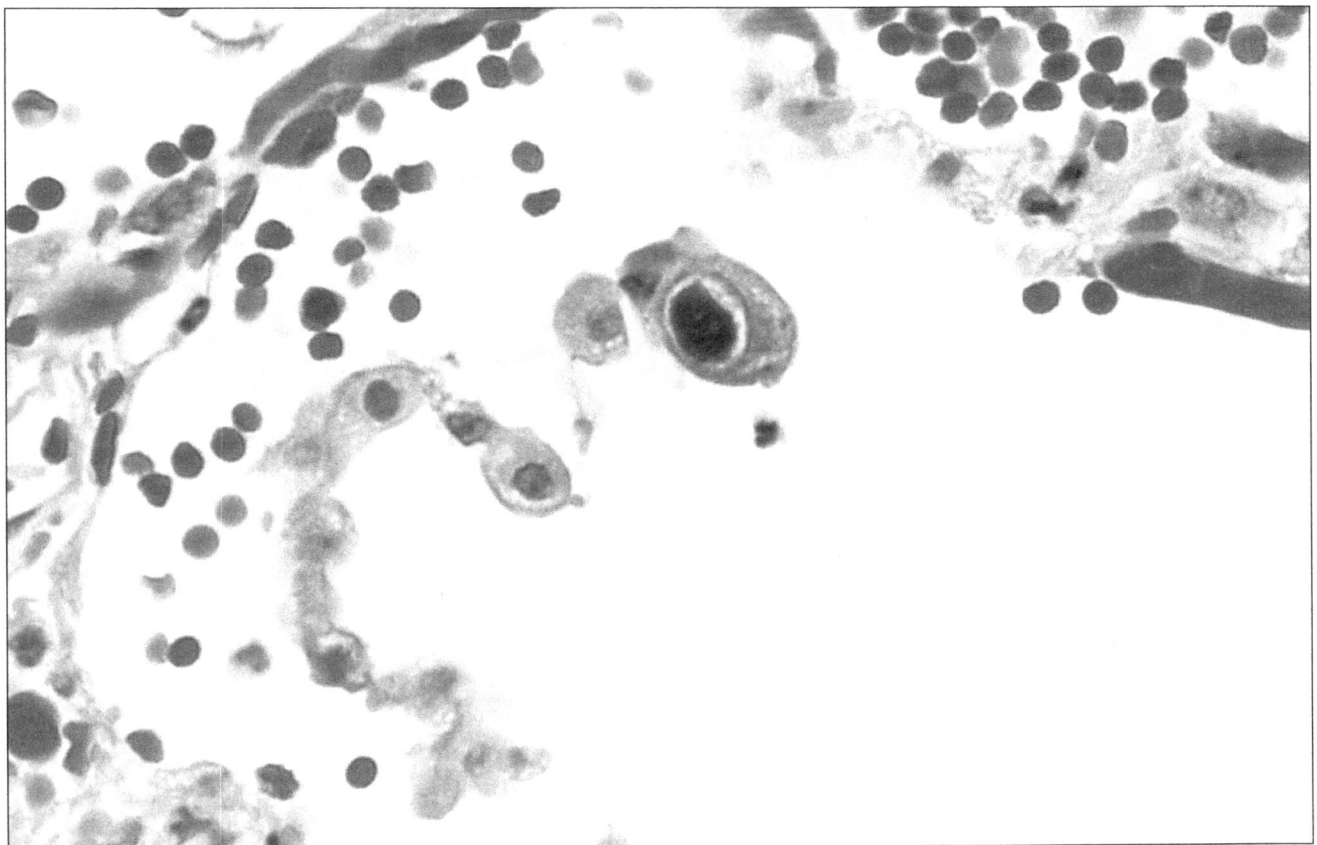

Typical "owl eye" intranuclear inclusion indicating CMV infection of a lung pneumocyte. Photo via Wikimedia Commons. [Public domain.]

antiretroviral therapy (HAART) to treat the human immunodeficiency virus and improve the immune function in the patient. Successful HAART may allow the CMV antiviral therapy to be discontinued, but the patient must be carefully monitored for relapse of the CMV infection.

Retinal detachment is another complication arising from cytomegalovirus retinitis. It may occur even in those undergoing successful antiviral treatment. Surgical intervention is required to restore functional vision in these cases.

PERSPECTIVE AND PROSPECTS

The term *cytomegalia* was first used in 1921 to describe the condition of an infant with intranuclear inclusions in the lungs, kidney, and liver. This condition in an adult was first attributed to a virus of the herpes group in 1925. Twenty-five cases of apparent cytomegalic inclusion disease had been described by 1932. Cytomegalovirus was pursued and isolated in the mid-1950s by researcher Margaret Smith. Around the same time, independently and serendipitously, groups in Boston, Massachusetts, and Bethesda, Maryland, also isolated the virus.

Development of new antiviral drugs and measures to reduce the immunocompromised state should continue to progress and improve the outcomes for patients infected with CMV.

—*Nancy Handshaw Clark, PhD and H. Bradford Hawley, MD*

Further Information

A.D.A.M. Medical Encyclopedia. "Cytomegalovirus Infections." *MedlinePlus*, 2 May 2013.

A.D.A.M. Medical Encyclopedia. "Cytomegalovirus Retinitis." *MedlinePlus*, 6 Dec. 2011.

Bellenir, Karen, and Peter D. Dresser, editors. *Contagious and Noncontagious Infectious Diseases Sourcebook*. Omnigraphics, 1996.

National Center for Immunization and Respiratory Diseases, Division of Viral Diseases. "Cytomegalovirus (CMV) and Congenital CMV Infection." *Centers for Disease Control and Prevention*, 6 Dec. 2010.

Roizman, Bernard, editor. *Infectious Diseases in an Age of Change: The Impact of Human Ecology and Behavior on Disease Transmission*. National Academy Press, 1995.

Roizman, Bernard, Richard J. Whitley, and Carlos Lopez, editors. *The Human Herpesviruses*. Raven Press, 1993.

Scheld, W. Michael, Richard J. Whitley, and Christina M. Marra, editors. *Infections of the Central Nervous System*. 3rd ed., Lippincott Williams & Wilkins, 2004.

Wagner, Edward K., and Martinez J. Hewlett. *Basic Virology*. 3rd ed., Blackwell Science, 2008.

Epstein-Barr virus

Category: Diseases/Disorders
Also known as: Human herpesvirus 4 (HHV-4)
Anatomy or system affected: Blood, cells, glands, immune system, lymphatic system, mouth, muscles, nose, throat
Specialties and related fields: Cytology, hematology, immunology, microbiology, oncology, pathology, pediatrics, virology
Definition: An extensively occurring virus that infects almost all humans during their lifetime, often remaining latent in their systems but sometimes causing malignant tumors and various types of cancer.

KEY TERMS

antibodies: protein molecules that detect antigens and destroy infected host cells

antigens: viral proteins that attract antibodies, which the immune system designs to attack them

B cells: also known as B lymphocytes; white blood cells that create antibodies

oncoviruses: viruses causing the growth of cancerous cells

replication: the viral insertion of genetic information into host cell nuclei to create additional similar viruses

T cells: also known as cytotoxic T lymphocytes; white blood cells that destroy cells hosting antigens or infected by pathogens, which eluded antibodies

virion: a viral particle that contains genetic information inside a protective structure

CAUSES AND SYMPTOMS

Present only in humans, Epstein-Barr virus was the first documented oncovirus. The virus, resembling other human herpesviruses, consists of sphere-shaped, barbed virions approximately 120 to 220 nanometers in diameter. Each Epstein-Barr virus genome contains two strands of deoxyribonucleic acid (DNA). A protein shell protects the genome, and an envelope surrounds the protein shell. Various Epstein-Barr virus strains have evolved that can infect an individual at the same time.

The Epstein-Barr virus typically infects salivary gland cells or B cells. Usually, Epstein-Barr viral infections are transmitted through saliva. Seeking host cells in order to replicate, the Epstein-Barr virus proliferates, creating approximately one hundred types of antigens, including nuclear antigen EBNA1, which the Epstein-Barr virus uses to put its DNA into new cells created during cell division.

T cells fight Epstein-Barr virus antigens by destroying infected host cells. T cells and antibodies stay in the immune system to continue protecting against infection, regulating latency, and developing immunity. EBNA1 is necessary for the Epstein-Barr virus genomes to endure being latent. T cells cannot detect the antigen EBNA1 and attack those host cells, which results in the Epstein-Barr virus often being invisible to immune protection. Latent infec-

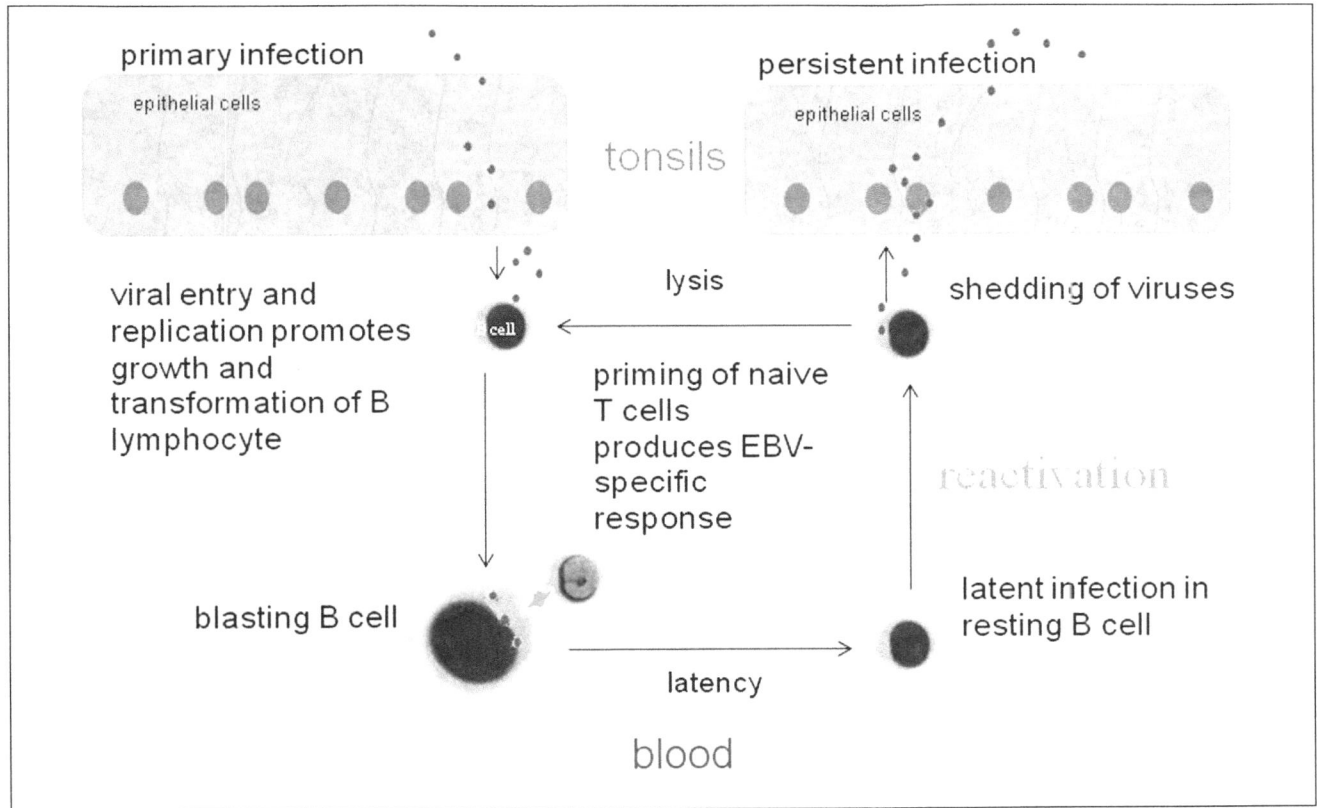

EBV infection cycle in healthy humans. Image by Graham Beards, via Wikimedia Commons. [CC 3.0.]

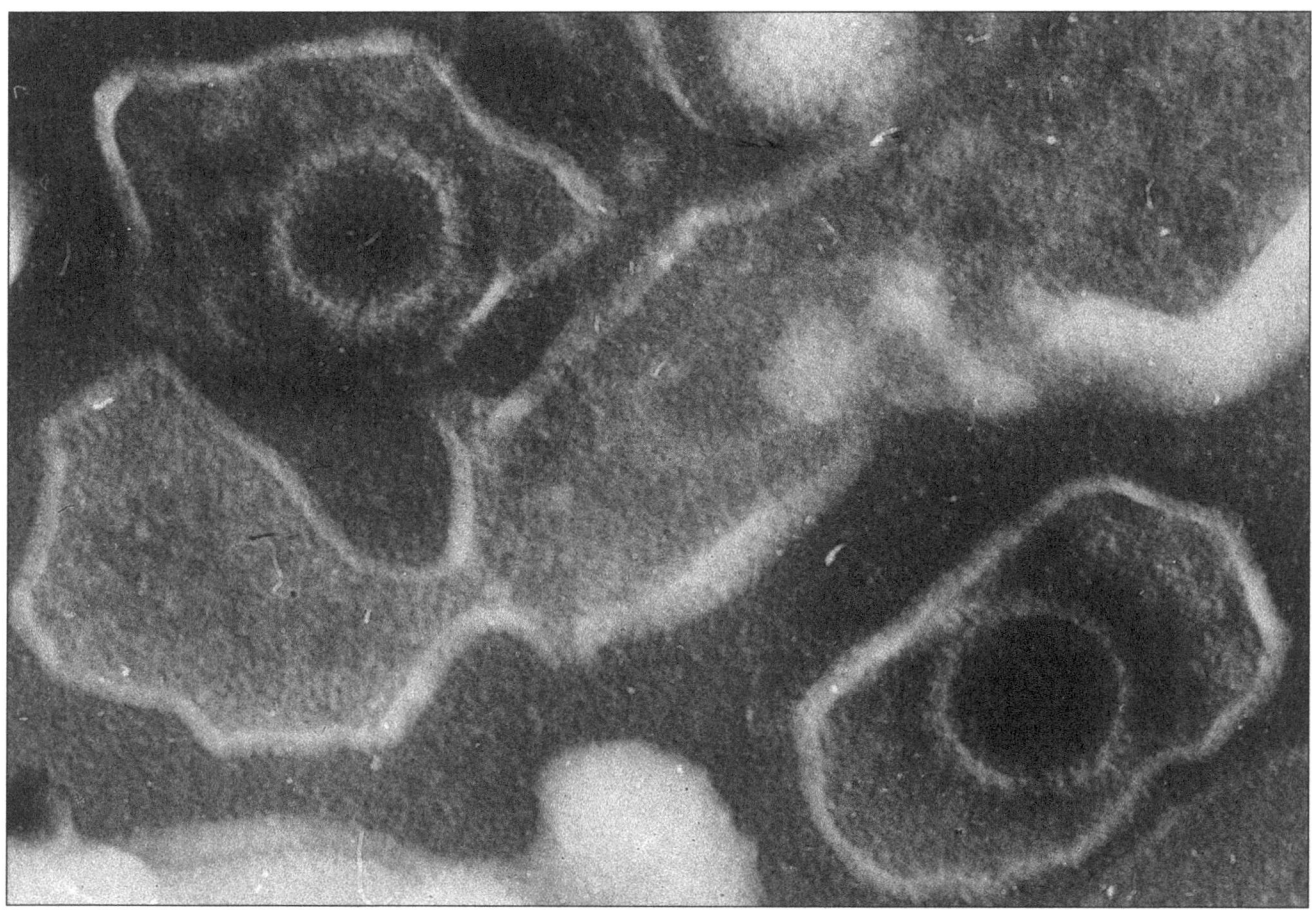

Electron microscopic image of two Epstein-Barr virus virions (viral particles) showing round capsids (protein-encased genetic material) loosely surrounded by the membrane envelope. Photo by Liza Gross, via Wikimedia Commons. [CC 2.5.]

tions are not apparent, usually remaining passive, but they can become active, potentially resulting in tumors and diseases.

The Epstein-Barr virus usually infects throat, blood, or immune system cells. Infectious mononucleosis, also known as glandular fever, is the most widely known Epstein-Barr viral infection. Physicians determine if people have been infected by Epstein-Barr virus by performing laboratory tests analyzing blood samples to detect if any of the antibodies to combat Epstein-Barr virus antigens are present and, if so, how many are present. Such antibodies might have existed for years and are not proof of an active infection.

People can contract the virus as children, adolescents, or adults, depending on geographic location and socioeconomic factors. Some infants are born with the virus transmitted by their mothers. The Epstein-Barr virus usually infects people when they are children, without obvious signs. Often, these individuals never know that they are infected. Approximately half of the people who contract the Epstein-Barr virus as an adolescent or at an older age, however, develop infectious mononucleosis.

Activated Epstein-Barr virus can result in several serious diseases, and people with suppressed immune systems are vulnerable to developing such malignancies as cancerous tumors in smooth muscle tissue, stomach carcinomas, lymphomas, and sarcomas. Epstein-Barr virus often causes nasal and throat cancers known as nasopharyngeal carcinoma. In some individuals with acquired immunodeficiency syndrome (AIDS), Epstein-Barr virus replicates in tongue cells, resulting in oral hairy leukoplakia. Epstein-Barr virus has also been associated with leukemia.

Weak immune systems cause people to be vulnerable to Epstein-Barr virus infections, particularly after organ transplantation and the use of immunosuppressive drugs to lower the immune reaction and to encourage acceptance of the new organ. In those cases, Epstein-Barr virus sometimes causes posttransplant lymphoproliferative disease to occur.

When it infects the nodes, Epstein-Barr virus might be a factor in people affected by Hodgkin disease. Researchers have considered a possible role of Epstein-Barr virus in the development of multiple sclerosis and breast cancer. They have eliminated it as a factor in chronic fatigue syndrome.

TREATMENT AND THERAPY

Approximately 90 to 95 percent of humans globally at any time have been infected with Epstein-Barr virus, which remains latent and endures in their bodies until death. There is currently no way to eliminate the virus once infection has occurred. Treatment focuses instead on the diseases that Epstein-Barr virus causes.

Researchers have attempted to develop antiviral vaccines to stop the replication of Epstein-Barr virus. In the early twenty-first century, scientists at Queensland Institute of Medical Research developed a vaccine prototype to strengthen T cells combatting Epstein-Barr virus antigens.

PERSPECTIVE AND PROSPECTS

The Epstein-Barr virus was located as a result of researchers seeking viruses possibly associated with

> **INFORMATION ON EPSTEIN-BARR VIRUS**
>
> **Causes**: Viral infection spread primarily through saliva
>
> **Symptoms**: In children, usually none; in adolescents and adults, often mononucleosis; associated with a number of cancers and other diseases
>
> **Duration**: Acute and then chronic
>
> **Treatments**: None for viral infection; chemotherapy and radiation for resulting cancers

cancer in humans. In 1961, London researcher M. Anthony Epstein attended a lecture at which Denis P. Burkitt discussed his work with tumors, later called "Burkitt lymphoma," in African children's facial bones. Epstein, experienced with investigating viruses causing animal tumors, wanted to examine Burkitt lymphoma tumor tissues to detect any viruses. The British Empire Cancer Campaign funded Epstein's travel to Uganda to acquire a consistent supply of tumor samples for his Middlesex Hospital Medical School laboratory. Epstein tried unsuccessfully to locate a virus for a couple of years.

The U.S. National Cancer Institute presented Epstein $45,000 for his investigations, and he hired doctoral student Yvonne M. Barr and colleague Bert G. Achong to expand his laboratory work attempting to culture viruses. The trio successfully grew a Burkitt lymphoma cell line in culture. When cells from that sample were examined with an electron microscope, the London scientists saw viral particles with structural elements of herpesvirus. Scrutinizing the virions, the trio declared that they had isolated a previously unknown human herpesvirus. They published their results in a 1964 *Lancet* article. After Epstein-Barr virus was identified, additional investigators studied the virus to expand knowledge of its structure, replication, and the diseases associated with it, determining that it was an oncovirus.

Research into ways to fight Epstein-Barr virus is ongoing. Scientists at the European Molecular Biology Laboratory and Institut de Virologie Moléculaire et Structurale have focused on controlling a protein molecule known as ZEBRA that accompanies Epstein-Barr virus, helping activate it from the latent phase.

—*Elizabeth D. Schafer, PhD*

Further Information

Cohen, Jeffrey I., et al. "The Need and Challenges for Development of an Epstein-Barr Virus Vaccine." *Vaccine*, vol. 31, Apr. 2013, pp. B194-B196.

Epstein, M. Anthony, and Bert G. Achong, editors. *The Epstein-Barr Virus*. Springer, 1979.

Ford, Jodi L., and Raymond P. Stowe. "Racial-Ethnic Differences in Epstein-Barr Virus Antibody Titers Among U.S. Children and Adolescents." *Annals of Epidemiology*, vol. 23, no. 5, May 2013, pp. 275-80.

Jackson, Alan C. *Viral Infections of the Human Nervous System*. Springer, 2013.

Odumade, Oludare A., Kristin A. Hogquist, and Henry H. Balfour, Jr. "Progress and Problems in Understanding and Managing Primary Epstein-Barr Virus Infections." *Clinical Microbiology Review*, vol. 24, no. 1, Jan. 2011, pp. 193-209.

Robertson, Erle S., editor. *Epstein-Barr Virus*. Caister Academic Press, 2010.

Tselis, Alex C., and Hal B. Jenson, editors. *Epstein-Barr Virus*. Taylor & Francis, 2006.

Umar, Constantine S., editor. *New Developments in Epstein-Barr Virus Research*. Nova Science, 2006.

Wilson, Joanna B., and Gerhard H. W. May, editors. *Epstein-Barr Virus Protocols*. Humana Press, 2001.

GOITER

Category: Diseases/Disorders
Anatomy or system affected: Endocrine system, glands, neck
Specialties and related fields: Endocrinology
Definition: An enlargement of the thyroid gland that is non-cancerous and not caused by a temporary condition such as inflammation.

KEY TERMS

goitrogenic: referring to a factor (typically food or chemicals) that produces goiter
hypersecretion: the excess production and secretion of a hormone or other chemical

CAUSES AND SYMPTOMS

Goiter is often a painless medical condition. Its only visible symptoms may be a slight but visible enlargement of the thyroid that creates a swelling at the base of the neck. In severe cases, the swelling becomes massive. The patient experiences difficulty breathing or swallowing as the enlarged thyroid compresses against the windpipe or esophagus. Other symptoms that may indicate goiter include weight loss, increased heart rate, elevated blood pressure, hair loss, and tremors. An ultrasound scan of the thyroid, blood tests for abnormal levels of thyroxine or thyroid-stimulating hormone, or low rates of iodine excretion in the urine confirms the diagnosis of goiter.

The several types of medical goiter fall into two broad categories: simple goiter and toxic goiter. A dietary deficiency of iodine causes simple goiter. In response, one or both lobes of the thyroid gland enlarge to produce more of the iodine-containing hormone thyroxine. Two types of simple goiter are recognized: endemic goiter and sporadic goiter.

INFORMATION ON GOITER

Causes: Of simple goiter, iodine deficiency or hormonal changes (adolescence, pregnancy); of toxic goiter, excessive production of thyroxine from oversecretion of thyroid-stimulating hormone by the pituitary

Symptoms: Thyroid enlargement ranging from slight to massive, with difficulty breathing or swallowing

Duration: Acute or chronic

Treatments: Iodine tablets, sometimes surgical removal of all or part of the thyroid

Endemic goiter typically occurs in landlocked geographic regions or in areas where farm soils are iodine-depleted. Simple goiter was once common in central Asia, central Africa, and the so-called Goiter Belt of the United States, which extended from the Great Lakes to the Intermountain West (between the Rockies and the Sierras).

Simple goiter most often appears in adolescence, but it may sometimes occur during pregnancy. This condition should be corrected in pregnant women to ensure the healthy development of the fetus and the birth of a healthy infant. Simple goiter readily responds to treatment via iodine tablets. Still, surgical removal of all or part of the enlarged thyroid may be necessary for some patients. Public health measures undertaken to eliminate or prevent simple goiter include adding iodine to table salt and water reservoirs in certain areas.

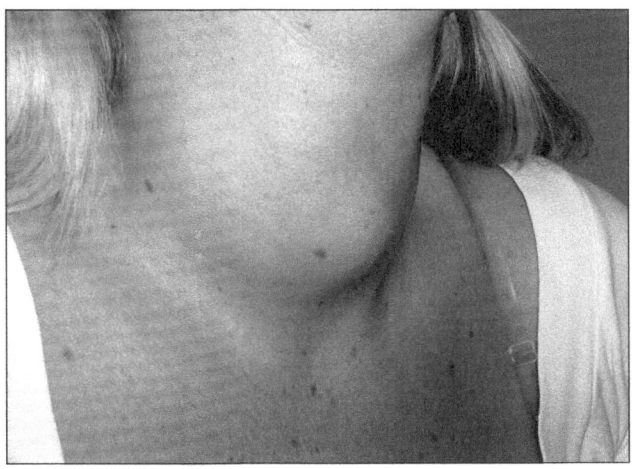

Goiter class 1. Photo by Drahreg01, via Wikimedia Commons. [CC 3.0.]

Sporadic goiter occurs in some individuals because of excessive goitrogenic (goiter-causing) foods such as cabbage, soybeans, spinach, and radishes. Sporadic goiter has also been linked with exposure to certain medications, such as aminoglutethimide or lithium. Although this type of goiter is considered nontoxic, it does produce impaired thyroid activity. Sporadic goiter can be treated by limiting the consumption of goitrogenic foods.

Toxic goiter is caused by excessive production of thyroxine hormone by the thyroid gland. This type of goiter is also called "hyperthyroid goiter," "exophthalmic goiter," or "Graves' disease." Toxic goiter results from an oversecretion (hypersecretion) of thyroid-stimulating hormone by the pituitary. In turn, the thyroid gland responds by enlarging and secreting excess amounts of thyroxine, resulting in goiter. Symptoms of Graves' disease include elevated metabolic rate, higher body temperature, rapid weight loss, nervousness, and irritability. In some patients, this type of goiter results in protrusive eyeballs and the appearance of staring.

Euthyroid goiter occurs when dietary levels of iodine are only slightly below normal. The pituitary gland responds to lowered thyroxine levels in the blood by producing additional thyroid-stimulating hormone. The thyroid gland responds to the ele-

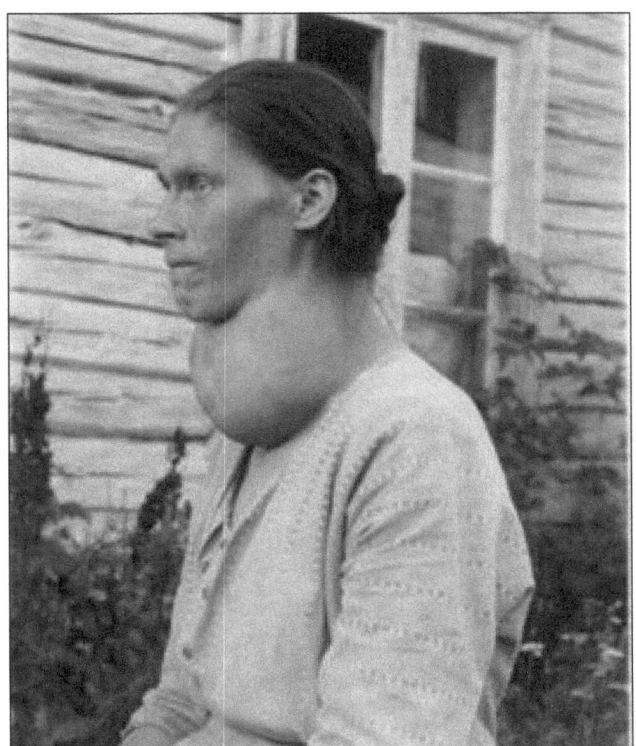

Goiter class 2. Photo by Martin Finborud, via Wikimedia Commons. [Public domain.]

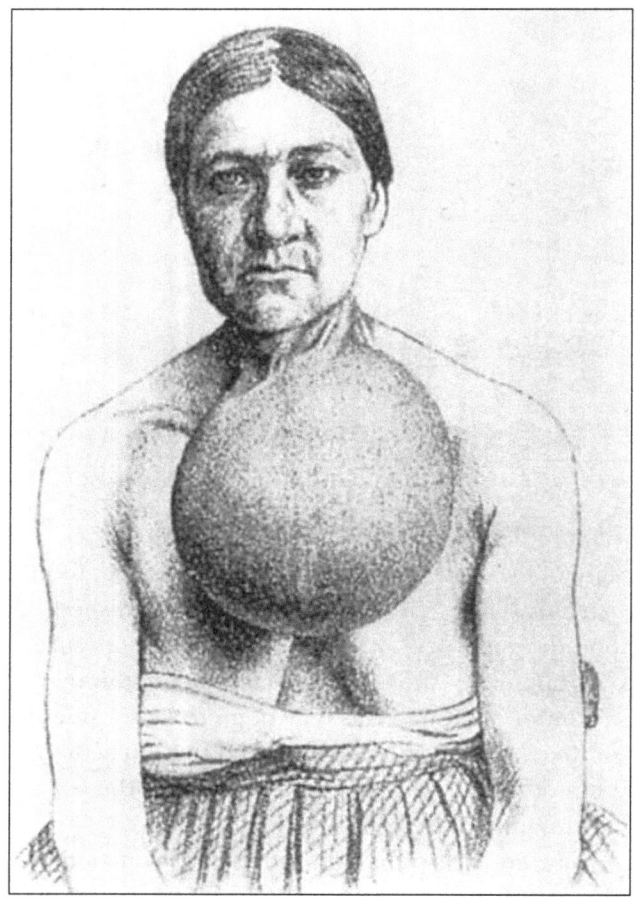

Goiter class 3. Image via Wikimedia Commons. [Public domain.]

vated thyroid-stimulating hormone by enlarging to increase thyroxine production.

TREATMENT AND THERAPY

Most goiters can be treated effectively through dietary supplements of iodine. The administration of iodine supplements must be very carefully regulated to prevent a so-called thyroxin storm resulting from excess thyroxine production by the enlarged thyroid gland. Some patients may choose alternative natural herbal therapies taken in tablet form. Still, these substances should be used only in consultation with a physician.

—*Dwight G. Smith, PhD*

Further Information

Cakir, Mehtap. *Differential Diagnosis of Hyperthyroidism*. Nova Science, 2010.

DeMaeyer, E. M. *The Control of Endemic Goiter*. World Health Organization, 1988.

Gaitan, Eduardo, editor. *Environmental Goitrogenesis*. CRC, 1989.

Hall, R., and J. Köbberling, editors. *Thyroid Disorders Associated with Iodine Deficiency and Excess*. Raven Press, 1985.

Hamburger, J. I. *Nontoxic Goiter: Concept and Controversy*. Charles C. Thomas, 1973.

Icon Health. *Goiter: A Medical Dictionary, Bibliography, and Annotated Research Guide to Internet References*. Author, 2004.

Jameson, J. Larry, and Leslie J. DeGroot. *Endocrinology: Adult and Pediatric*. Elsevier Saunders, 2010.

McDermott, Michael T. *Endocrine Secrets*. 6th ed., Elsevier Saunders, 2013.

IMPETIGO

Category: Diseases/Disorders
Anatomy or system affected: Immune system, skin
Specialties and related fields: Bacteriology, dermatology, emergency medicine, family medicine, internal medicine, microbiology, pediatrics, sports medicine
Definition: A superficial bacterial infection of the skin.

KEY TERMS

pruritic: an unpleasant condition provoking an urge to scratch

methicillin-resistant Staphylococcus aureus: a strain of the common skin microorganism *S. aureus* that has acquired new genes that render it resistant to standard antibiotics and more virulent

vesicopustules: a blister filled with pus

CAUSES AND SYMPTOMS

Impetigo is a superficial bacterial skin infection usually caused by group A streptococcus, *Staphylococcus aureus*, or a mixture of both. Group A streptococcus was originally the predominant pathogen, but recently *S. aureus* has become the most common strain. Impetigo caused by either of these bacteria is clinically identical.

Children are most commonly affected by impetigo, and infection is often preceded by minor trauma such as insect bites. Outbreaks predominantly occur during the summer months when the climate is hot and humid. Impetigo is very contagious and easily spread in crowded conditions such as families, schools, the military, and athletics. Poverty and poor personal hygiene can also predispose individuals to infection.

A typical infection first develops as multiple vesicopustules, which rupture and form a characteristic golden-yellow crust. The lesions are painless but commonly pruritic (itchy), and scratching can serve to spread infection. Systemic symptoms are rare, but there can be local lymphadenopathy. The face, particularly the region around the mouth, is a common site of infection.

> **INFORMATION ON IMPETIGO**
>
> **Causes**: Bacterial infection
>
> **Symptoms**: Skin inflammation, blisters, itchiness, scabbing
>
> **Duration**: Acute
>
> **Treatments**: Injection of antibiotics (penicillin, erythromycin)

TREATMENT AND THERAPY

Topical and oral antibiotics have been used for the treatment of impetigo. Historically, the treatment of choice was penicillin or ampicillin. However, the treatment regimen has changed as the most predominant bacteria are now *S. aureus* instead of group A streptococcus, which almost universally produces a beta-lactamase that makes them resistant to penicillin. It is now recommended to use beta-lactamase-resistant penicillins such as oxacillin, nafcillin, dicloxacillin or a first-generation cephalosporin such as cephalexin. Doxycycline is recommended if the patient is allergic to penicillins.

Topical antibiotics such as mupirocin 2 percent (three times daily) or retapamulin 1 percent (twice daily) ointments for five days are very effective treatments for isolated lesions. Topical antibiotics are as effective and have fewer side effects, making them a better choice in less severe cases. Oral antibiotics are a better choice for multiple lesions. Oral cephalexin (four times a day) for seven days is the standard regimen in such cases.

If methicillin-resistant *Staphylococcus aureus* (MRSA) is the suspected cause of impetigo, the physician must prescribe more powerful treatments.

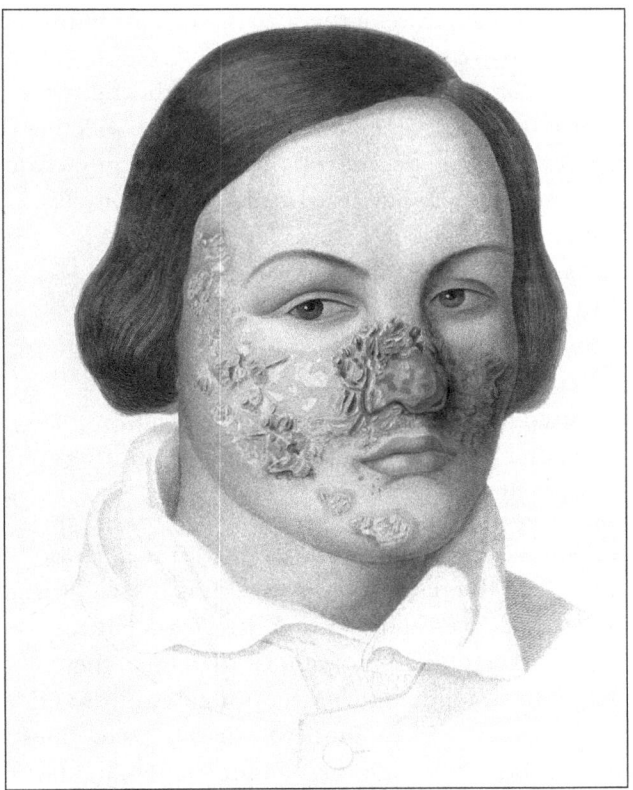

Illustration of a woman with severe facial impetigo. Photo by Wellcome Images, via Wikimedia Commons. [CC 4.0.]

These include a seven-day course of oral sulfa drugs (trimethoprim/sulfamethoxazole) twice a day, oral doxycycline twice a day, or oral clindamycin, three times a day. Oral antibiotics are preferred in cases with multiple lesions or outbreaks that affect multiple people.

Gentle cleansing of the area with soap and water or chlorhexidine can be helpful. Health-care providers should discuss personal hygiene with their patients to help prevent recurrence of infection. Frequent hand washing and not sharing bath linens can help prevent the spread of the bacteria. The lesions usually heal without scarring.

—Jeffrey B. Roberts, MD, Jeffrey R. Bytomski, DO, and Michael A. Buratovich, PhD

Further Information

Bhumbra, Nasreen A., and Sophia G. McCullough. "Skin and Subcutaneous Infections." *Update on Infectious Diseases*, edited by Richard I. Haddy and Karen W. Krigger, W. B. Saunders, 2003.

Dinulos, James G. H. *Habif's Clinical Dermatology: A Color Guide to Diagnosis and Therapy*. 9th ed., Elsevier, 2020.

"Impetigo." *Mayo Clinic*, 21 Apr. 2021, www.mayoclinic.org/diseases-conditions/impetigo/symptoms-causes/syc-20352352. Accessed 29 Aug. 2021.

Larsen, Laura, editor. *Childhood Diseases and Disorders Sourcebook*. Omnigraphics, 2012.

Plaza, Jose A., and Victor G. Prieto. *Inflammatory Skin Disorders*. Demos Medical Publishing, 2012.

Swartz, Morton N., and Mark S. Pasternack. "Cellulitis and Subcutaneous Tissue Infection." *Mandell, Douglas, and Bennett's Principles and Practice of Infectious Diseases*, edited by Gerald L. Mandell, John E. Bennett, and Raphael Dolin, 7th ed., Churchill Livingstone/Elsevier, 2010.

Taylor, Julie Scott. "Interventions for Impetigo." *American Family Physician*, vol. 70, 9, 1 Nov. 2004.

Van Schoor, Jacky. "Superficial Skin Infections in the Pharmacy." *SAPA*, vol. 13, no. 1, 2013, pp. 39-40.

Zappi, Eduardo. *Dermatopathology: Classification of Cutaneous Lesions*. Springer, 2013.

INFLUENZA

Category: Diseases/Conditions
Anatomy or system affected: Lungs, muscles, nose, respiratory system, throat
Also known as: The flu, grip, grippe, seasonal flu
Definition: A viral disease that affects the respiratory system.

KEY TERMS

antigenic drift: the gradual accumulation of point mutations during the circulation of influenza virus. It results from the high error rates associated with ribonucleic acid (RNA)-dependent RNA polymerase during virus replication

antigenic shift: a process by which two or more different strains of a virus combine to form a new strain that has a mixture of the surface antigens of the two or more original strains

hemagglutinin: a surface glycoprotein of the influenza virus that causes red blood cells to clump together.

neuraminidase: an enzyme on the surface of influenza viruses that catalyzes the breakdown of complex sugars that contain neuraminic acid.

orthomyxovirus: a family of negative-sense RNA viruses that infect animal species

Reye's syndrome: a rare but serious condition characterized by the swelling in the liver and brain, caused when children or adolescents take aspirin or other nonsteroidal anti-inflammatory drugs while infected by viruses

Influenza (commonly known as the flu) is a disease that affects the respiratory system. It is caused by a variety of viruses in the Orthomyxovirus family. Influenza infections are not unique to people; they also occur in other animals, most notably birds and pigs. Infection with an influenza virus leads to illness that can be mild or life-threatening, depending on the person's age, general health, and immunity to the particular infecting virus. Every year, the influenza viruses that infect people can differ from those that infected people the previous year.

CAUSES

There are two significant types of influenza viruses: A and B (influenza virus type C causes minor infections). Each influenza A or B virus carries on its outer surface two types of protein: hemagglutinin (H) and neuraminidase (N). Influenza A viruses are classified into subtypes based on the type of HA and NA proteins they carry. There are sixteen types of HA and nine types of NA. When scientists talk about H1N1 influenza, they mean an influenza type A virus that carries HA type 1 and NA type 1 on its surface.

Influenza B viruses, and influenza A subtypes, are further classified into strains. There are hundreds of influenza virus strains, but not all can infect people.

The genes that code for the H and N proteins tend to mutate (change) somewhat each year. The accumulation of these mutations as influenza circulates causes "antigenic drift." Antigenic drift changes the virus enough so that it reduces a person's natural immunity to it. Antigenic drift explains why new flu vaccines must be made each year.

Every few decades or so, an influenza A virus will undergo an antigenic shift. This significant change in the virus leads to the appearance of a completely new flu virus, against which people have no immunity. The emergence of H1N1 influenza in 2009 probably resulted from such a shift. Viruses that appear because of antigenic shifts may cause pandemics (worldwide epidemics), as did the 2009 H1N1 influenza virus. (The word "pandemic" does not mean "severe illness." It means the infecting microbe can easily cause illness that spreads across the globe.)

Viruses are generally specific to a species. Thus, the bird flu (avian influenza) virus usually cannot cause infection in a human. There have been several cases, however, in which bird flu viruses have infected humans. The best-known avian influenza virus is H5N1, which has caused more than five hundred confirmed cases in humans. Of these cases, 297 were fatal, making H5N1 the deadliest bird flu virus in humans.

The virus is transmitted to humans only by handling sick or uncooked dead birds. Health authorities worldwide remain concerned that if the virus develops the ability to jump among people (instead of, only, from birds to people), it will cause a major pandemic with many deaths.

RISK FACTORS

For the seasonal flu, people younger than age five or older than sixty-five years are most at risk of contracting the flu, as are health-care workers. Crowding increases the risk of virus transmission between people.

In addition, several groups of people are at high risk for complications from the flu. According to the Centers for Disease Control and Prevention (CDC), high-risk groups include pregnant women, people with certain chronic medical conditions (for example, heart disease or diabetes), people whose immune system is weakened or suppressed, young children, and people older than age fifty years.

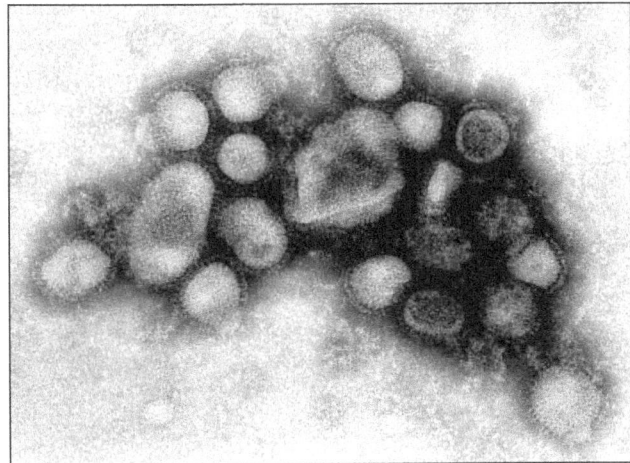

Swine influenza extracted in 2009. Photo by C.S. Goldsmith and A. Balish. Image courtesy of the CDC, via Wikimedia Commons. [Public domain.]

H5N1 avian influenza remains a problem in certain parts of the world. People living or traveling in areas where the virus is active are at risk if they handle sick birds or eat uncooked birds infected.

SYMPTOMS

It can take up to four days (in adults) from the infection until symptoms appear. The classic symptoms of the flu are fever and chills, sore throat, cough, runny nose, muscle aches, and headache. The headache can be severe enough to cause sensitivity to light. Muscle aches are most common in the legs, though they can appear anywhere in the body. Extreme fatigue is another common symptom.

Nausea, vomiting, and diarrhea can occur in people with the flu and are especially common in children and people infected with the 2009 H1N1 flu strain. Most flu symptoms disappear in five to six days, though full recovery takes longer; the fatigue may last several weeks.

Pneumonia is a common complication of influenza. It can be primary (caused by the flu virus) or secondary (caused by another virus or bacteria). Because influenza weakens the body and its immune system, infections by other microbes can colonize a person who is fighting the flu. Symptoms of pneumonia include a cough that gets worse instead of better, difficulty breathing, and, sometimes, bloody phlegm. A person who is recovering from the flu and redevelops fever and cough most likely has bacterial pneumonia.

People with chronic medical conditions should watch for signs that their condition is worsening because of the flu. Severe disease, unfortunately, is not uncommon, especially in people with heart disease or respiratory conditions such as asthma or emphysema.

SCREENING AND DIAGNOSIS

Most of the time, the flu is inferred from the symptoms, and no special testing is required. There are some situations in which knowing the exact subtype of flu virus can influence treatment decisions. Sometimes doctors need to determine if an outbreak of respiratory illness in the population was due to influenza. For that purpose, rapid testing is available.

There are eleven approved rapid tests in the United States. These tests give results in fifteen minutes, but their sensitivity and accuracy vary. Rapid testing is usually done using a swab from nose or throat secretions. (The location of the swab may also affect the test's accuracy in some tests.) Rapid testing can be done only within the first four days of symptom appearance.

The most accurate way of testing for the specific type of flu virus is through reverse transcription-polymerase chain reaction (RT-PCR). Testing with RT-PCR can take up to four hours and is not always available for diagnostic tests.

Medical technologists can culture the influenza virus from swabs taken from affected persons. In a viral culture, the virus obtained from the persons is allowed to multiply in the laboratory, where large quantities allow for typing. Viral cultures are not used to determine treatment because they take three to ten days to grow and provide results. However, viral cultures can determine what type of flu is circulating in a given population.

A test for the presence of the H5 flu virus is available to state and public health authorities. The test, known as influenza A/H5 (Asian lineage) virus real-time RT-PCR primer and probe set, is available when suspected human cases of avian influenza appear in the United States. It takes four hours to get the results. If the H5 virus is detected, further testing is needed to determine if the virus is indeed the H5N1 avian flu virus.

TREATMENT AND THERAPY

For most people who are otherwise healthy, the treatment of influenza consists of treating the symptoms. Treatment includes pain relievers for body aches and headaches and medicine to reduce fever. Many over-the-counter (OTC) multisymptom flu treatments are available. They treat the worst cold symptoms and can bring relief, though they will not cure the flu. OTC products contain a mixture of medications. To avoid overdosing, one should know what medicines the OTCs contain. For example, many OTC products contain acetaminophen, the active ingredient in Tylenol. People who take acetaminophen in addition to multisymptom OTC treatments risk building up a dangerous level of acetaminophen in their bodies.

Children younger than eighteen years of age who might have influenza should not take aspirin. Aspirin in children can cause Reye's syndrome, a potentially fatal disorder that often follows a viral infection. Medications against the flu virus are called "antiviral medications." Two classes of antivirals are available against the flu virus: Neuraminidase inhibitors are effective against influenza A and B. They interfere with the release of the virus from infected cells. Three drugs are available in this class: oseltamivir (Tamiflu), zanamivir (Relenza), and Peramivir (Rapivab). Two drugs are available in this class: amantadine (Symmetrel) and rimantadine (Flumadine). Amantadines are effective against (some) influenza A viruses only, and viral resistance to this class of antivirals is high. Finally, baloxavir (Xofluza) is the first polymerase acidic endonuclease inhibitor class of anti-influenza drugs. This drug inhibits influenza ribonucleic acid (RNA) replication.

Taking these medications within the first forty-eight hours after symptoms appear will reduce the length and severity of the symptoms. Treatment with antiviral drugs is essential in people at high risk for complications. This type of treatment reduces or prevents such complications. Antiviral drugs can also prevent the flu if a person has been exposed to it. However, these medications are not substitutes for influenza vaccines.

Of the neuraminidase inhibitors, zanamivir is given through an inhaler. Because inhaling the medicine can cause intense airway spasms, zanamivir is not recommended for people with certain airway diseases, such as asthma. Use of the inhaler can be problematic for older adults or people with certain physical or mental limitations.

Oseltamivir is Food and Drug Administration (FDA)-approved for treating uncomplicated acute influenza in anyone older than two years and for influenza prophylaxis in patients at least one-year-old. It is the preferred treatment of influenza in pregnant women, hospitalized patients, and outpatients with a severe, complicated, or progressive illness. To mitigate the stomach upset that oseltamivir causes, patients should take this drug with food. Finally, this medication has a bitter taste that puts children off. Mixing the contents of oseltamivir capsules with a thick, sweetened liquid makes it more attractive to children.

Zanamivir is FDA-approved for treating uncomplicated acute influenza in patients at least seven years old and influenza prophylaxis in patients at least five years old. Zanamivir is contraindicated in patients with milk protein allergies. Nor is it recommended for use in patients with severe influenza or underlying airway diseases.

Peramivir is given intravenously and is FDA-approved for treating uncomplicated acute influenza in otherwise healthy patients two years old or older. It is not approved for influenza prevention. Baloxavir is FDA-approved for the treatment of uncomplicated acute influenza in patients at least twelve years old. It also protects those who were recently exposed (within 48 hours) to influenza. Taking baloxavir with dairy products, calcium-fortified beverages, or laxatives prevents drug absorption.

Amantadine and rimantadine are approved for the prevention of flu in people one year of age and older. Amantadine is also approved for flu treatment in persons one year and older. Rimantadine is approved for treating persons aged thirteen years and older. Because of the widespread resistance of extant influenza virus strains to these drugs, they are rarely prescribed.

While drug resistance to amantadines has been a growing problem, resistance to oseltamivir is a newer phenomenon. Because oseltamivir is the most used antiviral flu treatment, resistance is a worrisome development. It is, therefore, more important than ever to limit the use of antiviral flu drugs to high-risk groups.

People often ask about taking elderberry for prevention and treatment of influenza. Drug stores and chain supermarkets sell elderberry-containing products that are promoted for relief of cold and flu symptoms and as an immune system booster. However, the is no acceptable evidence that elderberry is effective for prevention or treatment of influenza. Furthermore, its safety is unclear. The bark, stems, leaves, and root of the elderberry plant contain a compound called "sambunigrin," which can release cyanide.

PREVENTION AND OUTCOMES
Vaccination is the best protection against the flu. In early 2010, the CDC's Advisory Committee on Immunization Practices recommended a universal influenza vaccine every year for everyone age six months and older. (The previous recommendation called for yearly vaccinations for children six months to eighteen years of age and certain high-risk groups.)

Because the flu viruses that circulate in the population change every year, getting the flu vaccine each year is crucial. The vaccines change each year according to early testing results that show what virus subtypes are starting to appear. Vaccination is vital in people who are at high risk of severe complications from influenza. It is also important that people who care for or live with a person in any risk group be vaccinated to prevent giving the disease to the high-risk person. Health-care workers are also strongly encouraged to receive the vaccine every year to protect themselves and their patients.

There are four types of influenza vaccines:
- a killed virus vaccine grown in eggs and given by injection
- a live, weakened virus given as a nasal spray
- a killed virus vaccine grown in cultured cells
- and a recombinant influenza vaccine containing three times the amount of antigen used in older people.

The live virus vaccine is given to healthy (nonpregnant) persons between two and forty-nine years. The vaccine is marketed as FluMist or LAIV (live attenuated influenza vaccine). Side effects from the injected vaccine are usually mild and include redness and soreness in the injection area. Allergic reactions to the vaccine may also occur, though they are uncommon. Formerly, health-care workers advised against people allergic to eggs from receiving the injected flu vaccine. However, research has established people with egg allergies can safely receive egg-grown inactivated influenza vaccines. On rare occasions, some people who received the injected flu vaccine developed a paralysis disorder known as "Guillain-Barré syndrome."

Regardless of the type of vaccine, people have no protection against the flu until approximately two weeks after vaccination. People at high risk for flu complications (who receive the injected, killed vaccine) may be given antiviral drugs during the two weeks. The live vaccine can cause mild flu-like symptoms for several days.

Good hygiene is an integral part of protection against the flu. Washing hands frequently or using alcohol-based hand sanitizers will reduce the risk of getting the flu. It is imperative to wash hands before eating and touching areas on the face, especially the nose and mouth. People should be sure to wash their hands after blowing their nose or coughing into their hands. Covering the nose and mouth while coughing or sneezing reduces the risk of spreading influenza virus particles through the air.

—Adi R. Ferrara, BS, ELS and
Michael A. Buratovich, PhD

Further Information

"Antiviral Drugs for Influenza for 2020-2021." *Medical Letter on Drugs and Therapeutics*, vol. 62, no. 1610, 2020, pp. 169-73. A fine summary of the available drugs to treat and prevent influenza.

Barry, John M. *The Great Influenza: The Story of the Deadliest Pandemic in History*. Viking Penguin, 2005. Woven into this fascinating story of the world's deadliest flu pandemic is a look at the virus and the science of the flu. This book also provides an exciting look at the politics behind the response to major epidemics.

Beigel, John, and Mike Bray. "Current and Future Antiviral Therapy of Severe Seasonal and Avian Influenza." *Antiviral Research*, vol. 78, 2008, pp. 91-102. An article that discusses the use of antiviral medications against influenza viruses.

EBSCO Publishing. *Health Library: Flu*. www.ebscohost.com. A concise look at influenza.

"Elderberry for Influenza." *The Medical Letter on Drugs and Therapeutics*, vol. 61, no. 1566, 2019, p. 32. An authoritative look at elderberry and its lack of efficacy as a treatment for influenza.

"Influenza." *The Merck Manual Home Health Handbook*, edited by Robert S. Porter et al., 3rd ed., Merck Research Laboratories, 2009. A concise easily understood look at all aspects of influenza.

"Influenza Vaccines for 2020-2021." *Medical Letter on Drugs and Therapeutics*, vol. 62, no. 1607, 2020, pp. 145-50. Excellent summary of the influenza vaccines for the 2020-2021 flu season.

Strauss, James, and Ellen Strauss. *Viruses and Human Disease*. 2nd ed., Academic Press/Elsevier, 2008. A detailed discussion of animal viruses with emphasis on those associated with human disease. Includes accounts of the history of human viruses.

INSECT-BORNE DISEASES

Category: Diseases/Disorders
Anatomy or system affected: All
Specialties and related fields: Bacteriology, biochemistry, biotechnology, critical care, environmental health, epidemiology, microbiology, preventive medicine, public health
Definition: Diseases transmitted by insects, which have significant health and economic impact worldwide, causing illness, disability, and death.

KEY TERMS

endemic: occurring naturally in a geographic area or population group

epidemic: any disease, injury, or health-related event occurring suddenly in numbers more than normal

mucous membranes: the inner lining of the mouth and nasal passages, as well as any membrane or lining containing mucus-secreting glands

parasite: an organism that obtains food and shelter from another organism or host

pathogen: a disease-producing microorganism such as bacteria, viruses, algae, and fungi

vector: an organism that transmits a disease from one host to another

CAUSES AND SYMPTOMS

Insects such as mosquitoes, black flies, tsetse flies, eye flies, houseflies, fleas, and lice are responsible for transmitting pathogens that inflict disease and illness on hundreds of millions of people each year. Mosquitoes and blackflies are the most medically and economically destructive of bloodsucking insects. Mosquito-borne diseases kill more than one million people every year and infect hundreds of millions more. These diseases are generally one of three types. The first usually causes fever, rashes, joint pain, and occasionally fatal infections. The second type is hemorrhagic, which causes bleeding

> **INFORMATION ON INSECT-BORNE DISEASES**
>
> Causes: Transfer of pathogens or parasites via a bite or other contact with mosquitoes, flies, lice, and other insects
>
> Symptoms: Vary; may include fever, nausea, rashes, headache, swollen lymph glands, joint pain, bleeding, shock, blindness, and encephalitis
>
> Duration: Acute and sometimes fatal; may become chronic
>
> Treatments: Sometimes antibiotics, but often none; prevention through vaccines and biological and chemical control of vectors

from the mucous membranes and occasionally leads to fatal shock. The third type causes symptoms of encephalitis, an inflammation of the brain, and is identified with several epidemics.

The better-known mosquito-transmitted diseases include malaria, yellow fever, dengue fever, and West Nile virus. Malaria, responsible for the deaths of at least one million people in 2002, produces high fever and chills and does not provide lasting immunity to a relapse. The disease is treated with quinine, but patients can still develop the deadly blackwater fever. Yellow fever is more deadly than malaria and is endemic in Central and South America, the West Indies, and Africa. There is no treatment for yellow fever, although at-risk individuals can be vaccinated to prevent infection. Patients with yellow fever may contract hepatitis and suffer renal (kidney) failure, hemorrhage (blood loss), shock, and death.

Dengue fever, also called "breakbone fever," is rarely fatal. Still, it causes a high fever accompanied by severe pain and stiffness in the joints. The World Health Organization (WHO) estimates that between 50 and 100 million people are infected with Dengue fever annually; in 2010, there were a reported 1.6 million cases in the Americas. The disease is endemic in the tropics, where about 40 percent of the world's population lives. There is no vaccine or cure. Another form, hemorrhagic dengue, produces shock syndrome and follows a previous infection with dengue. The disease may infect people in as many as sixty-one countries.

West Nile virus was first reported in the United States in Queens, New York City, in 1999. In 2012, 5,674 human cases were reported, with 286 deaths. The virus also causes high mortality in many species of birds and results in numerous horse deaths. Most infected people are symptom-free, with mild cases causing flu-like symptoms such as fever, coughing, and weakness. Serious infections can progress to more severe headaches, high fevers, tremors, and partial paralysis, as well as encephalitis.

Biting black flies are a nuisance that can affect tourism, agriculture, forestry, and recreation. These bites can cause weight loss, stress-related illnesses, and reduced egg, milk, and meat production for animals. One of the most widespread blackfly diseases is onchocerciasis, or river blindness, which can be transmitted to humans, cattle, and other large mammals. The severe effects can occur long after the initial fly bite and are caused by a worm transmitted to the host. The worm curls up in lumps on the body, causing coarsening of the skin, depigmentation (loss of color), and intense itching that can drive a person to suicide in severe cases. If the worm enters the eyes, it can cause reduced peripheral vision, night blindness, and complete vision loss. Blackfly fever, found in the New England area of the United States, is a severe reaction to bites that causes fever, nausea, headaches, and swollen lymph glands.

Tsetse flies, houseflies, and eye flies are responsible for numerous infections and diseases. The tsetse fly's bite can transmit parasites and cause sleeping sickness, a West African disease in humans. The parasite causes enlarged glands, loss of appetite, and extreme lethargy. The patient eventually lapses into a coma, and the disease is fatal if not treated. A similar fatal disease called "nagana" occurs in animals,

Insect-Borne Viral Diseases

Disease	Principal Vectors
Encephalitis, California	Mosquitoes: *Culex tarsalis, Aedes species*
Encephalitis, Eastern equine	Mosquitoes: *Aedes sollicitans, Culiseta melanura*
Encephalitis, St. Louis	Mosquitoes: *Culex pipiens, C. p. quinquefasciatus, C. tarsalis*
Encephalitis, Venezuelan	Mosquitoes: *Aedes serratus, Ae. scapularis, Ae. taeniorhynchus, Anopheles aquasalis, Culex vomifer, C. taeniopus, Haemogogus species, Mansonia titillans, Psorophora confinnis, P. ferox*
Encephalitis, Western equine	Mosquitoes: *Culex tarsalis* and others
Pappataci or sandfly fever	Sandfly: *Phlebotomus papatasii*
Rift Valley fever	Mosquitoes: *Eretmapodites chrysogaster, Aedes caballus, Ae. deboeri, Ae. circumluteolus, Ae. tarsalis, Culex theileri*

mainly imported cattle and horses, cattle, goats, camels, and pigs.

Houseflies are nonbiting insects that can transfer pathogens from infected septic matter (feces) to human foodstuffs, sores, or mucous membranes. These pathogens can transmit cholera germs or cause diarrhea and eye infections. Eye flies drink fluid from the eyes or blood from sores, ulcers, and minor wounds on humans and animals. These tiny black flies transmit bacteria, especially to children, and spread eyesores such as conjunctivitis (pinkeye) and other infections.

Biting midges are small flies that can transmit several diseases. Sandfly fever causes a short illness with fever in humans. Bartonellosis, or Carrion's disease, occurs in South America in Peru, Ecuador, and Colombia in higher altitudes. Mild cases usually cause a slight fever, but severe cases can have an 80 percent mortality rate. After five to eight weeks, fever survivors develop large wart-like tumors all over the body, which cause pain and irritation. Leishmaniasis is a parasitic disease and ranges from a mild form with fevers and anemia to a disfiguring type with skin wounds to another form that can cause internal organ damage and death. Most forms infect animals and accidentally transfer to humans. The disease affects approximately twelve million people worldwide, with over one million new cases every year. Other biting midges transmit diseases such as the Oropouche virus, which is found in tropical America. Severe flu-like symptoms, with fever and vomiting, can last for up to two weeks but are usually not fatal.

Flea-borne murine (mice) typhus produces a typhus-like fever, eye rash, headache, chills, and general achiness. The most infamous disease transmitted by fleas, however, is the plague, which killed a quarter of the population of Europe in the fourteenth century. People become infected by receiving a flea bite, handling infected animals, or breathing infected respiratory droplets. The plague causes fever, chills, seizures, and severe headaches, followed by swollen lymph glands (or buboes) in the armpit, groin, or neck. Untreated septicemic plague is initially difficult to diagnose because it invades the bloodstream directly, eventually spreading to the liver, kidney, spleen, lungs, eyes, and/or brain lining. This type of plague has a 40 percent mortality rate with treatment and a 100 percent fatality rate if untreated. Pneumonic plague, contracted by inhaling infected drops from another person or animal, causes severe, overwhelming pneumonia, shortness

Insect-Borne Bacterial and Rickettsial Diseases

Disease	Disease Agent	Principal Vectors
Anthrax	*Bacillus anthracis*	Various horse flies by mechanical transmission
Carrion's disease	*Bartonella bacilliformis*	*Phlebotomus* sandflies
Food poisoning	*Shigella* and *Salmonella*	Various flies by mechanical transmission
Plague	*Yersinia pestis*	*Xenopsylla cheopis* and some other fleas
Trench fever	*Rickettsia Quintana*	Human body louse *Pediculus humanus*
Tularemia	*Francisella tularensis*	Deer flies and ticks
Typhus, louse-borne	*Rickettsia prowazekii*	Human body louse *Pediculus humanus*
Typhus, murine	*Rickettsia mooseri*	Rat flea *Xenopsylla cheopis*; the rat louse *Polyplax spinulosa* is a zoonotic vector

of breath, high fever, and blood in the phlegm. Life-threatening complications include shock, high fever, problems with blood clotting, and convulsions. Untreated pneumonic plague is almost always fatal. However, treating the patient with intravenous gentamicin fifteen to eighteen hours after symptoms effectively cures the disease.

Lice are responsible for several diseases, including louse-borne typhus, which comes from louse feces. Infection occurs through a scratch, contact with mucous membranes, or inhalation. Symptoms include fatigue, muscle aches, headache, coughing, rapid onset of fever, and a blotchy rash on the chest or abdomen. If untreated, the disease can cause delirium, low blood pressure, coma, and possibly death. Treatment with antibiotics usually provides a prompt cure. Brill-Zinsser disease is similar to a mild form of typhus. It is a reoccurrence of louse-borne typhus, sometimes waiting as much as thirty years between outbreaks.

Symptoms of louse-borne relapsing fever include head and muscle aches, nausea, appetite loss, dizziness, coughing, vomiting, and the abrupt onset of fever. Severe infections cause the liver and spleen to swell and make breathing painful. Trench fever, or Wolhynian fever, occurred in Central Europe during World War I and II and is generally rare and seldom fatal. There may be no symptoms or headaches, muscle aches, fever, and nausea.

Chagas' disease occurs in South and Central America. Transmission of bacteria occurs through infected feces, and symptoms range from mild and flu-like to severe chronic cardiac or digestive system disease. Estimations indicate that Chagas' disease affects eight to eleven million people living in Mexico, Central America, and South America. Between 10 and 30 percent of infected people will develop chronic, life-threatening symptoms or heart failure, and about will fifty thousand die each year from infection. There is no vaccine for Chagas' disease. The medications that treat it have profound side effects, and patients must take them for extended periods.

TREATMENT AND THERAPY

For most insect-borne diseases, treatment includes medical intervention such as antibiotics and vaccines to prevent transmission. As of 2013, vaccines for most diseases were still under development, and some of the diseases have no known cure. Educating people on how to avoid infection and treat the symptoms is essential.

Insect-Borne Protozoan Diseases

Disease	Disease Agent	Principal Vectors
Chagas' disease	*Trypanosoma cruzi*	Assassin bugs: *Panstrongylus megistus* and many species of *Triatoma*
Kala-azar	*Leishmania donovani*	Sandflies: *Phlebotomus chinensis, P. major, P. argentipes, P. perniciosus*
Leishmaniasis, American mucocutaneous	*Leishmania braziliensis*	Sandflies: *Phlebotomus intermedius, P. longipalpus, P. pessoai*
Leishmaniasis, Mexican	*Leishmania Mexicana*	Sandfly: *Phlebotomus flaviscutellatus*
Malaria, benign tertian	*Plasmodium vivax*	Mosquitoes: species of *Anopheles*
Malaria, malignant tertian	*Plasmodium falciparum*	Mosquitoes: *Anopheles stephensi, A. labranchiae*
Malaria, ovale tertian	*Plasmodium ovale*	Mosquitoes: *Anopheles gambiae, A. furestus*
Malaria, quartan	*Plasmodium malariae*	Mosquitoes: many species of *Anopheles*
Nagana (cattle, etc.)	*Trypanosoma brucei*	Tsetse fly: *Glossina morsitans*
Oriental sore	*Leishmania tropica*	Sandflies: *Phlebotomus papatasii* and *P. sergenti*
Sleeping sickness, East African	*Trypanosoma rhodesiense*	Tsetse flies: *Glossina morsitans* and *G. swynnertoni*
Sleeping sickness, West African	*Trypanosoma gambiense*	Tsetse flies: *Glossina tachinoides* and *G. palpalis*
Surra (camels, etc.)	*Trypanosoma evansi*	Horseflies in the family *Tabanidae*

Bacterial insect-borne diseases are usually treatable, provided the patient seeks treatment at the earlier stages of the disease. Doxycycline effectively treats most rickettsial diseases. Augmentin, ciprofloxacin, ceftriaxone, or chloramphenicol effectively treat bartonellosis. Intravenous gentamicin effectively treats both tularemia and plague. Ciprofloxacin, trimethoprim/sulfamethoxazole, or azithromycin treats disease caused by many strains of *Shigella*. However, in the Asian subcontinent and Africa, *Shigella* infections have a high risk of multidrug resistance. In these cases, physicians usually prescribe third-generation cephalosporins, such as ceftriaxone or cefixime. The same antibiotics also effectively treat *Salmonella* infections.

Protozoan infections sometimes require more toxic drugs. Amoeba infections respond to metronidazole, tinidazole, iodoquinol, or paromomycin. Leishmaniasis requires liposomal amphotericin B (first line) or alternative medications, including sodium stibogluconate, meglumine antimonate, paromomycin, or miltefosine. Leishmaniasis treatment must continue for about four weeks. Trypanosome treatment differs between species. Sixty days of benznidazole or 90 days of nifurtimox effectively treat *Trypanosoma cruzi*, the cause of Chagas' disease. *Trypanosoma brucei gambiense* (West African trypanosomiasis) and *T. b. rhodesiense* (East African trypanosomiasis) cause African sleeping sickness. African sleeping sickness has two stages, an earlier hemolymphatic stage, and a later central nervous system stage. Treatment of African sleeping sickness depends on the infecting trypanosome species and the stage of the disease. Treatment of the hemolymphatic stage of West African trypanosomiasis requires intramuscular (IM) injections of pentamidine or intravenous (IV) suramin. Late disease with central nervous system (CNS) involvement is treated with IV eflornithine or IV eflornithine plus oral nifurtimox, with IV melarsoprol as a viable alternative treatment. For the hemolymphatic stage of East African trypanosomiasis, however, IV suramin is the drug of choice. The later CNS involved stages use IV melarsoprol.

Plasmodium protozoans cause malaria. Malaria treatment depends on the area where the disease resides. Drug resistance patterns of Plasmodium parasites vary between locales, but some generalizations emerge. First, all travelers should use insect repellents and insecticide-treated bed nets as protective measures against mosquito bites. Second, the drug combination of atovaquone/proguanil (Malarone) is highly effective for malaria prevention and well-tolerated. Alternatives for malaria prevention in most areas include doxycycline, mefloquine, and tafenoquine. Primaquine or tafenoquine can prevent relapses of *P. vivax* malaria. Chloroquine and mefloquine are safe for use during pregnancy.

Tapeworm infections effectively respond to praziquantel, niclosamide (although the availability of this drug in the United States remains problematic), and, in some cases (e.g., echinococcus), albendazole. Filariasis, which causes elephantiasis and river blindness, is treated with diethylcarbamazine or ivermectin.

Biological control involves reducing a target population by introducing a predator, pathogen, parasite, competitor, or toxin produced by a microorganism. This control method was used as early as 1889 in California and became popular in the early twentieth century. Insecticides (or pesticides) replaced biological control and proved to be very successful in eliminating insect vectors. Early pesticides were composed of natural botanicals (plant products) such as nicotine, rotenone, and pyrethrum mixed with chemicals such as lime sulfur, arsenic, mercuric chloride, and soaps. The scientific development of insecticides began as early as 1867, and the structures of botanical insecticides were known in the 1920s. In 1939, the insecticide properties of the first synthetic insecticide, dichlorodiphenyltrichloroethane (DDT), were discovered. DDT has provided a significant benefit in controlling typhus, trench fever, and malaria, and it is still used in indoor insecticides for malaria control.

Pesticides may lose their effectiveness as the parasites become resistant to a specific toxin or insecticide. The focus in the early twenty-first century is on developing pesticides known as third-generation insecticides, mainly aimed at affecting mosquito development. Since these insecticides are developed for mosquitoes, they are less disruptive to the environment and less toxic to humans and other organisms.

Other preventive measures include insect growth regulators (IGRs), species-specific, and prevent larvae from developing. Genetic control, which involves introducing sterile males to the population or releasing insects with only male-producing properties, results in so few females that the population declines. Genetic control methods also may involve population replacement in which the genetic structure is modified in a particular species of insect to prevent disease transmission. A gene can be inserted that would cause the insect to die after breeding and would be passed to offspring. A different gene insertion would kill the females, the bloodsuckers in most species, but not the males.

Applying pesticides and insecticides over large areas effectively controls insect populations. However, an equally effective insect control method includes eliminating insect breeding and gathering areas. General measures to prevent infection include using personal repellents on people and livestock, wearing light-colored clothing and long sleeves and pants during feeding times, stabling livestock during peak biting periods, managing sewage and fecal waste, using netting or fine mesh screening, reducing the number of strays and wild animals that can act as hosts, and keeping the air moving with fans.

PERSPECTIVE AND PROSPECTS
Insect-borne diseases have been infecting people throughout history. Malaria was noted in ancient times and written about before the first century CE. Over time, some people speculated about a connection between insects and illness. However, the scientific equipment and knowledge were not yet available to prove the existence of the pathogens. Initial observations led to improved hygiene and better housing, which greatly reduced plague and typhus. Malaria and yellow fever, however, did not respond to these developments.

In 1877, Sir Patrick Manson discovered that some mosquitoes could carry a parasite that infects people. This discovery and subsequent work by many others stimulated the research into insect-borne diseases. The insect transmission of plague and typhus took ten to twelve years to understand, and others took decades. There were no specific drugs or vaccines for these diseases until 1925, except for quinine for malaria, which did not always work.

Research continues to find successful preventive and control measures, including developing more effective pesticides, insecticides, and genetic controls. Public health and veterinary medicine professionals must pay attention to illnesses in humans and animals and the potential insect connection to fight existing diseases and recognize new or mutating ones. For example, some researchers speculate that bloodsucking stable flies may have caused the initial human immunodeficiency virus (HIV) spread from chimpanzees to humans.

Although many insect-borne diseases were significantly reduced by 1970, they made a dramatic recovery in warm areas of the world, perhaps because of the evolution and adaptation of the pathogens. In addition, social problems such as poverty, famine, and war, which often result in overcrowded and unsanitary conditions, offer ideal breeding areas and easy transmission for numerous insect-borne illnesses and diseases.

—*Virginia L. Salmon and Michael A Buratovich, PhD*

Further Information
"Advice for Travelers." *Medical Letter on Drugs and Therapeutics*, vol. 61, 2019, pp. 153-60.
Busvine, James R. *Disease Transmission by Insects: Its Discovery and Ninety Years of Effort to Prevent It.* Springer, 1993.
Carlson, Emily. "Taking the 'Bite' Out of Vector-Borne Diseases." *National Institute of General Medical Sciences*, 15 May 2013.
"Dengue and Severe Dengue." *World Health Organization*, Nov. 2012.
"Drugs for Parasitic Infections: Treatment Guidelines from the Medical Letter." *Medical Letter on Drugs and Therapeutics*, vol. 11 (suppl.), no, 143, 2013, pp. e1-e31.
Harder, Ben. "Don't Let the Bugs Bite: Can Genetic Engineering Defeat Disease Spread by Insects?" *Science News*, vol. 166, no. 7, 2004, p. 104.
Marquardt, William C., editor. *Biology of Disease Vectors*. 2nd ed., Academic Press/Elsevier, 2005.
O'Hanlon, Leslie Harris. "Tinkering with Genes to Fight Insect-Borne Disease: Researchers Create Genetically Modified Bugs to Fight Malaria, Chagas, and Other Diseases." *The Lancet*, vol. 363, 2004, p. 1288.
Spielman, Andrew, and Michael D'Antonio. *Mosquito: A Natural History of Our Most Persistent and Deadly Foe.* Hyperion, 2001.
Turkington, Carol A., and Rebecca J. Frey. "Malaria." *The Gale Encyclopedia of Medicine*, edited by Jacqueline L. Longe, 3rd ed., Thomson Gale, 2006.
"West Nile Virus: What You Need to Know." *Centers for Disease Control and Prevention*, 12 Sept. 2012.

MEASLES

Category: Diseases/Conditions
Anatomy or system affected: All
Specialties and related fields: Dermatology, epidemiology, hematology, immunology, internal medicine, microbiology, neurology, ophthalmology, otorhinolaryngology, pulmonary medicine, virology
Also known as: Rubella, rubeola
Definition: A highly contagious viral infection that causes fever, cough, and a rash.

KEY TERMS

coryza: runny nose caused by hay fever or infections
Koplik spots: small, white spots on the inside of the cheeks early in the course of measles
subacute sclerosing panencephalitis: a very rare, but fatal central nervous system disease caused by measles virus infection

CAUSES

The measles virus is spread by direct contact with nasal or throat secretions of infected people and by airborne transmission (less frequently). Measles is communicable from one to two days before onset of symptoms, three to five days before the rash, and four days after the appearance of the rash.

RISK FACTORS

The factors that increase the chance of developing measles include being unvaccinated or inadequately vaccinated, living in crowded or unsanitary conditions, and traveling to developing countries where measles is common. Also, measles is most common in winter and spring.

Other risk factors include compromised immunity (e.g., untreated human immunodeficiency virus infection), even if vaccinated; being born after 1956 and having received no diagnosis of measles; and receiving a vaccine before 1968, without additional vaccination.

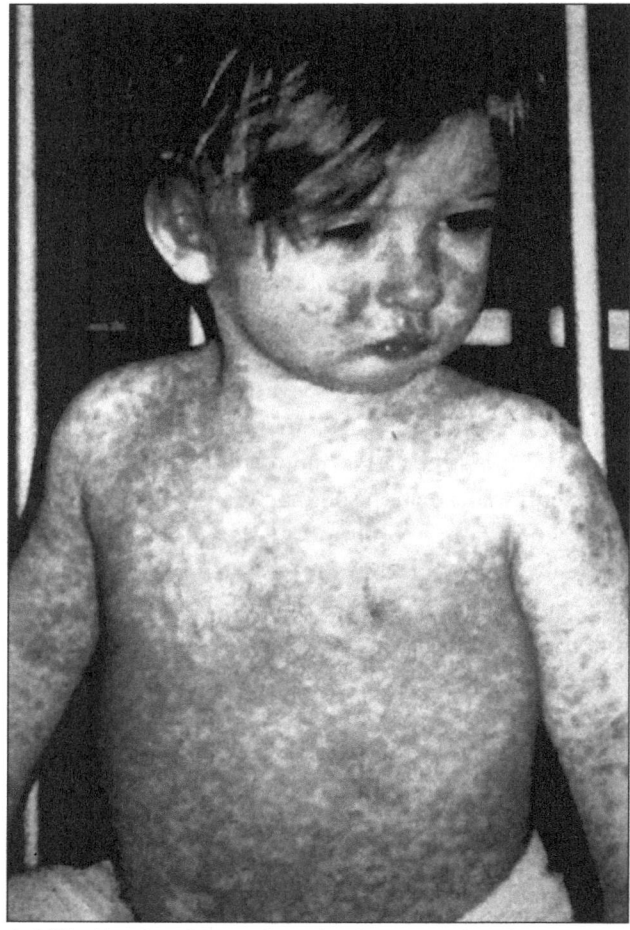

A child with a four-day measles rash. Photo via Wikimedia Commons. [Public domain.]

SYMPTOMS

Symptoms, which usually occur eight to twelve days following exposure, include a fever (often high), runny nose, red eyes, hacking cough, sore throat, exhaustion, and small spots inside the mouth (two to four days after initial symptoms). Three to five days after initial symptoms appear, a raised, itchy rash will start around the ears, face, and side of the neck and then generally spread to the arms, trunk, and legs over the next two days (and then last about four to six days). Full recovery, without scarring, generally takes seven to ten days from the onset of the rash.

SCREENING AND DIAGNOSIS

Diagnosis is made from the symptoms and the appearance of the rash. Laboratory tests are usually not needed to diagnose measles.

TREATMENT AND THERAPY

Measles is caused by a virus, so it cannot be treated with antibiotics. The focus of treatment is on relieving symptoms. Gargling with warm salt water will often relieve the sore throat. Using a humidifier can provide some relief.

A high fever can be treated with nonaspirin medication, which includes acetaminophen. Aspirin is not

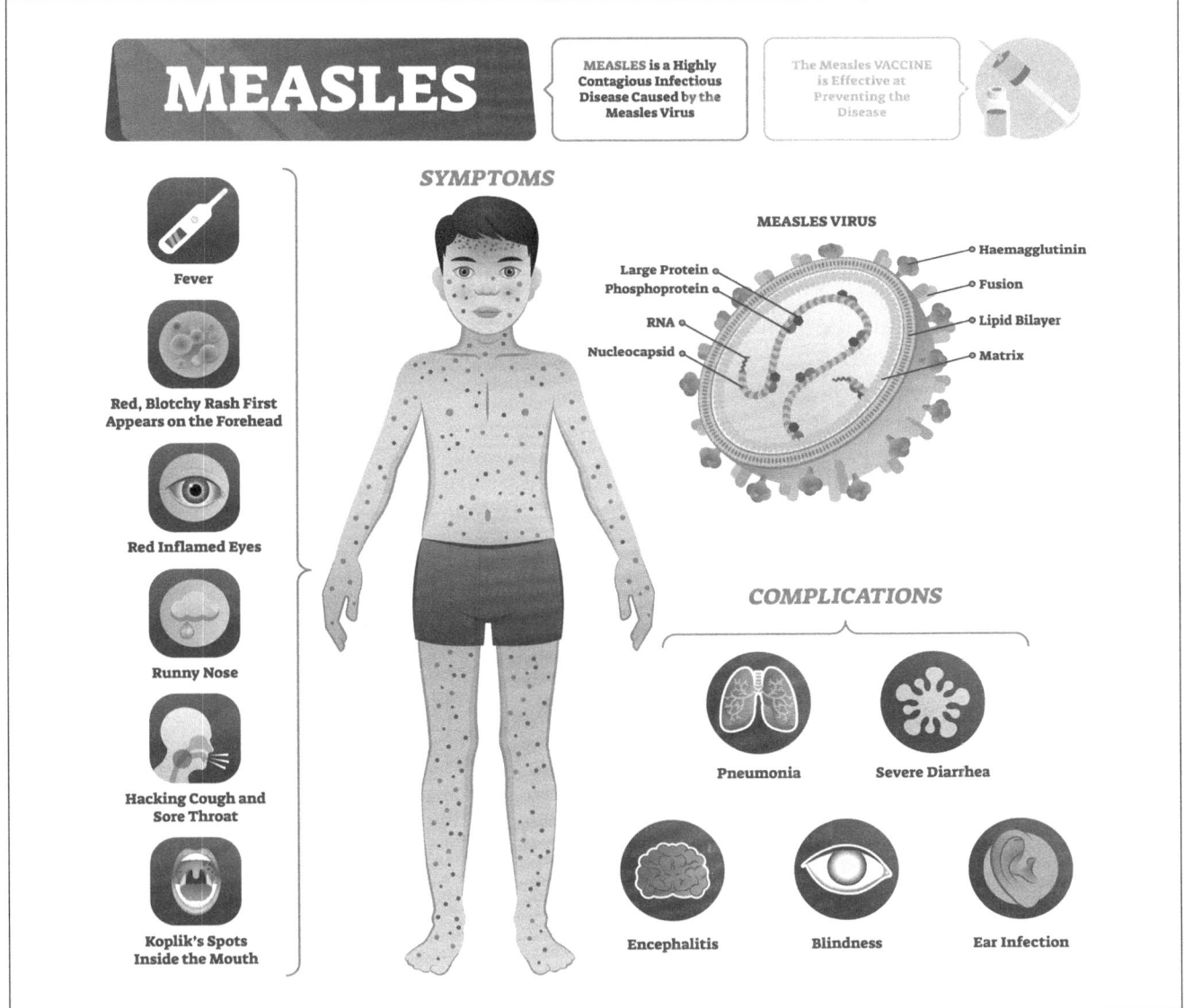

Measles. Image via iStock.com/VectorMine. [Used under license.]

> **FACTS: MEASLES**
>
> - Measles is one of the leading causes of death among young children even though a safe and cost-effective vaccine is available.
> - In 2008, there were 164,000 measles deaths globally: nearly 450 deaths per day, or 18 deaths per hour.
> - More than 95 percent of measles deaths occur in developing countries with inadequate health-care infrastructures.
> - Measles vaccination led to a 78 percent drop in measles deaths between 2000 and 2008 worldwide.
> - In 2008, about 83 percent of the world's children received one dose of measles vaccine by their first birthday through routine health services, up from 72 percent in 2000.

recommended for children or teens with a current or recent viral infection because of the risk of Reye's syndrome. One should consult the doctor about medicines that are safe for children.

Other treatment includes getting extra rest, drinking increased amounts of liquids, and eating a soft, bland diet. Cold sponge baths may also help with symptoms.

In most cases, complications are rare, but persons with severe cases may need to be hospitalized. Complications may include encephalitis (inflammation of the brain) and bacterial pneumonia (a lung infection).

PREVENTION AND OUTCOMES

Getting vaccinated is the best way to prevent measles, as the vaccine contains live viruses that can no longer cause disease. The vaccine is usually given in combination form and includes vaccines against measles, mumps, and rubella (MMR). The MMR vaccine is given twice: at age twelve to fifteen months and at age four to six years (or at age eleven to twelve years).

The U.S. Centers for Disease Control and Prevention (CDC) recommends that all children get two doses of MMR vaccine. Children should receive the first dose at twelve to fifteen months of age, and the second dose at four to six years of age. The MMRV vaccine protect against measles, mumps, rubella, and varicella (chickenpox). MMRV vaccine is licensed for children twelve months to twelve years old.

In some cases, the vaccine is given within three days after exposure. This can prevent or reduce symptoms. Immunoglobulin is given to certain unvaccinated people within six days of exposure. This is usually for infants and pregnant women.

In general, one should avoid the vaccine if he or she has had severe allergic reactions to vaccines or vaccine components, is pregnant (a woman should avoid pregnancy for one to three months after receiving the vaccine), has a weakened immune system, or has a high fever or severe upper respiratory tract infection. If not vaccinated, one should avoid contact with anyone who has measles.

—*Rick Alan*

Further Information

Bernstein, David, and Gilbert Schiff. "Viral Exanthems and Localized Skin Infections." *Infectious Diseases*, edited by Sherwood L. Gorbach, John G. Bartlett, and Neil R. Blacklow, Saunders, 2004.

Centers for Disease Control and Prevention. "Vaccine Safety: Measles, Mumps, and Rubella (MMR) Vaccine." www.cdc.gov/vaccinesafety.

EBSCO Publishing. *Health Library: Measles Vaccine.* www.ebscohost.com.

"Measles." *Epidemiology and Prevention of Vaccine-Preventable Diseases*, edited by W. Atkinson et al., 11th ed., Public Health Foundation, 2009.

Peter, G., and P. Gardner. "Standards for Immunization Practice for Vaccines in Children and Adults." *Infectious Disease Clinics of North America*, vol. 15, 2001, pp. 9-19.

Pickering, Larry K., et al., editors. *Red Book: 2009 Report of the Committee on Infectious Diseases*. 28th ed., American Academy of Pediatrics, 2009.

Weedon, David. *Skin Pathology*. 3rd ed., Churchill Livingstone/Elsevier, 2010.

Nasopharyngeal disorders

Category: Diseases/Disorders
Anatomy or system affected: Nose, respiratory system, throat
Specialties and related fields: Family medicine, occupational health, otorhinolaryngology
Definition: Disorders of the nose, nasal passages (sinuses), and pharynx (mouth, throat, and esophagus).

KEY TERMS

acute disease: a short and sharp disease process
chronic disease: a lingering illness
esophagus: the tube that leads from the pharynx to the stomach
larynx: the organ that produces the voice, which lies between the pharynx and the trachea; commonly called the "voice box"
nasopharyngeal: referring to the nose and pharynx (the upper part of the throat that leads from the mouth to the esophagus)
trachea: a tube that leads from the throat to the lungs; commonly called the "windpipe"

CAUSES AND SYMPTOMS

Nasopharyngeal disorders are all the diseases that can be present in the nasal cavity and the pharynx. These include the common cold, pharyngitis (sore throat), laryngitis (inflammation of the larynx), epiglottitis (inflammation of the lid over the larynx), tonsillitis (inflammation of the lymph nodes at the rear of the mouth), sinusitis (inflammation of the sinus cavities that surround the nose), otitis media (earache that is often associated with nasopharyngeal infection), nosebleed, nasal obstruction, halitosis (bad breath), and various other disorders.

The common cold is one of the most prevalent diseases that afflict humankind. Pharyngitis, or sore throat, often accompanies the common cold, or it may appear by itself. Acute infections can be caused by viruses or bacteria, often by certain streptococcus strains. The common term for the disorder is "strep throat." Acute pharyngitis can also be caused by chemicals or radiation. As a chronic disorder, pharyngitis can be caused by a lingering infection in other organs such as the lungs and sinuses. It can be attributable to constant irritation from smoking, drinking alcohol, or breathing polluted air. The usual symptoms of pharyngitis include sore throat, difficulty swallowing, and fever. The infected area appears red and swollen.

Ordinarily, pharyngitis is not severe. However, if certain strains of streptococcus are the cause, the infection may progress to rheumatic fever. This disease appears to be the result of an immune system reaction to some streptococcus bacteria. It can have painful effects in many parts of the body, including the joints, and can permanently damage parts of the heart. In rare cases, rheumatic fever can be fatal.

A viral infection usually causes acute laryngitis. However, bacteria, outside irritants, or misuse of the voice are other causes. Ordinarily, the vocal cords produce sounds by vibrating in response to the air passing over them. When inflamed or irritated, they swell, distorting the sounds produced. The affected person's voice becomes hoarse and raspy and may even diminish to a whisper. This sound distortion is the main symptom of laryngitis; other possible symptoms include a sore throat and congestion that causes constant coughing. The condition generally resolves itself and requires no treatment. Chronic laryngitis has the same symptoms but does not go away spontaneously. An infectious agent may cause it but more likely is attributable to some irritant activity, such as constantly misusing one's voice, smoking, drinking alcohol, or breathing contaminated air.

The epiglottis is a wafer-like tissue covered by a mucous membrane that sits on top of the larynx. It can become infected by such microorganisms as the bacteria *Haemophilus influenzae* type b, causing epiglottitis. Although the symptoms of epiglottitis can resemble those of pharyngitis, the infection can quickly progress to a severe, life-threatening disorder. Epiglottitis usually afflicts children from two to four years of age, but adults can also be affected. The infection can begin rapidly, causing the epiglottis to swell and obstruct the airway to the lungs, creating a major medical emergency. Within twelve hours of the onset of symptoms, 50 percent of patients require hospitalization and intubation (insertion of a breathing tube into the trachea). The symptoms are high fever, severe sore throat, difficulty breathing, difficulty swallowing, and general malaise. As the airway becomes more and more occluded, the patient begins to gasp for air. The lack of oxygen may cause cyanosis (blue color in the lips, fingers, and skin), exhaustion, and shock.

Another disease associated with the larynx is croup or laryngotracheobronchitis. As the medical name indicates, croup involves the larynx, the trachea, and the bronchi (the large branches of the lung). A virus usually causes it, but some cases are attributable to bacterial infection. Children from three to five years of age are the usual victims. This disease causes the airways to narrow due to inflammation of the inner mucosal surfaces. Inflammation causes coughing, but the narrowed airway causes the cough to be sharp and brassy, like the barking of a seal. Croup is usually relatively benign, but sometimes it progresses to a severe disease requiring hospitalization.

Various other disorders can afflict the larynx, such as damage to the vocal cords because of infection by bacteria, fungi, or other microorganisms. Vocal cord damage can result from misusing one's voice, smoking, or breathing contaminated air. Polyps (masses of tissue growing on the surface), nodes (tiny knots of tissue), or so-called singer's nodules may develop. Sores called "contact ulcers" might form on the vocal cords.

Tonsillitis is an inflammation of the tonsils, two large lymph nodes located at the back of the throat. It may also involve the adenoids, lymph nodes located at the top of the throat. The function of these lymph nodes is to remove harmful pathogens (disease-causing organisms) from the nasopharyngeal cavity. At times, the load of microorganisms they absorb becomes more than they can handle, and they become infected. The tonsils and adenoids may then become enlarged. A sore throat develops, along with a headache, fever, and chills. Glands of the neck and throat feel sore and may become enlarged. Young adults can also suffer from quinsy or peritonsillar abscesses. In this condition, one of the tonsils becomes infected, and pus forms between the tonsil and the soft tissue surrounding it. Quinsy causes pain in the throat or the soft palate, pain when swallowing, fever, and a tendency to lean one's head toward the affected side.

The nasal sinuses are four pairs of cavities in the bone around the nose. There are two maxillary sinuses, so-called because they are in the maxilla or upper jaw. Slightly above and behind them are the ethmoid sinuses, and behind them are the sphenoid sinuses. Sitting over the nose in the lower part of the forehead are the two frontal sinuses. All these sinuses are lined with a mucous membrane and have

---

INFORMATION ON NASOPHARYNGEAL DISORDERS

Causes: May include bacterial or viral infection, nasal obstruction (polyps), environmental allergens or toxins

Symptoms: Sore throat; inflamed lymph nodes, larynx, and sinus cavities; earache or ear infection; nosebleeds; nasal obstruction; fever; difficulty breathing or swallowing; general malaise; bad breath

Duration: Acute to chronic

Treatments: Antibiotics, over-the-counter medications, surgery; if severe, emergency intubation

small openings that lead into the nasal passages. Air moves in and out of the sinuses and allows mucus to drain into the nose. In acute sinusitis, infection builds up in the mucous membrane of any or all of the sinuses. The membrane lining the sinus swells and shuts the opening into the nasal passages. At the same time, membranes of the nose swell and become congested. Mucus and pus build up inside the sinuses, causing pain and pressure. Most often, sinusitis accompanies the common cold: the mucous membrane that lines the nose extends into the sinuses, so the cold infection can readily spread into the sinuses. The various viruses responsible for the common cold may be involved, as well as a broad group of bacteria. Chronic sinusitis results from repeated infections that have allowed scar tissue to build up, closing the sinus openings and impeding mucus drainage, or may result from allergies.

According to the Centers for Disease Control and Prevention (CDC), chronic sinusitis is the most common long-term illness in the United States, surpassing the rates for asthma, arthritis, and congestive heart disease and causing nearly fourteen million doctor's office visits per year. For unknown reasons, sinusitis sufferers are often beset with inflammation of the ducts, trapping mucus, bacteria, and viruses inside and allowing nasal polyps to develop. Researchers have been very interested in finding causes and effective treatments for sinusitis. In the late twentieth century, ear, nose, and throat physicians treated most chronic cases of sinusitis with fiber-optic surgery that allowed access to the cramped sinus passageways. However, patients often returned within weeks or months with ongoing problems. This fact has prompted reconsideration of the cause and nature of sinusitis. Some medical experts suspect that inflammation or the immune system's responses are the culprit but note that additional research must be completed before any definitive answers are found.

Tissues in the nasopharyngeal cavity may be affected by conditions occurring in other parts of the body. For example, vocal cord paralysis may be caused by vascular accidents, certain cancers, tissue trauma, and other events.

Some infections in the nasopharyngeal cavity can spread to the ear through the eustachian tubes that connect the two areas. Chief among the diseases of the ear that can be associated with nasopharyngeal disorders are the various forms of acute otitis media, an earache occurring in the central part of the ear. There are four basic types of otitis media. There is usually no infection in the first type, serous otitis media, but fluid accumulates inside the middle ear because of the blockage of the eustachian tube or the overproduction of fluid; the condition is usually mild with some pain and temporary loss of hearing. The second type is otitis media with effusion; with this condition comes both infection and accumulation of fluid. The third form is acute purulent otitis media, the most severe type. Pus builds up inside the middle ear, and its pressure may rupture the eardrum, allowing discharge of blood and pus. The fourth type is secretory otitis media, which usually occurs after several bouts of otitis media. Cells within the middle ear start producing a thicker fluid than usual and more of it.

Chronic otitis media is bacterial in origin, characterized by a perforation of the eardrum and chronic pus discharge. The eardrum is a flat, pliable disk of tissue that vibrates to conduct sounds from the outside to the inner-ear structures. The perforation in chronic otitis media can be one of two types: a relatively benign perforation occurring in the central part of the eardrum or a potentially dangerous perforation occurring near the edges of the eardrum. The latter perforation can be associated with hearing loss, increased discharge of pus and other fluids, facial paralysis, and the spread of infection to other tissues. When the perforation of chronic otitis media is near the edges of the eardrum, something called a "cholesteatoma" develops. This accumulation of matter grows in the inner ear and can be destructive to bone and other tissue.

The same organisms that cause otitis media can be responsible for a condition called "mastoiditis." The mastoid process is a bone structure lined with a mucous membrane. Infection from otitis media can spread to this area and, in severe cases, can destroy the bone. Mastoiditis used to be a leading cause of death in children.

Nosebleeds are common and often result from a blow to the nose, but colds, sinusitis, and breathing dry air can also cause them. The septum (the cartilaginous tissue that separates the nostrils) and the surrounding intranasal mucous membrane contain many tiny blood vessels that are easily ruptured. If an individual receives a blow to the nose, these vessels can break and bleed. They can also rupture due to irritation from a cold or other conditions. Breathing dry air sometimes causes the nasal mucous membrane to crust over, and bleeding can follow. Nosebleeds are not usually serious, but sometimes they indicate an underlying condition, such as hypertension (high blood pressure), a tumor, or another disease.

Nasal obstruction is common during colds and allergy attacks. However, it can also result from a deviated septum, a malformation in the cartilage between the nostrils that can be congenital or caused by a blow to the nose. Nasal obstruction can also be attributable to nasal polyps, nasal tumors, or swollen adenoids. A common source of nasal obstruction is the overuse of nasal decongestants. These agents relieve nasal congestion by reducing intranasal inflammation and swelling. However, if used too often or for too long, they can cause the very problem they were intended to cure: intranasal blood vessels dilate, the area swells, secretions increase, and the nose becomes blocked. This condition is known as rebound congestion or, in medical terminology, rhinitis medicamentosa (nasal inflammation caused by medication).

Halitosis, or bad breath, is a nasopharyngeal disorder because it can originate in the mouth. Diseases of the teeth or gums can cause it. Nevertheless, the most common causes are smoking or eating aromatic foods such as onions and garlic. Bad breath may also be a sign of disease conditions in other parts of the body, such as certain lung disorders or cancer of the esophagus. Hepatic failure, a liver dysfunction, may be accompanied by a fishy odor on the breath. Azotemia, the retention of nitrogen in the blood, may give rise to an ammonia-like odor. A sweet, fruity odor on the breath of diabetic patients may accompany ketoacidosis. This condition occurs when there are high levels of glucose in the blood. Sometimes, young children stick foreign objects or other materials into their noses; these materials can fester, causing severe halitosis. Bad breath is rarely apparent to the individual who has it, however offensive it may be to others. An excellent way to check one's breath is to lick the back of one's hand and smell the spot; malodor, if it exists, will usually be apparent.

TREATMENT AND THERAPY
Nasopharyngeal disorders are most often mild illnesses that are treated at home. For example, acute pharyngitis, or sore throat, is easily managed most of the time. Health-care workers advise the patient to rest, gargle with warm salt water several times a day, and soothe the pain with lozenges or anesthetic gargles. If a virus causes the infection, it usually will clear without further treatment. Suppose the physician suspects that the infection is bacterial in origin. In that case, throat smears can identify the infecting organism. If the throat smear shows a bacterial infection, then the physician prescribes antibiotics to eradicate the pathogens. Antibiotic therapy is essential if certain strains of streptococcus bacteria cause the infection. In this case, it is vital to destroy the or-

ganism to avoid the development of rheumatic fever. Bacterial pharyngitis and tonsillitis infections resolve with intramuscular injections of benzathine penicillin, oral penicillin VK, amoxicillin, cephalexin, azithromycin, or clindamycin if the patient has a penicillin allergy.

Most sinusitis cases result from viral infections. Therefore, antibiotics, in most cases, are superfluous. However, antibiotics are warranted if the sinusitis lasts for longer than ten days or if the patient has a fever and pus-filled nasal discharge for three to four days. The drugs of choice for mild to moderate bacterial sinusitis include oral Augmentin (amoxicillin/clavulanic acid) or doxycycline for seven days in adults and fourteen days in children. If this treatment regimen fails, the physician prescribes high-dose Augmentin (2 grams, twice a day), levofloxacin, or moxifloxacin. In cases of severe disease that require hospitalization, the patient receives intravenous ampicillin/sulbactam, ceftriaxone, levofloxacin, or moxifloxacin.

In acute laryngitis caused by a viral infection, the patient should rest their voice, inhale steam, and drink warm liquids. If bacteria are the cause of laryngitis, their physician initiates antibiotic therapy. In treating chronic laryngitis, the physician must discover the cause and remove it. If allergy is the cause, antihistamine therapy could help. If the cause is bacterial, antibiotic therapy is used. If smoking or drinking alcohol is the problem, all health care and social workers who serve this patient counsel them to stop. The simple palliative measures used for acute laryngitis—resting the voice, drinking warm liquids, and breathing steam—are also beneficial for chronic laryngitis.

Symptoms of epiglottitis are often similar to those of sore throat. Suppose there is any evidence of difficulty in breathing. In that case, however, the patient should be seen by a physician quickly, as an emergency may be developing. If epiglottitis obstructs the airway, the patient should go to the hospital and receive treatment in an intensive care setting. Antibiotics must be given to the patient to treat the infection. It is vital to make an airway for the patient. It may be necessary to insert a tube into the trachea to allow the patient to breathe. To treat bacterial epiglottitis, physicians usually prescribe intravenous ceftriaxone or Unsyn (ampicillin/sulbactam). Levofloxacin is an excellent alternative for patients with a penicillin allergy. If staphylococcal species are the confirmed infecting agent, then intravenous vancomycin, clindamycin, or cefazolin effectively treat it.

Before the age of antibiotics, tonsillitis was often treated surgically, with both tonsils and adenoids removed. This procedure is now rare, as the infection usually responds to antibiotic therapy. Similarly, in the case of peritonsillar abscess or quinsy, antibiotics usually clear the condition satisfactorily. In some cases, a surgeon may remove accumulations of pus. If the abscesses return, it may be advisable to remove the tonsils.

As a rule, a child with croup is treated at home. Because viruses usually cause the disease, antibiotics are unhelpful unless bacteria are involved. Steam helps liquefy mucus deposits on the interior walls of the trachea, the larynx, and the bronchi. The patient is given warm liquids to drink, and a family member watches them closely for any signs that the condition is getting worse will be detected. The following symptoms should alert the caregiver to the possibility that an emergency is developing and that medical help is needed quickly: drooling, difficulty breathing or swallowing, inability to bend the neck forward, blue or dark color in the lips, high-pitched sounds when inhaling, rapid heartbeat, and loss of consciousness.

The main goals of therapy for sinusitis are to control infection, relieve the blockage of the sinus openings to permit drainage, and relieve pain. When sinusitis is known to be of bacterial origin, the prescription of an appropriate antibiotic eradicates the organism. Often, however, sinusitis is attributable to viral infection, and other procedures treat it. Inhaling steam thins secretions and promotes drainage, as do mucolytic agents such as guaifenesin. Decongestant sprays and oral decongestants reduce swelling and open passages. Analgesics can be given for pain. In certain circumstances, surgeons drain the sinuses surgically.

Acute otitis media is most often diagnosed with the aid of an otoscope, an instrument that the doctor uses to look at the eardrum and surrounding tissues. The eardrum will be a dull red color, bulging, and perhaps perforated. While a viral infection may precede otitis media, the causative microorganisms and related ear infections, such as mastoiditis, are usually bacteria. For otitis media, the causative microorganisms include the following bacterial species: *Streptococcus pneumoniae*, *Haemophilus influenzae*, *Moraxella catarrhalis*, *Streptococcus pyogenes*, and *Staphylococcus aureus*. Antibiotics treat infections and prevent the spread of disease to other areas. For otitis media, physicians usually prescribe oral antibiotics. Suppose the patient has had no antibiotics in the last month. In that case, amoxicillin (875 mg) is prescribed twice a day for five to seven days. Suppose the patient has had antibiotics in the last month. In that case, the physician prescribes twice a day Augmentin, cefuroxime, cefpodoxime, or once daily cefdinir for five to seven days. Another alternative is an intramuscular injection of ceftriaxone for three days. Suppose the patient has a severe penicillin allergy. In that case, a viable alternative treatment is clindamycin, three times a day for five to seven days, or azithromycin as a Z-Pak. Sometimes pus and other fluids and solid matter build up in the inner ear. It may be necessary to pierce the eardrum to remove these deposits. A topical vasoconstrictor applied in the nose may reduce the swelling of blood vessels and relieve the blockage of the eustachian tubes. Antihistamines could be helpful to patients with allergies but are otherwise not indicated.

Mastoiditis is a complicated infection to treat. Because relatively hardy microorganisms cause mastoiditis, physicians prescribe more potent antibiotics. If staphylococci cause mastoiditis, then intravenous vancomycin effectively treats it. Intravenous ceftriaxone treats *Haemophilus influenzae* mastoiditis. Mastoiditis caused by *Pseudomonas aeruginosa* requires antibiotics specialized for this dangerous microorganism. *P. aeruginosa* mastoiditis requires intravenous cefepime or piperacillin/tazobactam. Should the patient have a severe penicillin allergy, then the physician uses the monobactam antibiotic aztreonam.

It is necessary to clean both the outer ear canal and the middle ear thoroughly for chronic otitis media. Patients wash their ears with a mild acetic acid solution with a corticosteroid for a week to ten days. Meanwhile, aggressive oral antibiotic therapy eradicates the pathogen. Surgeons can repair perforated eardrums associated with chronic otitis media with little or no loss of function. Likewise, surgeons must remove cholesteatomas.

Simple nosebleeds can be treated by pinching the nose with the fingers and breathing through the mouth for five or ten minutes to allow the blood to clot. Also, insert a plug of absorbent paper or cloth into the bleeding nostril. A physician should see patients with nosebleeds that do not stop quickly.

Nasal obstruction resulting from colds or allergies is treated by appropriate medications, decongestants for colds, and antihistamines for allergies. The only therapy for rhinitis medicamentosa, or rebound congestion caused by overuse of nasal decongestants, is to stop the medication and endure the congestion for as long as it takes the condition to clear. A deviated septum may require surgery. Sometimes it is necessary to consult a physician.

For simple halitosis caused by smoking or food, breath fresheners (with or without "odor-fighting" chemicals) are often used, even though they usually simply replace a "bad" odor with a "good" one.

Some people believe that chewing parsley or other leaves rich in chlorophyll will counteract the smell of garlic. When halitosis is attributable to tooth or gum disease, it will persist until the condition is cured. Halitosis may be of diagnostic value in certain situations where a characteristic odor could alert the physician to the possibility of a disease condition.

PERSPECTIVE AND PROSPECTS

Diseases and infections of the nasal cavity and throat have always been common among human populations, as have therapies to deal with them. Some of these disorders were quite serious until the advent of antibiotics, especially in young children, but modern medications and surgeries, where appropriate, have greatly lessened the danger. Many over-the-counter drugs combat sore throats, sinus congestion, and other nasopharyngeal symptoms of the common cold. However, colds themselves remain incurable because of the hundreds or thousands of different microorganisms that may be responsible.

The widespread use of a vaccine against Haemophilus influenzae type b, the most common causative organism of epiglottitis, has made this life-threatening disease a rarity.

The treatments available to physicians and patients for the symptoms of nasopharyngeal disorders are many. However, despite the numerous available medications, more severe infections or diseases, such as chronic tonsillitis or laryngitis, require a doctor's care, with more potent prescription drugs and surgery if needed. Still, the search continues for better drugs and perhaps preventive measures such as vaccinations to address the causes of these conditions.

—*C. Richard Falcon and Michael Buratovich, PhD*

Further Information

Friedman, Ellen M., and James P. Barassi. *My Ear Hurts! A Complete Guide to Understanding and Treating Your Child's Ear Infections*. Diane, 2004.

Greene, Alan R. *The Parent's Complete Guide to Ear Infections*. People's Medical Society, 1999.

Kimball, Chad T. *Colds, Flu, and Other Common Ailments Sourcebook*. Omnigraphics, 2001.

Levin, Brian J. *EMRA Antibiotic Guide*. 19th ed., Emergency Medicine Residents' Association, 2020.

Litin, Scott C., editor. *Mayo Clinic Family Health Book*. 4th ed., HarperResource, 2009.

PDxMD. *PDxMD Ear, Nose, and Throat Disorders*. Author, 2003.

Wagman, Richard J., editor. *The New Complete Medical and Health Encyclopedia*. 4 vols. J. G. Ferguson, 2002.

OSTEOARTHRITIS

Category: Diseases/Disorders

Anatomy or system affected: Bones, hands, hips, immune system, joints, knees, legs, musculoskeletal system

Specialties and related fields: Internal medicine, orthopedics, physical therapy, rheumatology

Definition: A group of more than one hundred inflammatory diseases that damage joints and their surrounding structures, resulting in symptomatic pain, disability, and systemwide inflammation.

KEY TERMS

anti-inflammatory drugs: drugs to counter the effects of inflammation locally or throughout the body; these drugs can be applied locally or introduced by electric currents (in a process called "iontophoresis"), by injections into the joint or into the muscles, or by mouth; the three classes of these drugs are steroidal, immunosuppressant, and nonsteroidal

cartilage: material covering the ends of bones; it does not have a blood supply or nerve supply but may swell or break down

inflammation: the body's defensive and protective responses to trauma or foreign substances by dilution, cellular efforts at destruction, and the walling-off of irritants; characterized by pain, heat, redness, swelling, and loss of function mediated through a chemical breakdown

physical modalities: the physical means of addressing a disease, which include heat, cold, electricity, exercises, braces, assistive devices, and biofeedback

rehabilitation: a physician-led program to evaluate, treat, and educate patients and their families about the sequelae of birth defects, trauma, disease, and degenerative conditions, with the goals of alleviating pain, preventing complications, correcting deformities, improving function, and reintegrating individuals into the family and society

synovium: the cellular lining of a joint, having a blood supply and a nerve supply; the synovium secretes fluid for lubrication and protects against injury and injurious agents

CAUSES AND SYMPTOMS

Approximately one in six people (more than 15 percent) suffers from one of approximately one hundred varieties of arthritis, and 2.6 percent of the population suffers from arthritis that limits their activities. Although many people over seventy-five years of age experience arthritis, the disease can occur in the young as a result of infections, rheumatic conditions, or birth defects. Young and middle-aged adults experience the disease as a result of trauma, infections, and rheumatic or immune reactions. Arthritis may be located in joints, joint capsules, the surrounding muscles, or diffusely throughout the body. Inflammation of the joint lining (synovium) can similarly afflict the linings of other organs: the skin, colon, eyes, heart, and urinary passage. Those suffering from the disease may therefore suffer from psoriasis and rashes, spastic colitis and diarrhea, dryness of the eyes, inflammations of the conjunctiva or iris, frequent urination, discharge, and burning upon urination, and other symptoms.

The collagen-type arthritic diseases involve the binding materials in the body or connective tissues and may be rheumatologic, generally more diffuse and in the distal joints (as in juvenile rheumatoid arthritis and rheumatic fever), or located in the skin and muscles (dermatomyositis). Psoriatic arthritis causes severe punched-out defects in the joints. Reiter's and Sjögren's syndromes involve the eyes and the joints. Genetic conditions, such as Gaucher's disease, frequently run in families. Metabolic disturbances, such as gout, can leave uric acid deposits in the skin and the joints. Gout sufferers experience very painful, hot, tender, and swollen joints—often in the large toe. Immunologically mediated arthritides may be associated with infections, liver diseases, bowel disturbances, and immune deficiencies. Localized infections may be bacterial, viral, or fungal. "Miscellaneous disorders," a basket category, include conditions that do not fit into any of the aforementioned categories: Psychogenic disorders and arthritis associated with cystic disorders are examples. Arthritis may also be associated with tumors that grow from cartilage cells, blood vessels, synovial tissue, and nerve tissue. Blood abnormalities may give rise to hemorrhages into joints (a side effect of sickle cell disease and hemophilia) and can be disabling and very painful, sometimes requiring surgery. Traumatic and mechanical derangements—sports and occupational injuries, leg-length disparity, and obesity—may elicit acute synovial inflammation with subsequent degenerative arthritis. Finally, wear-and-tear degeneration can occur in joints after years of trauma, repetitive use, and (especially in the obese) weight-bearing. The most common types of arthritis are rheumatoid arthritis (also called "atrophic or proliferative arthritis"), osteoarthritis, hypertrophic arthritis, and degenerative arthritis.

The inflammatory reactions in response to injury or disease consist of fluid changes—the dilation of blood vessels accompanied by an increase in the permeability of the blood vessel walls and consequent outflow of fluids and proteins. Harmful substances are immobilized with immune reactions and removed by the cellular responses of phagocytosis and digestion of foreign materials, resulting in the pro-

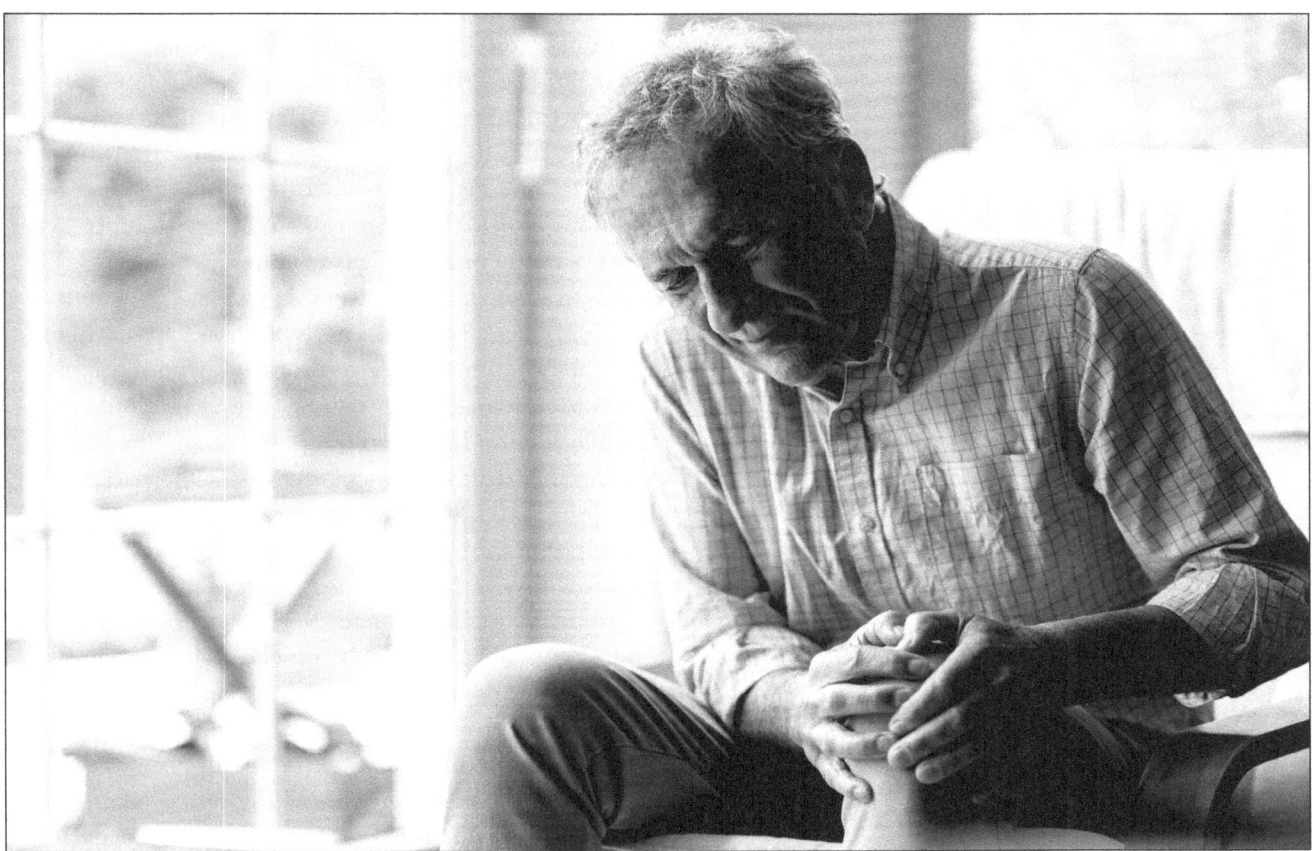
Osteoarthritis. Photo via iStock.com/PIKSEL. [Used under license.]

liferation of fibrous cells to wall off the damaging substances, leading to scar formation and deformities. The chemical reactions to injury commence with the degradation of phospholipids when enzymes are released by injured tissue. Phospholipids—fatty material that is normally present—break down into arachidonic acid, which is further broken down by other enzymes, lipoxygenase, and cyclooxygenase, resulting in prostaglandins and eicosanoid acids. Most anti-inflammatory medications attempt to interfere with the enzymatic degradation process of phospholipids and could be damaging to the liver and kidneys and the body's blood-clotting ability.

The physician bases the diagnosis of arthritic disease on the patient's medical history and a physical examination. Specific procedures such as joint aspiration, laboratory studies, and X-ray or magnetic resonance imaging (MRI) may help to establish the diagnosis and the treatment. The history will elicit the onset of pain and its relation to the time of day and difficulties performing the activities of daily living. A functional classification has evolved that is similar to the cardiac functional classification: Class 1 patients perform all usual activities without a handicap; class 2 patients perform normal activities adequately with occasional symptoms and signs in one or more joints but still do not need to limit their activities; class 3 patients find that they must limit some activities and may require assistive devices; class 4 patients are unable to perform activities, are largely or wholly incapacitated, and are bedridden

> **INFORMATION ON ARTHRITIS**
>
> Causes: Infection, rheumatic conditions, birth defects, trauma, immune reactions, wear-and-tear degeneration
>
> Symptoms: Joint pain, psoriasis, and rashes, spastic colitis and diarrhea, dryness of the eyes, frequent urination
>
> Duration: Chronic
>
> Treatments: Anti-inflammatory drugs; application of heat, cold, or electricity; exercise; biofeedback; assistive devices

or confined to a wheelchair, requiring assistance in self-care.

A person's medical history or surgical conditions and the medications that he or she is taking can influence the physician's diagnosis and prescription for treatment. Patients may present a gross picture of the body to the physician showing the joints involved in their symmetry (whether distal or proximal, and whether weight-bearing or posttraumatic in distribution). Physicians may ask (verbally or by questionnaire) for a history of other system complaints, which can then be checked more thoroughly. During a physical examination, the physician will check the joints, skin, eyes, abdomen, heart, and urinary tract. The neuromuscular evaluation may reveal localized tenderness of the joints or muscles, swelling, wasting, weakness, and abnormal motions. Joints may have weakened ligamentous, muscle, and tendon supports that could give rise to instability or grinding of joints, with subsequent roughening of cartilage surfaces. The arthritides are frequently associated with muscular pains, called "fibrositis" and "myofascial pain syndromes."

Fibrositis is a diffuse muscular pain syndrome with tenderness in the muscles, no muscle spasm, and no limitations in motion; all laboratory tests are within normal limits. It is frequent in postmenopausal women who have a history of migraines, cold extremities, spastic colitis, softening of the bone matrix accompanied by loss of minerals, and irritability. Myofascial trigger points can be found in both men and women, at all ages, with acutely tender nodules or cords felt in muscles. The pain of these trigger points is referred to more distal areas of the muscles that may not be tender to touch. Physicians may frequently miss the acutely tender trigger points. Tests will show whether pain occurs when muscles are contracted with motion, when muscles are contracted without motion, or when motion is carried out passively by the examiner without muscular effort by the patient.

Joint pathology is generally associated with some limitation in the range of motion. Sensation testing, muscle strength, and reflex changes may also indicate nerve tissue damage. Nerves occasionally pass close to joints and may be pinched when the joint swelling encroaches upon the passage opening. This condition may result in carpal tunnel syndrome, in which the median nerve at the wrist becomes pinched, causing pain, numbness, and weakness in the hand. Pinched nerves may also be associated with tarsal tunnel syndrome, in which the nerve at the inner side of the ankle joint may be compressed and cause similar complaints in the feet. Other nerves may be constricted in exiting from the spine and when passing through muscles in spasm.

The medications used to treat arthritis can involve the nervous system. An evaluation and estimation of the severity of the disease can be obtained by electrical testing, as in electroneuromyography. The nerves are stimulated, and their rate of transmitting the stimulus is measured. The normal transmission rate for nerves is forty-five meters per second. Delays at areas of impingement can be determined by measuring the transmission rate of a stimulus from different points along the nerve paths. Abnormal or damaged muscles will cause muscle fibers to contract spontaneously, or fibrillate. Chest expansion during inspiration and after expiration may be limited because of arthritis in the spine or because of lung pathology. Involvement of the spine can also be measured by the posture, the ability to move the neck, and the ability to move the lower back.

Arthritis of the spine leads to a progressive loss in motion. The amount lost can be measured by comparing the normal motion with the restricted motion of the patient. The neck may be limited in all directions, rotation of the head to the sides can restrict the driving view, and the head may gradually tilt forward. The lower back may also exhibit restriction in all directions; for example, it may be limited in forward bending because of spasms in the muscles in the back. Tilting backward of the trunk may be limited and painful when the vertebral body overgrowth of osteoarthritis or degenerative arthritis restricts the space for the spinal cord. The nerves pinched in their passage from the vertebrae may thus cause radiculitis, irritation of the nerves as they exit from the spine that leads to pain and muscle involvement. Circumferential measurements of the involved joints and the structures above and below can confirm swelling, atrophy from disuse or inaction, or atrophy from a damaged nerve supply. When measurements are repeated, they can indicate improvement or deterioration. One type of arthritis that most often affects the spine, ankylosing spondylitis, occurs predominantly in males in their late teenage and early adult years.

Testing of blood for cells, chemicals, or enzymes is helpful. The simplest test—the sedimentation (or "sed") test—measures the rate at which blood cells settle out of the plasma. Normally, women have a more rapid rate of sedimentation than men. When this rate exceeds the normal range, active inflammation in the body is indicated. Comparisons of sed tests performed at different stages can reveal the disease's rate of progression or improvement. The chemicals tested may include uric acid for gout and sugar for diabetes. Blood tests for immune substances and antibodies are also possible, although the American College of Rheumatology recommends avoiding broad testing of antibodies. The joint fluid can be aspirated and analyzed, particularly for appearance, density, number of blood cells, and levels of sugar. Cloudy fluid, the tendency to form clots, a high cell count, and lower-than-normal levels of sugar in the joint fluid (compared to the overall blood sugar level) indicate abnormalities. With inflammatory arthritides, the X-rays will show the results of synovial fluid and cellular overabundance. Clumps of pannus break off and may destroy the cartilage and bone. Bones about these joints, because of increased vascularity and blood flow, have fewer minerals and will appear less dense, a condition known as osteoporosis.

Deformities in inflammatory arthritis may be the result of unequal muscle pulls or the destruction or scarring of tissues; such deformities can occasionally be prevented by the use of resting splints, which are most important for the hands.

Degenerative and posttraumatic arthritis show joint narrowing, thinning of the cartilage layer, hardening of the underlying bone (called "eburnation"), and marginal overgrowth of the underlying bone (called "osteophytes"), resulting in osteoarthritis. Osteophytes, or marginal lipping in the back, may enhance symptoms of lower back pain. The cushions between the vertebrae, called "discs," are more than 80 percent water, a figure which diminishes with aging, bringing the joints in the back (the facets) closer together and compressing the facet joints between the vertebrae. Irritation and arthritis of these joints are the results. Other organ structures may be involved as well.

A diagnosis of rheumatoid arthritis should include two to four of the following criteria: morning stiffness, three or more joints involved symmetrically (especially the hands), six weeks or longer in duration, rheumatoid nodules that can be felt under the skin, blood tests showing a serum rheumatoid factor, and the radiographic evidence described above.

TREATMENT AND THERAPY

Treatment of arthritis may vary from home treatment to outpatient treatment to hospitalization for acute, surgical, and/or rehabilitative care. Educating patients as to their condition, prognosis, treatment goals, and the methods of treatment are necessary. Patients must be made aware of warning signs of progression, drug effects, local and systemic side effects of drug therapy, and diet associated with relieving pain, stiffness, and inflammation. If surgery is contemplated for joint replacement or other reasons, patients should be fully informed as to expectations and rate of functional activities. Postoperative restrictions in the range of motion must be given; in hip replacement, for example, hip bending should not exceed ninety degrees. The rotation and overlapping of legs must be limited initially after surgery.

Some physicians provide a questionnaire that outlines the activities of daily living and recommends how a patient should perform such activities and how much time should be spent at rest. The goals generally are to maintain function, alleviate pain, limit the progression of deformities, prevent complications, and treat associated and secondary disease states. In patients with degenerative arthritis—most often the elderly, who are at risk for other organ failures—arthritides associated with systemic diseases and other organ involvements may require care. Patients with rheumatoid arthritis, for example, frequently are anemic. Anti-inflammatory drugs, normally used to treat arthritis, may cause blood loss through the gastrointestinal tract and even ulcerations. The physician may therefore prescribe alternative therapies.

Other therapies can include assistive devices, counseling patients and their families regarding home management, medicinal regimen and compliance, behavior modification, sexual advice, and biofeedback. The aim is to reduce the need for and frequency of medical care, through a balance between

---

IN THE NEWS: GLUCOSAMINE AND CHONDROITIN

Medical, surgical, and rehabilitative techniques have been used in the treatment of arthritis. Recently more people have turned to complementary and alternative medicine for the treatment of medical disorders, including arthritis. Two nutritional supplements that have been widely used to treat osteoarthritis are glucosamine (a substance involved in cartilage formation and repair) and chondroitin sulfate (which provides cartilage with elasticity). While these substances are produced naturally by the human body, when marketed as dietary supplements glucosamine is usually derived from shellfish, while chondroitin comes from either cow or shark cartilage. Because dietary supplements are not regulated by any federal agency, consumers must be sure to deal with a reputable manufacturer to assure product quality.

A large-scale study of glucosamine and chondroitin in treating osteoarthritis of the knee was undertaken at sixteen rheumatology centers in the United States with funding from the National Institutes of Health. The first phase of the Glucosamine/Chondroitin Arthritis Intervention Trial (GAIT) compared five groups taking 1,500 milligrams of glucosamine, 1,200 milligrams of chondroitin sulfate, 1,500 milligrams of glucosamine with 1,200 milligrams chondroitin sulfate, 200 milligrams of a COX-2 inhibitor (a nonsteroidal anti-inflammatory drug, or NSAID, available by prescription to treat osteoarthritis), and a placebo. All substances used in this study were assessed to ensure their purity and quality. For patients who suffered moderate to severe pain (but not those suffering mild pain), the combination of glucosamine and chondroitin sulfate provided greater pain relief than did the placebo or the COX-2 inhibitor. Phase two of GAIT found that glucosamine and chondroitin were no more effective than a placebo at preventing joint damage caused by arthritis; the supplements did not slow the destruction of cartilage that leads to narrowing in knee joints.

Based on this study, the Arthritis Foundation suggests that these nutritional supplements should be used in conjunction with prescription medications and with exercise, weight control, and possibly surgery. Individuals considering glucosamine/chondroitin therapy should be aware that glucosamine is contraindicated for people with shellfish allergies and that it may affect blood sugar levels in diabetics. Chondroitin may affect blood-clotting ability in individuals taking anticoagulants. Research into the usefulness of glucosamine and chondroitin sulfate continues.

—*Robin Kamienny Montvilo, RN, PhD*

rest and activity and between effective drug dose, toxicity, and physical modalities. To protect joints and allow function, various braces and assistive devices may be needed. Scarring of a wrist joint can be alleviated by avoiding positions that inhibit function. Shoulders should not be left with arms close to the body, since frozen shoulders aggravate neck and arm problems.

Physicians may offer physical therapy, occupational therapy, assistive devices for self-care, ambulation, or home and automobile modifications. Assistive devices may include reachers, an elongated shoehorn handle, thickened handles for utensils, walkers, canes, crutches, and wheelchairs. Homes may require ramps for easier access, widened doors to allow wheelchair passage, grab bars in bathtubs, or raised toilet seats for easier transference from a wheelchair.

Heat therapy may reduce the pain, loosening and liquefying tightened tissues. Somewhat like gelatin, tissue liquefies when heated and solidifies when cooled. Patients frequently will be stiffer after protracted rest periods (for example, on waking) and feel better after some activity and exercise. Heated pools offer an excellent heating and exercise modality. The type of heat modality used will depend upon the depth of heating desired. Hot packs and infrared lamps will heat predominantly the skin surface areas and some underlying muscles. Diathermy units heat the muscular layers, and ultrasound treatments heat the deepest bony layers. Ultrasound (but not diathermy) can even be used in patients who have metallic implants such as joint replacements.

Transcutaneous electrical nerve stimulation can be used to alleviate pain. The units can regulate the frequency of electrical impulses. The usual starting rate is 100 cycles, which can alleviate pain in a few minutes; this rate is later changed to 4 cycles, which will give hours of relief even when discontinued. The intensity can also be varied. The sensation desired is a slight tingle. The effect described induces an increase in the release of beta-endorphin, a substance naturally produced by the body with effects similar to those of morphine. Endorphin is produced by other physical therapy procedures as well: hypnosis, acupuncture, suggestion, and stress, among others.

Patients in chronic pain may show a reduced level of beta-endorphin and an increase in substance P, and they may find no relief of pain with physical therapy. Substance P is a small peptide that increases the nerves' sensitivity to stimuli, producing greater pain. Patients with chronic pain may show depression, hysteria, and hypochondriasis on the Minnesota Multiphasic Personality Inventory and may require antidepressants. Exercise programs can help to increase endorphin levels. These exercises may range from simple movements performed by a therapist (the patient remaining passive) to active exertion against loads for strength. Stretching or gentle, intermittent traction may gradually decrease contractures, but neck traction should not be used in patients with rheumatoid arthritis of the neck.

Surgery may occasionally be necessary to alleviate pain, to replace joints, or to alleviate contractures. Isometric or static exercises can mobilize muscles without joint movement and maintain muscle viability during joint pain. Individuals can, however, be trained to perform activities more efficiently and effectively, thus saving energy. Posture training may alleviate postural muscle fatigue. In acute stages of inflammation, the treatment choices are rest, ice, compression, and proper positioning, and medicines for pain and inflammation. Heat modalities should not be used in acute cases, since the speed of chemical reactions increases on heating; the chemical enzyme activity of collagenase that destroys cartilage could increase the rate and extent of the damage. The simplest way to prepare cold applications is to fill a plastic container with water and refrigerate it. Physicians may also use fluoromethane or other refrigerant sprays. The hot packs sold in pharmacies can similarly be soaked in water and placed in the refrigerator to create an ice pack.

The medicinal approach utilizes nonsteroidal anti-inflammatory drugs (NSAIDs)—such as aspirin, indomethacin, ibuprofen, naproxen, piroxicam, and nabumetone—and adds other drugs as necessary. NSAIDs effectively treat osteoarthritis pain, but they can cause gastrointestinal, renal, and cardiovascular side effects, especially in older adults, and should not be used long-term. When possible, consider topical NSAIDs for knee or hand pain in place of oral NSAIDs since topical agents have fewer adverse effects than oral medications. COX-2 selective NSAIDs, such as celecoxib, only inhibit inflammation-induced cyclooxygenase and neither interferes with platelet function nor cause gastrointestinal toxicity. However, although celecoxib may increase the risk of clots in small blood vessels, its cardiovascular safety profile at commonly prescribed dosages is about the same as naproxen and ibuprofen. Acetaminophen is generally less effective than NSAIDs but is better tolerated at doses =4 g/day. Above at doses =4 g/day, acetaminophen causes severe hepatotoxicity.

Other medications for osteoarthritis include the serotonin and norepinephrine reuptake inhibitor duloxetine. While duloxetine is also Food and Drug Administration (FDA)-approved for anxiety, it is also approved for neuropathic and osteoarthritic pain. Duloxetine, however, is only modestly effective. Additionally, it has side effects that include headache, nausea, sleepiness, insomnia, dry mouth, constipation, diarrhea, decreased appetite, excessive sweating, and elevated blood pressure.

Opioids, such as tramadol, relieve osteoarthritis pain. Surprisingly, opioids only provide slightly more relief than placebos in clinical trials. Furthermore, continued use of opioids can lead to dependence and the development of tolerance to their effects. Opioids should not be considered first-line treatments for osteoarthritis pain but reserved as last resort medications for patients with intractable osteoarthritis pain.

Injections of corticosteroids (methylprednisolone or triamcinolone) into the joint capsules are generally safe and effective for local treatment of osteoarthritis. Such treatments provide pain relief that diminishes by two months after administration, but most clinicians wait at least three months between injections. These treatments can accelerate cartilage destruction in affected joints.

Injections of commercially available hyaluronic acid preparations into the joint space may increase the viscosity and elasticity of synovial fluid. Increased joint lubrication may, in turn, prevent degradation of articular cartilage. The FDA has approved intra-articular injections of hyaluronic acid for osteoarthritis of the knee. However, it has only modest beneficial effects. No reliable data shows that hyaluronic acid injections slow the progression of osteoarthritis.

PERSPECTIVE AND PROSPECTS
Historically, arthritis was treated with electric eels (as the source of electric shocks) and warm baths or sands. Some experimental treatments presently being tried include electric current to joints to bring about reductions in intra-articular pressures and the fluid and cellular content in joints. Acupuncture seems to increase beta-endorphin levels and relieve pain. Unfortunately, extensive reviews of controlled clinical trials have shown that acupuncture has little or no impact on arthritis. Topical use of capsaicin, an extract from peppers, is reported to counteract substance P. One group is attempting the experimental procedure of washing out inflamed joints with a saline-type solution. Turmeric, though widely promoted for pain relief and joint mobility, has not been approved by the FDA for any indication. Exercises continue to maintain and improve strength, dexterity, range of motion, and endurance. Good health habits-including adequate rest, good

nutrition, and nutritional supplements can be beneficial.

—*Eugene J. Rogers, MD, Victoria Price, PhD, and Michael A. Buratovich, PhD*

Further Information

Aesoph, Lauri M. *How to Eat Away Arthritis*. Prentice, 1996.

Flynn, John A., and Lora Brown Wilder, editors. *Recipes for Arthritis Health*. Rebus, 2003.

Fries, James F. *Arthritis: A Take-Care-of-Yourself Health Guide to Understanding Your Arthritis*. 5th ed., Addison, 1999.

Hunder, Gene G. *Mayo Clinic on Arthritis*. Rev. ed., Mayo Clinic, 2002.

Lane, Nancy E., and Daniel J. Wallace. *All About Osteoarthritis: The Definitive Resource for Arthritis Patients and Their Families*. Oxford UP, 2002.

Lorig, Kate, and James F. Fries, editors. *The Arthritis Helpbook: A Tested Self-Management Program for Coping with Arthritis and Fibromyalgia*. Updated ed., Da Capo, 2007.

McAlindon, T. E., M. P. LaValley, W. F. Harvey, et al. "Effect of Intra-articular Triamcinolone vs. Saline on Knee Cartilage Volume and Pain in Patients with Knee Osteoarthritis: A Randomized Clinical Trial." *JAMA*, vol. 317, no. 19, 2017, pp. 1967-75, doi:10.1001/jama.2017.5283.

MedlinePlus. "Arthritis." *MedlinePlus*, 24 Apr. 2013.

Nelson, Miriam E., et al. *Strong Women and Men Beat Arthritis*. Putnam, 2003.

Ramos, Alexis et al. "Acupuncture for rheumatoid arthritis." ("Acupuntura para el tratamiento de la artritis reumatoide.") *Medwave*, vol. 18, no. 6, 2018, p. e7284, doi:10.5867/medwave.2018.06.7283.

Shlotzhauer, Tammi L., and James L. McGuire. *Living with Rheumatoid Arthritis*. 2nd ed., Johns Hopkins UP, 2003.

Weinblatt, Michael E. *The Arthritis Action Program: An Integrated Plan of Traditional and Complementary Therapies*. Fireside, 2001.

Rashes

Category: Diseases/disorders
Anatomy or system affected: Skin
Specialties and related fields: Dermatology
Definition: General eruptions of the skin that are often associated with communicable diseases and most often temporary; most are some shade of red.

KEY TERMS

pruritic: itchy
systemic: affecting the whole body
wheal: a flat, firm, and raised area of the skin

CAUSES AND SYMPTOMS

Rashes may have many different causes: infection, inflammation, irritation, an allergic reaction, and systemic disease. Rashes usually vary in color from pale pink to red. They take many different forms: flat, raised, puffy, scaly, blistery, or crusted. They may be pruritic. Rashes may involve a small portion of the skin or cover much of the body. They may come in characteristic shapes, such as a bull's-eye, or may appear irregular. A rash may be accompanied by other signs and symptoms that help the healthcare provider determine the cause. Alternatively, a rash may form part of a constellation of signs and symptoms diagnostic of another disease or disorder.

Bacteria, viruses, or fungi may cause infectious rashes. For example, impetigo is caused by either staphylococcal or streptococcal bacteria, a herpes virus causes cold sores, and a fungus causes athlete's foot. Some infectious rashes are highly contagious among children or family members and others.

INFORMATION ON RASHES

Causes: Allergies, infection, disease, environmental toxins, inflammation, irritation

Symptoms: Skin lesions that may be flat, raised, puffy, scaly, blistery, or crusted

Duration: Acute to chronic

Treatments: Depends on the type; may include antibiotics, topical steroids, adding moisture to or drying affected area

Rashes associated with inflammation include allergic responses to drugs, certain foods, stings, and poison ivy. Allergic rashes are typically red and itchy. They may be flat or may arise as wheals. Many allergic rashes are merely annoying, but some can be part of a life-threatening condition called "anaphylaxis." Symptoms of anaphylaxis include blockage of the airways, a rash, and cardiac problems. Children can go into anaphylactic shock after eating a food to which they are highly allergic (such as shellfish, peanuts, or strawberries) or after being stung by a bee.

A common, but not usually serious, rash in infants is heat rash or miliaria rubra. It is also called "prickly heat." This rash is most common in hot and humid environments and on areas of the body covered by tight clothing.

Many so-called childhood diseases are characterized by fever and rash: measles, rubella (German measles), chickenpox, and fifth disease. The rash associated with each of these has distinctive features that help in the diagnosis of the disease. For example, the child with fifth disease has bright red cheeks, the so-called slapped cheek phenomenon, and a fine lacy rash on the trunk and extremities. The rash of rubella begins on the face and spreads rapidly to the trunk, arms, and legs. Scarlet fever, on the other hand, is a streptococcal infection accompanied by a rash. Again, the characteristics of the rash help in making the diagnosis: It has a fine sandpaper-like feeling when touched. All these childhood diseases are related to systemic viral infections.

TREATMENT AND THERAPY

The treatment of rashes depends on the cause. A common rule of thumb is that if a rash is wet, the treatment is to dry it, and vice versa. For example, an oozing rash caused by poison ivy may be relieved

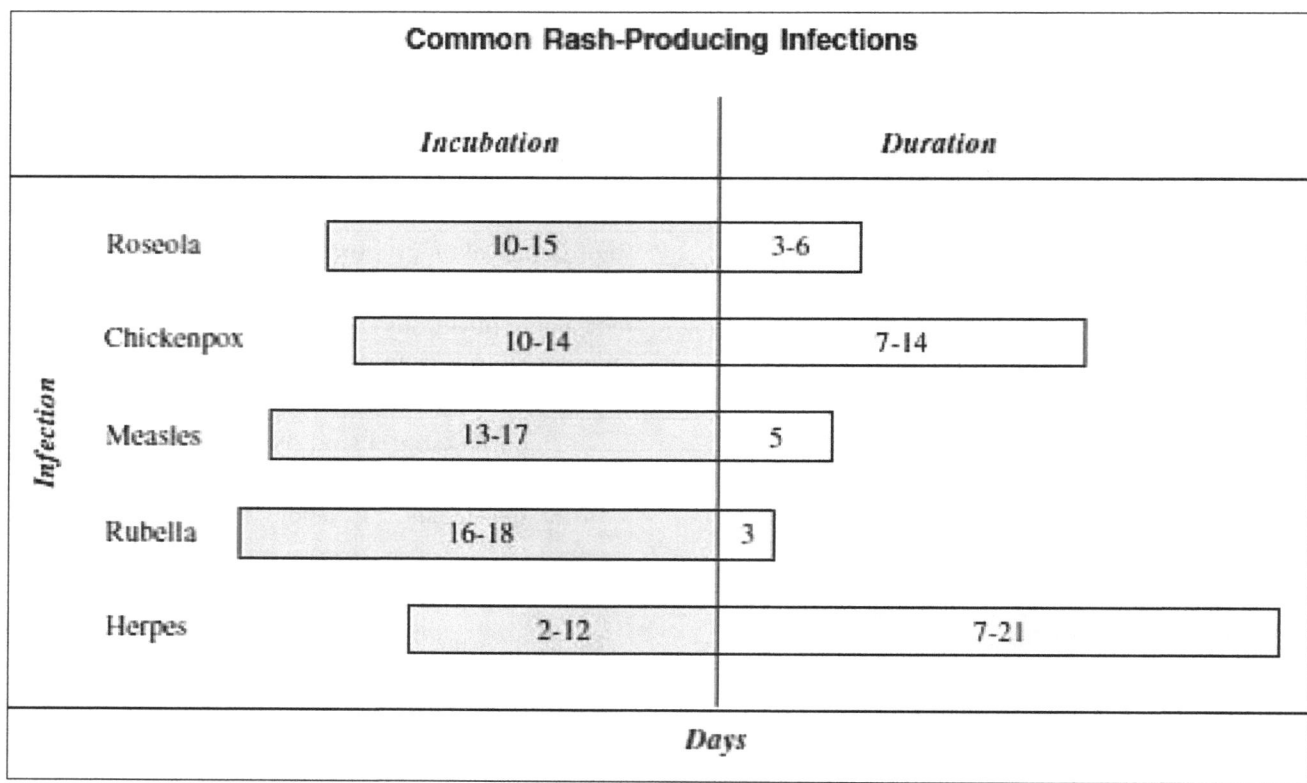

by a drying paste that relieves itching. In contrast, a dry rash may be best treated with an ointment or by an oatmeal bath.

Some rashes will resolve on their own. The main job of parents and health care providers is to relieve a child's unpleasant symptoms, such as itching, that go along with the rash. Patients with rashes that itch need to receive medications to relieve itching, such as antihistamines, so that they will not complicate their condition by scratching the affected skin. Most antihistamines, however, cause the side effect of sleepiness. Soothing oatmeal baths or moisturizing lotions can relieve itching without causing sleepiness.

Treatments for rashes can be either topical or systemic. Topical treatments are put directly on the skin. For example, athlete's foot is treated with topical ointments or powders containing antifungal agents that kill the fungus that causes the condition. Impetigo, on the other hand, is usually treated with systemic antibiotics to kill the causative bacteria.

A mainstay of dermatological treatment is steroid medications. Topical steroids such as hydrocortisone cream or ointment are applied directly to the skin and may be covered with a dressing. In some cases, as in a severe case of poison ivy, steroids may be given orally or by injection. Steroids have potentially serious adverse effects, so most health-care providers use them sparingly. They should seldom be used on the face or eyelids unless so prescribed by a physician.

PERSPECTIVE AND PROSPECTS

Rashes are a widespread problem in childhood and adolescence. Parents can often diagnose rashes themselves and treat them with appropriate over-the-counter products. Rashes associated with other symptoms, whose origin is unclear, or that fail to clear up in a reasonable amount of time should be evaluated and treated by a qualified health care provider.

—*Rebecca Lovell Scott, PhD, PA-C*

Further Information

Goldsmith, Lowell A., Gerald S. Lazarus, and Michael D. Tharp. *Adult and Pediatric Dermatology: A Color Guide to Diagnosis and Treatment*. F. A. Davis, 1997. A well-written, richly illustrated, user-friendly book with an appealing layout. The authors have admirably succeeded in producing a valuable resource of knowledge for any dermatologist.

Litin, Scott C., editor. *Mayo Clinic Family Health Book*. 4th ed., HarperResource, 2009. Perhaps the best general medical text for the layperson, this book covers the entire medical field. While the information is derived from various highly technical sources, the articles are written to be easily understood by a general audience.

Middlemiss, Prisca. *What's That Rash? How to Identify and Treat Childhood Rashes*. Hamlyn, 2002. A comprehensive guide to the identification and treatment of childhood rashes.

Porter, Robert S., et al., editors. *The Merck Manual Home Health Handbook*. Merck Research Laboratories, 2009. A best-selling medical reference book is now available in a new home edition. Easy to understand and full of updated information, this volume contains over fifteen hundred pages on diseases, causes, treatments, and drugs. Includes over three hundred drawings.

Schmitt, Barton D. *Your Child's Health: The Parents' One-Stop Reference Guide to Symptoms, Emergencies, Common Illnesses, Behavior Problems, Healthy Development*. Rev. ed., Bantam Books, 2005. Offers parents complete and authoritative advice from one of the nation's leading pediatricians in a step-by-step, quick-reference format.

Turkington, Carol, and Jeffrey S. Dover. *The Encyclopedia of Skin and Skin Disorders*. 3rd ed., Facts On File, 2007. More than one thousand entries on skin-related topics, including diseases, treatments, resources and organizations, skin cancer, acne treatment, Food and Drug Administration (FDA) approvals of new treatments, and remedies for wrinkled skin.

Weedon, David. *Skin Pathology*. 3rd ed., Churchill Livingstone/Elsevier, 2010. Text with extensive photographs, covering tissue reaction patterns; the epidermis, dermis, and subcutis; the skin in systemic and miscellaneous diseases; infections and infestations; and tumors, among other topics.

Rhinitis

Category: Diseases/Disorders
Also known as: Runny nose, hay fever, nasal allergies
Anatomy or system affected: Nose, respiratory system, throat
Specialties and related fields: Family medicine, immunology, otorhinolaryngology, pediatrics
Definition: A discharge from the nose caused by inflammation of the internal nasal structures.

KEY TERMS

allergic rhinitis: acute or seasonal nasal stuffiness and sneezing that follows the exposure to allergens such as pollen or animal dander; hay fever is one form of allergic rhinitis

mast cells: cells filled with basophilic granules, distributed throughout connective tissue that releasing histamine and other substances during inflammatory and allergic reactions

nonallergic rhinitis: acute nasal stuffiness produced because of the common cold or flu

postnasal drip: the discharge of nasal mucus into the back of the throat

CAUSES AND SYMPTOMS

Rhinitis can have various causes, including infection by a rhinovirus or certain bacteria and exposure to cold air or nasal allergens. Foreign bodies in the nose and certain structural deformities can also cause rhinitis.

When the nasal symptoms are due to allergies, the condition is called "allergic rhinitis." A partial list of allergens that can produce allergic rhinitis includes pollen, dust, molds, wool, feathers, tobacco smoke, airborne environmental pollutants, strong odors, spicy foods, and animal dander.

When the nasal symptoms are not due to allergies, the condition is called "nonallergic rhinitis" or nonallergic vasomotor rhinitis. A viral or bacterial infection can cause nonallergic rhinitis, exposure to cold air, structural deformities, certain endocrine disorders such as hypothyroidism or emotional stress, occasionally observed during the first trimester of pregnancy. Nonallergic rhinitis usually begins with a feeling of irritation in the nose or throat. The irritation is followed by sneezing, and mucus discharge as the nasal air passageways become more obstructed.

Atrophic rhinitis, a chronic form of nonallergic rhinitis, is a condition often seen first at puberty; the condition tends to run in families because of a genetic component. The causes of atrophic rhinitis are not fully understood, although deficiencies in iron and vitamins A and D may contribute. In this condition, a thin crusty surface that can be foul-smelling replaces the moist, pink, thick lining of the inside of the nose. Although the nasal cavity is wide open, people often complain of a feeling of stuffiness. Nosebleeds sometimes accompany the condition.

All forms of rhinitis usually include nasal dripping and sneezing. The discharge can be clear and watery or thicker and more viscous. It can be colorless; if there is a color, it is often white or less often green or yellow. Postnasal drip occurs when the discharge is into the back of the throat. This condition can result in a dry, usually nonproductive cough.

TREATMENT AND THERAPY

The treatment for rhinitis is an attempt to manage symptoms. The most effective treatment for allergic rhinitis is to remove the source of the irritation. Keeping the windows closed, using an air conditioner, and filtering the circulating air can reduce allergen exposure in the home. The use of saline irrigation can reduce nasal symptoms. When symptoms persist despite these efforts, treatment focuses on minimizing the allergic response. Drugs treatments that diminish symptoms of allergic rhinitis include antihistamines, steroids, or antileukotrienes.

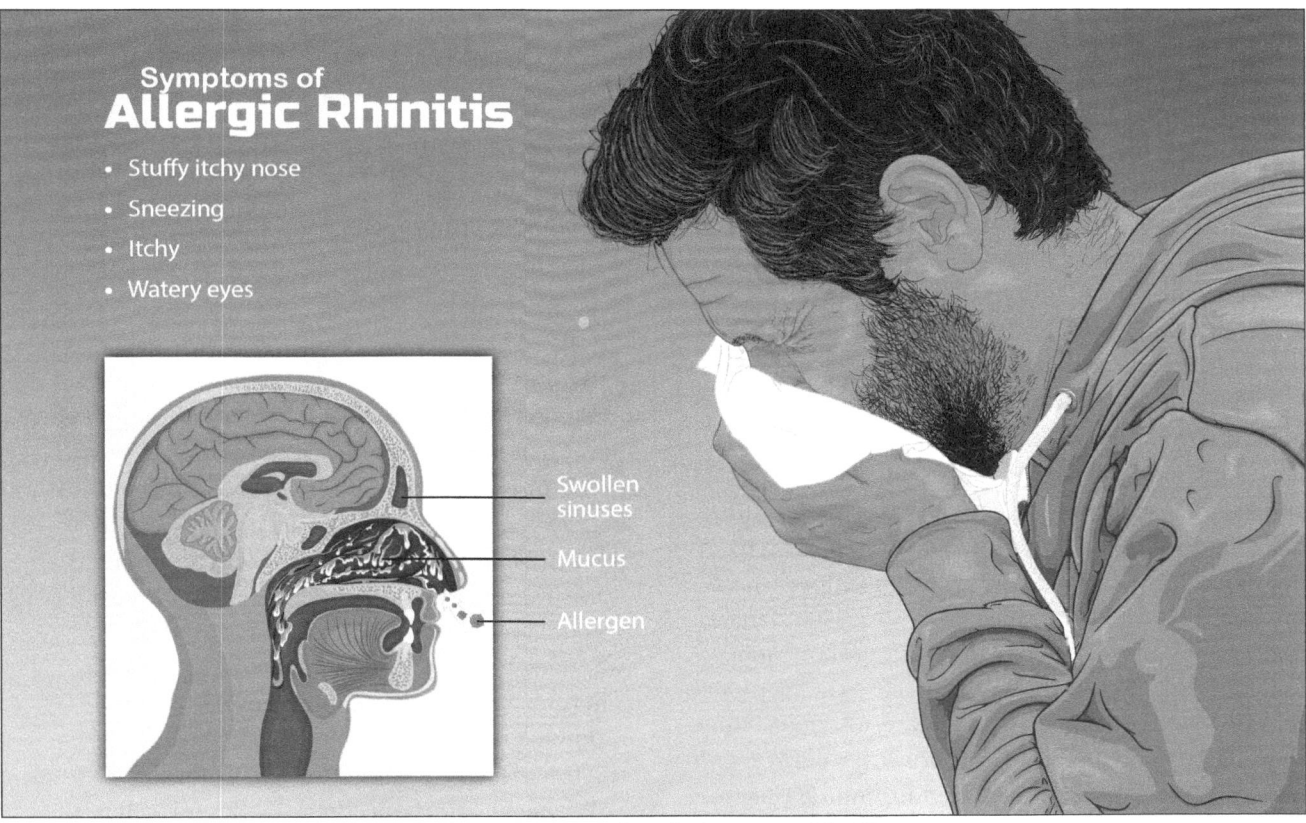

Rhinitis illustration. Image by https://www.myupchar.com/en, via Wikimedia Commons. [CC 4.0].

When the body encounters an allergen, B lymphocytes produce a specific antibodies subtype known as immunoglobulin E (IgE). When IgE molecules are attached to tissue cells, called "mast cells," that encounter the allergen, the mast cells release compounds called "mediators." Histamine is perhaps the best known of these mediators. The mediators trigger the nasal symptoms. Most of the drugs used to treat allergic rhinitis are designed to inhibit the actions of the mediators. Antihistamines block the action of histamine and so significantly reduce swelling and discharge. Likewise, antileukotrienes work by blocking leukotrienes, another immune system mediator. The mechanism by which nasal steroids (usually given as a spray) work is less clear, but they can provide temporary relief.

People have intermittent allergic rhinitis if symptoms occur less than four days a week or four weeks of the year. Persistent allergic rhinitis occurs if people have symptoms more than four times per week and more than four weeks of the year. If someone's allergic rhinitis symptoms do not affect their quality of life, their condition is mild. However, if their symptoms affect their quality of life, their condition is moderate or severe. The preferred treatments for mild intermittent allergic rhinitis are second-generation or intranasal antihistamines. Oral second-generation antihistamines include cetirizine (Zyrtec, generic), desloratadine (generic, Clarinex), fexofenadine (generic, Allegra), levocetirizine (Xyzal), and loratadine (Alavert, Claritin, generic). Intranasal antihistamines include azelastine and olopatadine (Patanase). The most effective single treatment for allergic rhinitis is intranasal corticosteroids. These drugs include beclomethasone dipropionate (Beconase, Qnasl), budesonide (Rhinocort), ciclesonide (Omnaris, Zetonna), flunisolide, fluticasone furoate (Flonase Sensimist), fluticasone propionate (generic, Flonase), mometasone furoate (Nasonex), Triamcinolone acetonide (Nasacort). When combined with intranasal or oral antihistamines, intranasal corticosteroids effectively treat moderate to severe symptoms.

Other options include intranasal ipratropium bromide if corticosteroids and antihistamines fail to relieve someone's allergic rhinitis symptoms. This antimuscarinic agent does not efficiently pass into the systemic circulation and does not readily cross the blood-brain barrier. Ipratropium reduces nasal discharge but does not relieve sneezing, nasal itching, or congestion. This drug dries the nasal and oral cavities. Therefore, it can increase the incidence of nose bleeds and sore throats. A second alternative agent is intranasal cromolyn sodium. Cromolyn sodium inhibits mast cell-mediated histamine release, preventing allergic rhinitis symptoms. People should use cromolyn sodium nasal sprays one to two weeks before exposure to the allergen and three to four times daily. When administered before allergen exposure, such as visiting a house full of cats, it can diminish the acute allergic response. However, cromolyn sodium is effective than intranasal corticosteroids. It is relatively side-effect-free, but it can cause nasal stinging. Finally, if all other treatments fail, a monoclonal antibody against IgE called "omalizumab" (Xolair) can provide allergy patients the relief they so desperately desire. Allergy patients receive subcutaneous injections of omalizumab every two to four weeks. It effectively relieves symptoms of even the most stubborn types of allergic rhinitis.

Mast cells release not only histamine, a relatively short-acting mediator, but longer-acting mediators called "leukotrienes." Leukotrienes cause significant nasal congestion, itching, and sneezing. The oral

> **INFORMATION ON RHINITIS**
>
> **Causes**: Irritants, infections, cold air
>
> **Symptoms**: Stuffiness or irritation in nose often accompanied by mucus discharge
>
> **Duration**: Usually acute but can be chronic
>
> **Treatments**: Removal of irritation, resolution of infection, antihistamines, nasal steroids

leukotriene receptor antagonist montelukast (Singulair) relieves the symptoms of seasonal and perennial allergic rhinitis. It modestly relieves allergic rhinitis symptoms about as well and a second-generation oral antihistamine, but less well as an intranasal corticosteroid. The Food and Drug Administration (FDA) continues receiving rare but consistent reports of suicidal behavior and other neuropsychiatric events from patients on montelukast. Therefore, the FDA recommends restricting montelukast use to those from whom other treatments have been ineffective or intolerable.

When the symptoms do not respond well to the above treatments, immunotherapy is required. For this treatment, it is necessary to determine the allergens to which the person is sensitive. To identify the offending allergen, skin or blood tests are the most commonly utilized methods. After identifying the specific allergen, desensitizing the immune system by carefully administering allergen challenges raises the tolerance level necessary to produce the nasal symptoms. Allergen-specific immunotherapy can alter the natural history of allergic respiratory disease and induce long-term remission.

If the cause of nonallergic rhinitis was exposure to cold air, then going into a warmer environment usually eliminates the symptoms. If the cause is the common cold or the flu, symptoms are sometimes relieved by decongestants or antihistamines. Some of these drugs are available over the counter, while others require a prescription. Unless there is a primary or secondary bacterial infection accompanying the rhinitis, antibiotics are not effective. Drinking lots of fluids, getting bed rest, and breathing humidified air can reduce the discomfort. With any viral or bacterial infection (especially H1N1 influenza infections), affected individuals should consult a medical professional as soon as possible if breathing becomes a problem. Muscle aching and the general feeling of malaise accompanying nonallergic rhinitis can often be relieved by over-the-counter medications such as aspirin or ibuprofen.

Irrigating the nasal cavity with sterile saline can provide short-term relief of allergic rhinitis symptoms. If a bacterial infection is present, then antibiotics are indicated. Nasal douches effectively treat associated nasal crusting. In severe cases, atrophic rhinitis is treated by Young's operation. This surgical procedure reduces the size of the nasal cavity.

When the cause of rhinitis is a foreign body or structural deformity, removing the foreign body or surgically changing the nose's internal structure often eliminates the symptoms.

PERSPECTIVE AND PROSPECTS

Considerable financial and personal costs are associated with rhinitis since it is such a common condition. Because rhinitis is so common, considerable effort is going into completely understanding this disease. As a result, new treatments with fewer side effects should become available.

—*David Hornung, PhD and Michael A. Buratovich, PhD*

Further Information

Baraniuk, James N., and Dennis Shusterman, editors. *Nonallergic Rhinitis.* Informa Healthcare, 2007.

Busse, William W., and Stephen T. Holgate, editors. *Asthma and Rhinitis.* Wiley-Blackwell, 2000.

Carson-DeWitt, Rosalyn. "Allergic Rhinitis." *Health Library*, 31 Oct. 2012.

"Drugs for Allergic Rhinitis and Allergic Conjunctivitis." *Medical Letter on Drugs and Therapeutics*, vol. 63, no. 1622, 2021, pp. 57-64.

Dykewicz, Mark S., et al. "Rhinitis 2020: A Practice Parameter Update." *The Journal of Allergy and Clinical Immunology*, vol. 146, no. 4, 2020, pp. 721-67, doi:10.1016/j.jaci.2020.07.007.

Henochowicz, Stuart I. "Allergic Rhinitis." *MedlinePlus*, 17 Jun. 2012.

Henochowicz, Stuart I. "Vasomotor Rhinitis." *MedlinePlus*, 17 Jun. 2012.

Scadding, Glenis K., and Wytske J. Hokkens. *Rhinitis.* Health Press, 2007.

RHINOVIRUSES

Category: Diseases/Disorders
Anatomy or system affected: Cells, chest, lungs, nose, respiratory system, throat
Specialties and related fields: Biochemistry, biotechnology, cytology, epidemiology, genetics, histology, immunology, otorhinolaryngology, pathology, preventive medicine, public health, serology, virology
Definition: Disease-causing agents that are responsible for more common colds than any other respiratory virus.

Key terms

antigen: a proteinaceous, membrane-bound, cell surface component that stimulates the production of antibodies, which subsequently provoke an immune response

endothelial cell: cells that line blood and lymph vessels

Enterovirus: a genus of viruses similar to rhinoviruses

leukocyte: a white blood cell

picornavirus: the family of viruses that includes the *enterovirus* and *rhinovirus* genera

receptor: a membrane-bound protein that normally mediates interactions between the cell in which it is bound and specific, external signals, such as hormones

serotype: a group of viruses that can be characterized by common cell surface antigens

CAUSES AND SYMPTOMS
Rhinoviruses have been identified as the virus most often responsible for the common cold. Rhinoviruses have also been implicated in complications of asthma. Rhinoviruses are transmitted through sneezing and coughing, which expels droplets of moisture-laden with the virus. Once introduced into the respiratory system, the virus enters cells by interfacing with the intercellular adhesion molecule-1 (ICAM-1) receptor. As its name implies, ICAM-1 provides adhesion between endothelial cells and leukocytes after injury or stress. Still, it also facilitates the entry of rhinoviruses into cells, where they can replicate. The subsequent immune response is responsible for most of the symptoms of the common cold.

Colds occur more often in winter than in other seasons, although they can occur year-round. This seasonal effect is thought to result from an increase in time spent in closer contact with other people who may carry a rhinovirus.

> **INFORMATION ON RHINOVIRUSES**
>
> **Causes**: Transmitted through sneezing and coughing
>
> **Symptoms**: Sneezing, coughing, nasal and sinus drainage, congestion, fluid in the ears, headache, fever; in more severe cases, wheezing and pneumonia
>
> **Duration**: Approximately seven days for infection; two or more weeks for symptoms
>
> **Treatments**: Zinc lozenges, rest; preventive measures (handwashing with soap or antiseptic such as alcohol-based sanitizer, disinfection of surfaces commonly touched by people, covering coughs and sneezes with tissue or article of clothing)

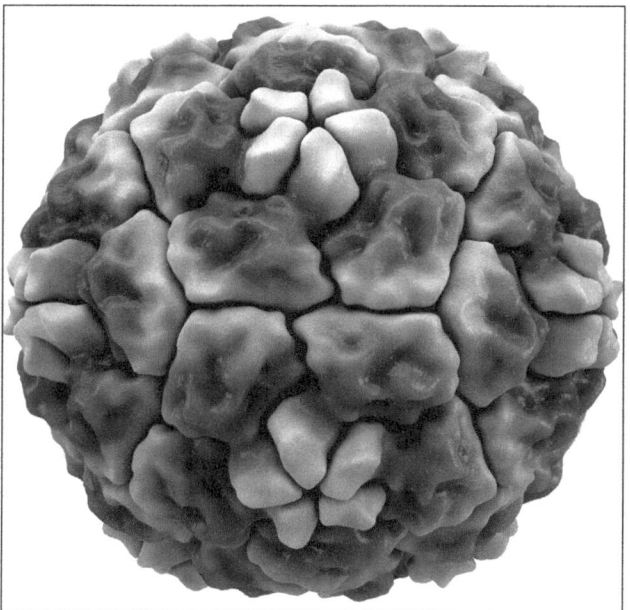

Isosurface of a human rhinovirus, showing protein spikes. Image by Thomas Splettstoesser, via Wikimedia Commons. [CC 4.0].

TREATMENT AND THERAPY
No cure exists for the treatment of rhinoviruses once contracted, and no vaccine exists to inoculate against infection with rhinoviruses. However, many strategies exist for reducing the transmission of viruses between infected individuals. Traditional home remedies such as chicken soup, bed rest, and drinking a lot of fluids may increase the comfort level of the sufferer. However, they do not shorten the course of the disease. Additionally, while vitamin C and echinacea may help reduce cold symptoms and the length of the cold, there has not been extensive evidence as to their helpfulness in preventing or getting rid of a cold. Antibiotics are not effective against rhinoviruses. Preventive measures are the best methods for reducing infection rates, including breastfeeding infants and frequent handwashing. Increased vitamin D levels may also be associated with a lowered risk of infection.

Studies conducted on zinc lozenges as a treatment for the common cold have produced mixed results. In test tubes, positively charged zinc inhibits the processing of viral proteins by several different mechanisms. One analysis of previous studies suggested that differences in the effectiveness of zinc lozenges could be explained by the ligand or ligands bound to the zinc. Zinc lozenges with only one ligand, such as zinc acetate or zinc gluconate lozenges, were more effective in reducing cold duration than zinc lozenges with more ligands though even they were not effective in all studies. The ineffectiveness of intranasal zinc application was hypothesized to result from an electrical potential difference of 60 to 120 millivolts between the nose and mouth, which results in the repulsion of charged particles such as ionized zinc.

There are ninety-nine known serotypes of rhinoviruses. This variety of cell surface antigens makes developing a vaccine that is effective against multiple rhinoviruses difficult. In the twenty-first century's first decade, virologists identified a region of the rhinoviral P4 protein that is very common between the different serotypes. Future efforts to synthesize a vaccine may focus on this common element.

PERSPECTIVE AND PROSPECTS

The common cold has been known for millennia and was first given this name in the sixteenth century. Evidence exists across cultures demonstrating knowledge of the cold, extending as back as far as ancient Egypt. In the eighteenth century, Benjamin Franklin's *Definition of a Cold* (1773) demonstrated insightful speculation about the airborne nature of cold transmission and suggested methods for preventing the disease.

The Rhinovirus was first isolated in 1956. During successive decades was identified as the virus best associated with the common cold. As technology improved, so did the detection and identification of different viruses responsible for the common cold. Simple culturing methods led to reverse transcriptase-polymerase chain reaction (RT-PCR) assays, which were more sensitive in detecting and characterizing specific rhinoviruses. In various campaigns to find a treatment for the common cold, antiviral drugs, and interferon effectively protect against rhinoviruses, attempts to translate these results into treatment have not been successful.

The Common Cold Research Unit (CCRU), initially established in Great Britain at the outset of World War II as the Harvard Hospital, operated from 1946 to 1989 and was devoted to researching the causes of the common cold as well as possible treatments for the disease. There, coronaviruses, which can also be responsible for causing the common cold, were first isolated in 1965.

—*Andrew J. Reinhart, MS*

Further Information
Carson-DeWitt, Rosalyn, and Brian Randall. "Common Cold." *Health Library*, 9 Jan. 2013.
"Common Cold." *MedlinePlus*, 23 Apr. 2013.
"Common Colds: Protect Yourself and Others." *Centers for Disease Control and Prevention*, 11 Mar. 2013.
Eccles, Ronald, and Olaf Weber, editors. *Common Cold: Birkhäuser Advances in Infectious Diseases*. Birkhäuser Basel, 2009.
"Rhinovirus Infections." *HealthyChildren.org*. American Academy of Pediatrics, 11 May 2013.
Tyrrell, David, and Michael Fielder. *Cold Wars: The Fight Against the Common Cold*. Oxford UP, 2002.
Yin-Murphy, Marguerite, and Jeffrey W. Almond. "Picornaviruses-Classification and Antigenic Types." *Medical Microbiology*, edited by Samuel Baron, U of Texas Medical Branch, 1996.

ROSEOLA

Category: Diseases/Disorders
Also known as: Roseola infantum, exanthem subitum, sixth disease
Anatomy or system affected: Abdomen, arms, brain, immune system, legs, skin
Specialties and related fields: Family medicine, pediatrics

Definition: A disease characterized by mild fever and a rash that mainly affects young children.

KEY TERMS

human herpesvirus-6 (HHV-6): human herpesvirus 6 (HHV-6) is a set of two closely related herpes viruses known as HHV-6A and HHV-6B. HHV-6B infects nearly 100% of human beings, typically before the age of three, and often results in fever, diarrhea, and sometimes with roseola.

lymph glands: a small bean-shaped structure that filters substances that travel through the lymphatic fluid; lymph glands contain lymphocytes (white blood cells) that help the body fight infection and disease

CAUSES AND SYMPTOMS

Roseola is caused by the human herpesvirus-6 (HHV-6), to which most children have been exposed by age four. Immunity passed from mother to fetus usually protects infants from contracting roseola before they are six months old. Although the precise period during which patients are contagious is unknown, health professionals have determined that the virus incubates for as many as ten days after exposure. Patients usually are contagious only during the fever phase of roseola.

A child with roseola develops a fever that can reach 106 degrees Fahrenheit and persist for two to five days. The lymph glands in the throat may become swollen, and upper respiratory congestion may

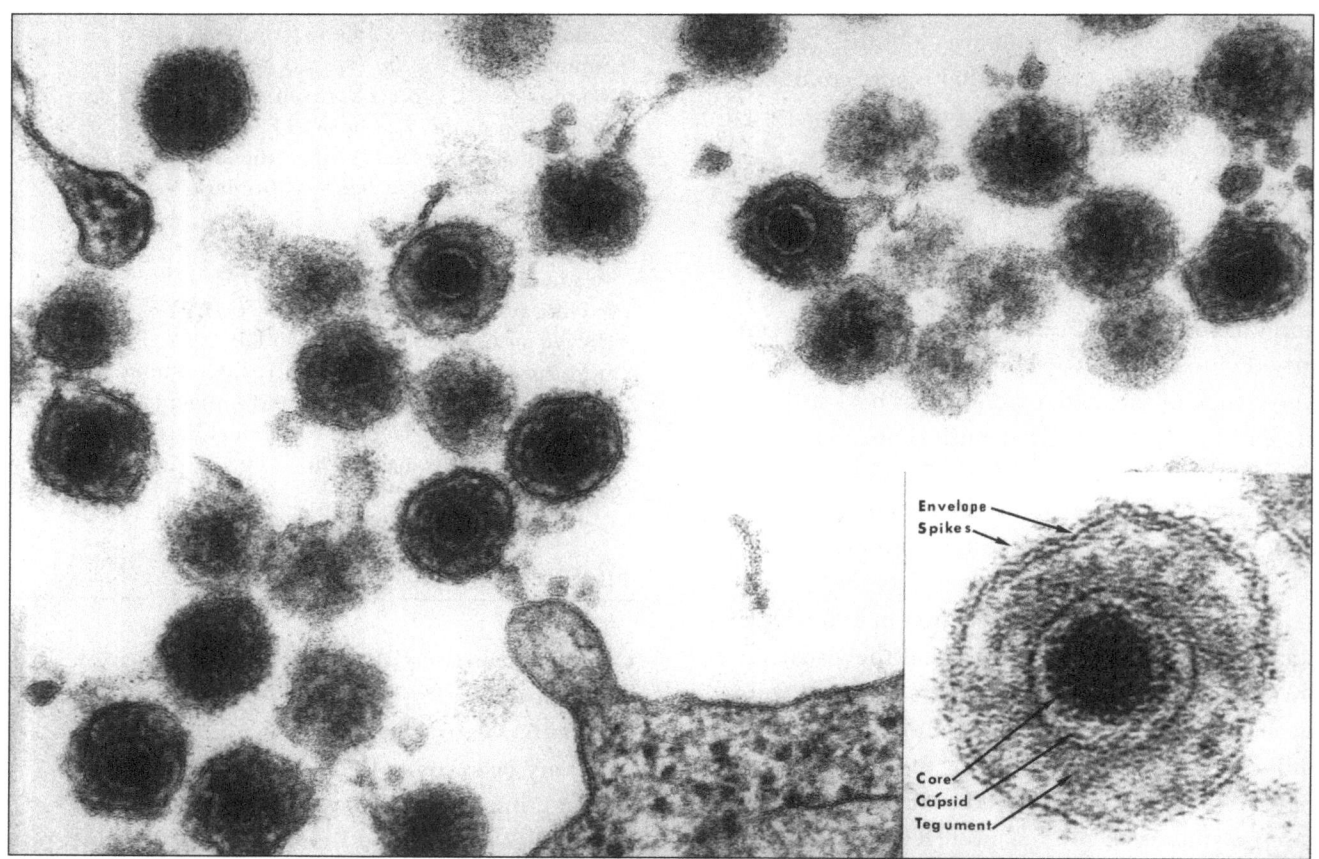

An electron micrograph of HHV-6, a double stranded DNA virus of the herpes family known to infect t-cells and is the cause of the childhood rash "roseola" and some cases of mononucleosis. Photo via Wikimedia Commons. [Public domain.]

occur. Some children appear agitated, while others do not behave in an ill manner and continue normal activities. Lethargy, lack of appetite, and diarrhea may accompany the fever. The fever occasionally causes febrile seizures as the brain reacts to sudden and extreme temperature changes. Approximately 5 to 15 percent of roseola patients experience these convulsions, which last several minutes and usually are not harmful.

When the fever ceases, a red or pink rash appears on most patients 'bodies and remains for several hours to three days. When pressed, the rash blanches. It does not blister, cause pain or itch. Occasionally, a roseola patient is feverish and never develops a rash or has a rash without a preceding fever. A rash may appear prematurely during the fever phase or be delayed until after the fever has subsided. Some children infected with roseola never display any symptoms. Rarely, roseola can precede encephalitis and aseptic meningitis.

TREATMENT AND THERAPY
In healthy children, roseola usually is a benign disease that resolves spontaneously and does not require specific therapy. Treatment for roseola consists of methods to soothe symptoms. Pediatricians recommend baths and acetaminophen, and ibuprofen if the child is old enough to lower the fever. Health professionals also advise patients to drink fluids to prevent dehydration. The patient should be isolated until the fever is gone.

A child who has convulsions should be examined by medical professionals immediately. Patients with dark purple rashes should also be seen by physicians, as should children whose rashes do not blanch when touched or remain more than several days. Blisters and itchy or painful rashes also demand professional attention. Children with roseola who seem unusually sick should also be examined, as should children with prolonged fevers that do not improve with medication and baths.

> **INFORMATION ON ROSEOLA**
>
> Causes: Herpesvirus infection
>
> Symptoms: Red or pink rash, high fever, swollen lymph nodes, lethargy, lack of appetite, diarrhea, sometimes febrile seizures
>
> Duration: A few weeks
>
> Treatments: Alleviation of symptoms; may include baths, acetaminophen, and ibuprofen, adequate fluid intake, the isolation during the fever stage

Most patients recover fully. Although the resulting antibodies are present in most adults, roseola can be reactivated if the immune system is weakened.

Treating roseola patients with antiviral drugs is necessary if the infection goes to the brain or heart. Such infections cause increased death rates. When necessary, the preferred antiviral medications for HHV-6 infections include ganciclovir, foscarnet, or cidofovir. Cidofovir damages the kidneys, and therefore, is the least preferred of these three drugs.

PERSPECTIVE AND PROSPECTS
Roseola has been referred to in medical literature since the mid-nineteenth century. Early twentieth-century investigators unsuccessfully attempted to identify the disease's pathogen. By 1988, medical professionals determined that the HHV-6 causes roseola. Two strains, A and B, have been identified, with strain B causing most roseola cases in children. The human herpesvirus-7 (HHV-7) has been linked to cases occurring in older patients.

—*Elizabeth D. Schafer, PhD*

Further Information
Gershon, Anne A., Samuel L. Katz, and Peter J. Hotez, editors. *Krugman's Infectious Diseases of Children*. 11th ed., Mosby, 2004.
Grossman, Leigh B., editor. *Infection Control in the Child Care Center and Preschool*. 8th ed., Silverchair Science, 2012.

Hoekelman, Robert A., editor. *Primary Pediatric Care.* 4th ed., Mosby, 2001.

Marks, Julie, "Roseola." *Health Library,* 30 Aug. 2018, www.healthline.com/health/roseola. Accessed 1 Sept. 2021.

Parker, James N., and Phillip M. Parker. *Roseola: A Medical Dictionary, Bibliography, and Annotated Research Guide to Internet References.* Icon Health, 2004.

"Roseola." *MedlinePlus,* 5 Aug. 2021, medlineplus.gov/ency/article/000968.htm. Accessed 1 Sept. 2021.

SHINGLES

Category: Diseases/Conditions
Anatomy or system affected: Peripheral nervous system, skin
Specialties and related fields: Dermatology, epidemiology, immunology, internal medicine, microbiology, neurology, oncology, ophthalmology, public health, virology
Also known as: Herpes zoster infection
Definition: A painful viral infection of the nerves and skin.

KEY TERMS

herpes zoster: chickenpox

postherpetic neuralgia: lasting pain after resolution of shingles in the same patches of the skin that formerly suffered from shingles

varicella-zoster virus (VZV): the virus that causes chickenpox or herpes zoster and shingles

CAUSES

Shingles is caused by the varicella-zoster virus (VZV), the same virus that leads to chickenpox. Shingles occurs in people who have had chickenpox. After causing the first chickenpox infection, the virus does not leave the body. Instead, it settles in nerve roots near the spinal cord. Once reactivated, the virus travels along nerve paths to the skin, where it causes shingles, manifested as pain and a rash.

RISK FACTORS

Only 20 percent of people who have had chickenpox eventually develop shingles, so researchers are trying to determine what makes some people more likely than others to develop the condition. Some of the factors that make people more likely to develop shingles include excessive emotional or physical stress and extreme fatigue. People with certain medical conditions, including a weakened immune system, are more likely to develop shingles. Conditions that increase the risk include a history of childhood cancer; current cancer, especially Hodgkin's disease, lymphoma, leukemia; and human immunodeficiency virus (HIV) infection or acquired immunodeficiency syndrome (AIDS). People older than sixty years of age are about three times more likely to develop shingles than are younger people, and Caucasians are four times more likely than African Americans to develop shingles.

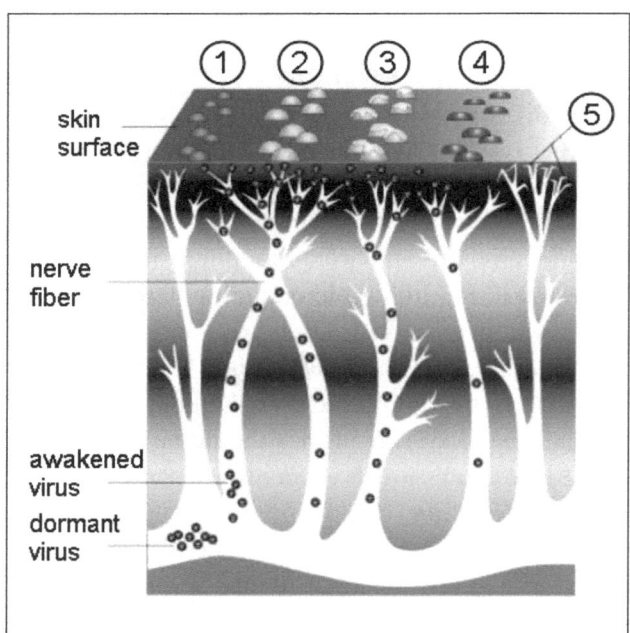

Progression of shingles. A cluster of small bumps (1) turns into blisters (2). The blisters fill with lymph, break open (3), crust over (4), and finally disappear. Postherpetic neuralgia can sometimes occur due to nerve damage (5). Image by Renee Gordon, via Wikimedia Commons. [Public domain.]

Certain medications or medical treatments increase the risk for shingles. Radiation therapy and immunosuppressant drugs (for organ transplants, cancer, and autoimmune diseases), chemotherapy, and immunosuppressive medications increase susceptibility for shingles. Other medications that increase the risk of shingles include cyclosporine, azathioprine, cyclophosphamide, chlorambucil, and cladribine.

SYMPTOMS
Shingles usually begins with an unpleasant itching, burning, tingling, or painful sensation in a band-like area of the skin. The skin rash of shingles begins to appear three to four days after noticing these sensations. The prodromal period is the time (about three to four days) before the rash occurs. During this time, one might have the following symptoms: fever, muscle aches, fatigue, anxiety, nervousness, and discomfort in the skin, usually on one side of the face, torso, trunk, back, or buttocks. This discomfort feels like numbness, itching, burning, stinging, tingling, shooting pain, electric shock, or sharp pain. Another symptom is extreme sensitivity to even light touch.

Active shingles begins when the patient notices the rash in the same place where they felt the original skin sensations. The rash begins as a reddish band or individual bumps running in a line. The bumps develop fluid-filled centers. Within seven to ten days, the bumps start to dry and crust over. Pain or itching, or both, in the area of the rash, may begin, and the pain may be severe. Suppose the rash develops on the side of the nose or elsewhere on the face. In that case, the eye is affected, and you should contact a doctor immediately.

About 20 to 30 percent of patients =60 years old who have had a bout of shingles develop a condition called "postherpetic neuralgia" (PHN). PHN is a lasting pain in those areas of the skin where the patient had shingles. It results from nerve damage caused by VZV, and the pain can last for months to years after the resolution of shingles. The pain associated with PHN can be severe and debilitating.

SCREENING AND DIAGNOSIS
Screening tests are usually administered to people without current symptoms but at high risk for certain diseases or conditions. However, there are no screening tests or screening guidelines for the early detection of shingles.

Generally, the characteristic discomfort, pain, and distinctive rash make shingles easily diagnosable. A doctor may scrape some skin from a blister or collect some of its fluid to confirm that one has shingles. The physician sends these samples to a laboratory for testing. The tests can detect the presence of the varicella-zoster virus. These tests include microscopic examination, viral culture, immunofluorescence, and polymerase chain reaction techniques. It may take several weeks to obtain test results.

TREATMENT AND THERAPY
There are no treatments to cure shingles. Treatments involve lifestyle changes, medications, and alternative and complementary therapies to lessen symptoms. Treatment attempts to shorten the length of the illness; prevent shingles by getting the shingles vaccine; prevent complications, such as PHN; relieve and reduce pain and discomfort, and prevent the rash from becoming infected. There are no surgical procedures for the treatment of shingles.

Itching and pain may be relieved with calamine lotion, wet compresses, frequent oatmeal baths, over-the-counter pain relievers (such as acetaminophen, ibuprofen, and naproxen); and capsaicin, a topical substance that comes from hot peppers. The doctor may prescribe drugs to relieve pain that does not respond to over-the-counter remedies.

Certain antiviral medications may control shingles by changing how the virus reproduces in nerve cells.

These medications include acyclovir (Zovirax), famciclovir (Famvir), and valacyclovir (Valtrex). Antiviral therapy may shorten a shingles episode, but patients must being treatment within forty-eight to seventy-two hours of the first development of symptoms. These medications can also reduce the severity and duration of PHN and are recommended for patients with the highest risk for this condition (persons older than age fifty-five years). Taking antiviral medications before PHN develops is the most effective way to reduce its severity. The doctor may also prescribe a short course of oral steroid medication (such as prednisone) if the patient's immune system is functioning normally.

Food and Drug Administration (FDA)-approved treatments for treating the pain associated with PHN include gabapentin (*Neurontin*, and others), pregabalin *(Lyrica)*, a 5 percent lidocaine patch, and an eight percent capsaicin patch *(Qutenza)* are FDA-approved for the treatment of pain associated with PHN. In 2019, the FDA approved a 1.8 percent lidocaine patch *(ZTlido)* to treat PHN pain. ZTlido works just as well as 5 percent lidocaine (Lidoderm and generics). Second-line treatments include tricyclic antidepressants, such as amitriptyline and nortriptyline, but if these drugs are used off-label. Opioid analgesics are effective for moderate to severe pain associated with PHN. Transcutaneous electrical nerve stimulation or transcutaneous electrical nerve stimulation (TENS) machines, a device that generates low-level pulses of electrical current on the skin's surface, can mitigate PHN pain. Nerve blocks are injections near nerves that provide temporary pain relief and are a last resort.

PREVENTION AND OUTCOMES
There is no proven way to prevent shingles. Stress and fatigue may contribute to an outbreak. Future cases of shingles should decrease as more children are vaccinated against chickenpox.

Zostavax, a live-attenuated VZV vaccine, was FDA-approved by the U.S. Food and Drug Administration to prevent shingles in those aged sixty years and older. Unfortunately, it was withdrawn from the market in 2020. *Shingrix*, an adjuvanted, recombinant vaccine, was licensed for herpes zoster prevention in adults ≥50 years old in 2017. The adverse effects of Shingrix included muscle aches, fatigue, headache, shivering, fever, upset stomach, and local injection-site pain, redness, and swelling. In 2021, the FDA approved Shingrix for adults of any age who have disease- or therapy-induced immunodeficiency or immunosuppression.

—*Rosalyn Carson-DeWitt and Michael A. Buratovich, PhD*

Further Information

Bennett, John F., Raphael Dolin, and Martin J., editors. *Mandell, Douglas, and Bennett's Principles and Practice of Infectious Diseases*. 9th ed., Churchill Livingstone/Elsevier, 2019. This book has a chapter that discusses the virus that causes chickenpox and shingles.

Mounsey, Anne L., Leah G. Matthew, and David C. Slawson. "Herpes Zoster and Postherpetic Neuralgia: Prevention and Management." *American Family Physician*, vol. 72, 2005, pp. 1075-80. A clinical guide to preventing and treating shingles and postherpetic neuralgia.

"Shingrix—An Adjuvanted, Recombinant Herpes Zoster Vaccine." *Medical Letter on Drugs and Therapeutics*, vol. 59, no. 1535, 2017, pp. 195-96.

Tyring, S. K. "Management of Herpes Zoster and Postherpetic Neuralgia." *Journal of the American Academy of Dermatology*, vol. 57, no. 6, suppl., 2007, pp. S136-S142. Preventing and treating shingles and postherpetic neuralgia from the perspective of dermatology.

Weaver, Bethany A. "Herpes Zoster Overview: Natural History and Incidence." *Journal of the American Osteopathic Association*, vol. 109, 2009, pp. S2-S6. An overview of herpes zoster, or shingles.

Sinusitis

Category: Diseases/Disorders
Anatomy or system affected: Nose, respiratory system
Specialties and related fields: Family medicine, internal medicine, otorhinolaryngology
Definition: Irritation and swelling of the sinuses.

KEY TERMS

deviated septum: a condition that causes a shift of the bones and cartilage from the middle of the nose to either side, making one side of the nasal passages much smaller than the other

nasal polyps: noncancerous growths inside the nose; usually associated with allergies or asthma, which can block the sinus drainage tract

orbit: the bones and other tissues that surround the eye, commonly known as the eye socket

CAUSES AND SYMPTOMS

The sinuses are airspaces in the skull's forehead just above the eyes, on either side of the nose below the eyes, and in the area just above the nose and in between the eyes. Mucus and tiny hairs, called "cilia," line the sinuses. Cilia trap inhaled particles and bacteria and move them back out through the nose, eliminating these potential irritants inhaled during normal breathing. The tracts through which the sinuses drain are relatively small and easily blocked by swelling of the area. Sinus blockage impairs drainage and cause the buildup of normal sinus secretions.

The term "sinusitis" refers to irritation or swelling of the sinuses and their membranes. Typical symptoms may include a feeling of congestion or pressure in the nose or face and a runny nose with secretions that may vary in color from clear to yellowish-green to bloody. The facial pressure is often worse when bending forward.

> **INFORMATION ON SINUSITIS**
>
> **Causes**: Common cold; allergies; environmental exposure to smoke or air pollution; blockage from nasal polyps, deviated septum, or pregnancy
>
> **Symptoms**: Irritation or swelling of sinuses, congestion or pressure in nose or face, runny nose with secretions varying from clear to yellowish-green to bloody, decreased sense of smell, productive cough, fever, tooth pain, bad breath
>
> **Duration**: Acute
>
> **Treatments**: Increased fluid intake, antihistamines, anti-inflammatory drugs, decongestants, humidified air, nasal irrigation, oral or nasal allergy medications, antibiotics if needed

Most often, sinusitis is precipitated by the common cold. Another frequent cause is allergies, with typical symptoms of sneezing, runny nose, and itchy, watery eyes. An allergic patient sensitive to a particular airborne substance (pollen, ragweed, dust, animal dander) has a particularly vigorous response when these particles land in the nose and enter the sinuses. Increased production of mucus and the body's natural immune defenses combine to produce thick and copious nasal secretions that can fill the sinuses in an attempt to eliminate the offending agent.

Another factor predisposing a patient to sinusitis is environmental exposure to smoke or air pollution that irritates the sinuses. Problems that cause a blockage of the sinus drainage system, including nasal polyps, a deviated septum, or pregnancy (which leads to swelling of the nasal membranes due to hormonal changes), can interfere with mucus drainage from the sinuses. Finally, other genetic diseases such as cystic fibrosis or immune system disorders can predispose patients to sinusitis.

Although viruses or allergies cause most cases of sinusitis, these can often lead to infection by bacteria if they do not resolve promptly. Bacterial sinusitis requires treatment with antibiotics to avoid the rare but severe complications of infection of the orbit or the brain and its surrounding tissues.

The distinction between bacterial and other causes of sinusitis depends on the patient's symptoms and a physical examination. A patient is more likely to have bacterial sinusitis if two or three of the following symptoms are present for at least seven days: facial pressure, nasal congestion, discolored nasal mucus, decreased sense of smell, productive or "wet" cough, fever, tooth pain on the upper jaw, or bad breath.

Sinus X-rays, done frequently in the past, are not considered a reliable diagnostic test for sinusitis. Though sinus computed tomography (CT) scans allow detailed visualization of sinus anatomy, they do not reliably distinguish bacterial sinusitis from other forms. They are helpful only in cases of long-standing, refractory symptoms for which sinus surgery is considered.

TREATMENT AND THERAPY
The initial sinusitis treatment involves extra fluids, anti-inflammatory drugs such as ibuprofen, antihistamines, short-term use of nasal decongestant sprays (no longer than three days), and oral decongestants such as pseudoephedrine. Humidified air (e.g., steam from a hot shower) and nasal irrigation with water or saline can offer short-term symptom relief.

If allergies are the cause of sinusitis, then oral or nasal allergy medications are appropriate. Examples are nonprescription antihistamines such as chlorpheniramine, brompheniramine, or diphenhydramine; they can cause drowsiness in some patients. Loratadine, fexofenadine and cetirizine, and other related, newer generation antihistamines are also available over the counter. They offer once-daily dosing and are significantly less sedating. Other nasal sprays such as topical steroids are available by prescription and provide significant relief.

Most sinusitis cases result from viral infections that do not require antibiotics. Symptomatic treatments include saline nasal washes, intranasal corticosteroids, and over-the-counter analgesics (e.g., acetaminophen, ibuprofen, aspirin, etc.). Nasal decongestants may help viral sinusitis cases, but there is no credible evidence that decongestants help with bacterial sinusitis infections.

If symptoms persist longer than ten days, then antibiotic therapy may be necessary, and a health-care provider evaluation is warranted. Other indications that antibiotics are warranted include the presence of pus-filled nasal discharge, facial pain for three to four days, or if symptoms improve after an upper respiratory viral infection and then become worse five to six days later. Many different types of antibiotics are effective for sinusitis, and prescription practices vary. Acute sinusitis treatment also differs from chronic sinusitis treatments. For mild to moderate acute sinusitis, the standard treatment is *Augmentin* twice a day for fourteen days. The alternative treatment is doxycycline, twice a day, for seven days. If these initial treatments fail, then the patient is given one of three options: (1) high-dose *Augmentin* (2 grams) twice a day for fourteen days; (2) levofloxacin daily for seven days, or (3) moxifloxacin once daily for seven days. These treatment regimens are for

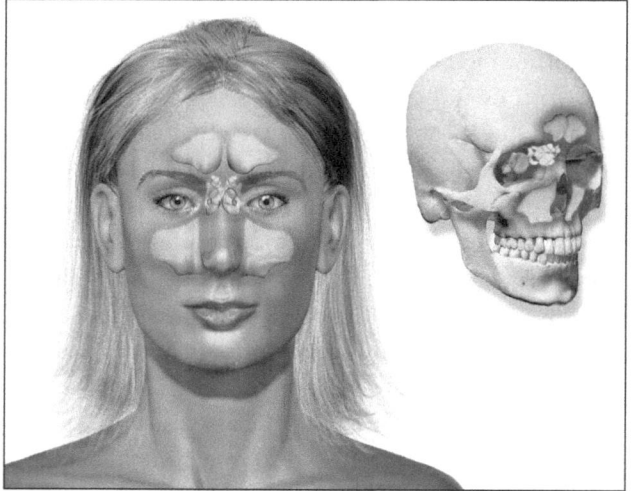

Illustration depicting sinusitis. Image by Bruce Blaus, via Wikimedia Commons. [CC 3.0.]

> **IN THE NEWS:**
> **BALLON SINUPLASTY**
>
> In late 2005, the Acclarent Company received permission from the Food and Drug Administration (FDA) to market a device to clear blocked sinuses similar to that used to clear blocked arteries in the heart. A flexible catheter tube inserted into the nostril guides a balloon into the targeted sinus. The balloon is inflated, spreading the bones of the passageway sufficiently to permit accumulated mucus or pus to drain. A minimally invasive outpatient procedure, balloon sinuplasty, is performed under local anesthesia and takes one to two hours. Patients report little or no pain and can often return to regular activity within twenty-four hours. The sinuplasty devices cost from $1,200 to $1,500 and are not reusable. Total costs for the procedure run from $4,000 to $6,800; some private insurance plans cover the procedure.
>
> If the patient has nasal polyps, the surgeon must remove them before they have balloon sinuplasty. Nevertheless, it provides a possible alternative for sinusitis sufferers who do not need or prefer not to undergo surgical procedures involving cutting away bone or other tissue to open the blocked sinus. Surgeons using the devices praised them. The American Rhinologic Society was more cautious in its October 2006 position statement, asserting that the technology had limited indication at the time. In November 2006, the California Blue Cross labeled the procedure investigational and not medically necessary. Since the FDA's clearance was based on the devices' comparability to already approved methods, it did not require safety or effectiveness data submission. The most extensive 2006 clinical trial, which claimed that the procedure was safe and effective, followed 109 patients over twenty-four weeks. Longer-term efficacy remains unknown.
>
> —*Milton Berman, PhD*

outpatient cases. If the patient suffers from severe sinusitis that requires hospitalization, then they are administered intravenous antibiotics.

PERSPECTIVE AND PROSPECTS

Before the antibiotic era, sinusitis treatment involved drainage of the sinuses by extracting a tooth, puncturing the roof of the mouth, or entering the nose and creating a drainage tract to drain the sinuses and subsequently irrigate them with fluid for cleansing. Given the invasiveness of these procedures, they have become uncommon with the development of effective antibiotic therapy.

The development of tiny, high-resolution cameras known as "endoscopes" in the 1950s created a revolution in the understanding of sinus disease. Direct visualization of the nasal passages and sinus drainage tracts allowed a better understanding of the sinus anatomy. It thus led to the use of this equipment to facilitate surgical treatment.

Occasionally, patients with recurrent symptoms require surgical removal of infected sinus tissue and enlargement of the natural drainage tracts to minimize sinus obstruction. A specialist in otorhinolaryngology can perform such surgery using an endoscope without the need for general anesthesia. Patients do not typically require hospitalization, and complications are rare.

—*Gregory B. Seymann, MD and*
Michael A. Buratovich, PhD

Further Information

"Acute Sinusitis." *Mayo Clinic*, 27 Aug. 2021, www.mayoclinic.org/diseases-conditions/acute-sinusitis/symptoms-causes/syc-20351671. Accessed 27 Aug. 2021.

Beers, Mark H., et al., editors. *The Merck Manual of Diagnosis and Therapy.* 18th ed., Merck Research Laboratories, 2006.

Brook, Itzhak, editor. *Sinusitis: From Microbiology to Management.* Taylor & Francis, 2006.

Kennedy, David W., and Marilyn Olsen. *Living with Chronic Sinusitis: A Patient's Guide to Sinusitis, Nasal Allergies, Polyps, and Their Treatment Options.* Hatherleigh Press, 2007.

McCaffrey, Thomas. "Functional Endoscopic Sinus Surgery: An Overview." *Mayo Clinic Proceedings*, vol. 68, 1993, pp. 571-77.

Mickelson, Samuel, and Michael Benninger. "The Nose and Paranasal Sinuses." *Textbook of Primary Care Medicine*, edited by John Noble, 3rd ed., Mosby, 2001.

"Sinus Infection (Sinusitis)." *Cleveland Clinic*, 6 Apr. 2020, my.clevelandclinic.org/health/diseases/17701-sinusitis. Accessed 28 Aug. 2021.

Younis, Ramzi T., editor. *Pediatric Sinusitis and Sinus Surgery.* Taylor & Francis, 2006.

SKIN DISORDERS

Category: Diseases/Disorders
Anatomy or system affected: Skin
Specialties and related fields: Dermatology, family medicine, occupational health
Definition: Diseases and conditions that affect the skin, ranging from harmless to life-threatening.

KEY TERMS

benign: in reference to a neoplasm, having a nonmalignant character

dermatology: the study of the skin, its chemistry, physiology, histopathology, cutaneous lesions, and the relationships of these lesions to systemic disease

malignant: in reference to a neoplasm, having the property of uncontrollable growth and dissemination, recurrence after removal, or both

melanin: dark brown or black molecules of pigment that generally occur in the skin, hair, pigmented coat of the retina, and pupil of the eye, and selected cells of the brain

metastasis: the shifting of a disease, or its local manifestations, from one portion of the body to another; in cancer, the appearance of neoplasms in parts of the body remote from the primary tumor

ANATOMY OF THE SKIN

The skin is the largest organ of the body. It provides a barrier between the external and internal worlds: It protects against external contamination and helps maintain the inner body's sterility. The skin also assists in temperature regulation; humans can survive only within a narrow temperature range. The skin has nerve receptors that supply the brain with information, providing an interface with the world. There are specialized receptors for touch, temperature, vibration, and position in space (proprioception).

Appendages to the skin are fingernails, toenails, and hair. They are mainly of psychological importance. Nails protect the tips of fingers and toes in humans but are not needed for protection as claws are in lower animals. Hair is analogous to feathers. In birds, tiny muscles attached to the base of each feather cause them to ruffle; this creates air pockets and allows birds to conserve heat and keep warm. The same muscles persist in humans, causing "goose flesh," but they do not serve any other function. The primary importance of these appendages is cosmetic. For example, people spend billions of dollars on hair care products each year. The motivation for this activity is psychological.

The two main layers in the skin are the epidermis and dermis. The epidermis is the upper or outermost layer, and cells are continually formed at its base. As new cells form, they push existing cells toward the surface of the skin. These cells gradually lose their watery central contents, causing them to dry out (desiccate) and become flattened. This process typically spans approximately a month. Thus, the surface of the body is composed mainly of dead cells that have become flattened. These cells usually are lost continually and create dandruff when shed from the scalp. Sloughed cells provide excellent conditions for bacterial growth on other body parts, accounting for the unpleasant odors that accompany poor hygiene habits.

Two other important types of cells are in the epidermis: melanocytes and Langerhans cells. Melanocytes contain melanin and provide all the variations of pigmentation found in the human species. They multiply when stimulated by the ultraviolet radiation in sunlight. Melanocyte proliferation causes the skin to become darker, a protective mechanism against damage from ultraviolet radiation. Langerhans cells contain surface receptors for immunoglobulins. They play a central role in skin allergic reactions, such as contact dermatitis or delayed hypersensitivity reactions.

The dermis is an inner layer of skin located beneath the epidermis. Its principal function is protection. Within the dermis are highly specialized cells containing microscopic filaments. These cells impart tensile strength to the skin in the same way fibers strengthen fiberglass or reinforcing steel mesh strengthen concrete. Because they are so dense, they also serve as a barrier to most pathogens and many chemicals. Eccrine sweat glands are in the dermis throughout the entire body. These produce a salty secretion (essentially saltwater) that assists in thermoregulation through evaporative cooling. They are also sensitive to emotional stress. Apocrine sweat glands are primarily in the armpits (axilla) and groin and produce a milky secretion. When bacteria break down these secretions on the skin's surface, they produce a characteristic odor. The bases of hair follicles are also in the dermis. The small sebaceous, or oil-secreting, gland associated with most hair follicles soften and moisturize the hair.

Hair covers most surfaces of the body; exceptions are the palms of the hands, the soles of the feet, and the glans penis in men. The texture and length of the hair vary with location on the body, gender, genetic heritage, and age. Dramatic increases in the growth and distribution of hair occur at puberty. With increasing age, hair typically thins from the scalp and other body parts. It also changes color, assuming a gray or white color because of the loss of melanin at the base of the hair follicle.

COMPLICATIONS AND DISORDERS

When normal skin anatomy and physiology are upset, several common diseases or disorders result. When breaks occur in the skin, bacteria, viruses, fungi, and other pathogens can invade the body, leading to infections. Locally, these infections can cause inflammation (redness and pain) of the skin; if widespread, they can lead to systemic infections. When the cells and other substances found in the skin become irregular or are abnormal, skin disorders or conditions result.

Skin disorders and conditions. Pigmentation of the skin results from the presence of melanocytes, cells that manufacture and contain melanin. Most humans have pigmentation over their entire bodies; the degree of pigmentation varies with different racial and ethnic groups. Local areas of increased color have a range of names depending on the size of the pigmented area. A freckle is small and discrete. A nevus is a larger area of hyperpigmentation. These conditions are attributable to underlying variations in the distribution of melanocytes. They are genetic in origin and permanent; sunlight exposure tends to accentuate them. Melasmas are irregular, flat, light brown areas on the neck, cheeks, or forehead. They are caused by hormonal changes associated with pregnancy or contraceptive pills and by exposure to sunlight. Melasmas fade with the reduction of excess hormones. There are also color changes in the labia of females during pregnancy; these changes are both harmless and permanent.

Generalized increases in skin coloration can occur with some metabolic diseases. Addison's disease involves an increase in melanocyte-stimulating hormone (MSH). Increased MSH levels lead to an overall bronzing of the body, with accentuation increases of the palms and soles. The condition subsides with the treatment of the underlying cause of the disease. Similar pigment increases are associated with some forms of lung cancer, hemochromatosis, and chronic arsenic exposure. The latter two conditions result from the deposition of iron (hemochromatosis) and arsenic in the skin.

Generalized decreases in skin coloration can also occur. Suppose melanocytes fail to migrate to the skin during embryologic development. In that case, hair follicles will lack color, resulting in a condition called "piebaldism." Characteristically, this is a white patch in the hair of the forehead. An immunologically mediated loss of melanocytes causes vitiligo. If not adequately and promptly treated, individuals with phenylketonuria (PKU) experience a generalized depigmentation of hair and eye color, in addition to mental retardation. An albino lacks melanocytes; because melanin is also responsible for eye color, albinos have red eyes. The loss of hair is called "alopecia." It can occur because of aging, sustained pulling on the hair with some hairstyles, and genetics. Women do not usually experience much alopecia until after menopause. Conversely, some men start to lose their hair during their twenties.

Skin diseases. "Eczema" or "dermatitis" is a general term that describes a skin disease involving vesicles that ooze fluid. A rash usually characterizes these conditions; they are inflammatory reactions commonly caused by chemical or plant material contact. They can be caused by an adverse reaction to a drug or by sunlight. Bacteria, yeasts, or other fungi on the skin can cause eczema. Most rashes itch or burn; scratching can spread them. Athlete's foot is a typical example of eczematous dermatitis.

Maculopapular diseases encompass several common skin conditions, such as red measles (rubeola), German measles (rubella), and scarlet fever. Viruses that land on the skin cause these diseases. They are characterized by relatively large, localized areas of changed skin color (macules) that are also raised (papules) but not fluid-filled. After they run their clinical course, they disappear without leaving a scar. The more dangerous toxic shock syndrome also belongs to this group of diseases caused by a toxin from the bacteria *Staphylococcus aureus*.

Thickening of the skin and forming red to purple areas with sharply defined borders characterize papulosquamous skin diseases. The most common example is psoriasis. Other examples are pityriasis and ichthyosis. The pathology responsible for psoriasis is an alteration in the normal development of skin cells. In individuals with psoriasis, new skin cells develop and migrate to the surface in only five days instead of the usual thirty. This fact alone explains the flaking (rapid cell turnover), redness (thinner skin and a rich blood supply for new skin), and pain and itching (less protection for sensory nerve endings) experienced. Pityriasis includes a group of different conditions caused by other viruses. Patches or large spots develop on the skin. They usually resolve within a few weeks. Aside from being locally photosensitive, they typically are not serious. Ichthyosis describes a group of genetic conditions characterized by extreme scaling of the skin.

> **INFORMATION ON SKIN DISORDERS**
>
> **Causes**: Infection, disease, allergies, environmental factors (e.g., ultraviolet radiation), hormonal changes, irritation, clogged sweat glands, eczema
>
> **Symptoms**: May include inflammation, infection, flaking, pain, itching, redness, rashes, lesions, bleeding
>
> **Duration**: Acute to chronic
>
> **Treatments**: Topical ointments, antibiotics, corticosteroids, surgery, chemotherapy, radiation therapy

Vesiculobullous diseases have fluid-filled blisters that can vary in size from relatively minor (vesicles) to relatively large (bullae). Insect bites, herpes, and some bacterial infections lead to the formation of vesicles or bullae. Such conditions are attributable to an immune reaction that leads to blisters at the junction between the epidermis and dermis. They can be accompanied by intense pruritus (itching); scratching often leads to scarring.

Pustular diseases of the skin include acne, folliculitis, and candidiasis. They are characterized by the inflammation of hair follicles caused by surface bacteria or yeasts. Adequate personal hygiene is the most effective method of prevention. These diseases are usually not serious, but prolonged or repeated attacks can result in scarring and disfigurement. The sebaceous glands, which secrete oil at the base of hair follicles, can increase in size. The subsequent increase in oil output worsens the condition.

Clogged sweat glands can lead to acne. While this is primarily a problem for teenagers, it can affect individuals of any age. Exposure to cutting oils and other hydrocarbons such as gasoline and paint thinners can cause a similar condition called "chloracne." Chloracne is characterized by inflammation in the base of hair follicles found on exposed skin in areas such as the nape of the neck, forearms, and face. The inability to sense temperature and regulate body heat through sweating is called "anhidrosis." This condition can cause shock and potentially death.

Other diseases can affect the skin. Five such diseases are mentioned: leprosy, scleroderma, lupus, atherosclerosis, and diabetes mellitus. Leprosy, or Hansen's disease, is caused by *Mycobacterium leprae*, a relative of the bacteria that cause tuberculosis. In leprosy, the causative organism accumulates in the skin and peripheral nerves. The lepromatous disease causes disfigurement and loss of sensation, the latter being similar to that experienced by an uncontrolled diabetic. Disfigurement is responsible for the stigma associated with leprosy since ancient times: loss of fingers and toes and mutilation of the nose and ears. Leprosy is caused by long-term association with the organism and can be adequately treated with appropriate antibiotics.

Scleroderma (literally, "hard skin") is an uncommon disease characterized by fibrosis of the skin and involvement of visceral organs. The skin involvement can range from an isolated, hardened patch to a life-threatening, generalized condition described as an ever-tightening case of steel. The skin becomes stretched tightly over the underlying skeleton. Skin tone is lost with restriction of movement.

Systemic lupus erythematosus is a disease of unknown etiology characterized by inflammation in many different organ systems. The skin is usually involved, as nearly all individuals with lupus develop a characteristic butterfly-shaped rash on their faces. This red coloration covers the cheeks and nose. Persons with lupus are also sensitive to sunlight, and many develop alopecia. Most of those affected are female. The disease waxes and wanes; treatment depends on the particular organs involved.

Atherosclerosis and diabetes can block the arteries supplying the skin's nerves, leading to a loss of sensory input. When the patient cannot experience pain, cuts and other abrasions on the skin go unnoticed. Untreated, these lesions can lead to gangrene, sometimes requiring amputation of a body part.

Skin cancer. The most commonly diagnosed form of cancer is that involving the skin. It is not the most fatal form, but millions of cases are discovered annually. The origin of most skin cancers can be traced to excessive exposure to radiation from the sun. They can occur on any surface of the body, although they are more common in areas usually exposed to the sun, such as the face, the backs of the hand, and the neck. Skin cancers can arise in the epidermis or dermis. The majority are noncancerous or benign. Epidermal nodules are characterized by local thickening of the epidermis, often accompanied by scaling of the skin in the affected area. Nodules in the dermis may appear as lumps with no alteration of the epidermis above them.

There are three malignant forms of skin cancer. Basal cell carcinoma arises from cells deep in the epidermis. This form of tumor rarely spreads (metastasizes), but it can be extensive and destructive locally. Squamous cell carcinoma is less common but can be invasive (involving adjacent tissues) and can metastasize. Melanoma is relatively uncommon but can grow exceptionally rapidly; it can be fatal in a matter of months. It involves the uncontrolled growth of melanocytes. Melanomas have irregular borders and color or pigmentation. Any pigmented lesion or suspicious change in the skin should be evaluated by a medical professional promptly.

Prevention is the preferred method of dealing with skin cancer. When outside, loose-fitting clothing can protect from the sun, and a hat can protect the head. When exposure is unavoidable, a product with a sun-blocking agent will reduce exposure. Limiting exposure to the sun until the body has reacted by producing additional melanocytes (tanned) is recommended.

Prolonged exposure to the sun also accelerates changes in the skin associated with aging. Collagen fibers provide the characteristic firm feel to the skin of a young person. With aging, the skin becomes less firm, losing its tone, and begins to sag. Inadequate moisture also contributes to the loss of skin tone. Excessive exposure to the sun hastens both of these processes.

—*L. Fleming Fallon Jr., MD, PhD, MPH*

Further Information

Barker, Jonathan, et al., editors. *Rook's Textbook of Dermatology*. 9th ed., Wiley-Blackwell, 2016. This is a core text in dermatology that will appeal to professionals and members of the general public who want a concise introduction to the subject. The book aims to integrate basic science with clinical practice.

Frankel, David H., editor. *Field Guide to Clinical Dermatology*. 2nd ed., Lippincott Williams & Wilkins, 2006. Frankel, a noted internist, and dermatologist has enlisted widely respected and talented colleagues to help produce this book. It is a uniquely organized and easily readable field guide complete with 220 pages of excellent color illustrations.

Freinkel, Ruth K., and David T. Woodley, editors. *Biology of the Skin*. Parthenon, 2001. Covers the basic biology of the skin, how the skin functions, effects of the environment, the molecules that direct cutaneous function, genetic influences, and methods in cutaneous research.

Goldsmith, Lowell A., Gerald S. Lazarus, and Michael D. Tharp. *Adult and Pediatric Dermatology: A Color Guide to Diagnosis and Treatment*. F. A. Davis, 1997. This book provides excellent pictures to accompany good descriptions of dermatologic diseases.

Grob, J. J., et al., editors. *Epidemiology, Causes, and Prevention of Skin Diseases*. Blackwell Science, 1997. This well-written book presents data on large groups of people. The sections on skin cancer are especially noteworthy.

Mueller, Heidi, editor. *Principles and Practice of Dermatology*. Foster Academics, 2016. An interesting compendium of medical knowledge about the skin, its care, and the pathology of skin diseases.

Weedon, David. *Skin Pathology*. 3rd ed., Churchill Livingstone/Elsevier, 2010. Text with extensive photographs, covering tissue reaction patterns; the epidermis, dermis, and subcutis; the skin in systemic and miscellaneous diseases; infections and infestations; and tumors, among other topics.

Medications

Divided into two parts, this section discusses common prescription medications and alternative therapies designed to either strengthen the immune system in the case of immunodeficient conditions, or suppress the immune system in the case of an autoimmune condition. The sixteen essays in this section cover familiar medications like antihistamines, corticosteroids, and antiviral drugs as well as biological therapy (treatment that uses living organisms to fight disease) and immunotheraphy (stimulating the immune system by gradually increasing doses of an allergic substance). This section also covers natural treatments for allergies, asthma, lupus, and rheumatoid arthritis.

Prescription Medications
Anti-inflammatory drugs 409
Antihistamines 414
Antiviral drugs: Mechanisms of action 418
Antiviral drugs: Types 422
Biological therapies 426
Corticosteroids 433
Decongestants 438
Immunotherapy 440
Sublingual immunotherapy 447
Theophylline 450

Natural Products, Herbal Supplements, and Other Alternatives
Idiopathic environmental intolerances 455
Immune support 458
Natural treatments for allergies 460
Natural treatments for asthma 464
Natural treatments for lupus 470
Natural treatments for rheumatoid arthritis 472

Prescription Medications

Anti-inflammatory drugs

Category: Treatment
Anatomy or system affected: All
Specialties and related fields: Dermatology, endocrinology, family medicine, internal medicine, ophthalmology, orthopedics, otorhinolaryngology, rheumatology, vascular medicine.
Definition: Medicines used to relieve inflammation, pain, redness, and swelling; generally grouped into two categories: nonsteroidal anti-inflammatory drugs (NSAIDs) and corticosteroids (steroid hormones that have anti-inflammatory effects).

KEY TERMS

arthritis: a painful condition that involves inflammation of one or more joints

bursitis: inflammation of the sac of lubricating fluid located between joints

hormone: a substance made by the body that travels through the bloodstream to reach its target organ and have its effect

inflammation: the body's response to injury that may include redness, pain, swelling, and warmth in the affected area

salicylates: a group of drugs (including aspirin) derived from salicylic acid, used to relieve pain, reduce inflammation, and lower fever

steroids: a class of hormones produced by the adrenal glands; can also be made synthetically

tendinitis: inflammation of a tendon, a tough band of tissue that connects muscle to bone

INDICATIONS

Nonsteroidal anti-inflammatory drugs (NSAIDs) relieve painful conditions such as arthritis, bursitis, gout, menstrual cramps, tendonitis, sprains, and strains. The best known NSAID is aspirin, a very commonly used pain reliever. Additionally, aspirin is commonly prescribed to prevent a myocardial infarction, and to patients who have had one myocardial infarction (heart attack) to decrease the risk of a second. While some NSAIDs require a prescription, many are sold over the counter.

These drugs can come in the form of capsules, caplets, tablets, liquid suspensions, and suppositories. Ofirmev is an intravenous form of acetaminophen.

Common NSAIDS

Generic drug	Trade name
Acetaminophen	Generics (OTC), Tylenol, Ofirmev, Mapap
Nonselective NSAIDs	
Aspirin	Generic (OTC)
Diclofenac	Generic (OTC), Zorvolex, Voltaren
Etodolac	Lodine
Fenoprofen	Generic, Xspire
Flurbiprofen	Ansaid
Ibuprofen	Generics, Motrin, Advil, Rufen, Nuprin (OTC)
Ketoprofen	Generic
Meclofenamate	Generic
Meloxicam	Generic, Mobic, Vivlodex
Nabumetone	Relafen
Naproxen	generics, Naprosyn, Anaprox, Aleve (OTC)
Salsalate	Generic
Oxaprozin	Daypro
Selective COX-2 Inhibitor	
Celecoxib	Generic, Celebrex

NSAIDs inhibit the enzyme cyclooxygenase (COX). COX enzymes catalyze the conversion of a fatty acid found in cell membranes called "arachidonic acid" to prostaglandin H2. Prostaglandins are signaling molecules that induce inflammation. Prostaglandin H2 is the first prostaglandin made in a series of distinct prostaglandins that mediate different aspects of inflammation. By inhibiting an early stage in the synthesis of prostaglandins, NSAIDs inhibit the onset of inflammation. There are three types of COX enzymes: COX-1, COX-II, and COX-III. Many different tissues constantly express COX-1 at low levels. COX-1 mediates housekeeping functions that dilate blood vessels in the kidneys, prevent clotting in small blood vessels around the heart, and maintain the health of the inner mucosal layer of the stomach. Several different cell types make COX-2 in response to tissue damage. Therefore, while cells tend to make COX-1 constitutively, a subset of cell types induce COX-2 synthesis under specific circumstances. Only the brain makes COX-3, and this brain-specific enzyme mediates pain reception in the brain.

Corticosteroids make up the second group of anti-inflammatory drugs used to ameliorate the symptoms associated with conditions such as asthma, lupus, arthritis, psoriasis (with and without phototherapy), and allergic reactions. Like NSAIDs, corticosteroids are available in various forms including inhalants, creams, ointments, and oral (systemic) medications.

Corticosteroids pass directly through cell membranes and bind to steroid receptors inside the cell. The steroid receptor-corticosteroid complex enters the nucleus and elicits changes in gene expression. Corticosteroid-induced changes in gene expression decrease inflammation and pain. In the respiratory tract, inhaled corticosteroids decrease mucous production, prevent airway remodeling, and diminish bronchoconstriction in the airways.

Commonly used inhaled corticosteroids to treat asthma include beclomethasone (QVAR Redihaler),

> **IN THE NEWS:**
> **DANGERS OF COX-2 INHIBITORS**
>
> In a 2001 issue of the *Journal of the American Medical Association*, Debabrata Mukherjee and coauthors summarized the results of two major randomized trials of COX-2 inhibitors: the Vioxx Gastrointestinal Outcomes Research Study (VIGOR), with 8,076 patients, and the Celecoxib Long-Term Arthritis Safety Study (CLASS), with 8,059 patients, as well as several smaller trials of these drugs. The VIGOR study found that treatment with rofecoxib (trade name Vioxx), a popular pain reliever for arthritis, increased the risk of developing a thrombotic cardiovascular event (myocardial infarction, unstable angina, cardiac thrombus, resuscitated cardiac arrest, sudden or unexplained death, ischemic stroke, and transient ischemic attacks) by twofold over naproxen treatment. Myocardial infarction rates for COX-2 inhibitors were found to be significantly higher than for the placebo group in both large studies. Other smaller-scale studies are consistent with the findings from the VIGOR and CLASS trials.
>
> Some of these adverse effects of Vioxx could be mitigated by simultaneous treatment with aspirin; however, such an approach significantly detracts from the utility of nonsteroidal anti-inflammatory drugs (NSAIDs) such as Vioxx, since one would experience the same degree of stomach irritation from the aspirin that NSAIDs are prescribed to avoid. In September 2004, the pharmaceutical company Merck pulled Vioxx off the market because of the preponderance of evidence suggesting that it poses serious risks of heart attack and stroke. It has been estimated that as many as 30,000 to 100,000 patients have had heart attacks or strokes because of taking Vioxx.
>
> —*Michael R. King, PhD*

budesonide (Pulmicort Flexhaler, Pulmicort Respules), ciclesonide (Alvesco), mometasone furoate (Asmanex HFA, Asmanex Twisthaler), fluticasone furoate (Arnuity Ellipta), and fluticasone propionate (Flovent Diskus, Flovent HFA, ArmonAir Digihaler). Treatments for chronic allergic rhinitis, the itchy, runny nose caused by seasonal allergies, use nasal sprays that administer many of the same corticosteroids used to treat asthma but at a lower dose. Several nasal corticosteroids designed specifically for children include Children's Qnasi (beclomethasone), Children's Rhinocort Allergy (budesonide), Children's Flonase Sensimist Allergy Relief (fluticasone furoate), Children's Flonase Allergy Relief (fluticasone propionate), and Children's Nasacort Allergy (triamcinolone acetonide).

Steroids prescribed to treat inflammatory bowel diseases include oral prednisone (Deltasone, Orasone), methylprednisolone (Medrol), prednisolone (Oraped, Prelone, Pediapred), and budesonide (Entocort and an extended-release tab, Uceris). Rectal steroids include budesonide foam (Salix), hydrocortisone foam (Cortifoam), and hydrocortisone enema (Colocort, Cortenema, Cortifoam).

Osteoarthritis patients who fail to respond to more traditional treatments sometimes receive intra-articular injections of methylprednisolone acetate (Depo-Medrol) and triamcinolone acetonide (Kenalog, Zilrettta).

COMPLICATIONS

Although used across many medical specialties and for a plethora of reasons, NSAIDs are not without their dangers. When used in the short term and occasionally, NSAIDs are relatively safe. With extended use, however, NSAIDs interfere with platelet function and prolong bleeding (except for salsalate and celecoxib), gastrointestinal toxicity (dyspepsia, gastrointestinal ulcers, perforation, and bleeding), renal toxicity (hypertension and fluid retention), and increased risk of heart attacks.

Excessive use of aspirin or other products that contain salicylic acid, including aspirin, methyl salicylate (Oil of Wintergreen), and bismuth subsalicylate (such as in Pepto-Bismol), causes salicylism. The symptoms of salicylism include fast breathing rates (tachypnea and hyperpnea), ringing in the ears (tinnitus), nausea and vomiting, altered mental status, and high body temperature (hyperthermia). Salicylic acid interferes with energy production in mitochondria, which increases heat production. It also irritates the gastric mucosae. Because salicylic acid is a weak acid, it causes metabolic acidosis. The body responds by accelerating the breathing rate to rid the body of acid. However, in its unionized form, salicylic acid crosses the blood-brain barrier, decreasing brain glucose levels and disrupting ionic concentration in the brain, culminating in confusion, altered mental status, seizures, and coma.

Women who are pregnant should not take NSAIDs, since NSAID use during pregnancy increases the risk of miscarriage. If used during the third trimester, NSAIDs can cause persistent hypertension or other cardiac malformations. NSAIDs are largely safe for breastfeeding mothers. Anyone with stomach or intestinal problems, liver disease, heart disease, high blood pressure, bleeding diseases, diabetes, Parkinson's disease, or epilepsy should consult their physicians before taking NSAIDs. It is important to note that children should not be given aspirin if they are recovering from a viral infection as it can lead to Reye's syndrome -a potentially fatal condition that results in swelling of the liver and brain.

Corticosteroid therapy produces dramatic, immediate relief from pain, swelling, and inflammation due to arthritis. Small amounts of steroids may be injected directly into the inflamed joint or taken orally. However, the beneficial effects tend to be temporary and long-term use can lead to the development of cataracts, osteoporosis, glaucoma, increased blood sugar which can worsen a person's diabetes, weight gain, reduced resistance to infections, as well as gastrointestinal ulcers and bleeding. Topical use of corticosteroids long-term increases the risk of skin atrophy, skin thinning and decreased healing of skin lesions. It follows that the advent of other highly effective alternatives has led to less frequent use of steroids to treat arthritis. Other risks of long-term corticosteroid use include acne, hirsutism, insomnia, mood disorders, and Cushing's syndrome.

Topical Corticosteroids

Drug	Strength	Vehicle
Super-High Potency		
Betamethasone dipropionate (generic, Diprolene)	0.05%	Ointment
Clobetasol propionate (generic, Clobex, Olux, Olux-E, Temovate, Cormax)	0.05%	Cream, lotion, ointment, gel, foam, shampoo, solution
Fluocinonide (generic, Vanos)	0.1%	Cream
Halobetasol (generic, Ultravate, Bryhali, Lexette)	0.05% & 0.01%	Cream, ointment, lotion, foam
High Potency		
Amcinonide (generic)	0.1%	Ointment
Betamethasone dipropionate augmented (generic)	0.05%	Cream
Betamethasone dipropionate (generic)	0.05%	Ointment
Clobetasol propionate (Impoyz)	0.025%	Cream
Desoximetasone (generic, Topicort)	0.25%	Cream, ointment spray
Desoximetasone (generic)	0.05%	Gel
Fluocinomide (generic)	0.05%	Ointment, gel, cream, solution
Halcinomide (Halog)	0.1%	Cream, ointment
Mometasone furoate (generic)	0.1%	Ointment
Medium-High Potency		
Amcinonide (generic)	0.1%	Cream, lotion
Betamethasone dipropionate (generic)	0.05%	Cream
Betamethasone valerate (generic)	0.1%	Ointment, cream
Desoximetasone (generic)	0.05%	Cream
Diforasone diacetate (generic)	0.05%	Cream
Fluocinonide emollient (generic)	0.05%	Cream
Fluticasone propionate (generic)	0.005%	Ointment
Triamcinolone acetonide	0.5%	Ointment, cream
Medium potency		
Betamethasone dipropionate (Sernivo)	0.05%	Spray
Betamethasone valerate (generic, Luxiq)	0.12%	Foam
Fluocinolone acetonide (generic, Synalar)	0.025%	Ointment
Flurandrenolide (generic, Cordran)	0.05%	Ointment
Hydrocortisone valerate (generic)	0.2%	Ointment
Mometasone furoate (generic, Elocon)	0.1%	Cream
Triamcinolone acetonide (generic, Triderm, Trianex))	0.1% and 0.05%	Ointment, cream

Topical Corticosteroids (continued)

Drug	Strength	Vehicle
Medium-Low Potency		
Betamethasone dipropionate (generic)	0.05%	Lotion
Betamethasone valerate (generic)	0.1%	Cream
Desonide (generic)	0.05%	Ointment
Fluocinolone acetonide (generic, Synalar)	0.025%	cream
Flurandrenolide (generic, Cordran, Nolix)	0.05%	Cream, lotion
Fluticasone propionate (generic, Cutivate)	0.05%	Cream, lotion
Hydrocortisone butyrate (generic, Locoid, Locoid Liprocream)	0.1%	Cream, ointment, solution
Hydrocortisone probutate (Pandel)	0.1%	Cream
Hydrocortisone valerate (generic)	0.2%	Cream
Prednicarbate (generic, Dermatop)	0.1%	Ointment, cream
Triamcinolone acetonide (generic)	0.025% & 0.1%	Ointment, lotion
Low Potency		
Alclometasone dipropionate (generic)	0.05%	Cream, ointment
Betamethasone valerate (generic)	0.1%	Lotion
Clocortolone pivalate (generic, Cloderm)	0.1%	cream
Desonide (generic, Desowen, Desonate, Verdeso)	0.05%	Cream, lotion, gel, foam
Fluocinolone acetonide (generic)	0.01%	Cream, solution
Triamcinolone acetonide (generic)	0.025%	Cream, lotion
Lowest Potency		
Hydrocortisone (generic, Aquanil-HC, Nu-Derm Tolereen)	0.5%, 1.0% & 2.5%	Ointment, cream, lotion

Additionally, corticosteroids are a common treatment for persons suffering from more serious asthmatic conditions or when treatment with bronchodilators has not proven effective. Corticosteroids, which are not bronchodilators and do not open the airways, instead work to reduce inflammation to allow the lungs to function properly. They should be used regularly and for the complete course as prescribed to achieve full benefits. Corticosteroids may be sprayed into the nose to relieve stuffy nose, irritation, hay fever, or other allergies, while oral corticosteroids primarily prevent asthma attacks. Oral corticosteroids can increase the risk of oral thrush and hoarseness. After using an oral corticosteroid, patients should always wash their mouths out with water.

Ophthalmic anti-inflammatory medicines can reduce problems that occur during or following eye surgery by alleviating eye inflammation. These can be obtained only with a doctor's prescription. Corticosteroids also relieve inflammation of the temporal arteries, the blood vessels that run along with the temples. Inflammation here can disrupt the blood supply and result in blindness, partial loss of vision, strokes, and even heart attacks. Extended use of ocular corticosteroids increases the risk of glaucoma.

Individuals with medical conditions such as allergies, diabetes, pregnancy, osteoporosis, glaucoma, infections, thyroid problems, liver disease, kidney disease, heart disease, or high blood pressure should discuss these conditions with their physician before taking corticosteroids. Short-term use of corticosteroids rarely causes side effects. However, report breathing problems or tightness in the chest, pain, rash, swelling, extreme exhaustion, irregular heartbeat, or wounds that do not heal to a physician. Do not abruptly stop steroids without consulting a physician, especially if the steroids have been taken for a long time, as the body requires a weaning process to adapt.

PERSPECTIVE AND PROSPECTS

The bark of the willow tree, which contains salicylates, was known in eighteenth-century England to reduce fever and aches. In 1876, scientists reported the first successful treatment of acute arthritis with sodium salicylate (aspirin). In the 1970s, pharmacologist John Vane amassed evidence of the effectiveness of NSAIDs.

The earliest demonstration of the importance of corticosteroids as anti-inflammatory agents occurred in the 1940s regarding rheumatoid arthritis. The challenge of corticosteroid therapy lies in achieving the desired results with a minimum of side effects.

—Mary Hurd, Lillian Dominguez, MD
and Michael A. Buratovich, PhD

Further Information

American Medical Association. *American Medical Association Family Medical Guide.* 4th ed., John Wiley & Sons, 2004.
"Anti-Inflammatories and Corticosteroids." *American Association for Respiratory Care*, 2013.
"Drugs for Osteoarthritis." *The Medical Letter on Drugs and Therapeutics*, vol. 62, no. 1596, 20 Apr. 2020, pp. 57-62.
Liska, Ken. *Drugs and the Human Body, with Implications for Society.* 8th ed., Pearson/Prentice Hall, 2009.
Lupi, Chiara, et al. "Medicines for Headache Before and During Pregnancy: A Retrospective Cohort Study (ATENA Study)." *Neurological Sciences: Official Journal of the Italian Neurological Society and of the Italian Society of Clinical Neurophysiology*, vol. 42, no. 5, 2021, pp. 1895-1921, doi:10.1007/s10072-020-04702-0.
"NSAIDs: Nonsteroidal Anti-Inflammatory Drugs." *American College of Rheumatology*, Aug. 2012.
Subak-Sharpe, Genell J., and Thomas O. Morris, editors. "Drug Therapy." *The Columbia University College of Physicians and Surgeons Complete Home Medical Guide.* 3rd ed., Crown, 1995.
"What Is an Inflammation?" *PubMed Health*, Jan. 2015.

ANTIHISTAMINES

Category: Treatment
Anatomy or system affected: Chest, circulatory system, ears, eyes, head, immune system, lungs, nose, psychic-emotional system, respiratory system, throat, skin
Specialties and related fields: Family medicine, immunology, otorhinolaryngology, pharmacology, preventive medicine, pulmonary medicine
Definition: Over-the-counter and prescription-type drugs that are commonly prescribed for allergy symptoms to reduce the early effects of allergies caused by histamines.

KEY TERMS

allergic rhinitis: an uncomfortable condition of the nose resulting from the sensitivity of the nasal passageway to pollen or other substances
arrhythmias: problems with the rhythm of the heart, such as irregular heartbeat
decongestants: drugs that are taken to reduce swelling of the nasal passages and decrease the production of mucus, the fluids commonly found in the sinuses during allergic reactions and colds

drug synergy: a process by which drugs taken in combination with each other interact and can have a greater effect than the drugs taken separately

histamines: proteins released by the immune system as part of allergic reactions

mucous membranes: the lining covering the parts of the body in the major air passageways and in the alimentary tract

INDICATIONS AND PROCEDURES

Every day, we inhale untold quantities of visible and invisible compounds and entities. Visible components include dust, dirt, allergens, and human skin. Dust consists of tiny particles of waste matter or earth that form a fine, dry powder that alights on surfaces, or the ground. Dirt refers to loose soil particles. Allergens are pollens or other small particles of plant and animal products. Finally, dead human skin cells are a significant component (about 80 percent) of dust. About 90 percent of airborne particles are too small to see and consist of bacteria, viruses, molds, and volatile organic compounds (VOCs).

The upper respiratory tract is coated with mucous glands that secrete a layer of mucous that acts as a sticky layer that traps inhaled particles. The trachea is lined with cells that have hair-like extensions called "cilia." Cilia beat in synchrony, like oars on a Viking ship, to move the constantly synthesized mucous upward, to the pharynx, where it is expectorated or swallowed. This system, the mucociliary escalator, clears the respiratory tract of inhaled materials.

In some individuals, the immune system recognizes inhaled allergens as foreign substances and mounts an immune response against them. Wandering cells called "dendritic cells" gobble up inhaled allergens and take them to the closest lymph node. There, the dendritic cell processes and presents the allergens to special white blood cells called "lymphocytes." Specifically, a type of lymphocyte called a "B cell" makes antibodies against these allergens. Antibodies bind to foreign substances and inactivate them, clump them, and make them easier to dispose of or destroy. Under the influence of secreted signaling molecules such as interleukin-4 (IL-4) and interleukin-13 (IL-13), which are made by another type of lymphocyte called a "T cell," the B cells synthesize an antibody subtype called "immunoglobulin E (IgE)." IgE plays a unique role in allergies.

Several bodily tissues are junction points between the external environment and the body's internal environment. Examples of such tissues include the skin, gastrointestinal tract, respiratory tract, eyes, hair follicles, and so on. Such junctional tissues contain many interspersed cells called "mast cells." Like other blood cells, mast cells come from the bone marrow, but after their release into the peripheral circulation, they do not fully mature until a junctional tissue recruits them, and they become lodged there. IgE molecules, made by B cells in response to allergen exposure, bind en masse to receptors on the surfaces of mast cells.

When exposed to allergens, they bind to the IgE-decorated mast cells. The cross-linking of allergens on the surfaces of mast cells by surface-bound IgEs sends a powerful signal to the mast cells and they release a bevy of powerful chemical mediators. The most significant two mediators include histamine, which acts quickly, and leukotriene, which acts slowly. Histamine causes the endothelial cells that line blood vessels to shrink and the blood vessel to leak. Leaking blood vessels cause local swelling. Second, histamines cause smooth muscles, especially those that line the bronchial tubes to contract, leading to wheezing. Third, histamine increase the secretion of mucous glands in the upper respiratory tract, which can cause the nose and eyes to run. Fourth, histamine sensitizes pain receptors in tissues so that pain sensations are heightened.

Antihistamines are the drug of choice for intermittent rhinitis symptoms, including nasal itching, sneezing, and rhinorrhea (runny nose). Ocular antihistamines reduce the itching, tearing, and redness associated with allergic conjunctivitis. Histamine exerts its biological effects by binding to a receptor called the "H1 receptor." Antihistamines obstruct the H1 receptor and prevent histamine from binding to it and inducing its effects.

Antihistamines provide a rapid form of treatment for controlling histamine-based physical reactions, including cold and allergy symptoms, rashes and hives, and insect bites and stings. They are also especially helpful for the allergic condition known as hay fever, which is related to seasonal allergies and allergic rhinitis. Antihistamines decrease the discomfort and symptoms caused by histamine reactions. Symptoms of histamine reactions may include sneezing, itchy skin, rashes, a swollen throat, watery or itchy eyes, and a runny nose. In reducing these effects, antihistamines may also be useful in helping to decrease the risk of additional infections caused by the swelling of sensitive mucous membranes in the body, particularly in the sinuses, nose, and throat. Typically, if such membranes remain swollen, the passageways of the body, such as the sinuses, can become congested, making it easier for infections to develop.

Antihistamines are typically administered orally, in pill form, one or more times per day, but they are also available in the form of eye drops, nose sprays, and liquids. They are also combined frequently with other drugs such as decongestants to ameliorate further any uncomfortable cold symptoms and to prevent consequent problems such as sinus infections. Antihistamines alone are generally considered to be ineffective at reducing nasal congestion. Examples of antihistamine/decongestant combinations include Claritin-D, Allegra D, Clarinex-D, and Zyrtec-D, which contain loratadine, fexofenadine, desloratadine, and cetirizine, respectively, combined with pseudoephedrine.

USES AND COMPLICATIONS

In addition to reducing histamine reactions, first-generation antihistamines have several side effects, including dry mouth, drowsiness, dizziness, nausea and vomiting, blurred vision, restlessness in some children, confusion, and difficulty urinating. Because first-generation antihistamines tend to be fat-soluble molecules, they cross the blood-brain barrier and cause sedation and confusion, particularly in the elderly. Consequently, some antihistamines (e.g., doxylamine), therefore, can treat insomnia and motion sickness (e.g., meclizine). Newer, or second-generation antihistamines (e.g., loratadine, desloratadine, fexofenadine, cetirizine, levocetirizine), cause significantly less drowsiness.

Nasal antihistamines can cause nasal itching and burning, nose bleeds, changes in taste, dry mouth, and headaches. However, these adverse effects are rare. Ocular antihistamines can cause burning, itching, or redness of the eyes. Headaches may also occur, but these drugs are also usually well tolerated.

Furthermore, any drug, including antihistamines, can be abused if used in larger quantities than prescribed or recommended. For instance, some individuals may use high quantities of antihistamines to experience a more pronounced sedating effect or other psychoactive effects. Overuse of antihistamines or any substance outside its recommended use is dangerous, particularly in situations requiring safety (for instance, driving, operating machinery, being around strangers, being in strange places) may lead to unexpected negative consequences. Of the side effects mentioned, drowsiness is most problematic, since people who need to take the drugs more than once a day may have their daytime activities interrupted by feeling sleepy. Additionally, combining antihistamines with other substances, prescription drugs, or others such as alcohol, then drug synergies can occur. With sedating drugs such as alcohol, for instance, the onset of drowsiness can hasten and its strength can be greater than might be expected with

Antihistamines

Drug	Formulation
First-generation antihistamines	
Diphenhydramine Generic, Benadryl Allergy, Children's Benadryl Allergy, Banophen	25, 50 mg capsule; 25 mg tablet; 12.5 mg per 5 mL solution; 50 mg/mL injection
Chlorpheniramine generic, Chlor-Trimeton	4 mg tablet
Carbinoxamine Generic Ryvent	4 mg tablet; 4 mg / 5 mL solution 6 mg tablet
Cyproheptadine Generic	4 mg tablet; 2 mg/5 mL solution
Second-generation antihistamines	
Loratadine Generic, Claritin, Children's Claritin Alavert	10 mg tablets & capsules/10 mg disintegrating tablets 5 mg chewable tablets and 1 mg/mL syrup 10 mg disintegrating tablets
Desloratadine Generic Clarinex	5 mg tablets, 2.5, 5 mg disintegration tablets 5 mg tablets
Fexofenadine Generic, Allegra Allergy Children's Allegra Allergy	30, 60, 180 mg tablet 30 mg disintegrating tablet/ 30 mg/5 mL suspension
Cetirizine Zyrtec Allergy Children's Zyrtec Allergy Zerviate	5, 10 mg tablets and capsules; 10 mg disintegrating tablets 5 mg/mL syrup 0.24% ocular solution (1 drop, 2X/day)
Levocetirizine Xyzal Allergy 24 hour Children's Xyzal Allergy	5 mg tablets 2.5 mg/5 mL oral solution
Nasal Antihistamines	
Azelastine Generic Ophthalmic solution	0.1%, 0.15% nasal spray 0.05% ocular solution
Ocular antihistamines	
Olopatadine Generic, Pataday Nasal spray	0.1%, 0.2% ocular solution 0.6% nasal spray
Bepotastine Bepreve	1.5% ocular solution
Alcaftadine Lastacaft	0.25% ocular solution
Ketotifen Generic, Alaway	0.025% ocular solution
Epinastine generic	0.05% ocular solution
Emedastine Emadine	0.05% ocular solution

either the antihistamine or the alcohol alone. As such, the use of antihistamines, particularly in combination with other sedating drugs (opioids, barbiturates, anesthetics, benzodiazepines, sedating pain medications), or even sedating alternative medicines, is not advised in situations requiring attention and alertness, such as driving or operating machinery.

Because of issues such as drug interactions and how the drug may affect the body, antihistamines should be taken cautiously. They also should not be used by women who are pregnant or breastfeeding, people with liver or kidney problems, acute glaucoma, or enlarged prostate unless directed by a provider. Other contraindications may exist as well. The advice of a physician or pharmacist is best followed when taking any drug.

PERSPECTIVE AND PROSPECTS

Antihistamines have been paired with substances such as decongestants so that they may relieve more symptoms. In the past, however, some additions have come with both advantages and disadvantages. The addition of pseudoephedrine to antihistamine medications, for example, increased their ability to address symptoms and decreased some of the drowsiness. Pseudoephedrine, however, has stimulating properties that have been identified as problematic, and it was removed from many types of medications.

Antihistamine development is also driven by a desire to make them more specific. For instance, one person may need an antihistamine to reduce nasal irritation while another may need one to alleviate itchy eyes. As such, it is expected that antihistamines will be developed to have much more specific effects on the body and to have little to no sedating or other side effects while still being effective at reducing allergy and cold symptoms. Nevertheless, some of the familiar antihistamines known today are likely to remain available, as they are generally useful. Also, mildly sedating medicines, such as antihistamines taken at a normally recommended dose, may continue to have a place in medicine, as they serve as a good substitute for individuals needing nonaddictive sleep medication and who are unlikely to abuse these substances.

—*Nancy Banasiak, MSN, APRN*

Further Information

"Antihistamines: Understanding Your OTC Options." *American Academy of Family Physicians*, Feb. 2012.

Bozek, A. "Pharmacological Management of Allergic Rhinitis in the Elderly." *Drugs & Aging*, Jan. 2017.

"Drugs for Allergic Rhinitis and Allergic Conjunctivitis." *The Medical Letter on Drugs and Therapeutics*, vol. 63, no. 1622, 2021, pp. 57-64.

Hossenbaccus, L., S, Linton, S. Garvey, et al. "Towards Definitive Management of Allergic Rhinitis: Best Use of New and Established Therapies." *Allergy Asthma Clin Immunol*, vol. 16, no. 39, 2020, doi.org/10.1186/s13223-020-00436-y.

Sur, D. K., and M. L. Plesa. "Treatment of Allergic Rhinitis." *American Family Physician*, Dec. 2015.

Web MD, www.webmd.com/allergies/antihistamines-for-allergies. Accessed 20 Sept. 2017.

ANTIVIRAL DRUGS: MECHANISMS OF ACTION

Category: Treatment

Anatomy or system affected: Blood, brain, eyes, gastrointestinal system, intestines, liver, lungs, lymphatic system, mouth, reproductive system, respiratory system, skin, throat

Specialties and related fields: Dermatology, epidemiology, gynecology, hematology, internal medicine, microbiology, neurology, oncology, ophthalmology, osteopathic medicine, otorhinolaryngology, pathology, pharmacology, public health, pulmonary medicine, virology

Definition: Drugs that prevent the replication of viruses in the cells of the human body.

KEY TERMS

highly active antiretroviral therapy (HAART): the use of a combination of three or four anti-human immunodeficiency virus (HIV) drugs in an HIV-positive individual to suppress replication of new HIV particles and slow the progression to full-blown acquired immunodeficiency syndrome (AIDS)

lentivirus: a classification of retroviruses characterized by a very long incubation period (ten to twenty years) before symptoms of a disease appear

opportunistic infection: an infection caused by any type of pathogen in individuals who have an impaired immune system

pneumocystis pneumonia: a form of pneumonia caused by the fungus *Pneumocystis carinii* and commonly seen in persons with AIDS

protease inhibitors: any of several drugs that inhibit the HIV protease, an enzyme encoded by the HIV genome that cleaves proteins into smaller polypeptide changes, and prevents the assembly of HIV virions

retrovirus: a virus with ribonucleic acid (RNA) as its genetic material that produces a deoxyribonucleic acid (DNA) copy of the RNA to be integrated into a chromosome of the host cell, from which it will make new infectious copies of the RNA during the viral life cycle

reverse transcriptase: an enzyme encoded by the genomes of retroviruses that makes DNA copies of RNA molecules

T4 cells: also called "CD4 cells" or "T-helper cells"; a specific type of white blood cell (lymphocyte) which regulates the entire immune system and is the preferred target for HIV infection, resulting in immunodeficiency

viral load: a measurement of the amount of HIV present in the blood; often used to monitor the effectiveness of anti-HIV therapy

viral tropism: the tendency of or efficiency with which a specific virus productively infects a particular cell type or tissue.

INTRODUCTION

Viruses, the smallest agents of infection, consist of either deoxyribonucleic acid (DNA) or ribonucleic acid (RNA) and typically are enclosed within a protein coat (capsid). Viruses lack their own metabolism, so to replicate, they must infect a living organism (host) and coopt that host's cellular machinery.

The viral life cycle is similar for most viruses. Attachment to the host cell is achieved through interaction between viral and host surface proteins. The virus crosses the host cell membrane (entry), the capsid proteins protecting the viral genome are shed (uncoating), and the genome is transcribed into mRNAs (messenger RNA), which are translated by the host cell's protein synthesis machinery. After uncoating, retroviruses can convert their RNA genome to DNA, a process called "reverse transcription," and integrate into the host genome (strand transfer). After genome replication, the virus self-assembles and is released from the cell by lysis or budding.

THERAPIES AGAINST VIRAL INFECTION

Therapies for viral infections can be classified into agents (antivirals) that inhibit viral replication within the cell, agents (antibodies, virucides) that block viral infection of the host cell, and agents (immunomodulators) that modulate the host response to the viral infection. To selectively inhibit viral replication, drugs exploit the differences between viral and human proteins. Most antiviral drugs target viral nucleic acid synthesis.

INHIBITION OF ATTACHMENT, ENTRY, AND UNCOATING

Human immunodeficiency virus (HIV) infection involves a "handshake" between proteins on the surface of host cells and viral envelop glycoproteins. The viral envelop glycoproteins gp120 and gp41 form a complex that binds to the CD4 protein complexed to the chemokine receptor CCR5.

Strains of HIV that infect CCR5-expressing cells (e.g., macrophages) are called "M-tropic" or "R5 viruses." Other HIV strains infect cells that express the alpha-chemokine receptor CXCR4 and are called "T-tropic" or "X4 viruses." Patients with long-term HIV infections may experience a so-called tropism switch in which their infecting HIV strains change from M-tropic viruses to T-tropic viruses.

The HIV drugs enfuvirtide and maraviroc are small molecules that inhibit the entry of a virus to its target cell by interacting with viral surface glycoproteins. Enfuvirtide (Fuzeon) is a peptide that blocks the conformational change in gp41 required for fusion and entry. Maraviroc (Selzentry) binds to the HIV protein gp120, which prevents its interaction with the host chemokine receptor CCR5. Maraviroc is ineffective against X4 viruses and patients with long-term HIV infections should have their endogenous HIV typed with the Trofile test that distinguishes between R5 and X4 HIV strains. An anti-CD4 monoclonal antibody called "ibalizumab" (*Trogarzo*) inhibits HIV from binding and entering host cells. It is administered intravenously for multidrug-resistant HIV-1 (MDR-HIV) and is Food and Drug Administration (FDA)-approved for HIV patients who have failed to achieve proper suppression of HIV infection with other treatment regimens. An oral medication called "fostemsavir" (Rukobia) binds to gp120 on the surface of HIV and prevents its interaction with CD4 and viral entry into host cells. The drug *n*-docosanol is a 22-carbon saturated fatty acid that appears to block the entry of lipid-enveloped viruses into target cells.

The anti-influenza virus drugs amantadine, and rimantadine target the viral uncoating step by blocking matrix protein that forms a transmembrane proton channel in the influenza A lipid envelope. After fusion with the host cell endosome, the passage of hydrogen ions through the proton channel into the virion acidifies the interior, which alters interactions among nucleocapsid proteins and initiates viral uncoating.

INHIBITION OF GENOME REPLICATION AND EXPRESSION

Drugs that inhibit viral polymerases target viral replication. Nucleoside and nucleotide analog drugs are substrates for the viral polymerase, the enzyme that links nucleotide monomers covalently into DNA or RNA. Nucleotides contain one or more phosphate groups, whereas nucleosides require intracellular phosphorylation before incorporation into the nucleic acid strand.

For example, acyclovir, an analog of the nucleoside guanosine, inhibits replication of herpes simplex virus (HSV) types 1 and 2 and varicella-zoster virus (VZV). It lacks the 3-hydroxyl group needed to create a bond to the next nucleotide in the growing nucleic acid chain; therefore, it is a chain terminator of viral DNA elongation. Because it prevents the binding of the usual substrate to the enzyme, it is a competitive inhibitor. Valacyclovir, an orally administered and more bioavailable form of acyclovir, is inactive until chemically converted within the cell (that is, as a prodrug of acyclovir). Other guanosine/guanine inhibitors include penciclovir, whose prodrug form is famciclovir; ganciclovir, whose prodrug form is valganciclovir, which has increased activity against cytomegalovirus (CMV) infections; and ribavirin, which inhibits viral RNA polymerase activity and inhibits the 5' capping of viral mRNA. Ribavirin also appears to enhance the host T-cell-mediated immune response and to inhibit the host inosine monophosphate dehydrogenase, thereby decreasing the intracellular pool of guanosine triphosphate needed for viral replication and acting like a virus mutagen.

Penciclovir, another guanine analog, is sometimes incorporated into DNA (unlike acyclovir), and is active against VZV, HSV, and Epstein-Barr virus

(EBV). Other nucleoside/nucleotide analogs include cidofovir, a cytosine analog that is used to treat eye infections caused by CMV; vidarabine, an adenosine analog that treats eye infections caused by HSV-1 and HSV-2; and the thymidine analogs brivudine, an anti-VZV treatment, and trifluridine (Lonsurf), which was FDA-approved for recurrent, metastatic gastric and gastroesophageal junction adenocarcinoma.

The reverse transcriptase of retroviruses, such as HIV, are inhibited by nucleotide/nucleoside inhibitors, and non-nucleoside reverse transcriptase inhibitors. Nucleoside reverse transcriptase inhibitors (NRTIs) include zidovudine (the first antiretroviral drug approved for HIV treatment), emtricitabine, abacavir, tenofovir, didanosine, and lamivudine. Non-nucleoside reverse transcriptase inhibitors (NNRTIs) include nevirapine, efavirenz, delavirdine, and rilpivirine. An NRTI and an NNRTI are often combined as part of a highly active antiretroviral treatment (HAART) regimen.

Additionally, retroviruses also require an enzyme called "integrase" for stable integration of the viral DNA into the host genome. Highly effective Integrase inhibitors have revolutionized HIV treatment. Raltegravir (Isentress) is the first integrase inhibitor approved for clinical use. Other integrase inhibitors include dolutegravir (Tivicay), elvitegravir, which is combined with other drugs and is not available alone, bictegravir (available in Biktavy, a combination medication with bictegravir and the NRTIs emtricitabine and tenofovir alafenamide), and cabotegravir (Vocabria).

Viral replication can also be blocked by noncompetitive inhibition of the polymerase, as in the case of NNRTIs and reverse transcriptase. Foscarnet is a pyrophosphate analog that binds the pyrophosphate-binding site of herpesvirus DNA polymerase and HIV reverse transcriptase. Foscarnet blocks pyrophosphate cleavage from nucleotides, preventing their incorporation into the DNA chain.

Hepatitis C virus (HCV) encodes two proteins that replicate HCV genomic RNAs. The first, NS5A, is a zinc-binding, phosphoprotein involved in HCV RNA replication. The second, NS5B, is an RNA-dependent RNA polymerase (RdRp). The RdRp replicates genomic HCV RNAs that are packaged into capsids to form infective virions. Several drugs that treat HCV infections inhibit NS5B, preventing its replication. Elbasvir, ledipasvir, pibrentasvir, and ombitasvir are NS5A inhibitors. Sofosbuvir and dasabuvir are NS5B inhibitors. These medications are usually combined with other medicines to form combination drugs that are prescribed to hepatitis C patients.

Baloxavir marboxil (Xofluza) is an anti-influenza drug that inhibits polymerase acidic (PA) endonuclease. This drug is administered orally and is a single-dose treatment for acute uncomplicated influenza in patients twelve-years old and older.

INHIBITION OF VIRAL MATURATION AND RELEASE

For many viruses, the maturation of viral proteins by a protease is essential before the virions are released. Several drugs have been developed that inhibit the HIV protease by binding to its active site; they include tipranavir, indinavir, saquinavir, nelfinavir, and fosamprenavir.

HCV begins its life cycle by binding to the plasma membrane of liver cells and inducing the liver cell to "swallow" it. Once within the liver cell, HCV uncoats within the lysosome, and the genomic RNA is translated into a large, precursor protein that is clipped into individual viral proteins by the HCV protease. Several anti-HCV drugs directly inhibit the HCV protease and prevent productive HCV infection and spread. Grazoprevir, glecaprevir, voxilaprevir, and paritaprevir are HCV protease inhibitors.

Viral release is targeted by anti-influenza medications that include the oral medication oseltamivir, the intravenously administered drug peramivir, and an inhaled medication called "zanamivir." These medications are sialic acid analogs that are competitive reversible inhibitors of neuraminidase, an enzyme expressed on the surface of influenza A and B viruses. Viral neuraminidases cleave sialic acid residues on host receptors recognized by viral hemagglutinin, which releases new viruses from the infected cell, allowing them to spread and infect other cells. Neuraminidase inhibitors, therefore, limit the spread of the virus. All three work best if taken within forty-eight hours of the onset of symptoms and they shorten the duration of the disease by eighteen to thirty hours and decrease the risk of severe disease.

IMPACT

Considerable progress has been made in the development of effective therapies for viral infections. Better understandings of the physiology of viral replication will reveal more drug targets and increase the therapeutic options for viral infections, especially for emerging viruses such as coronavirus and chronic viral diseases such as hepatitis B and C.

—*Kathleen LaPoint, MS*

Further Information

Driscoll, John S. *Antiviral Drugs*. John Wiley & Sons, 2006. Presents the most commonly used antiviral drugs and discusses the mechanisms by which the drugs exert their therapeutic effects.

Mahy, Brian W. J., and Marc H. V. van Regenmortel, editors. *Desk Encyclopedia of Human and Medical Virology*. Academic Press/Elsevier, 2010. Describes common and rare viruses in detail, along with their treatments.

Neal, M. J. *Modern Pharmacology at a Glance*. 6th ed., Wiley-Blackwell, 2009. An introduction to pharmacology that explains how drugs, including antiviral drugs, work.

Wagner, Edward K., and Martinez J. Hewlett. *Basic Virology*. 3rd ed., Blackwell Science, 2008. An undergraduate text covering issues of virology and viral disease, properties of viruses and virus-cell interaction, working with viruses, and replication patterns of specific viruses.

ANTIVIRAL DRUGS: TYPES

Category: Treatment

Anatomy or system affected: Blood, brain, eyes, gastrointestinal system, intestines, liver, lungs, lymphatic system, mouth, reproductive system, respiratory system, skin, throat

Specialties and related fields: Dermatology, epidemiology, gynecology, hematology, internal medicine, microbiology, neurology, oncology, ophthalmology, osteopathic medicine, otorhinolaryngology, pathology, pharmacology, public health, pulmonary medicine, virology

Definition: Medications used to prevent the replication of viruses in the cells of the human body during infection.

KEY TERMS

highly active antiretroviral therapy (HAART): the use of a combination of three or four anti-human immunodeficiency virus (HIV) drugs in an HIV-positive individual to suppress replication of new HIV particles and slow the progression to full-blown acquired immunodeficiency syndrome (AIDS)

lentivirus: a classification of retroviruses characterized by a very long incubation period (ten to twenty years) before symptoms of a disease appear

protease inhibitors: any of several drugs that inhibit the HIV protease, an enzyme encoded by the HIV genome that cleaves proteins into smaller polypeptide changes, and prevent the assembly of HIV virions

retrovirus: a virus with ribonucleic acid (RNA) as its genetic material that produces a deoxyribonucleic acid (DNA) copy of the RNA to be integrated into a chromosome of the host cell, from which it will make new infectious copies of the RNA during the viral life cycle

reverse transcriptase: an enzyme encoded by the genomes of HIV or hepatitis B virus (HBV) that synthesizes a DNA copy of an RNA template

seroconversion: the detection of anti-HIV antibodies in the blood of an HIV-infected person, who is then said to be HIV-positive

syndrome: a collection of symptoms associated with a particular disease state; an individual patient may show some, but not necessarily all, of these symptoms

T4 cells: also called "CD4 cells" or "T-helper cells"; a specific type of white blood cell (lymphocyte) which regulates the entire immune system and is the preferred target for HIV infection, resulting in immunodeficiency

viral load: a measurement of the amount of HIV present in the blood; often used to monitor the effectiveness of anti-HIV therapy

HIV AND AIDS MEDICATIONS

Antivirals targeted at the human immunodeficiency virus (HIV) make up more than one-half of the available antivirals. These antivirals can be divided into six subclasses: nucleoside reverse transcriptase inhibitors (NRTIs), non-nucleoside reverse transcriptase inhibitors (NNRTIs), protease inhibitors (PIs), integrase strand transfer inhibitors (INSTIs), CCR5 antagonists, and fusion inhibitors. Each class targets a different HIV enzyme or receptor.

Nucleoside reverse transcriptase inhibitors. NRTIs are competitive substrate inhibitors that complete with naturally occurring deoxynucleotides. NRTIs inhibit the enzyme, reverse transcriptase, thereby blocking the transcription of viral ribonucleic acid (RNA) to host deoxyribonucleic acid (DNA), preventing HIV from replicating, and preventing incorporation into the host genome. Available NRTIs include zidovu-

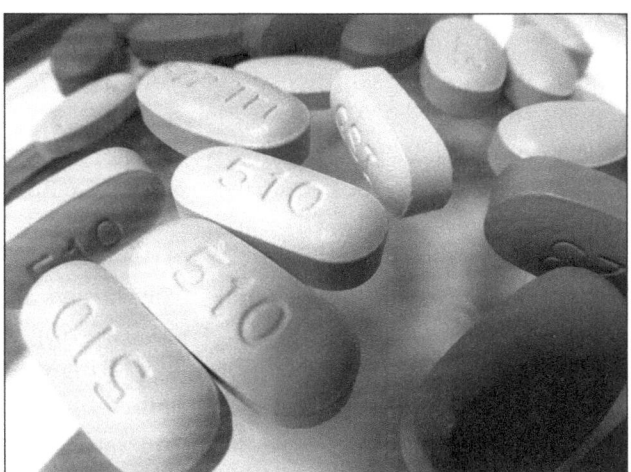

Antiretroviral Drugs to Treat HIV Infection. Photo by the National Institute of Allergy and Infectious Diseases (NIAID), via Wikimedia Commons.

dine, didanosine, stavudine, lamivudine, abacavir, and emtricitabine.

Non-nucleoside reverse transcriptase inhibitors. NNRTIs prevent viral RNA from being converted into DNA through the inhibition of reverse transcriptase. Available NNRTIs include efavirenz, nevirapine, delavirdine, and etravirine.

Protease inhibitors. HIV protease is an enzyme that exerts its effect after HIV has successfully entered the host cell and been incorporated into the host genome. Protease is responsible for breaking large protein strands called "polyproteins" into smaller viral particles, which then mature and become infectious to the host. Protease inhibitors prevent this cleaving of polyproteins and, therefore, prevent HIV particles from maturing and replicating. Available protease inhibitors include atazanavir, darunavir, fosamprenavir, indinavir, lopinavir/ritonavir, nelfinavir mesylate, ritonavir, saquinavir, and tipranavir.

Integrase strand transfer inhibitors. Integrase is an enzyme that facilitates integration of viral HIV DNA into the host cell genome. By preventing incorporation of HIV DNA, the provirus does not form and, therefore, no viral reproduction occurs within the host. The available integrase strand transfer inhibitors are raltegravir (Isentress), dolutegravir (Tivicay), elvitegravir (Vitekta), cabotegravir (Vocabria), and bictegravir.

CCR5 antagonists. The cell surface protein, CCR5, along with its coreceptor, CD4, are the major receptors that facilitate the entry of HIV into the host cells. CCR5 is the major coreceptor involved in viral entry for "CCR5-tropic" strains of HIV. CCR5-tropic HIV-1 strains, or M-strains, predominate during the early stages of infection and remain dominant in 50 to 60 percent of late-stage disease. During late-stage disease, a patient's endogenous HIV strains undergo a "tropism shift" whereby the patient's HIV strains shift from CCR5-tropic strains to CXCR4-tropic or T-strains. The oral mediation maraviroc (Selzentry) binds to the CCR5 coreceptor, preventing the virus from entering the host cell. Like raltegravir, it is active against HIV strains resistant to other antiretroviral drugs. CCR5 antagonists inhibit CCR5, changing the conformation of the coreceptor and, therefore, preventing fusion of the host cell membrane and HIV. Maraviroc does not inhibit CXCR4-tropic HIV strains.

Fusion inhibitors. Fusion inhibitors bind to the viral envelope glycoprotein and block the conformational change that, if carried out, would result in the fusion on the HIV viral and host cell membrane. Enfuvirtide (Fuzeon) is a peptide that is given subcutaneously. Ibalizumab (Trogarzo) is an intravenously administered monoclonal antibody that binds to CD4 and blocks HIV binding and entry. Finally, an oral medication, fostemsavir (Rukobia), binds to gp120 and prevents HIV from interacting with CD4, thereby preventing viral binding and host cell entry.

Highly active antiretroviral therapy (HAART) always includes drug combinations that inhibit multiple HIV processes. These combination medications decrease the risk of developing resistant strains and more effectively decrease viral load.

COMBINATION HIV MEDICATIONS

Trade name	Drug Combination
Atripla and generic	Efavirenz/emtricitabine/tenofovir
Biktarvy	Bictegravir/emtricitabine/tenofovir
Cabenuva	Cabotegravir/rilpivirine
Cimduo	Lamivudine/tenofovir
Complera	Emtricitabine/rilpivirine/tenofovir
Delstrigo	Doravirine/lamivudine/tenofovir
Dovato	Dolutegravir/lamivudine
Genvoya	Elvitegravir/cobicistat/emtricitabine/tenofovir
Juluca	Dolutegravir/rilpivirine
Odefsey	Emtricitabine/rilpivirine/tenofovir
Pifeltro	Doravirine/lamivudine/tenofovir
Stribild	Elvitegravir/cobicistat/emtricitabine/tenofovir
Symfi, Symfi Lo and generic	Efavirenz/lamivudine/tenofovir
Symtuza	Darunavir/cobicistat/emtricitabine/tenofovir
Temixys	Lamivudine/tenofovir
Triumeq	Abacavir/dolutegravir/lamivudine
Trizivir	Abacavir/lamivudine/zidovudine

INFLUENZA MEDICATIONS

Four antiviral medications are available, either as treatment or prophylaxis, for influenza A or B. These drugs can be divided into M2 inhibitors and neuraminidase inhibitors.

M2 inhibitors prevent uncoating of the influenza A virus, thereby blocking entrance of the virus into the host. Available M2 inhibitors include amantadine and rimantadine. M2 inhibitors provide prophylactic protection against influenza or for treatment of influenza A. However, the Centers for Disease Control and Prevention (CDC) recommends against the use of M2 inhibitors for influenza A due to high levels of resistance among circulating strains.

Neuraminidase inhibitors are the drug of choice for current influenza strains and are active against both A and B strains. Both are approved for both prophylaxis and treatment. Neuraminidase enzyme is an enzyme that plays a role in preparing the glycoproteins to which the influenza virus can attach. Available neuraminidase inhibitors are an inhaled drug called "zanamivir" (Relenza), an intravenously administration medication called "peramivir" (Rapivab), and an oral medication, oseltamivir (Tamiflu).

Baloxavir (Xofluza) inhibits the influenza viral polymerase acidic endonuclease, a protein that plays a critical role in influenza virus RNA replication. Baloxavir is given orally and tends to be better tolerated than oseltamivir.

HERPESVIRUS MEDICATIONS

Another virus that can lead to a variety of symptoms and complications is the herpes simplex virus (HSV). HSV can be divided into two types, HSV-1 and HSV-2. Additional viruses within the herpes family include cytomegalovirus (CMV), Epstein-Barr virus (EBV), and varicella zoster virus (VZV). The herpesvirus can cause an array of infections affecting various body structures, including genital, orolabial, dermatologic, and ocular. Agents used to treat HSV-1 and HSV-2 include acyclovir, famiciclovir, and valacyclovir. Acyclovir and related agents work by inhibiting DNA polymerase, stopping viral DNA synthesis.

HEPATITIS MEDICATIONS

Hepatis B infections are susceptible to reverse transcriptase inhibitors since hepatitis B virus (HBV) uses reverse transcriptase in its infective life cycle. The reverse transcriptase inhibitors tenofovir, lamivudine, adefovir, and entecavir treat hepatitis B infections. Interferon-a2b and peginterferon-a2a are also used in the treatment of hepatitis B.

COMBINATION MEDICATIONS USED IN ORAL TREATMENT REGIMES

Trade name	Drug combinations
Epclusa and generic	Sofosbuvir/velpatasvir
Zepatier	Elbasvir/grazoprevir
Harvoni and generic	Ledipasvir/sofosbuvir
Mavyret	Glecaprevir/pibrentasvir
Vosevi	Sofosbuvir/velpatasvir/voxilaprevir
Viekira Pak	Ombitasvir/paritaprevir/ritonavir/dasabuvir

Originally, hepatitis C treatment includes a regimen of pegylated interferon alpha-2a in combination with ribavirin, an antiviral. Ribavirin inhibits viral protein synthesis by preventing both replication of viral genome and elongation of RNA fragments. Interferons are signaling molecules that induce antiviral responses within noninfected cells, making them more difficult for the virus to infect them and spread. Unfortunately, these regimens are poorly tolerated and while they reduce viral load, they almost never cure the disease.

The advent of direct acting antivirals revolutionized hepatis C treatment. Oral medications that inhibit hepatitis C viral replication and protein processing can completely drive the hepatitis C virus (HCV) from the body.

There are three categories of direct acting antivirals: (1) NS5B inhibitors; (2) NS5A inhibitors; and (3) HCV protease inhibitors. NS5A and NS5B are two HCV-encoded proteins that form an RNA dependent RNA polymerase that replicate HCV genomic RNA. The HCV protease processes the initially synthesized large HCV "polyprotein" into smaller, functional proteins that drive HCV replication and infection. Inhibition of either the HCV RNA-dependent RNA polymerase or the HCV protease shuts down viral replication. NS5B inhibitors include sofosbuvir and dasabuvir. Velpatasvir, ledipasvir, pibrentasvir, and ombitasvir are the available NS5A inhibitors, HCV protease inhibitors include grazoprevir, glecaprevir, voxilaprevir, and paritaprevir. There are also combination medications that conveniently combine these drugs into combination oral treatment regimens.

IMPACT

The antivirals covered here represent some of the most common antivirals used. Viral diseases that respond to antiviral treatment include HIV and AIDS, influenza, HSV, and viral hepatitis. Mechanisms of action vary among agents, even those used to treat a specific virus. It is important that the differentiation between bacterial and viral pathology is made by clinicians to correctly treat ailments that may have similar presentations.

—*Allison C. Bennett, PharmD*

Further Information

Aberg, Judith A., Jonathan E. Kaplan, and H. Libman. "Primary Care Guidelines for the Management of Persons Infected with Human Immunodeficiency Virus." *Clinical Infectious Diseases*, vol. 49, no. 5, 2009, pp. 651-81. Comprehensive guidelines for the treatment of HIV, including treatment-naïve and treatment-experienced regimens. Includes first-line agent recommendations and drug information of the treatments covered.

Clerq, Eric De. "Antiviral Drugs in Current Clinical Use." *Journal of Clinical Virology*, vol. 30, 2004, pp. 115-33. Thorough discussion of the mechanism of action of antivirals used for various disease states. Includes chemical compound structure and some pharmacokinetic and pharmacodynamic information.

Driscoll, John S. *Antiviral Drugs*. John Wiley & Sons, 2006. Presents the most commonly used antiviral drugs and discusses the mechanisms by which the drugs exert their therapeutic effects.

Gallagher, Jason C., and Conan MacDougall. *Antibiotics Simplified*. 4th ed., Jones and Bartlett Learning, 2016. A beautifully organized and easily understood compendium of antibiotics and how to use them.

Mahy, Brian W. J., and Marc H. V. van Regenmortel, editors. *Desk Encyclopedia of Human and Medical Virology*. Academic Press/Elsevier, 2010. Describes common and rare viruses in detail, along with their treatments.

Whalen, Karen. *Pharmacology*. (Lippincott Illustrated Reviews Series). 7th ed., Lippincott Williams & Wilkins, 2018. Designed as a refresher for people already familiar with the basics of pharmacology, but also has a very good section on antiviral agents.

Yost, Raymond, et al. "A Coreceptor CCR5 Antagonist for Management of HIV Infection." *American Journal of Health-System Pharmacy*, vol. 66, no. 8, Apr. 2009, pp. 715-26. Covers the pharmacology of maraviroc, including mechanism of action, pharmacology, pharmacokinetics, and clinical efficacy. Also covers its place in therapy in the treatment of HIV/AIDS.

BIOLOGICAL THERAPIES

Category: Treatment
Also known as: Biological agents, biological response modifiers, biotherapy, immunotherapy
Anatomy or system affected: Blood, cells, immune system, lymphatic system
Specialties and related fields: Alternative medicine, biotechnology, genetics, hematology, immunology, oncology, pathology
Definition: Treatments that use natural substances from the immune system to fight disease or infections or to overcome side effects from other treatments.

KEY TERMS

cancer: any malignant cellular tumor
cytokine: small proteins released by cells that have specific effects on cell-cell interactions, communication, and behavior of other cells
immunotherapy: therapy using antibodies or other immune system components or using antigens designed to stimulate an immune response to a tumor

INDICATIONS AND PROCEDURES

Biological therapies are treatments designed to improve or restore the ability of the immune system to fight disease and infection and help protect the body from the side effects of other treatments. The immune system includes different types of cells that fight diseases such as cancer, diabetes, rheumatoid arthritis, and Crohn's disease. The immune system consists of organs and structures that include the spleen, lymph nodes, bone marrow, tonsils, and white blood cells. The different types of white blood cells play an especially important role in fighting disease. They include B and T lymphocytes and natural killer (NK) lymphocytes. B-cell lymphocytes produce antibodies that attack other cells, and T-cell lymphocytes directly attack diseased cells and signal other immune system cells to defend the body. The NK cells make chemicals that bind to and kill foreign invaders in the body.

In addition to B, T, and NK cells, the immune system has white blood cells called "monocytes" that engulf and digest foreign invaders. Dendritic cells transport and deliver foreign cells to other immune system cells. Lymphocytes and monocytes are produced in the bone marrow and are later distributed into the bloodstream to be available to every part of the body. They allow for the protection from cancer and other diseases and invaders to the body. The immune system secretes two types of substances to fight disease: antibodies and cytokines. Antibodies respond to foreign invaders that they recognize, called "antigens." An antibody is found to match or recognize a specific antigen and attach itself to the antigen to give an immune response. Cytokines are proteins produced by the immune system to directly attack cells and are considered messenger cells, as they communicate with other cells to form a response. This type of therapy, therefore, is designed in part to boost the immune response, both directly and indirectly, to make the immune system respond to sick or tumorous cells.

There are four goals of biological therapy. The first is to make the immune system better able to recognize abnormal cells to destroy them, prevent them from spreading or make them more like healthy cells. The second is to stop the process that converts normal cells to cancer cells. The third is to improve the body's ability to repair or replace damaged cells. The fourth is to stop side effects caused by other forms of cancer treatments, such as chemotherapy and radiation.

USES AND COMPLICATIONS

There are different types of biological therapies whose method of treatment will vary depending on what type of cancer or other disease is involved, how far the disease has spread, and what other treatments are used. The types of biological therapies that are utilized today are predominately for treating cancer patients. These therapies include monoclonal antibodies, cancer vaccines, growth factors, cancer growth inhibitors, anti-angiogenics, interferons and interleukins, and gene therapy.

Monoclonal antibodies are specific antibodies developed in a laboratory that recognize only a single type of antigen or foreign invader in the body. Antigens are typically found on the surface of various cancer cells, and by producing specific antibodies for these antigens, one can selectively attack cancer cells of interest. A monoclonal antibody can also be programmed to act against cell growth factors, thereby interfering with the growth of cancer cells. Monoclonal antibodies can be developed to react with anticancer drugs or other toxins by attaching to the cancer cell and aiding in the destruction of that cell. Monoclonal antibodies can also carry radioisotopes that, when attached to a cancer cell, will identify that cell and the specific cancer type. Examples of monoclonal antibodies approved by the Food and Drug Administration (FDA) include rituximab (Rituxan) and trastuzumab (Herceptin). Rituxan treats non-Hodgkin's lymphomas, and Herceptin is

Different Types of Therapeutic Monoclonal Antibodies for Autoimmune Diseases

Trade Name	International Non-proprietary Name (INN)	Target	Therapeutic Indication(s)
Amjevita®	Adalimumab	TNFα	Ankylosing spondylitis, rheumatoid arthritis, ulcerative colitis, Crohn's disease; psoriatic arthritis, psoriasis
Zinplava™	Bezlotoxumab	*C. difficile* toxin B	Enterocolitis, pseudomembranous
Dupixent®	Dupilumab	IL-4Rα	Asthma; dermatitis
Ocrevus™	Ocrelizumab	CD20	Multiple sclerosis
Siliq	Brodalumab	IL-17RA	Psoriasis
Cinqair™	Reslizumab	IL-5	Asthma
Portrazza	Necitumumab	EGFR	Carcinoma, non-small-cell lung
Inflectra	Infliximab	TNFα	Ankylosing spondylitis, rheumatoid arthritis, ulcerative colitis, Crohn's disease; psoriatic arthritis, psoriasis
Anthim®	Obiltoxaximab	PA component of *B. anthracis* toxin	Anthrax infection
Cosentyx™	Secukinumab	interleukin-17A	Psoriatic arthritis, psoriasis, ankylosing spondylitis
Nucala	Mepolizumab	IL-5	Asthma
Praluent	Alirocumab	PCSK9	Dyslipidemias
Praxbind®	Idarucizumab	dabigatran etexilate	Hemorrhage
Repatha®	Evolocumab	LDL-C/PCSK9	Dyslipidemias; hypercholesterolemia
Entyvio®	Vedolizumab	Integrin-α4β7	Ulcerative colitis, Crohn's disease
Lemtrada®	Alemtuzumab	CD52	Multiple sclerosis
Remsima®	Infliximab	TNF-alpha	Ankylosing spondylitis, rheumatoid arthritis, ulcerative colitis, Crohn's disease; psoriatic arthritis, psoriasis
ABthrax®	Raxibacumab	*Bacillus anthracis* protective antigen	Prevention and treatment of inhalation anthrax
Benlysta®	Belimumab	BLyS	Systemic lupus erythematosus (SLE)
Xgeva®	Denosumab	RANKL	Prevention of SREs in patients with bone metastases from solid tumors
Prolia®	Denosumab	RANKL	Osteoporosis
RoActemra®	Tocilizumab	IL-6 receptor	Rheumatoid arthritis
Ilaris®	Canakinumab	IL-1ß	Cryopyrin-associated periodic syndromes including familial cold autoinflammatory syndrome and Muckle-Wells syndrome; tumor necrosis factor receptor-associated periodic syndrome (TRAPS), hyperimmunoglobulin D Syndrome (HIDS)/mevalonate kinase deficiency (MKD), and familial Mediterranean fever (FMF)

Different types of therapeutic monoclonal antibodies for autoimmune diseases (continued)

Trade Name	International Non-proprietary Name (INN)	Target	Therapeutic Indication(s)
Simponi®	Golimumab	TNFα	Rheumatoid arthritis, psoriatic arthritis, ankylosing spondylitis
Stelara®	Ustekinumab	IL-12/IL-23	Plaque psoriasis
Cimzia®	Certolizumab pegol	TNFα	Crohn's disease; rheumatoid arthritis
Soliris®	Eculizumab	Complement C5	Paroxysmal nocturnal hemoglobinuria
Lucentis®	Ranibizumab	VEGF-A	Neovascular (wet) age-related macular degeneration, macular edema following retinal vein occlusion
Tysabri®	Natalizumab	VLA-4	Multiple sclerosis (relapsing), Crohn's disease
Xolair®	Omalizumab	IgE	Asthma
Erbitux®	Cetuximab	EGFR	Head and neck cancer, colorectal cancer
Raptiva®	Efalizumab	CD11a	Psoriasis
Humira®	Adalimumab	TNFα	Ankylosing spondylitis, rheumatoid arthritis, ulcerative colitis, Crohn's disease; psoriatic arthritis, psoriasis
Remicade®	Infliximab	TNFα	Ankylosing spondylitis, rheumatoid arthritis, ulcerative colitis, Crohn's disease; psoriatic arthritis, psoriasis
Synagis®	Palivizumab	F-protein of RS virus	Respiratory syncytial virus (RSV)
Daclizumab	Necitumumab	CD25 (a chain of IL2 receptor)	Reversal of transplantation rejection
Simulect®	Basiliximab	CD25 (a chain of IL2 receptor)	Reversal of transplantation rejection
ReoPro®	Abciximab	GPIIb/IIIa	High-risk angioplasty (prevention of blood clots)
Orthoclone OKT3®	Muromonab-CD3	CD3	Transplantation rejection

used to treat breast cancers that overproduce the HER2 (ERBB2) gene product.

Anti-inflammatory monoclonal antibodies treat autoimmune disorders. Antitumor necrosis factor-alpha antibodies, such as adalimumab, infliximab, golimumab, and certolizumab treat juvenile rheumatoid arthritis, psoriatic arthritis, rheumatoid arthritis, ulcerative colitis, Crohn's disease, psoriasis, psoriatic arthritis, and ankylosing spondylitis. Anti-interleukin-6 antibodies, such as tocilizumab (Actemra) and sarilumab (Kevzara) treat rheumatoid arthritis. Ustekinumab (Stelara) is an anti-interleukin-12 & -23 antibody that treats plaque psoriasis. Secukinumab (Cosentyx) and ixekizumab (Talz) are anti-interleukin-17A antibodies that treat plaque psoriasis.

Vaccines are another type of biological therapy that is widely used to prevent diseases, such as influenza, mumps, measles, and other infectious diseases. Vaccines are defined as substances that are used to help protect individuals from infection or disease. Cancer vaccines are currently being developed and are in use for only a few cancer types, such as human papillomavirus (HPV), which may give rise to cervical cancer, and Bacillus Calmette-Guérin (BCG), which is a vaccine typically used for tuberculosis but is a therapeutic vaccine for bladder cancer. Two other therapeutic cancer vaccines include sipuleucel-T (Provenge) for prostate cancer and talimogene laherparepvec (Imlygic) for melanoma. Sipuleucel-T consists of white blood cells isolated from the patient's peripheral blood that are exposed to an antigen found on the surfaces of prostate cancer cells. Reinfusion of the white cells into the patient provides their body with cells completely geared toward identifying and destroying prostate cancer cells. Talimogene is a genetically engineered herpes virus that infects and destroys cancer cells and marks the cancer cells for destruction by the immune system.

New biological vaccines for COVID-19 include mRNA-based vaccines that contain modified mRNAs encased in a lipid nanoparticle. The mRNAs encode the spike protein of SARS-CoV-2, the virus that causes COVID-19, and elicits a robust immune response against it. Other COVID-19 vaccines consist of genetically engineered adenoviruses that infect cells and express SARS-CoV-2 genes in the host cells. The immune system mounts an immune response against the SARS-CoV-2 gene products, which protects the patient from COVID-19.

The advantage of a vaccine is that it can trigger an immune response in the body. White blood cells in the body can make antibodies that will recognize the proteins in the vaccine, whether the vaccine is from a virus, bacterium, or cancer cell. The antibodies will then be available to fight those antigens and prevent or decrease the impact of the disease.

Growth factors are considered biological therapies because they are natural substances in the body that are used to stimulate the bone marrow to produce blood cells. Growth factors are used in conjunction with other types of cancer treatments, since chemotherapy devastates both the normal and the diseased population of blood cells in a cancer patient as its means of killing the cancer cells, thus depleting the blood cells needed for health. After chemotherapy, growth factors can be given to a patient to boost blood counts and help fight infection and disease. Examples of growth factors are filgrastim (Neupogen) and pegylated G-CSF (Neulasta).

Cancer growth inhibitors or blockers are natural substances that can block a growth factor that will otherwise trigger a cancer cell to divide and grow. Growth factors that reside on the surface of cancer cells include epidermal growth factor (EGF) and fibroblast growth factor (FGF), which control cell growth, and platelet-derived growth factor (PDGF), which controls blood vessel development and cell growth. Each of these growth factors has a specific receptor molecule on the cell surface of the cancer cell, such as epidermal growth factor receptor (EGFR). Most cancer cell inhibitors currently used block the signaling pathway of receptors, such as tyrosine kinase inhibitors and proteasome inhibitors. Examples of tyrosine kinase inhibitors are imatinib (Gleevec), used to treat chronic myeloid leukemia (CML), and bortezomib (Velcade), used to treat melanoma. Because CML cells have a fusion protein (BCR-ABL) not found in normal cells, tyrosine kinase inhibitors (TKIs) specifically inhibit CML without adversely affecting other cells. If the CML becomes resistant to imatinib, newer TKIs like dasatinib (Sprycel), nilotinib (Tasigna), bosutinib (Bosulif), and ponatinib (Iclusig) are designed to inhibit the mutant version of the fusion protein.

Anti-angiogenics are substances that block cancer blood vessel growth. Angiogenesis is the process of growing new blood vessels. Anti-angiogenic drugs prevent tumors from growing blood vessels. Since cancer cells need a blood supply to continue their growth and division process, blocking blood vessel growth starves the tumor for nutrients and oxygen. Anti-angiogenic drugs inhibit the growth factor vascular endothelial growth factor (VEGF) from reaching blood vessels, preventing remodeling of the blood supply to the tumor. Anti-angiogenic drugs include anti-VEGF monoclonal antibodies, such as bevacizumab (Avastin), ranibizumab (Lucentis), and brolucizumab (Beovu), and VEGF decoys, such as aflibercept (Eylea). Anti-VEGF medications also prevent the growth of extra blood vessels in patients with diabetic macular edema (DME), retinal vein occlusion, and diabetic retinopathy. One example of an anti-angiogenic drug is thalidomide, which affects the chemicals that cells use to signal one another. This drug has proven helpful in treating melanoma and other cancers.

Interferons and interleukins are substances that are part of the body's immune response, called "cytokines." These cytokines work by interfering with the growth and cell division of cancer cells, by stimulating an immune response and enhancing the ability of killer T cells and other cells to attack and kill cancer cells, and by encouraging the cancer cell to produce chemicals that attract the immune system to them. Interferons and interleukin-2 are used to treat cancers such as melanoma, multiple myeloma, and some types of leukemia. Interleukins made from genetically engineered cells include recombinant alpha interferons, such as alfa-2a (Roferon-A) or alfa-2b (Intron A), that treat chronic viral hepatitis. Recombinant beta-interferons, Avonex, Rebif, and Betaseron, treat multiple sclerosis. Modified alpha-interferons conjugated with polyethylene glycol (pegylated-interferon; PEG-Intron), in combination with ribavirin, treats chronic hepatitis C infections.

Gene therapies are currently experimental, but they have potential in the treatment of cancers and other diseases. Genes are made up of strands of deoxyribonucleic acid (DNA), which are coded messages for various functions in the body. Normal cells have a set of genes that are needed for normal growth, development, and maintenance of the body's systems and functions. Cancer cells differ from normal cells in that a genetic mutation has occurred that gives rise to uncontrolled cell growth and division. The advantage of gene therapy is that it targets specific cancer cells, thereby not affecting normal cells that would otherwise be destroyed by conventional therapies.

Presently available gene therapies include onasemnogene abeparvovec-xioi (Zolgensma), which is an adeno-associated virus vector-based gene therapy for children years old who have spinal muscular atrophy (SMA). SMA is an inherited disorder that causes degeneration of alpha motor neurons in the spinal cord leading to muscle weakness and atrophy. This treatment improves motor function and prolongs survival without the need for permanent assisted ventilation but the durability of this treatment remains uncertain. The second gene therapy for SMA is nusinersen (Spinraza), an antisense oligonucleotide that fixes the processing problems with SMN2 messenger RNAs, increasing the synthesis of SMN protein. A drug that works similarly to nusinersen is Risdiplam (Evrysdi), which also treats SMA. Finally, voretigene neparvovec-rzyl (Luxturna) is a treatment for inherited retinal dystrophy. This nonreplicating, recombinant adeno-associated virus serotype 2 vector infects retinal cells and drives the expression of the human *RPE65* gene. Inherited retinal dystrophies result from gene defects in photoreceptors and retinal pigment epithelial (RPE) cells. Mutations in over 200 different genes cause inherited retinal dystrophies. Two copies of mutations in the RPE65 gene affect about 1,000 to 3,000 persons in the United States. Injection of voretigene neparvovec-rzyl into the subretinal space can restore the expression of RPE65 in these retinal cells and the visual function of retinal cells.

Side effects are associated with each type of biological therapy. They vary depending on the individual's medical history, diagnosis, and type of therapy. Each person may react differently to specific treatments. Biological therapies often cause flu-like symptoms, such as chills, fever, muscle aches, nausea, vomiting and diarrhea, bone pain, loss of appetite, and fatigue. Other side effects may include rashes, bleeding or bruising easily, and low levels of blood cells. Swelling at the injection site is also common. Side effects may be severe, mild, or absent. If they are significant, then patients may need to stay in the hospital during treatment. Side effects do not often last long, and they usually go away after the completion of treatment. Allergic reactions may have additional symptoms.

Certain treatments can be given to control side effects, such as Neupogen or G-CSF to increase white blood cell counts and help prevent infection in patients who use chemotherapy; Procrit, Epogen, or erythropoietin to increase red blood cell counts in patients who develop anemia; and IL-11, interleukin-11, or Oprelvekin (Neumega) to increase platelet counts. Paracetamol or antihistamine given before the first treatment prevents an allergic reaction.

PERSPECTIVE AND PROSPECTS
Biological therapies have been investigated for many years as an important advance in the treatment of cancer and other diseases. It could be said that biological therapies have been in use for more than two hundred years with the discovery of immunization by Edward Jenner to treat a disease called "vaccinia," or cowpox. Around the beginning of the twentieth century, William B. Coley began treating cancer patients with bacteria to build an immune response. This approach, which became known as Coley toxins, was used for decades with great success. In 1908, Paul Ehrlich received the Nobel Prize in Physiology or Medicine for his work on biotherapies by discovering receptor molecules (antigens) that reside on cell surfaces that can attach to antibodies, triggering the release of antitoxins to fight disease. Work on biological therapies continued in the 1980s when clinical trials demonstrated the efficacy of interferon against hairy-cell leukemia. This treatment became FDA approved for this and other cancer disorders such as chronic myeloid leukemia, acquired immunodeficiency syndrome (AIDS)-related Kaposi's sarcoma, and genital warts. Further work on cytokines gave rise to interleukin treatment for kidney cancer, metastatic cancer, and AIDS.

Further developments have led to many treatments for cancer, viral diseases, and autoimmune disorders. With current technologies in genetics, more information about the genetic basis of cancer has led to advances in biological therapies for more than two hundred types of cancer. Most therapies to date do not target a specific genetic makeup. However, new treatments are arising that can target specific genetic mutations that have become known. For example, Herceptin can treat HER2-positive metastatic breast cancer, and MabThera treats non-Hodgkin's lymphoma. This individualized type of therapy will not only improve the management of different diseases but also decrease the toxicity of treatment that results from an individual's genetic makeup. Most of what is used today for biological therapies is just the beginning, with the future holding tremendous promise for continued success with these treatments.

—*Susan M. Zneimer, PhD, FACMG*

Further Information
An, Zhiqiang. Therapeutic Monoclonal Antibodies: From Bench to Clinic. Wiley, 2009.
Black Jacquelyn G., and Laura J. Black. Microbiology. 10th ed., Wiley, 2018.
Danquah, Michael K., and Mahato, Ram I., editors. Emerging Trends in Cell and Gene Therapy. Humana Press, 2013.

De Vita, Vincent T., Jr., Samuel Hellman, and Steven A. Rosenberg, editors. Principles and Practice of Oncology. 11th ed., Lippincott Williams & Wilkins, 2018.

Fischer, David S., et al. The Cancer Chemotherapy Handbook. 6th ed., Mosby, 2003.

Hawkins Robert E. Cellular Therapy of Cancer: Development of Gene Therapy Based Approaches. World Scientific, 2013.

Lattime, Edmund C., and Stanton L. Gerson. Gene Therapy of Cancer: Translational Approaches from Preclinical Studies to Clinical Implementation. Academic Press, 2013.

Rosenberg, Steven A., editor. Principles and Practice of the Biologic Therapy of Cancer. 3rd ed., Lippincott Williams & Wilkins, 2000.

Scherman, Daniel, editor. Advanced Textbook on Gene Transfer, Gene Therapy and Genetic Pharmacology: Principles, Delivery and Pharmacological and Biomedical Applications of Nucleotide-based Therapies. 2nd ed., World Scientific Publishing Europe Ltd., 2019.

Stern, Peter L., Peter C. L. Beverley, and Miles W. Carroll, editors. Cancer Vaccines and Immunotherapy. Cambridge UP, 2000.

Templeton, Nancy Smyth, editor. Gene and Cell Therapy: Therapeutic Mechanisms and Strategies. 4th ed., CRC Press, 2015.

Williams, J. "Principles of Genetics and Cancer." Seminars in Oncology Nursing, vol. 13, no. 2, 1997, pp. 68-73.

CORTICOSTEROIDS

Category: Biology
Also known as: Glucocorticoids, mineralocorticoids
Anatomy or system affected: Endocrine system, immune system
Specialties and related fields: Biochemistry, endocrinology, family medicine, immunology
Definition: Steroid hormones such as cortisol and aldosterone are synthesized and secreted by the adrenal cortex and the synthetic equivalents of adrenal steroids.

KEY TERMS

Addison's disease: a disease characterized by hypoadrenalism caused by cortisol deficiency

cortisol: a steroid hormone of the adrenal cortex that has many physiological actions

Cushing's syndrome: a disorder characterized by hyperadrenalism caused by an excess secretion or exogenous administration of cortisol

glucocorticoid: a steroid hormone such as cortisol from the adrenal cortex that has many physiological actions, including the regulation of glucose metabolism

mineralocorticoid: a steroid hormone from the adrenal cortex that regulates salt and water balance

STRUCTURE AND FUNCTIONS

Corticosteroids are steroid hormones produced by the cortex of the adrenal glands. They have several physiological actions, including regulating glucose, lipid, and protein metabolism, regulating inflammation and the immune response, maintaining homeostasis during stress, and controlling water and electrolyte balance and blood pressure.

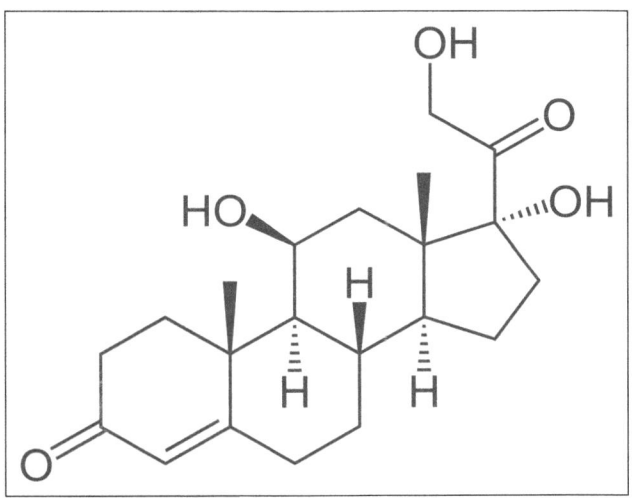

Cortisol (hydrocortisone), a corticosteroid with both glucocorticoid and mineralocorticoid activity and effects. Image via Wikimedia Commons. [Public domain.]

Corticosteroids that have their primary effects on glucose metabolism are glucocorticoids. Cortisol is the primary glucocorticoid, although the adrenal cortex also secretes significant amounts of corticosterone and cortisone. In contrast, those that control electrolyte and water balance are mineralocorticoids. Aldosterone is the primary mineralocorticoid.

Topical Corticosteroids

Potency	Corticosteroid
Super-high	augmented betamethasone dipropionate (0.05% ointment) clobetasol propionate (0.05% cream) fluocinonide (0.1% cream) halobetasol propionate (0.05% cream)
High	amcinonide (0.1% ointment) clobetasol propionate (Impoyz; 0.025% cream) desoximetasone (0.25% cream & 0.05% gel) diflorasone diacetate (0.05% ointment) fluocinonide (0.05% ointment, gel, cream, & solution) halcinonide (Halog; 0.1% cream & ointment) mometasone furoate (0.1% ointment).
Medium-high	amcinonide (0.1% cream) desoximetasone (0.05% cream) diflorasone diacetate (0.05% cream) fluocinonide emollient (0.05% cream) fluticasone propionate (0.005% ointment) triamcinolone acetonide (0.5% ointment)
Medium	betamethasone valerate (0.12% foam) fluocinolone acetonide (0.025% ointment) flurandrenolide (0.05% ointment) hydrocortisone valerate (0.2% ointment) triamcinolone acetonide (0.1% ointment & cream) triamcinolone acetonide (Trianex; 0.05% ointment)
Medium-Low	Desonide (0.05% ointment) Fluocinolone acetonide (0.025% cream) Flurandrenolide (0.05% cream) Fluticasone propionate (0.05% cream & lotion) Hydrocortisone butyrate (0.1% cream & ointment) Hydrocortisone probutate (0.1% cream) Hydrocortisone valerate (0.2% cream) Prednicarbate (0.1% cream & ointment)
Low	Alclometasone dipropionate (0.05% cream) Clocortolone pivalate (0.1% cream) Desonide (0.05% cream, lotion, and gel) Fluocinolone acetonide (0.01% cream) Triamcinolone acetonide (0.025% cream & lotion)

Glucocorticoids promote an increase in blood glucose by stimulating the synthesis of glucose (gluconeogenesis). They also stimulate the catabolism of lipids and proteins. Thus, glucocorticoids increase blood glucose and are antagonistic to insulin.

Adrenocorticotropic hormone (ACTH) produced by the pituitary gland controls the synthesis of corticosteroids. Corticotropin-releasing hormone (CRH) produced by the hypothalamus controls the secretion of ACTH. A feedback loop exists so that high cortisol levels inhibit the release of CRH and ACTH, and when cortisol levels are low, CRH and ACTH are released.

Aldosterone is primarily responsible for controlling salt and water balance by promoting the excretion of potassium and the retention of sodium and water. Through its effect on salt and water balance, aldosterone can increase blood pressure. Plasma levels of aldosterone are controlled by various mechanisms, including plasma volume and potassium ion concentration.

DISORDERS AND DISEASES

Addison's disease results from adrenal insufficiency (hypocortisolism). Although adrenal gland dysfunction (primary adrenal insufficiency) causes most cases, some are caused by a pituitary gland disorder (secondary adrenal insufficiency). An autoimmune disorder that destroys the adrenal cortex is the major cause of primary adrenal insufficiency. A lack of ACTH usually causes secondary adrenal insufficiency. Pituitary tumors, surgical removal of the pituitary, and loss of blood flow to the pituitary are the major causes of secondary adrenal insufficiency. The main symptoms of adrenal insufficiency include loss of appetite, weight loss, fatigue, muscle weakness, and hypotension. Endocrinologists diagnose Addison's disease by administering ACTH and monitoring the adrenal gland's response by measuring serum and urine cortisol levels. The oral administration of hydrocortisone, a synthetic form of cortisol, treats adrenal insufficiency. If aldosterone is also deficient, then fludrocortisone is administered.

Adrenal insufficiency is often caused by a mutation in one of the enzymes synthesizing cortisol. These cases are referred to as congenital adrenal hyperplasia (CAH). Since serum cortisol is low or absent, the pituitary gland stimulates the adrenal gland to produce more cortisol. The precursor steroids and their metabolic products can cause varying degrees of virilization of female fetuses and infants. Replacement therapy is the treatment of choice. Surgery to reconstruct the genital organs may be necessary in severe cases.

Diagnosis of Cushing's syndrome is most commonly made by determining the amount of cortisol in the urine. Hypercortisolism can lead to Cushing's syndrome. The main symptoms include obesity, osteoporosis, fatigue, hypertension, hyperglycemia, and amenorrhea (absence of menstruation). Cushing's syndrome may be caused by prolonged use of glucocorticoids or by an overproduction of glucocorticoids by the adrenal glands. The most frequent cause of glucocorticoid overproduction is pituitary and adrenal tumors. Physicians treat Cushing's syndrome by reducing administered glucocorticoids or destroying the tumor responsible for the disease by surgical removal, radiation, or chemotherapy.

Hypoaldosteronism is a condition in which the adrenal cortex does not produce an adequate amount of aldosterone, which results in an inability to control and regulate blood volume and blood pressure. Blood pressure can fall to dangerously low levels.

THE USE OF CORTICOSTEROIDS

Glucocorticoid hormones, in addition to regulating glucose metabolism, also possess pronounced anti-inflammatory properties. Therefore, synthetic corticosteroids such as prednisone, prednisolone, methylprednisolone, hydrocortisone, and dexamethasone have immunosuppressive effects and are used to treat a variety of chronic autoimmune and inflammatory diseases. They can reduce the pain, swelling, itching, inflammation, and redness associated with arthritis, asthma, bursitis asthma, dermatitis, eczema and psoriasis, lupus erythematosus, Crohn's disease, ulcerative colitis, and various ear, eye, and skin infections, and allergic reactions. Corticosteroids are administered orally, by inhalers and intranasal sprays, as eye drops, topical creams and ointments, and injection.

Oral and intranasal corticosteroids for asthma, allergic rhinitis, or chronic obstructive pulmonary disease include the following drugs:
- Beclomethasone dipropionate (QVAR Redihaler)
- Budesonide (Pulmicort Flexhaler)
- Ciclesonide (Alvesco),
- Fluticasone furoate (Arnuity Ellipta),
- Fluticasone propionate (Flovent Diskus; Flovent HFA; ArmonAir Respiclick; ArmonAir Digihaler)
- Mometasone furoate (Asmanex HFA; Asmanex Twisthaler)

Combinations of inhaled corticosteroids and bronchodilators (e.g., Advair, Breo Ellipta, Symbicort) also relieve the symptoms of respiratory ailments.

Topical corticosteroids come in different potencies ranging from super-high potency, to high, to medium-high, to medium, to medium-low, to low potency.

Oral corticosteroids include cortisone acetate, dexamethasone, hydrocortisone, methylprednisolone, prednisolone, and prednisone.

CORTICOSTEROID ADVERSE EFFECTS

Corticosteroids have few side effects if used short-term and at low dosages. If used long-term, however, they do carry a risk of significant side effects. Oral corticosteroids have the highest risk of system side effects, and locally applied corticosteroids, the lowest. Side effects and their severity always depend on the dose and how long the patient takes them. Side effects of oral corticosteroids include:

- fluid retention, particularly in the ankles
- increased blood pressure
- psychiatric effects (mood swings, memory issues, and other mental disturbances)
- upset stomach
- weight gain on the abdomen, face (moon face), and neck.

The long-term effects of oral corticosteroids longer term include:

- elevated pressure in the eyes (glaucoma)
- thin skin, bruising, and slower wound healing
- cataracts—a clouding of the lens in one or both eyes
- a round face (moon face)
- high blood sugar, exacerbating or triggering diabetes
- increased infection risk
- thinning bones (osteoporosis) and fractures
- suppressed adrenal gland function—leading to severe fatigue, loss of appetite, nausea, and muscle weakness

Inhaled and intranasal corticosteroids do not cause high blood corticosteroid blood concentrations. However, oral corticosteroids can increase the risk of oral candidiasis, also known as oral thrush, and hoarseness. Gargling with water after use decreases the risk of these side effects. Topical corticosteroids do not produce high blood corticosteroid levels. However, they can cause thinning of the skin, acne, and red skin lesions.

Corticosteroid injections into joints help relieve the pain associated with osteoarthritis or rheumatoid arthritis. Corticosteroid injections can cause pain at the site of injection (postinjection flare), thinning of the skin, skin discoloration, and loss of color in the skin. Other potential side effects include facial flushing, insomnia, and high blood sugar. Injected corticosteroids also diminish cartilage repair and deposition in joints. For these reasons and others, physicians typically limit corticosteroid injections to three or four a year.

Systemically, prolonged use of corticosteroids can lead to medically induced Cushing's syndrome, suppression of the immune system, hypertension, hypokalemia (low serum potassium), and hypernatremia (high serum sodium).

DRUG-DRUG INTERACTIONS WITH CORTICOSTEROIDS

The liver, and to a lesser degree the small intestine, metabolize most drugs we take. The liver contains a battery of enzymes that metabolize drugs and other foreign molecules (xenobiotics) that enter our bodies. Of these drug-metabolizing enzymes, cytochrome P450s are the most important. Cytochrome P450s constitute an enzyme family of closely related, albeit distinct enzymes that metabolize a vast array of organic chemicals. Generally, cytochrome P450s catalyze reactions that make drugs more water-soluble so that the body can more easily eliminate them.

Drug metabolism, however, is not as simple as it sounds. Some drugs inhibit specific cytochrome P450 enzymes. Enzyme inhibitors can prevent the metabolism of other medications, raising the serum concentrations of those drugs and cause drug toxicities. For example, the macrolide antibiotic erythromycin inhibits cytochrome P450 3A4. Combining any other drug metabolized by cytochrome P450 3A4 with erythromycin risks drug toxicity. Cytochrome 3A4 metabolizes endogenous steroid hormones and steroid drugs. Therefore, combining erythromycin with prednisone or other corticosteroids prevents their metabolism and increases drug toxicity.

Other sets of drugs induce cytochrome P450 enzymes. These drugs supercharge the metabolism of drugs, reducing their half-lives and serum concentrations, causing treatment failure. The antituberculosis antibiotic rifampin induces cytochrome P450 3A4. Therefore, combining rifampin with corticosteroids causes increased corticosteroid metabolism and treatment failure.

Also, dietary and herbal supplements can interact with corticosteroids. Some protect against the potential side effects of corticosteroids, and others augment the biological effects of corticosteroids. Several supplements seem to counteract at least some of the side effects of corticosteroids. For example, calcium and vitamin D supplements protect against osteoporosis brought on by corticosteroids. Likewise, clinical trials have demonstrated that topical aloe and licorice augment the effects of topical corticosteroids. Chromium supplements seem to improve blood sugar levels in persons with corticosteroid-induced diabetes. Creatine supplements may attenuate corticosteroid-induced muscle loss. Ipriflavone supplements treat osteoporosis and reduce the progress of corticosteroid-induced osteoporosis. Some supplements have dubious efficacy even though many people take them. For example, some people take dehydroepiandrosterone (DHEA) to protect against the side effects of corticosteroids, even though no evidence exists for this practice. Other supplements, such as licorice, interact unpredictably with corticosteroids and should be avoided when taking corticosteroids.

PERSPECTIVE AND PROSPECTS

In 1855, Thomas Addison became the first physician to describe the clinical symptoms of adrenal insufficiency. In the early 1930s, Frank Hartman, Wilbur Swingle, and Joseph Pfiffner were the first to prepare active adrenal extracts capable of treating the symptoms of adrenal insufficiency. By the mid-1930s, Pfiffner, Edward Calvin Kendall, Oskar Wintersteiner, and Tadeus Reichstein had isolated and crystallized some of the adrenal hormones. In 1944, Lewis Sarett became the first to synthesize cortisone. In the late 1940s, Philip Showalter Hench discovered that the administration of cortisone could alleviate arthritis symptoms.

In recent years, it has been shown that corticosteroids express their effect by modulating the expression of various genes involved in many physiological functions, including metabolism and the immune or inflammatory response.

—*Charles L. Vigue, PhD and Michael A. Buratovich, PhD*

Further Information

Dikago, Antan Riux. *Commonly Asked Questions About Cushing Syndrome Finally Answered*. Author, 2020.

Holt, Elizabeth H., Beatrice Lupsa, Grace S. Lee, Hanan Bassyouni, and Harry Peery. *Goodman's Basic Medical Endocrinology*. 5th ed., Elsevier, 2021.

Jackson, Daniel J., and Leonard B. Bacharier. "Inhaled Corticosteroids for the Prevention of Asthma Exacerbations." *Annals of Allergy, Asthma & Immunology*, S1081-1206(21)00572-X, 13 Aug. 2021, doi:10.1016/j.anai.2021.08.014.

Jain, Shreshta, et al. "Management of COVID-19 in Patients with Seizures: Mechanisms of Action of Potential COVID-19 Drug Treatments and Consideration for Potential Drug-Drug Interactions with Anti-seizure Medications." *Epilepsy Research*, vol. 174, 2021, p. 106675, doi:10.1016/j.eplepsyres.2021.106675.

Kleine, Bernhard, and Winfried G. Rossmanith. *Hormones and the Endocrine System: Textbook of Endocrinology*. Springer, 2016.

Lüdecke, Dieter K., George P. Chrousos, and George Tolis, editors. *ACTH, Cushing's Syndrome, and Other Hypercortisolemic States*. Raven Press, 1990.

Mahler, Donald A. *COPD: Answers to Your Most Pressing Questions about Chronic Obstructive Pulmonary Disease*. Johns Hopkins UP, 2022.

Riedemann, Therese, Alexandre Patchev, Kwangook Cho, and Osborne F. X. Almeida. "Corticosteroids." *Molecular Brain*, vol. 3, 2020, pp. 2-21.

"Steroids." National Health Service (UK), 14 Jan. 2020, www.nhs.uk/conditions/steroids/. Accessed 22 Aug. 2021.

Vinson, Gavin P., Barbara Whitehouse, and Joy Hinson. *The Adrenal Cortex*. Prentice Hall, 1992.

Wagner, Carina, et al. "Systemic corticosteroids for the treatment of COVID-19." *The Cochrane Database of Systematic Reviews*, vol. 8, CD014963, 16 Aug. 2021, doi:10.1002/14651858.CD014963.

"What Are Corticosteroids?" *healthychildren.org*, 21 Jan. 2020. www.healthychildren.org/English/health-issues/conditions/allergies-asthma/Pages/Corticosteroids.aspx. Accessed 22 Aug 2021.

Decongestants

Category: Treatment
Anatomy or system affected: Circulatory system, ears, nose, respiratory system, throat
Specialties and related fields: Family medicine, otorhinolaryngology
Definition: Oral and topical medications used to relieve nasal and sinus congestion and promote the opening of collapsed Eustachian tubes.

KEY TERMS

adjunctive: referring to the treatment of symptoms associated with a condition, not the condition itself

contraindication: a condition that makes a particular treatment not advisable; contraindications may be absolute (should never be used) or relative (should be used only with caution when the benefits outweigh the potential problems)

evidence-based medicine: a method of basing clinical medical practice decisions on systematic reviews of published medical studies

systemic: affecting the entire body; systemic treatments may be administered orally, directly into a vein, into the muscle, or through mucous membranes

topical: referring to treatments applied directly to the skin or mucous membranes that affect primarily the area in which they are applied

upper respiratory tract: the nose, sinuses, throat, ears, Eustachian tubes, and trachea

INDICATIONS AND PROCEDURES

Decongestants are used to shrink inflamed mucous membranes, promote drainage, or open collapsed Eustachian tubes. They are often used to temporarily relieve congestion caused by an upper respiratory tract infection (a cold), a sinus infection, hay fever, and other nasal allergies by promoting both nasal and sinus drainage. They are also often used as adjunctive therapy in treating middle-ear infection (otitis media) to decrease congestion around the openings of the Eustachian tubes. They may relieve the ear pressure, blockage, and pain experienced by some people during air travel. Careful scientific evaluation of the effectiveness of decongestants, however, has shown somewhat contradictory results.

Decongestants stimulate specific receptors in the smooth muscle of the upper respiratory tract, leading to constriction of the blood vessels and shrinkage of the mucous membranes. Decreased mucus production improves airflow through the upper respiratory tract and relieves the sensation of stuffiness.

USES AND COMPLICATIONS

Decongestants may be applied topically, like sprays or drops, or taken by mouth. Commonly used decongestants include ephedrine, epinephrine, naphazoline, oxymetazoline, phenylephrine, pseudoephedrine, tetrahydrozoline, and xylometazoline. Some of these drugs are available over the counter and some by prescription only.

Elderly patients must use oral preparations with caution, as should children and people with high blood pressure or other cardiac problems. If used as directed, decongestants do not usually cause excessive increases in blood pressure, overstimulate the heart, or change the distribution of blood in the circulatory system. Topical preparations are safer because they are less likely to cause side effects. Nevertheless, all decongestants, whether taken orally or administered topically, should be used cautiously.

The significant advantage of oral decongestants is their long duration of action. Topical decongestants work more quickly but last a shorter period and are more likely to irritate the tissues to which they are applied. If used too often or for too long (more than three to five days), nasal preparations may lead to a condition called "rhinitis medicamentosa" or "rebound congestion," in which the congestion may be worse than before the person started using the medication.

People who take a specific type of antidepressant medication called a "monoamine oxidase inhibitor" (MAOI) and those with severe high blood pressure or heart disease should not take decongestants at all. People with thyroid disease, diabetes mellitus, glaucoma, or an enlarged prostate gland should take these drugs only after consulting a health-care professional. Specific decongestants are contraindicated in infants and children.

People who take excessive doses of decongestants or who take them with other drugs that stimulate the

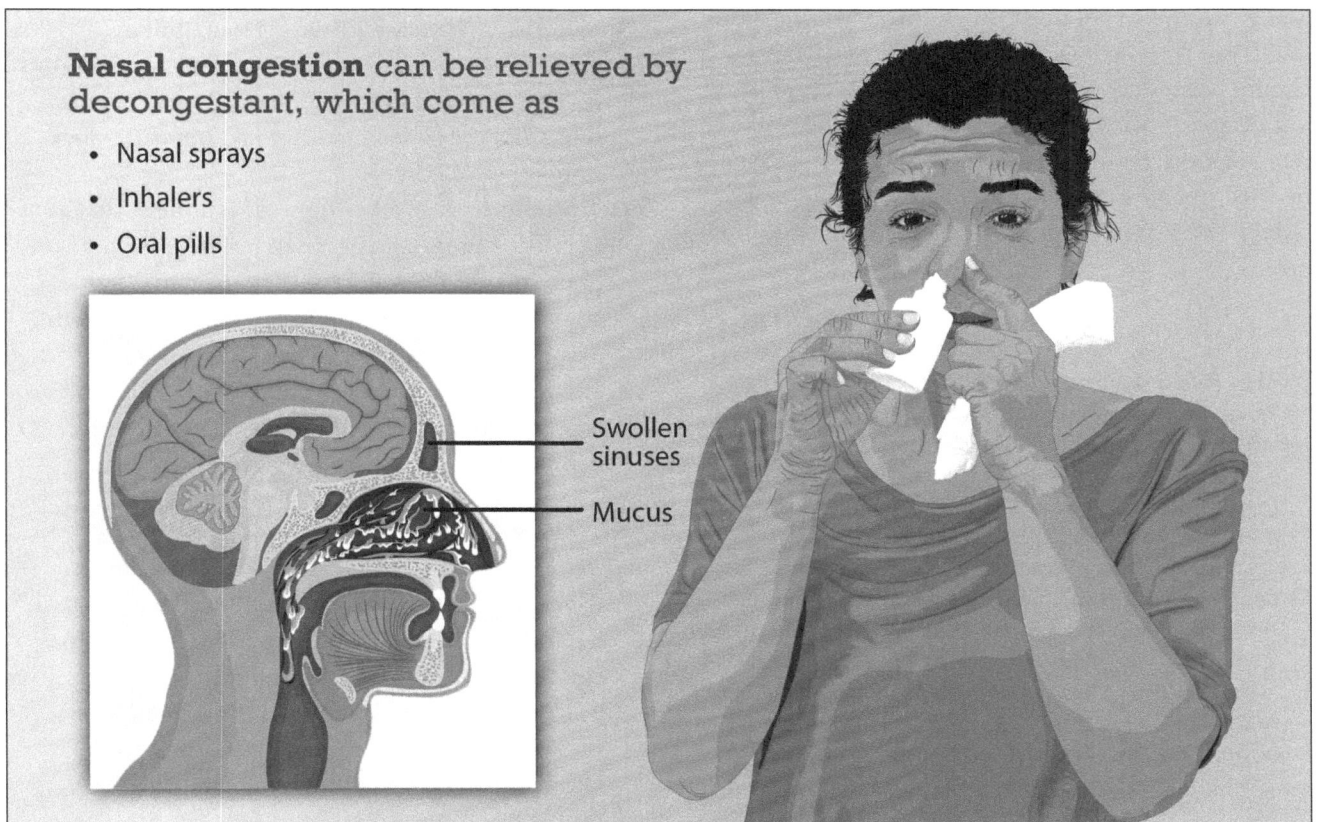

Person suffering from nasal congestion. Image by https://www.myupchar.com/en, via Wikimedia Commons. [CC 4.0.]

central nervous system may experience insomnia, restlessness, dizziness, tremors, or nervousness. Overdose or long-term use of high doses may lead to hallucinations, convulsions, cardiovascular collapse, or even death.

PERSPECTIVE AND PROSPECTS

Although decongestants have been widely used for decades, evidence-based medicine reveals few good studies indicating that decongestants do treat illnesses. Systematic and careful reviews of the scientific studies available in the medical literature suggest that a single dose of a decongestant may relieve the stuffiness associated with the common cold in adults. However, no evidence exists for the use of repeated doses. In people with a cough, a combination decongestant-antihistamine provides some relief in adults but not in children. In children with otitis media, there is a small statistical benefit from using a combination decongestant-antihistamine. Still, it is not clear that the children benefit clinically. An evidence-based medicine review suggests that they not be used in children, especially given the increased risk of side effects from these medications in this age group.

—*Rebecca Lovell Scott, PhD, PA-C*

Further Information

American Academy of Otolaryngology-Head and Neck Surgery. "Antihistamines, Decongestants, and Cold Remedies." *American Academy of Otolaryngology-Head and Neck Surgery*, Dec. 2010.

FamilyDoctor.org. "Decongestants: OTC Relief for Congestion." *FamilyDoctor.org*, Feb. 2012.

Flynn, C. A., G. Griffin, and F. Tudiver. "Decongestants and Antihistamines for Acute Otitis Media in Children." *The Cochrane Library*, Issue 4. John Wiley & Sons, 2003.

Komaroff, Anthony, editor. *Harvard Medical School Family Health Guide*. Free Press, 2005.

Lexicomp. *The Drug Information Handbook*. 26th ed., Lexi-Comp, 2017.

Marcdate, Karen, and Robert M. Kliegman. *Nelson Essentials of Pediatrics*. 8th ed., Elsevier, 2018.

Schroeder, K., and T. Fahey. "Over-the-Counter Medications for Acute Cough in Children and Adults in Ambulatory Settings." *The Cochrane Library*, Issue 4. John Wiley & Sons, 2003.

Taverner, D., L. Bickford, and M. Draper. "Nasal Decongestants for the Common Cold." *The Cochrane Library*, Issue 4. John Wiley & Sons, 2003.

IMMUNOTHERAPY

Category: Chemotherapy and Other Drugs
Also known as: Biological therapy, biotherapy
Anatomy or system affected: Blood, brain, eyes, gastrointestinal system, immune system, intestines, liver, lungs, lymphatic system, mouth, psychic-emotional system, reproductive system, respiratory system, skin, throat
Specialties and related fields: Dermatology, gastroenterology, gynecology, hematology, immunology, internal medicine, neurology, oncology, otorhinolaryngology, pathology, pharmacology, pulmonary medicine
Definition: Immunotherapy is a treatment that stimulates the immune system to fight cancer and reduce related side effects of the disease. Agents come from biological sources and may be given alone or combined with chemotherapy. Immunotherapies boost the patient's immune system to fight cancer cells, while chemotherapy drugs attack the cancer cells directly.

KEY TERMS

adoptive cell therapy: a type of immunotherapy in which T cells (a type of immune cell) are given to a patient to help the body fight diseases, such as cancer; also called cellular immunotherapy

immune modulator: a substance that stimulates or suppresses the immune system and may help the body fight cancer, infection, or other diseases

preventative vaccine: a vaccine to create immunity by introducing a weakened or killed form of a bacteria or virus, which the immune system uses to create antibodies

targeted antibodies: a form of cancer immunotherapy treatment that can disrupt cancer cell activity and alert the immune system to target and eliminate cancer cells

therapeutic vaccine: a vaccine administered after a disease or infection has already occurred; works by activating the immune system of a patient to fight an infection

CANCERS TREATED

Immunotherapy can treat a wide range of different cancers. To date, various types of immunotherapies Bladder cancer, brain, cancer, breast cancer, cervical cancer, childhood cancers, colorectal cancer, esophageal cancer, head and neck cancers, kidney cancers, leukemia, liver cancer, lung cancer, lymphoma, melanoma, multiple myeloma, myelomas, ovarian cancer, pancreatic cancer, prostate cancer, sarcoma, stomach cancer, skin cancer, and uterine (endometrial) cancer. Immunotherapy regimens for other cancers are currently under investigation.

SUBCLASSES OF THIS GROUP

Adoptive cell therapy or cellular immunotherapy uses the cells of our immune system to eliminate cancer. Cancer patients still maintain immune cells that can recognize and eliminate cancer cells. Solid tumors often turn immune cells off if they get too close. In such cases, the immune systems of cancer patients need to "relearn" how to recognize and kill cancer cells. Alternatively, immune cells need new weapons to battle cancers. Cellular immunotherapies take advantage of already existing immune cells in the bodies of cancer patients and redeploy them.

There are four main types of cellular immunotherapy: tumor-infiltrating lymphocyte (TIL) therapy, engineered T-cell receptor (TCR) therapy, chimeric antigen receptor (CAR) therapy, and natural killer (NK) cell therapy. TIL therapy harvests T cells that have already infiltrated patients' tumors and then, in the laboratory, activates and expands them and infuses them back into the patient. These activated T cells seek out and destroy tumors. TCR goes one step further than TIL. Instead of harvesting, activating, and reintroducing T cells, TCR gives those harvested T cells a set of genetically engineered T-cell receptor genes. Therefore, the harvested T cells acquire a new surface protein with which they can recognize the tumor cells, become activated, and destroy the tumor CAR cells stretch the boundaries of immunotherapy even further. Harvested T cells from the cancer patient are genetically engineered to make a receptor that sticks to a cancer cell-specific protein. When this chimeric receptor sticks, it stimulates the T cell to kill the tumor cell. Since chimeric receptors only recognize proteins on the surfaces of cancer cells, they are a specific weapon against cancers. Finally, NK cell therapy uses genetically engineered natural killer cells that express chimeric antigen receptors that empower them to recognize and kill cancer cells.

Cancer vaccines are preventative and therapeutic. Preventative vaccines prevent hepatitis B virus and human papillomavirus infections and, consequently, protect against the formation of HBV- and HPV-related cancers. Therapeutic cancer vaccines sensitize the body against so-called neoantigens expressed by cancer cells. Identify those neoantigens and sensitizing the patient's immune system to those neoantigens brings a new wing of the immune system into the body's fight against cancer.

Immune modulators target the immune system's "gas pedals" and "brake pedals" that cancer cells exploit to hide from the immune system. These include checkpoint inhibitors, cytokines, adjuvants, and agonists. Checkpoint inhibitors disable the brake pedals on the immune system that tumors use to shut it down. For example, tumor cells express molecules like PD-1L that binds to the PD-1 receptor on the surfaces of T cells and shuts them off. Immune modulators mask PD-1L and keep it from turning off T cells. Immune modulators free T cells to attack and destroy tumor cells. Cytokines are small proteins that regulate the immune response. Several cytokines also have profound inhibitor effects on some cancers. Agonists activate killer T cells to recognize and kill tumor cells. Adjuvants generally stimulate the immune response, promoting anticancer activities within the immune system.

Oncolytic viruses are genetically engineered viruses tuned to infect and destroy specific cancer cells. Since cancer cells have impaired antivirus systems, they are susceptible to viral infection. Viruses engineered to infect certain cancers will infect and kill only those rogue cells they are specified to kill.

Targeted antibodies can disrupt cancer cell activity and alert the immune system to target and eliminate tumors. There are three types of targeted antibodies: naked monoclonal antibodies, antibody drug-conjugates (ADCs), and bispecific antibodies. Naked monoclonal antibodies bind tightly to a cancer-specific surface protein. They mark the tumor cell for destruction by the host of phagocytic cells in the body and the complement system in the blood. ADCs have a toxic drug attached to them that is deployed when the antibody binds its target. ADCs bind to tumor-specific proteins and engage their poison, efficiently and specifically killing their tumor-based target. Bispecific antibodies have antigen-binding sites on both sides of the protein. These proteins serve as bridges between cancer cells and T-cytotoxic cells. Bringing the cancer cell to the T-cytotoxic cell activates the T-cytotoxic cell and has a ring-side seat for the destruction of the cancer cell.

DELIVERY ROUTES

Agents may be administered by mouth (orally), injection (subcutaneously-intramuscularly or intravenously).

Some vaccines are given into the skin (intradermal) or placed into the bladder in a liquid form (instillation). Agents may be taken at home or may require a visit to the physician's office or hospital. The schedule of administration varies with the agent.

HOW THESE DRUGS WORK

Cancer develops when normal cells change their genetic makeup over some time. As these changes occur, proteins are moved to the cell surface that the body does not recognize. The body's immune system activation against these unrecognized substances is called an "immune response" and is the principle of immunotherapy. Antibodies developed outside the body or substances that encourage the body to develop antibodies against antigens are the foundation for immunotherapy. An antigen is any substance that causes the immune system to produce antibodies. The immune system includes lymph nodes, the spleen, tonsils, bone marrow, and white blood cells.

Some of the goals of immunotherapy include: (1) increasing the immune system's sensitivity to cancer cells to improve the ability of the immune system to attack and kill such cells; (2) preventing normal cells from becoming malignant; (3) preventing the spread of cancer cells; (4) encouraging the body to repair damaged cells; and (5) and changing the activity of normal cells around tumors.

FDA-Approved CAR T-Cell Treatments

Treatment	Target
Axicabtagene ciloleucel (Yescarta)	CD19 – for lymphoma
Brexucabtagene autoleucel (Tecartus)	CD19 – for lymphoma
Idecabtagene vicleucel (Abecma)	BCMA – for advanced multiple myeloma
Lisocabtagene maraleucel (Breyanzi)	CD19 – for lymphoma
Tisagenlecleucel (Kyrmriah)	CD19 – for leukemia and lymphoma

TIL, TCR, and NK CAR therapies are available only through clinical trials. Some of the results in clinical trials have demonstrated the robust and durable response these therapies can provide to cancer patients.

In October 2017, the U.S. Food and Drug Administration (FDA) approved the first CAR T-cell therapy for adults with large B-cell lymphomas.

One of the advantages of CAR T cells is that they are not MHC restricted. CAR T-cell treatments also show memory in leukemia treatments. CAR-T cells directly recognize tumor surface proteins. When they bind to tumor surface proteins, they proliferate and kill tumor cells.

Of the cancer vaccines, there are four preventative and two therapeutic cancer vaccines.

Preventative Cancer Vaccines

Vaccine	Protective effects
Cervarix	Protects against two strains of HPV, types 16 and 18, that cause most cervical cancers
Gardasil	Protects against infection by HPV types 16, 18, 6, and 11
Gardasil-9	Protects against HPV types 16, 18, 31, 33, 45, 52, and 58
Hepatitis B (HBV) vaccine (HEPLISAV-B®)	Protects against infection by the hepatitis B virus and prevents the development of HBV-related liver cancer

HPV vaccines help prevent HPV-related anal, cervical, head and neck, penile, vulvar, and vaginal cancers. HPV infection is superficial, and the body does not form a robust immune response against it. HPV vaccines, however, generate excellent, wide-ranging immunity against HPV. This vaccine-generated immune response prevents infection by the most cancer-causing HPV strains and the cancers that they cause.

Therapeutic cancer vaccines include Bacillus Calmette-Guérin (BCG) and Sipuleucel-T (Provenge). BCG stimulates the cellular immune response against early-stage bladder cancers. Sipuleucel-T stimulates antigen-presenting cells in patients with prostate cancer to generate T cells that attack and destroy the tumor.

Immunomodulators are among the most successful immunotherapy agents. Checkpoint inhibitors block immune checkpoints that shut down the immune system. Since tumors frequently manipulate these signals to turn off the immune responses against them, checkpoint inhibitors turn the immune system back on.

Cytokines are used more frequently than any other type of immunotherapy, as they are employed at some point in most cancers. Because cancer treatments can cause serious side effects and complications, side effect control is an essential part of therapy. White blood cells fight infection in the body and are decreased by chemotherapy drugs, leading to neutropenia. Anemia, a decrease in red blood cells responsible for carrying oxygen to cells, can be life-threatening in cancer patients. Erythropoietin stimulates the release of mature red blood cells and is an essential part of cancer therapy. Colony-stimulating factors encourage the bone marrow to convert immune cells into neutrophils, critical to fighting infection. Cytokines are naturally produced in the body but can be developed in the laboratory using recombinant deoxyribonucleic acid (DNA) technology. Cytokines interact with receptors on immune cells to stimulate, for example, red blood cell production or inhibit or slow cancer cell growth. While some cytokines are not therapeutic for cancer, they are needed to allow patients to receive their full doses of immunotherapy and chemotherapy.

A group of cytokines called "interleukins" are therapeutic for cancer. In 1992, interleukin-2 (IL-2)

Checkpoint Inhibitors

Name	Anticancer Effects	Cancers Targeted
Atezolizumab (Tecentriq)	targets the PD-1/PD-L1 pathway	bladder cancer, breast cancer, liver cancer, lung cancer, and melanoma
Avelumab (Bavencio)	targets the PD-1/PD-L1 pathway	bladder cancer, kidney cancer, and Merkel cell carcinoma, a type of skin cancer
Cemiplimab (Libtayo)	targets the PD-1/PD-L1 pathway	approved for subsets of patients with cutaneous squamous cell carcinoma, basal cell carcinoma, and lung cancer
Dostarlimab (Jemperli)	targets the PD-1 pathway	uterine (endometrial) cancer
Durvalumab (Imfinzi)	targets the PD-1/PD-L1 pathway	bladder cancer and lung cancer
Ipilimumab (Yervoy)	targets the CTLA-4 pathway	melanoma, mesothelioma, liver cancer, and lung cancer
Nivolumab (Opdivo)	targets the PD-1/PD-L1 pathway	bladder cancer, colorectal cancer, esophageal cancer, gastric cancer, head and neck cancer, kidney cancer, liver cancer, lung cancer, lymphoma, melanoma, and mesothelioma
Pembrolizumab (Keytruda)	targets the PD-1/PD-L1 pathway	bladder cancer, breast cancer, cervical cancer, colorectal cancer, cutaneous squamous cell carcinoma, esophageal cancer, head and neck cancer, kidney cancer, liver cancer, lung cancer, lymphoma, melanoma, Merkel cell carcinoma, and stomach cancer

Cytokines

Name	Immune System Effects	Cancers Targeted
Aldesleukin (Proleukin)	targets the IL-2/IL-2R pathway	kidney cancer and melanoma
Granulocyte-macrophage colony-stimulating factor (GM-CSF)	an immunomodulatory cytokine	neuroblastoma
Interferon alfa-2a	targets the IFNAR1/2 pathway	leukemia and sarcoma
Interferon alfa-2b (Intron A)	targets the IFNAR1/2 pathway	leukemia, lymphoma, melanoma, and sarcoma
Peginterferon alfa-2b (Sylatron/PEG-Intron®)	targets the IFNAR1 pathway	melanoma

was the first immunotherapy approved for use alone in treating cancer. IL-2 is used for advanced kidney cancer and melanoma, either alone or with other chemotherapies or immunotherapies. Interleukin stimulates T cells and natural killer cells in the immune system. Interferons, which are also cytokines, are thought to work by slowing the growth of cancer cells and the blood vessels that supply the tumor. Interferons increase the production of antigens in the cancer cell, making it more visible to antibodies. The administration of interferon may also boost natural killer cells.

Available adjuvants include imiquimod and poly-ICLC. Imiquimod is a small molecule that activates the Toll-like receptor 7 (TLR7) and generally stimulates the immune system. Poly-ICLC targets

Therapeutic Antibodies

Antibody	Target	Cancer Treated
Monoclonal Antibodies		
Alemtuzumab (Campath)	targets the CD52 pathway	leukemia
Bevacizumab (Avastin)	targets the VEGF/VEGFR pathway inhibits tumor blood vessel growth	brain cancer, cervical cancer, colorectal cancer, kidney cancer, liver cancer, lung cancer, and ovarian cancer
Cetuximab (Erbitux)	targets the EGFR pathway	colorectal cancer, and head and neck cancer
Daratumumab (Darzalex)	targets the CD38 pathway	multiple myeloma
Denosumab (Xgeva)	targets the RANKL pathway	sarcoma
Dinutuximab (Unituxin)	targets the GD2 pathway	pediatric neuroblastoma
Elotuzumab (Empliciti)	targets the SLAMF7 pathway	multiple myeloma
Isatuximab (Sarclisa)	targets the CD38 pathway	multiple myeloma
Mogamulizumab (Poteligeo)	targets the CCR4 pathway	non-Hodgkin lymphoma, mycosis fungoides, and Sézary syndrome
Naxitamab-gqgk (Danyelza)	targets the GD-2 pathway	neuroblastoma
Necitumumab (Portrazza)	targets the EGFR pathway	lung cancer
Obinutuzumab (Gazyva)	targets the CD20 pathway	leukemia and lymphoma
Ofatumumab (Arzerra)	targets the CD20 pathway	leukemia
Olaratumumab (Lartruvo)	targets the PDGFRá pathway	sarcoma
Panitumumab (Vectibix)	targets the EGFR pathway	colorectal cancer
Pertuzumab (Perjeta)	targets the HER2 pathway	breast cancer
Ramucirumab (Cyramza)	targets the VEGF/VEGFR2 pathway inhibits tumor blood vessel growth	colorectal cancer, esophageal cancer, liver cancer, lung cancer, and stomach cancer
Rituximab (Rituxan)	targets the CD20 pathway	leukemia and lymphoma
Tafasitamab (Monjuvi)	targets the CD19 pathway	lymphoma
Antibody-Drug Conjugates		
Belantamab mafodotin-blmf (Blenrep)	targets the BCMA pathway and delivers toxic drugs to tumors	advanced multiple myeloma
Brentuximab vedotin (Adcetris)	targets the CD30 pathway and delivers toxic drugs to tumors	lymphoma
Enfortumab vedotin (Padcev)	targets the Nectin-4 pathway and delivers toxic drugs to tumors	advanced bladder cancer
Gemtuzumab ozogamicin (MyloTarg)	targets the CD33 pathway and delivers toxic drugs to tumors	leukemia
Ibritumomab tiuxetan (Zevalin)	targets the CD20 pathway and delivers toxic drugs to tumors	lymphoma
Inotuzumab ozogamicin (Besponsa)	targets the CD22 pathway and delivers toxic drugs to tumors	leukemia

Therapeutic Antibodies (continued)

Antibody	Target	Cancer Treated
Antibody-Drug Conjugates		
Loncastuximab tesirine (Zynlonta)	targets the CD19 pathway and delivers toxic drugs to tumors	lymphoma
Moxetumomab pasudotox (Lumoxiti)	targets the CD22 pathway and delivers toxic drugs to tumors	leukemia
Polatuzumab vedotin (Polivy)	targets the CD79b pathway and delivers toxic drugs to tumors	lymphoma
Sacituzumab govitecan-hziy (Trodelvy)	targets the TROP-2 pathway	breast cancer
Trastuzumab deruxtecan (Enhertu)	targets the HER2 pathway and delivers toxic drugs to tumors	advanced, HER2-positive breast cancer
Trastuzumab emtansine (Kadcyla)	targets the HER2 pathway and delivers toxic drugs to tumors	breast cancer
Bispecific Antibodies		
Amivantamab (Rybrevan)	targets EGFR and MET receptors on tumor cells	lung cancer
Blinatumomab (Blincyto)	targets CD19 on tumor cells as well as CD3 on T cells	leukemia

TLR3 and generally stimulates the immune response. Imiquimod is used in patients with basal cell carcinoma, and Poly-ICLC is approved for patients with squamous cell carcinoma.

Oncolytic viruses are genetically engineered, naturally occurring viruses, decreasing their ability to infect noncancerous cells and enhancing their ability to infect cancer cells. Likewise, oncolytic viruses can tag cancer cells with genes that make them more visible to the immune system. After infecting cancer cells, these oncolytic viruses can burst cancer cells, killing them and releasing cancer antigens. These cancer antigens can stimulate immune responses that find and eliminate any remaining tumor cells anywhere else in the body. Many oncolytic virus treatments are still experimental, but one commercially available product is called "T-VEC" (Imlygic). This modified herpes simplex virus infects specific tumors and destroys them. It is given to some patients with melanoma.

Monoclonal antibodies generally interrupt signals in the cell that cause it to become cancerous. Each monoclonal antibody is designed to bind to a specific antigen on the cell. Some monoclonal antibodies attack the blood supply of the tumor, called "antiangiogenesis." Monoclonal antibodies create so-called passive immunotherapy because they use antibodies made outside the body in large numbers. ADCs deliver toxic drugs into cancer cells, killing them. Bispecific antibodies link immune cells to cancer cells, accelerating their demise. Active immunotherapy occurs when the patient's body makes antibodies against antigens, such as in vaccine therapy. There are approximately twenty monoclonal antibodies approved for use in cancer treatment.

SIDE EFFECTS

Immunotherapy may cause flu-like symptoms, including fever, chills, nausea, vomiting, fatigue, headache, low blood count (anemia), inability to fight infection, bone pain, and muscle aches. If the agent is injected, then a rash or swelling may be noted at the site. Blood pressure can drop during administration. More severe but less common side effects include bleeding, difficulty breathing, edema leading to congestive heart failure, heart damage, and severe and potentially life-threatening reactions (such as anaphylaxis).

CAR T-cell therapies can cause tumor lysis syndrome (TLS). TLS results from many cancer cells dying within a short period, releasing their contents into the blood. Rapid cancer cell death releases excessive quantities of uric acid, potassium, and phosphorus into the bloodstream. The kidneys cannot excrete these molecules fast enough, causing TLS. Excess phosphorus binds to calcium, causing low blood calcium levels. Changes in blood levels of uric acid, potassium, phosphorus, and calcium adversely affect several organs, especially the kidneys, and heart, brain, muscles, and gastrointestinal tract.

—*Patricia Stanfill Edens, RN, PhD, FACHE, Catherine J. Walsh, PhD, and Michael A. Buratovich, PhD*

Further Information

Boldt, Clayton A. "TIL Therapy: 6 Things to Know." *MD Anderson Cancer Center*, 15 Apr. 2021, www.mdanderson.org/cancerwise/what-is-tumor-infiltrating-lymphocyte-til-therapy—6-things-to-know.h00-159460056.html. Accessed 29 Aug. 2021.

Chabner, Bruce A., and Dan L. Longo, editors. *Cancer Chemotherapy and Biotherapy: Principles and Practice*. Lippincott Williams & Wilkins, 2006.

Gullatte, M. M. *Clinical Guide to Antineoplastic Therapy: A Chemotherapy Handbook*. Oncology Nursing Society, 2005.

Polovich, M., J. M. White, and L. O. Kelleher. *Chemotherapy and Biotherapy Guidelines*. 2nd ed., Oncology Nursing Society, 2005.

Predergast, G. C., and E. M. Jaffee. *Cancer Immunotherapy*. 2nd ed., Academic Press, 2013. This book discusses the immune system's role in suppressing tumor development and provides basic and clinical cancer researchers with an overview of immunotherapy and chemotherapy in the fight against cancer.

Wang, X. Y., and P. B. Fisher, editors. *Immunotherapy of Cancer*. (Advances in Cancer Research). Vol. 128. Academic Press, 2015. This book provides information on cancer research with expert reviews and is directed towards students and researchers.

"What Is Cancer Immunotherapy?" *Cancer Research Institute*, Oct. 2020, www.cancerresearch.org/immunotherapy/what-is-immunotherapy. Accessed 29 Aug. 2021.

Yamaguchi, Y., editor. *Immunotherapy of Cancer: An Innovative Treatment Comes of Age*. Springer, 2016. A new book that summarizes the present status and future for cancer immunotherapy.

Zhao, Lijun, and Yu J. Cao. "Engineered T Cell Therapy for Cancer in the Clinic." *Frontiers in Immunology*, vol. 10, 2019, p. 2250, doi.org/10.3389/fimmu.2019.02250.

SUBLINGUAL IMMUNOTHERAPY

Category: Therapies/Techniques
Anatomy or system affected: Blood, immune system, lymphatic system, mouth, throat
Specialties and related fields: Allergists, hematology, immunology, otorhinolaryngology, pathology, pharmacology
Definition: Treating allergies by placing an allergen solution, such as pollen extract, under the tongue.

KEY TERMS

eosinophils: type of white blood cell that functions in allergies and worm infections
immunoglobulin E (IgE): an antibody subtype dedicated to parasite infections and allergies
immunotolerance: an active state of unresponsiveness to specific antigens
sublingual: placing something under the tongue

OVERVIEW

Sublingual immunotherapy (SLIT) is a method of treating allergies that closely resembles conventional "allergy shots." In both methods, small amounts of allergenic substances are administered periodically and over time through a route different from the way the body ordinarily encounters them. For example, plant pollens ordinarily cause their allergic reactions by being inhaled. With allergy shots, pollen extracts are injected under the skin. In SLIT, allergens are placed under the tongue.

The immune system has many components, and only one of them, the immunoglobulin E (IgE)/eosinophil system, produces typical allergic reactions. Allergen immunotherapy alters the immune response to allergens by promoting immunotolerance through repeated allergen-specific exposure. SLIT works the same way, but it introduces allergens into the bloodstream through the sublingual route. The intended effect of the alternate routes of administration is to "train" other branches of the immune system to become tolerant to allergens before the IgE/eosinophil system can react to their presence.

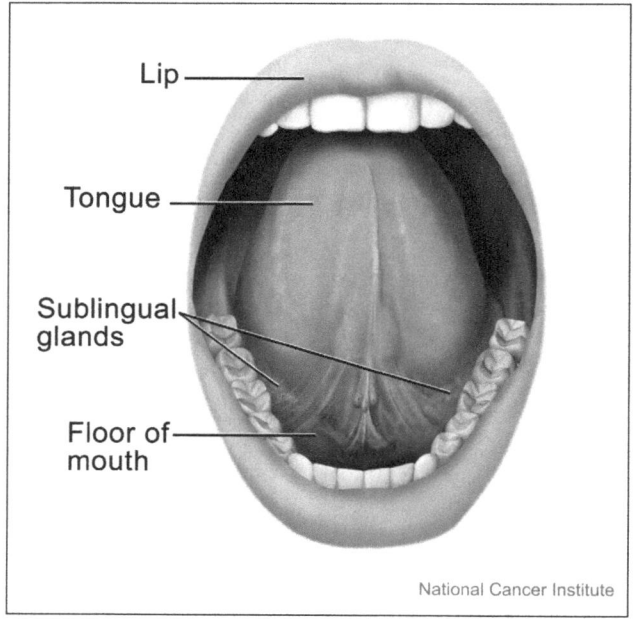

A diagram of the mouth and tongue area, highlighting the sublingual glands. Image by Alan Hoofring/NCI, via Wikimedia Commons. [Public domain.]

SLIT Allergen Immunotherapies

Palforzia	Peanut allergen powder
Grastek	Timothy grass pollen allergen extract
Odactra	House dust mite allergen extract
Oralair	Mixed grass pollens allergen extract
Ragwitek	Short ragweed pollen allergen extract

The tremendous potential advantage of SLIT over allergy shots is that SLIT does not involve needles; this makes it less unpleasant and capable of being done at home rather than at a doctor's office. The absence of needles may also explain why SLIT has long been categorized as an alternative rather than conventional medicine.

There are no universally accepted criteria by which treatment is classified as part of alternative rather than conventional medicine. Some treatments, such as acupuncture, fall in the alternative category because they belong to a system of medicine considerably unlike that of the modern conventional system; others, like traditional herbology, fall in the alternative category because they involve unprocessed "natural" substances rather than drugs; still, others are considered alternative simply because they have been rejected for one reason or another by conventional medicine or have been adopted by practitioners of other forms of alternative medicine.

SLIT is primarily in the last camp. Until approximately 2000, SLIT was most commonly the province of holistic or alternative practitioners. Therefore, health-care professionals viewed SLIT with skepticism by mainstream medicine. However, numerous well-designed studies of SLIT have been reported in recent years, causing the method to gain increasing acceptance among conventional allergists.

SCIENTIFIC EVIDENCE

Perhaps the best evidence for the effectiveness of SLIT involves the treatment of allergic rhinitis (hay fever). In a double-blind study of 855 adults with grass allergies, SLIT using grass pollen tablets for approximately eighteen weeks markedly reduced allergy symptoms, including nasal congestion and itchy eyes. Substantial benefits for most common hay fever symptoms were also seen in another double-blind study enrolling 634 people. In a third double-blind study involving 105 persons, SLIT significantly improved symptoms of rhinitis and conjunctivitis from grass and rye pollen allergies compared to placebos. Skin reactivity to these allergens, a more objective sign of allergy, also showed a more substantial reduction in persons using SLIT. Other studies have shown benefits for hay fever caused by grass pollen or other allergens, including dust mites and tree pollen.

However, in a 2008 comprehensive review of studies investigating SLIT for grass pollen and house dust-mite allergies, researchers could not substantiate claims of effectiveness, mainly because of the variable quality of the studies they uncovered.

As with conventional allergy shots for hay fever, it appears that if SLIT is, in fact, effective, patients must use it for a long time for best results. Three years of treatment may be better than two, and two years better than one. To provide benefits for grass allergy season, SLIT must begin a minimum of eight weeks before the onset of the grass allergy season; even longer lead times produce even better results. Putting all this evidence together, it appears that SLIT may work best if used every year and year-round.

One study suggests that SLIT is not only effective for treating allergy. However, a Cochrane review found that SLIT provides significant relief for some asthmatics. SLIT may help prevent the development of new allergies or mild persistent asthma in children with allergic rhinitis or intermittent asthma. SLIT has also shown promise for latex allergy and other forms of allergy.

Research Spotlight: Peanut Allergy in Children

Currently, there are no treatments available for people with peanut allergies. According to Duke University Medical Center and Massachusetts General Hospital researchers, a new treatment may be a safe and effective form of immunotherapy for children with peanut allergies. The double-blind, placebo-controlled study, funded in part by the National Center for Complementary and Alternative Medicine and published in the Journal of Allergy and Clinical Immunology, investigated the safety, clinical effectiveness, and immunologic changes with sublingual immunotherapy. This treatment involves administering tiny amounts of the allergen extract under a person's tongue.

Researchers randomly assigned eighteen children (aged one to eleven) with known peanut allergies to receive either peanut sublingual immunotherapy or placebo. Participants in the peanut group received increased doses of peanut extract every two weeks for six months. Following each dose increase, participants continued the same daily dose at home. Once a maximum dose of 2,000 micrograms of peanut protein was reached, participants continued to take this daily maintenance dose at home for approximately six more months.

After a total of twelve months of sublingual immunotherapy, participants underwent a food challenge, which involved taking increasing doses of peanut protein in the form of peanut flour mixed with food. The food-challenge placebo consisted of oat flour mixed with food given in the same increments. All experimental subjects received allergy skin-prick tests and had blood samples taken at different points throughout the study.

The researchers found that the participants who had received peanut sublingual immunotherapy could safely consume twenty times more peanut protein than those who had received the placebo (1710 milligrams [mg] versus 85 mg). This level of desensitization is clinically significant because it represents protection from accidental ingestion of peanuts, which is often less than 100 mg (or one peanut). In addition, allergy skin-prick tests showed a decreased allergic response to peanuts in the treatment group. The blood tests showed immunologic changes in the treatment group, suggesting a significant difference in the allergic response.

SAFETY ISSUES

SLIT appears to be safer than conventional allergy shots. The most frequently reported adverse effects include oral itching or swelling and gastrointestinal upset; in most cases, these side effects are mild and short-lived. In one study, 12 percent of persons with allergic rhinitis or asthma experienced worsening symptoms at some point in their treatment. Severe allergic reactions appear to occur rarely. SLIT trials in children with high-risk asthma show that people with asthma have no higher risk of side effects than the nonasthmatic control group.

—*EBSCO CAM Review Board*

Further Information

Cox, L. S., et al. "Sublingual Immunotherapy: A Comprehensive Review." *Journal of Allergy and Clinical Immunology*, vol. 117, 2006, pp. 1021-35.

Dahl, R., et al. "Sublingual Grass Allergen Tablet Immunotherapy Provides Sustained Clinical Benefit with Progressive Immunologic Changes Over Two Years." *Journal of Allergy and Clinical Immunology*, vol. 121, 2008, pp. 512-18.

Fortescue R., K. M. Kew, and MShiu Tsun. "Sublingual Immunotherapy for Asthma." *Cochrane Database of Systematic Reviews*, Issue 9, 2020, CD011293, doi:10.1002/14651858.CD011293.pub3.

Marogna, M., et al. "Preventive Effects of Sublingual Immunotherapy in Childhood." *Annals of Allergy, Asthma, and Immunology*, vol. 101, 2008, pp. 206-11.

Moore, Andrew. "Immunotherapy Can Provide Lasting Relief." *American Academy of Allergy, Asthma, and Immunology*, 28 Sept. 2020, www.aaaai.org/tools-for-the-public/conditions-library/allergies/immunotherapy-can-provide-lasting-relief. Accessed 28 Aug. 2021.

Nettis, E., et al. "Double-Blind, Placebo-Controlled Study of Sublingual Immunotherapy in Patients with Latex-Induced Urticaria." *British Journal of Dermatology*, vol. 156, 2007, pp. 674-81.

Pfaar, O., and L. Klimek. "Efficacy and Safety of Specific Immunotherapy with a High-Dose Sublingual Grass Pollen Preparation." *Annals of Allergy, Asthma, and Immunology*, vol. 100, 2008, pp. 256-63.

Rodriguez-Perez, N., et al. "Frequency of Acute Systemic Reactions in Patients with Allergic Rhinitis and Asthma Treated with Sublingual Immunotherapy." *Annals of Allergy, Asthma, and Immunology*, vol. 101, 2008, pp. 304-10.

"Sublingual Immunotherapy (SLIT) Allergy Tablets." *American Academy of Allergy, Asthma, and Immunology*, Mar. 2020, www.aaaai.org/Tools-for-the-Public/Drug-Guide/Sublingual-Immunotherapy-(SLIT)-Allergy-Tablets. Accessed 28 Aug. 2021.

Theophylline

Category: Drugs
Anatomy or system affected: Blood vessels, brain, heart, liver, lungs, psychic-emotional system, respiratory system
Specialties and related fields: Internal medicine, osteopathic medicine, otorhinolaryngology, pharmacology, pulmonary medicine
Definition: Once among the most common treatments for asthma, theophylline is no longer widely used, having been replaced by safer drugs.

KEY TERMS

cyclic adenosine monophosphate (cAMP): a small molecule made inside cells in response to specific stimuli that elicits changes in cell behavior and function

phosphodiesterase: an enzyme that degrades second messenger molecules like cAMP

second messenger: a small molecule made by cells after they are stimulated by hormones, physical stimuli, cytokines, or other types of cell signals

tachycardia: an excessively high heart rate, usually over 100 beats per minute for an adult

bronchodilation: relaxation of the smooth muscle surrounding the airways, increasing the diameter of the airways, and facilitating the passage of gases to and from the lungs

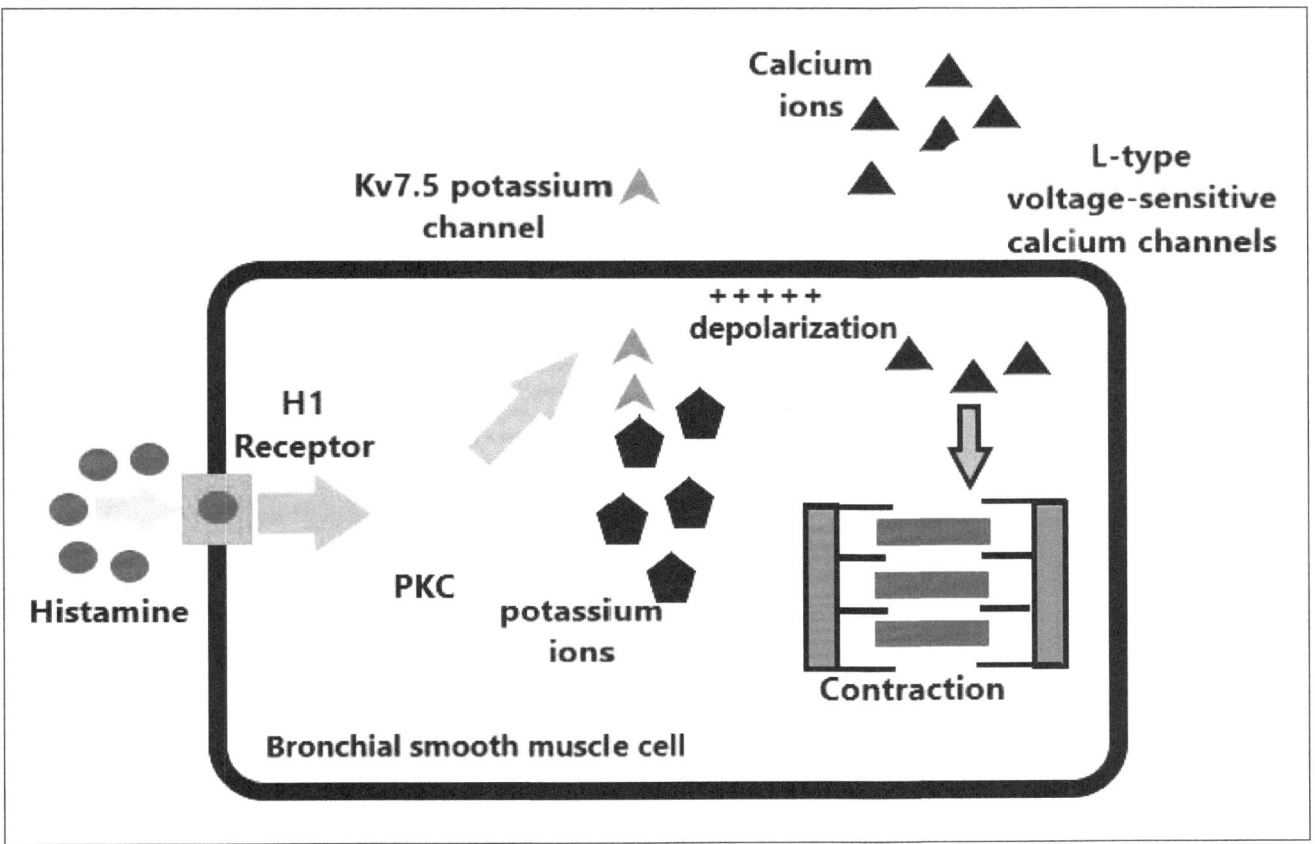

Calcium ions induce smooth muscle contraction of the airways, or bronchoconstriction, which leads to wheezing, and shortness of breath. By Michael Buratovitch. [Used with permission.]

MECHANISM OF ACTION

Allergies result from the exposure of the airways to irritants that elicit the release of histamine and leukotrienes from resident mast cells. Histamine binds to and activates H1 receptors on the surfaces of bronchial smooth muscle cells. Activation of H1 histamine receptors activates protein kinase C (PKC), and PKC inhibits the Kv7.5 potassium channel protein. The interruption of potassium ion (K+) efflux through the channels causes a positive change in membrane voltage (ΔV). The L-type voltage-sensitive calcium channels (VSCCs) sense this change in the membrane potential and open to allow an increased influx of calcium ions (Ca2+). Calcium ions induce smooth muscle contraction of the airways, or bronchoconstriction, which leads to wheezing, and shortness of breath.

The antiasthma medication theophylline, also known as aminophylline, Elixophyllin, Theo-24, Uniphyl, and generic, inhibits an intracellular enzyme called "phosphodiesterase III" (PDE III). PDE III typically degrades the second messenger cyclic adenosine monophosphate (cAMP). Inhibition of PDE III causes a rise in intracellular cAMP levels. cAMP is a potent activator of protein kinase A (PKA). When activated, PKA phosphorylates an enzyme called "myosin light chain kinase" (MLCK), inhibiting it. Myosin is a component of the contractile machinery of all muscle cells. Myosin contains two proteins, a heavy and a light chain. Without maintenance of the light chain by the MLCK, myosin stops mediating smooth muscle contraction. Theophylline, therefore, restrains smooth muscle contraction, promoting bronchodilation, and relieving wheezing and shortness of breath.

ADVERSE EFFECTS
Unfortunately, theophylline also affects PDE in other cell types besides bronchial smooth muscle. In cardiac muscle, theophylline raises cAMP levels, causing increased heart rates and more forceful contractions. In liver cells, increased intracellular levels of cAMP cause the degradation of glycogen and the release of glucose into the bloodstream, raising blood glucose levels. The availability of safer alternatives has reduced the use of theophylline except for those refractory asthma cases that are not controlled by other means. When used, blood theophylline levels are maintained between a narrow range of 10 to 15 mcg/mL.

The adverse effects of theophylline include nausea and vomiting, nervousness, headache, and insomnia. If blood theophylline levels climb above 15 mcg/mL, then patients can suffer from high blood glucose levels (hyperglycemia), low serum potassium levels (hypokalemia), an abnormally high heart rate (tachycardia), an irregular heartbeat (cardiac arrhythmias), seizures, and death.

DRUG-DRUG INTERACTIONS
Other caveats associated with theophylline include other medications that interact with it. Some drugs raise theophylline blood levels. Drugs that prevent the liver from properly metabolizing theophylline can raise its blood levels above the threshold of safe use and cause adverse effects. Examples of drugs that increase theophylline blood levels include the antigout medication allopurinol, oral contraceptives, the antiulcer medicine cimetidine, the antidepressant fluvoxamine, and fluoroquinolone (e.g., levofloxacin, and others), and macrolide antibiotics (e.g., erythromycin).

Other medications increase the rate of theophylline metabolism and lower its blood concentration, preventing it from working. For example, cigarette or cannabis smoking raises the activity of the liver and causes increased degradation of theophylline. Thus, at regularly prescribed dosages, theophylline fails to work in smokers. Other drugs that decrease blood theophylline levels include activated charcoal, the antiseizure medicine phenytoin, the antituberculosis drug rifampin, the antifungal ketoconazole, and barbiturates, which are used as sedatives and antiseizure agents.

Theophylline can increase the activity of other drugs in the body. The heart failure medicine riociguat has a mechanism of action that complements theophylline and taking these two medicines together can cause the blood pressure to decrease precipitously. Consequently, these two medications should never be taken together. Another agent that seriously interacts with theophylline is alcohol. Taking theophylline with alcohol increases the risk and severity of side effects and should be avoided.

Specific herbal and dietary supplements also interact with theophylline. Theophylline impairs the efficacy of vitamin B_6 supplements. To exert its effect on the body, vitamin B_6 is converted into pyridoxal 5'-phosphate (PLP), and theophylline interferes with this conversion. Some of the side effects of theophylline might be due, in part, to PLP depletion.

St. John's Wort is a common herbal remedy for depression and mood stabilization. However, St. John's Wort increases theophylline metabolism, decreasing its serum concentrations and preventing it from working.

Some people use the herbal supplement cayenne to aid their digestion, calm a sour stomach, or decrease gas production. Cayenne increases the absorption of theophylline and can increase blood theophylline levels above the safe threshold.

Finally, ipriflavone is taken by many people to increase their bone strength. This compound also increases theophylline levels in the body and increases the risk of theophylline toxicity.

—*Michael A Buratovich, PhD*

Further Information

Barnes, Peter J. "Theophylline." *American Journal of Respiratory and Critical Care Medicine*, vol. 188, no. 8, 2013, pp. 901-6.

Bass, Pat. "Is Theophylline a Good Choice for Treating Your Asthma?" *Verywell Health*, 24 Apr. 2020, www.verywellhealth.com/theophylline-201158.

Galanter, Joshua M., and Homer A. Boushey. "Drugs Used in Asthma." *Basic and Clinical Pharmacology*, edited by Bertram G. Katzung and Anthony J. Trevor, 13th ed., pp. 341-42, McGraw-Hill Education, 2015.

Jilani, T. N., C. V. Preuss, and S. Sharma. "Theophylline." StatsPearls Publishing, Jan. 2021 [Updated 2021 May 15], www.ncbi.nlm.nih.gov/books/NBK519024/.

"Theophylline (Oral Route) Side Effects." *Mayo Clinic*, Mayo Foundation for Medical Education and Research, 1 Feb. 2020, www.mayoclinic.org/drugs-supplements/theophylline-oral-route/side-effects/drg-20073599?p=1.

"Theophylline: MedlinePlus Drug Information." *MedlinePlus*, U.S. National Library of Medicine, 15 Nov. 2019, medlineplus.gov/druginfo/meds/a681006.html.

Natural Products, Herbal Supplements, and Other Alternatives

Idiopathic environmental intolerances

Category: Diseases/Disorders
Also known as: Multiple chemical sensitivity syndrome, reactive airway disease, sick building syndrome, environmental illness, universal allergy, twentieth-century disease, chemical hypersensitivity syndrome, total allergy syndrome, and cerebral allergy.
Anatomy or system affected: Brain, eyes, head, immune system, lungs, muscles, nerves, nervous system, respiratory system, skin
Specialties and related fields: Allergists, dermatology, environmental health, epidemiology, immunology, neurology, occupational health, public health, rheumatology, toxicology
Definition: The experience of multiple symptoms resulting from numerous and varied environmental chemical exposures without objective diagnostic physical findings or laboratory test results that define a specific illness.

KEY TERMS
clinical ecologist: proponents of the claim that exposure to low levels of certain chemicals harm susceptible people
immunotoxic: an event or substance that harms the immune system

CAUSES AND SYMPTOMS
Idiopathic environmental intolerance (IEI) is a subjective condition that formerly went by many different names. IEI refers to a phenomenon in which someone experiences multiple symptoms resulting from repeated and varied environmental chemical exposures. These symptoms occur without objective diagnostic physical findings or laboratory test results that define an illness. The inability of physicians to connect specific environmental chemicals with distinct clinical manifestations has hampered formal descriptions of IEI.

Because of the broad variability and highly subjective nature of IEI, it has no precise diagnostic criteria, laboratory test regimen, or clinical definition. A review of case reports shows that most IEI patients are adults and primarily female. Some people may report multiple symptoms that involve several organs. Still, many people receive a diagnosis of IEI even though they have few or no symptoms. The common thread between all IEI cases is that patients experience symptoms in response to environmental exposures of some sort.

Clinicians suspect IEI if patients report the onset of symptoms after moving into a new house, being exposed to chemicals in the workplace, or using pesticides in the home. Patients often describe an increasing intolerance to commonly encountered chemicals at concentrations tolerated by other people. Diagnosis is made when the following six criteria are met: repeated exposure reproduces symptoms, the condition is chronic, low chemical exposure levels cause symptoms, symptoms improve with the removal of offending chemicals, multiple unrelated chemicals trigger responses, and multiple systems are affected.

The sorts of chemicals to which IEI patients claim to be sensitive are extensive and continually grows. According to most case studies, patients identify the chemicals that trigger their symptoms by their smell. Unsurprisingly, patients identify perfumes and scented products, pesticides especially chlordane and chlorpyrifos), domestic and industrial solvents, new carpets and other renovation materials, carpet shampoo (lauryl sulfate) and other cleaning agents, isocyanates, car exhaust, adhesives and glues, fiberglass, carbonless copy paper, gasoline, kerosene, and diesel fumes, urban air pollution, fabric softener, cigarette smoke, plastics, natural gas, combustion products (poorly vented gas heaters, overheated batteries), and medications (dinitrochlorobenzene for warts, intranasally packed neo synephrine, prolonged antibiotics, and general anesthesia with petrochemicals), glutaraldehyde, and formaldehyde as potential symptomatic triggers. In other IEI cases, patients report symptoms because of exposure to some foods, food additives, and drugs. Still, other IEI cases report the onset of symptoms upon exposure to mercury in dental fillings and electromagnetic fields. Unfortunately, there are no dose-response studies of this phenomenon. However, IEI patients commonly report that certain chemicals trigger their symptoms at concentrations far below those commonly encountered daily. A further complication is that there are no relationships between the known toxicological characteristics of the triggering chemicals and the symptoms experienced by IEI patients. Also, the chemical concentrations at which IEI patients experience symptoms are far below those known to cause toxic effects.

> **INFORMATION ON**
> **IDIOPATHIC ENVIRONMENTAL INTOLERANCES**
>
> **Causes**: Environmental exposure to chemicals
>
> **Symptoms**: Symptoms vary but may include headaches (often migraine); chronic fatigue, musculoskeletal aching; chronic respiratory inflammation (rhinitis, sinusitis, laryngitis, asthma); attention-deficit disorder; hyperactivity (affecting younger children); food intolerance
>
> **Duration**: Acute to chronic
>
> **Treatments**: Alleviation of symptoms, supportive therapy

Analogies are sometimes made between asthma and IEI since some chemicals linked to IEI cases can also elicit asthmatic attacks. However, patients with asthma have detectable changes in their respiratory tracts, whereas IEI cases consist of subjective symptoms.

The commonly reported symptoms vary substantially, including headaches (often migraines), chronic fatigue, musculoskeletal aching, chronic respiratory inflammation (rhinitis, sinusitis, laryngitis, asthma), attention-deficit disorder, and hyperactivity in younger children. Other less commonly reported complaints include tremor, seizure, and mitral valve prolapse.

MECHANISMS

None of the available theories properly explain the cause of IEI. The main proposals invoke immunological, toxicological, psychological, or even sociological causes. Agreement on the mechanism of IEI remains elusive.

A group known as the "clinical ecologists" favor immunologic mechanisms. According to clinical ecologists, IEI results from presently unrecognized allergy or immunologic hypersensitivity to exceedingly low concentrations of certain chemicals. A variation on this theory is the "immunotoxic" theory. The immunotoxic theory postulates that exposure to low levels of specific chemicals elicits an autoimmune response in IEI patients.

A more recent proposal for IEI etiology is the neurotoxic theory. Accordingly, IEI patients experience symptoms because low levels of chemicals stimulate the olfactory-limbic system of the brain and hypothalamus. Alternatively, low levels of chemical irritants may cause oxidative damage to specific tissues. The tissues of IEI patients are somehow more sensitive to oxidative damage by these irritants.

Other physicians proposed that IEI is a psychiatric disease or personality disorder. Some have compared it to a panic disorder, mass hysteria, or even adult manifestations of childhood abuse. Others suggest that IEI manifests posttraumatic stress syndrome, behavioral conditioning, or other psychiatric conditions. Various researchers have noted a higher prevalence of psychiatric diagnoses among IEI patients. Clinical ecologists would interpret these findings as psychiatric conditions resulting from IEI and not the cause of IEI.

DIAGNOSIS
IEI diagnoses rely wholly on the patient's medical history. Unfortunately, there are no defining criteria, diagnostic symptoms, or objective physical signs to aid the clinician. While case studies report many different laboratory tests, brain scans, and immunologic markers, no laboratory or immunologic tests reliably detect IEI.

TREATMENT AND THERAPY
IEI treatment depends entirely on how the clinician views this condition. Clinical ecologists usually recommend avoiding exposure to irritating chemicals. Others may recommend supplementing the diet with specific micronutrients, vitamins, or other agents. Infrequently, physicians will recommend intravenous gamma globulin, coupled with sublingual immunotherapy. Unfortunately, evidence for the efficacy of this approach is lacking, and some studies even suggest that this type of treatment can make the patient worse.

Some more off-beat practitioners suggest "detoxification" programs that include forced sweating while replacing lost minerals with supplementation.

Finally, other practitioners recommend psychotherapy if the patient's history contains evidence of psychopathology. There is evidence for short-term benefits for this approach but no evidence of long-term benefits.

CONCLUSION
Is IEI a maladaptation to modern industrial society? Do some people have sensitivities to modern synthetic chemicals not found in most people? The wide range of symptoms described by IEI patients, and the absence of detectable physical abnormalities, make IEI a mysterious condition. Additionally, the highly subjective nature of IEI and the lack of proper diagnostic criteria make it impossible to define this condition with any precision.

Theories for IEI etiology range from the immunologic to the allergic, immunotoxic, neurotoxic, cytotoxic, psychologic, sociologic, and iatrogenic. However, there is a complete absence of scientific evidence establishing these mechanisms as the leading cause of IEI.

A clear connection between current and past psychopathologies exists in some IEI patients. Still, it seems unlikely that psychological factors explain all IEI cases.

A paucity of well-controlled studies that link IEI to the concentrations of specific chemicals continues to hamper research into this condition. Likewise, there is no hard evidence that IEI patients have any immunologic or neurologic abnormalities to date. Likewise, no form of therapy has yet been shown to alter the patient's illness in a favorable way. Without such foundational observations, IEI will remain a largely speculative condition that clinicians will address on a patient-by-patient basis.

—*Michael A. Buratovich, PhD*

Further Information
American Academy of Allergy, Asthma, and Immunology, Board of Directors. "Position Paper: Idiopathic Environmental Intolerances." *AAAI*, Jan. 1999, www.aaaai.org/Aaaai/media/Media-Library-PDFs/Allergist%20Resources/Statements%20and%20Practice%20Parameters/Idiopathic-environmental-intolerances-1999.pdf. Accessed 6 Sept. 2021.

American College of Physicians. "Position Paper: Clinical Ecology." *Annals of Internal Medicine*, vol. 111, 1989, pp. 168-78.

Barrett S. *MCS: Multiple Chemical Sensitivity*. American Council on Science and Health, 1994.

Board of the International Society of Regulatory Toxicology and Pharmacology. "Report of the ISRTP Board." *Regulatory Toxicology Pharmacology*, vol. 18, 1993, p. 79.

Committee on Environmental Hypersensitivities. *Report of the Ad Hoc Committee on Environmental Hypersensitivities Disorders*. Ministry of Health, 1985.

Council on Scientific Affairs, American Medical Association. "Clinical Ecology." *JAMA*, vol. 268, 1992, pp. 1634-35.

National Research Council. *Multiple Chemical Sensitivities*. National Academy Press, 1992.

Royal College of Physicians and Royal College of Pathologists. "Good Allergy Practice-Standards of Care for Providers and Purchasers of Allergy Services within the National Health Service." *Clinical and Experimental Allergy*, vol. 25, 1995, pp. 586-95.

IMMUNE SUPPORT

Category: Alternative and Complementary Medicine
Anatomy or system affected: Blood, eyes, gastrointestinal system, immune system, intestines, lungs, lymphatic system, mouth, respiratory system, skin, throat
Specialties and related fields: Dermatology, gastroenterology, hematology, immunology, internal medicine, ophthalmology, otorhinolaryngology, pharmacology, pulmonary medicine
Definition: Therapies to increase the effectiveness of the immune system in fighting infection.

KEY TERMS

immune system: a complex network of cells and proteins that defends the body against infection
immunomodulators: a substance that affects the functioning of the immune system

OVERVIEW

The body must contend with constant attacks by microscopic organisms. To defend itself, it has a wide range of defenses that together are called the "immune system." Persons with diseases that cause immune deficiency, such as acquired immunodeficiency syndrome (AIDS), are harmed by infectious microorganisms that a healthy person could ward off easily. However, even healthy people get sick from time to time, as infectious agents manage to sneak by the defenses. Also, some healthy people nonetheless get sick quite often. Any explanation of why it is so challenging to improve resistance to illness should include a discussion of the nature of immunity.

The immune system. The immune system consists primarily of various types of white blood cells and the chemicals they manufacture (such as antibodies). In certain conditions, such as AIDS, many of these white blood cells are damaged or dead. In such cases, the term "immune deficiency" is appropriate. The circumstance is analogous to an army that lacks, say, weaponry.

However, careful examination of most people who frequently get colds (or bladder infections or herpes attacks, for example) fails to turn up any visible deficits in the immune system. They have all the immune cells and antibodies they need in roughly the right amounts, and all the various parts appear to work just fine. It is not known why some people get sick so often.

One can hypothesize that in some people, the immune system fails to function appropriately for a relatively subtle, invisible reason, much as a well-equipped army might lose its fighting form because of apathy or disunity. However, even people who develop frequent colds manage to fight off thousands of other infections every day.

For this reason, an alternative hypothesis comes to mind: that oversusceptibility to a particular type of infection may be caused by something more specific than general immune weakness. For example, chronically inflamed mucous membranes might lead to frequent colds because an inflamed mucous membrane may be more porous to cold viruses. Similarly, a woman's bladder wall might allow easy attachment of bacteria, leading to frequent bladder infections. In reality, though, these are all speculations. It is not known why some people frequently develop minor infections. For this reason, it is challenging to find a way to fix the problem.

Immunomodulation. Many natural products are said to boost general immunity. However, while science can study the effect of a single treatment on a single illness, it is not known how a treatment strengthens the immune system in general. Scientists can measure the effects of an herb on individual white blood cell types and note activity changes. Nevertheless, they do not know how to interpret the results of those measurements as a whole. After all, the immune system is a system, and systems are notoriously complicated to analyze. Current knowledge does not allow science to predict the ultimate effect of subtle changes in the system's parts.

To acknowledge this limitation, scientists tend to use "immunomodulatory" rather than "immune-stimulating" when they refer to a substance that causes measurable alterations in immune function. This terminology notes a change (modulation) but does not assume the change is good, bad, or indifferent.

Hundreds or thousands of herbs have immunomodulatory effects. In many cases, these may represent nothing more than the body's reaction to the herb as a foreign presence-an immune reaction to the herb itself, in other words, with no unique benefits. In some cases, observed immunomodulatory effects could indicate an alteration in immune function with potential benefits under certain conditions, but it is impossible to know.

Theoretically, some natural substances could boost all aspects of immunity. However, if it did, it would be a hazardous substance. The immune system is finely balanced. An immune system that is too relaxed fails to defend against infections; an immune system that is too active attacks healthy tissues, causing autoimmune diseases (such as AIDS). A universal immune booster might cause lupus, Crohn's disease, asthma, Graves' disease, Hashimoto's thyroiditis, multiple sclerosis, or rheumatoid arthritis, among other problems.

Rather than preferring an immune booster, one might instead prefer a treatment that somehow fine-tunes the immune system. It is not known, however, if such a treatment exists.

NATURAL MEDICINE

Herbs and supplements. There is no doubt that good general nutrition is necessary for strong immunity. However, excessive intake of some nutrients (zinc, for example) may weaken immunity. Still, there is specific scientific evidence that multivitamin/multimineral supplements may help certain people stay well. Several herbs and supplements have shown promise for preventing or treating certain specific infections, including bladder infection, colds and flu, diarrhea, fungal infection, herpes infection, middle ear infection, and vaginal yeast infection.

Immunizations are widely used to strengthen the immune response to specific illnesses, such as influenza. However, some people (especially the elderly) may not respond adequately to immunizations. Certain natural products, such as ginseng, vitamin E, and multivitamin/multimineral supplements, may enhance the immune response. Echinacea is widely claimed to be an immune-strengthening herb. However, evidence suggests that its regular use does not help prevent colds or other infections. Echinacea may, however, help colds that have already begun. The fungi products *Coriolus versicolor*, active hexose correlated compound, maitake, reishi, and shiitake are widely believed to help support the immune system during cancer treatment. However, there is no reliable evidence to indicate that they are effective for this purpose. Substances that enhance the growth of friendly bacteria in the large intestine have been studied for their favorable effects on the immune system, with mixed results. Probiotics (such as acidophilus) consist of various bacterial species capable of rebalancing the healthy population of bacteria in the gut. Certain types of starches, called "prebiotics," are not fully digested and, therefore, remain in the intestine and feed healthy bacteria. There is some evidence that probiotics and, to a lesser extent, prebiotics may reduce allergic symptoms and possibly minor infections, especially in children.

Lifestyle issues. There is little doubt that if one lives a healthy lifestyle with good nutrition and plenty of exercise, one will approach more closely a state of optimum health. However, the key to this health is moderation. Too much exercise (as in marathon running) can weaken the immune system, leading to infections. (Heavy endurance exercise can benefit from the use of vitamin C, beta-sitosterol, and glutamine to prevent the "postmarathon sniffle.")

Although it is commonly said that high levels of sugar intake weaken immunity, there is no meaningful evidence to support this view. Similarly, while severe alcohol abuse damages immune function, there is no evidence that moderate alcohol consumption increases the risk of infection.

Some persons believe that getting cold causes colds, but this claim has not been proven. There is also no reliable evidence that reducing the intake of dairy products will prevent respiratory infections. Finally, contrary to popular belief, early antibiotic treatment of children with ear infections does not damage the child's immunity and thereby cause a greater rate of ear infections.

Alternative therapies. Various alternative therapies are said to be able to enhance overall health and thereby prevent illness in general. These include acupuncture, Ayurveda, chiropractic spinal manipulation, naturopathy, Reiki, Tai Chi, therapeutic touch, traditional Chinese herbal medicine, and yoga. However, there is little to no meaningful scientific evidence to indicate that these methods have any specific positive effect on immunity.

—*EBSCO CAM Review Board*

Further Information

Grimm, W., and H. Muller. "A Randomized Controlled Trial of the Effect of Fluid Extract of Echinacea purpurea on the Incidence and Severity of Colds and Respiratory Infections." *American Journal of Medicine*, vol. 106, 1999, pp. 138-43.

Jiang, M. H., L. Zhu, and J. G. Jiang. "Immunoregulatory Actions of Polysaccharides from Chinese Herbal Medicine." *Expert Opinion on Therapeutic Targets*, vol. 14, 2020, pp. 1367-1402.

Majdalawieh, A. F., and R. I. Carr. "In Vitro Investigation of the Potential Immunomodulatory and Anti-Cancer Activities of Black Pepper (Piper nigrum) and Cardamom (Elettaria cardamomum)." *Journal of Medicinal Food*, vol. 13, 2020, pp. 371-81.

Senchina, D. S., et al. "Herbal Supplements and Athlete Immune Function-What's Proven, Disproven, and Unproven?" *Exercise Immunology Review*, vol. 15, 2009, pp. 66-106.

Turner, R. B., D. K. Riker, and J. D. Gangemi. "Ineffectiveness of Echinacea for Prevention of Experimental Rhinovirus Colds." *Antimicrobial Agents and Chemotherapy*, vol. 44, 2000, pp. 1708-9.

Vonau, B., et al. "Does the Extract of the Plant Echinacea purpurea Influence the Clinical Course of Recurrent Genital Herpes?" *International Journal of STD and AIDS*, vol. 12, 2001, pp. 154-58.

Natural Treatments for Allergies

Category: Alternative and Complementary Medicine
Anatomy or system affected: Blood, eyes, gastrointestinal system, immune system, intestines, lungs,

lymphatic system, mouth, respiratory system, skin, throat
- **Specialties and related fields**: Dermatology, gastroenterology, hematology, immunology, internal medicine, ophthalmology, otorhinolaryngology, pharmacology, pulmonary medicine
- **Principal proposed natural treatments**: Butterbur, sublingual immunotherapy
- **Other proposed natural treatments**: Acupuncture, adrenal extract, antioxidants, Ayurvedic medicine, *Bacopa monniera* (brahmi), barberry, bee pollen, betaine hydrochloride, cat's claw, *Coleus forskohlii*, conjugated linoleic acid, enzyme potentiated desensitization, fish oil, gamma-linolenic acid, hops, hypnosis, methyl sulfonyl methane, nettle leaf, oligomeric proanthocyanidins, other flavonoids, including citrus bioflavonoids, probiotics, quercetin, rosmarinic acid/Perilla frutescens, royal jelly, soy sauce extract, spirulina, *Tinospora cordifolia*, topical capsaicin, traditional Chinese medicine, vitamin B_6, vitamin B_{12}, vitamin C, vitamin E
- **Definition**: Treatment for an allergic reaction best known as hay fever.

KEY TERMS

allergies: a damaging immune response to a substance, such as pollen, fur, food, or dust, to which it has become hypersensitive

herbs: any plant with leaves, seeds, or flowers used for flavoring, food, medicine, or perfume

IgE: an antibody subtype made by the immune system in response to allergens or worm infections

mast cells: a cell found throughout connective tissues, especially under the skin, near blood vessels and lymph vessels, in nerves, and in the lungs and intestines, filled with basophil granules that contain histamine and other immunomodulators

supplements: a manufactured of natural product that augments one's diet or medicines by taking a pill, capsule, tablet, powder, or liquid

INTRODUCTION

About 7 percent of all Americans have hay fever, an allergic condition that can cause runny nose, sneezing, and teary eyes. It is known officially as allergic rhinitis, allergic sinusitis, or allergic conjunctivitis, depending on whether symptoms manifest mainly in the nose, sinuses, or eyes, respectively. Hay fever usually peaks when particular plants are pollinating or when molds are flourishing. People who have year-round hay fever (perennial rhinitis) may be allergic to persistent allergens in the environment coming from such sources as dust mites, mice, and cockroaches.

In response to the foregoing triggers, a person prone to allergies develops an exaggerated immune response. Secreted glycoproteins called "immunoglobulin Es" (IgEs) flood the nasal passages; white blood cells called "eosinophils" arrive by the millions and billions; and inflammatory substances such as histamine, prostaglandins, and leukotrienes are released in massive amounts. The overall effect is the familiar one of swelling, dripping, itching, and aching.

The mechanism of allergic response is fairly well understood. Why allergic people react so excessively to innocent bits of pollen, however, remains a complete mystery. Conventional treatment for hay fever primarily involves nonsedating antihistamines and nasal steroids and is usually quite effective.

PRINCIPAL PROPOSED NATURAL TREATMENTS

The herb butterbur is best known as a promising new treatment for migraine headaches. However, butterbur may also be helpful for allergic rhinitis. In a two-week, double-blind, placebo-controlled study of 186 people with intermittent allergic rhinitis, the use of butterbur at a dose of three standardized tablets daily or one tablet daily reduced allergy symptoms compared with placebo. Significantly greater benefits were seen in the higher dose group. Such "dose dependency" is taken as a confirming sign that a treatment really works.

In another double-blind study, 330 people were given either butterbur extract (one tablet three times daily), the antihistamine fexofenadine (Allegra), or a placebo. The results showed that butterbur and fexofenadine were equally effective, and both were more effective than placebo. A two-week double-blind (and earlier) study of 125 persons with hay fever (technically, seasonal allergic rhinitis) compared a standardized butterbur extract with the antihistamine drug cetirizine. According to ratings by both doctors and patients, the two treatments proved equally effective. This study did not use a placebo group. Two much smaller studies produced inconsistent results.

An alternative to allergy shots known as sublingual immunotherapy (SLIT) involves using allergenic substances placed under the tongue. Numerous double-blind, placebo-controlled studies indicate that SLIT can improve all major symptoms of allergic rhinitis when the offending allergens are known. However, in a 2008 comprehensive review of SLIT for grass pollen and house dust mite allergies, researchers raised questions regarding the quality and consistency of these and other studies. If SLIT is effective, it may require two to three years for significant benefit to developing. One placebo-controlled study found that three years of treatment was more effective than two years. In addition, to provide benefits for grass allergy season, SLIT must be started at least eight weeks before the onset of the grass allergy season; even longer lead times lead to even better results. Putting all this evidence together, it appears that SLIT may work best if used year-round and year after year. One study suggests that SLIT is not only effective for treating allergy but also effective in preventing the development of new allergies or mild persistent asthma in children with allergic rhinitis or intermittent asthma.

While SLIT is well accepted in conventional medicine, another form of alternative allergy shots remains firmly in the alternative medicine field: enzyme potentiated desensitization (EPD). This method involves injections of allergens combined with certain enzymes. In one double-blind, placebo-controlled study, EPD failed to prove more helpful than placebo for seasonal allergic rhinitis.

THE BODY'S RESPONSE TO ALLERGENS
An allergic reaction occurs when foreign materials, or antigens, enter the body and encounter the immune system. Immune cells, called "B lymphocytes," secrete IgE antibodies against the antigens. The IgE antibodies bind to the surfaces of cells found throughout connective tissue called "mast cells." When the recently encountered antigens encounter the IgEs bound to the mast cell surfaces, they bind to them. The formation of antigen-antibody complexes on mast cell surfaces induces the mast cells to release their granules. These granules contain histamine and other immune modulators. Histamine causes the walls of capillaries to leak and smooth muscles in the respiratory tract to constrict. This accounts for the redness, swelling, heat, and pain associated with allergies.

OTHER PROPOSED NATURAL TREATMENTS
Several natural products have shown potential benefits for allergic rhinitis in one or more preliminary controlled trials. These include a water-extract of hops, a freeze-dried extract of stinging nettle, various probiotics, an extract of soy sauce (Shoyu polysaccharides), the herbs *Tinospora cordifolia* and *Astragalus membranaceus*, rosmarinic acid (a substance found in rosemary, and other herbs, including *Perilla frutescens*), and an Ayurvedic herbal formula containing *Commiphora mukul*, *T. cordifolia*, *Rubia*

cordifolia, *Emblica officinalis*, *Moringa pterygosperma*, and *Glycyrrhiza glabra*.

Traditional Chinese herbal medicine also has shown some promise for allergies. Another traditional Chinese treatment, acupuncture, is commonly recommended for allergies, but a controlled trial of forty people failed to find significantly more benefit with real acupuncture than with fake acupuncture. However, another study found benefits with real acupuncture plus real traditional Chinese herbs as opposed to placebo acupuncture and nonspecific Chinese herbs. Establishing the efficacy of acupuncture is difficult because designing a convincing placebo arm of the experiment is tedious and problematic. A carefully conducted review of seven placebo-controlled failed to find convincing evidence for acupuncture's effectiveness against allergic rhinitis.

One rather unusual study tested a nasal spray containing capsaicin, the "hot" in cayenne and other hot peppers. It is not clear how practical this spray would be (researchers had to use a local anesthetic in the nose before administering the spray). Preliminary evidence suggests that spirulina may counter allergic reactions of the type involved in hay fever. A sizable (112-participant) double-blind study of vitamin E at a dose of 800 milligrams daily for hay fever found modest benefits at best. A smaller study failed to find any benefits.

A twelve-week, double-blind, placebo-controlled study of forty people tested the supplement conjugated linoleic acid as a treatment for people with allergies to birch pollen and found some evidence of benefit. Vitamin C is often suggested as a treatment for allergies, but the research results are preliminary and somewhat contradictory.

Test tube studies suggest that flavonoids (biologically active compounds found in many plants) may help reduce allergy symptoms. A particular flavonoid, quercetin, seems to be one of the most active. Many natural medicine texts claim that quercetin works like the drug cromolyn (Intal) in that it prevents the release of allergenic mediators by mast cells. However, while there is direct evidence that cromolyn is effective, there have not been any published studies in which people were given quercetin, and their allergic symptoms decreased.

Tomato extract has been advocated for the treatment of allergic rhinitis, but the one double-blind study said to demonstrate benefit actually proves almost nothing because of major flaws in its statistical analysis.

Oligomeric proanthocyanidins (OPCs) from grape seed or pine bark are also often said to be effective. However, an eight-week double-blind trial of forty-nine persons found no benefit from grape seed extract (the dose was not stated).

The last several substances discussed (vitamins E and C, flavonoids, and OPCs) are antioxidants. One study failed to find evidence of benefit with a mixture of antioxidants: beta-carotene (9 mg per day), vitamin C (1,500 mg per day), vitamin E (130 mg per day), zinc (45 mg per day), selenium (76 mg per day), and garlic (150 mg per day). Adrenal extracts, bee pollen, *Bacopa monniera* (brahmi), barberry, vitamin B_6, vitamin B_{12}, cat's claw, *Coleus forskohlii*, methyl sulfonyl methane, and betaine hydrochloride are sometimes recommended for hay fever, but there is no significant evidence that they are effective. A 2009 review of six high-quality trials with more than one thousand children found that neither omega-3 nor omega-6 oil consumption prevented allergic diseases in high-risk children. Allergic diseases included eczema, asthma, allergic rhinitis, and food allergy, and omega-3 and omega-6 sources included gamma-linolenic acid, fish oil, canola oil, and borage oil.

It has often been suggested that the consumption of honey can reduce symptoms of hay fever. However, the one published study designed to test this suggestion failed to find a benefit. Another study failed to find the bee product royal jelly effective.

—*EBSCO CAM Review Board*

Further Information

Anandan, C., U. Nurmatov, and A. Sheikh. "Omega 3 and 6 Oils for Primary Prevention of Allergic Disease." *Allergy*, vol. 64, 2009, pp. 840-48.

Badar, V. A., et al. "Efficacy of *Tinospora cordifolia* in Allergic Rhinitis." *Journal of Ethnopharmacology*, vol. 96, 2004, pp. 445-49.

Brinkhaus, B., et al. "Acupuncture and Chinese Herbal Medicine in the Treatment of Patients with Seasonal Allergic Rhinitis." *Allergy*, vol. 59, 2004, pp. 953-69.

Cox, L. S., et al. "Sublingual Immunotherapy." *Journal of Allergy and Clinical Immunology*, vol. 117, 2006, pp. 1021-35.

Dahl, R., et al. "Sublingual Grass Allergen Tablet Immunotherapy Provides Sustained Clinical Benefit with Progressive Immunologic Changes over Two Years." *Journal of Allergy and Clinical Immunology*, vol. 121, 2008, pp. 512-18.

Douglas, R. M., et al. "Vitamin C for Preventing and Treating the Common Cold." *The Cochrane Database of Systematic Reviews*, vol. 3, no. CD000980, 2007, doi:10.1002/14651858.CD000980.pub3.

Giovannini, M., et al. "A Randomized Prospective Double-Blind Controlled Trial on Effects of Long-Term Consumption of Fermented Milk Containing *Lactobacillus casei* in Pre-school Children with Allergic Asthma and/or Rhinitis." *Pediatric Research*, vol. 62, 2007, p. 215.

Kobayashi, M., et al. "Shoyu Polysaccharides from Soy Sauce Improve Quality of Life for Patients with Seasonal Allergic Rhinitis." *International Journal of Molecular Medicine*, vol. 15, 2005, pp. 463-67.

Langewitz, W., et al. "Effect of Self-Hypnosis on Hay Fever Symptoms." *Psychotherapy and Psychosomatics*, vol. 74, 2005, pp. 165-72.

Magnusson, A. L., et al. "The Effect of Acupuncture on Allergic Rhinitis." *American Journal of Chinese Medicine*, vol. 32, 2004, pp. 105-15.

Marogna, M., et al. "Preventive Effects of Sublingual Immunotherapy in Childhood." *Annals of Allergy, Asthma, and Immunology*, vol. 101, 2008, pp. 206-11.

Matkovic, Z., V. Zivkovic, and M. Korica. "Efficacy and Safety of *Astragalus membranaceus* in the Treatment of Patients with Seasonal Allergic Rhinitis." *Phytotherapy Research*, vol. 24, 2010, pp. 175-81.

Pfaar, O., and L. Klimek. "Efficacy and Safety of Specific Immunotherapy with a High-Dose Sublingual Grass Pollen Preparation." *Annals of Allergy, Asthma, and Immunology*, vol. 100, 2008, pp. 256-63.

Rajan, T. V., et al. "Effect of Ingestion of Honey on Symptoms of Rhinoconjunctivitis." *Annals of Allergy, Asthma, and Immunology*, vol. 88, 2002, pp. 198-203.

Roberts, J., et al. "A Systematic Review of the Clinical Effectiveness of Acupuncture for Allergic Rhinitis." *BMC Complementary and Alternative Medicine*, vol. 8, 2008.

Shahar, E., G. Hassoun, and S. Pollack. "Effect of Vitamin E Supplementation on the Regular Treatment of Seasonal Allergic Rhinitis." *Annals of Allergy, Asthma, and Immunology*, vol. 92, 2004, pp. 654-58.

Yoshimura, M., et al. "An Evaluation of the Clinical Efficacy of Tomato Extract for Perennial Allergic Rhinitis." *Allergology International*, vol. 3, 2007, pp. 225-30.

NATURAL TREATMENTS FOR ASTHMA

Category: Alternative and Complementary Medicine

Anatomy or system affected: Blood, brain, eyes, gastrointestinal system, immune system, intestines, lungs, lymphatic system, mouth, respiratory system, skin, throat

Specialties and related fields: Dermatology, gastroenterology, hematology, immunology, internal medicine, ophthalmology, otorhinolaryngology, pharmacology, pulmonary medicine

Principal proposed natural treatments: *Boswellia, Coleus forskohlii, Tylophora*, ephedra (unsafe), vitamin C

Other proposed natural treatments: Acupuncture, adrenal extract, aloe, antioxidants, astha-15 (an Ayurvedic herbal combination), brahmi (*Bacopa monniera*), beta-carotene, betaine hydrochloride, butterbur, *Carum copticum* (ajwain), chamomile, coenzyme Q10, damiana, elecampane, elimination diet, essential fatty acids (omega-3 and omega-6 fatty acids), essential oil of eucalyptus, fish oil, flaxseed oil, food allergen elimination diet, garlic, gamma-linolenic acid from evening primrose oil, green-lipped mussel, grindelia, horehound, hyssop, hypnosis, ivy leaf, licorice, *Lobelia inflata*, magnesium, marshmallow, massage, melatonin, mullein, onion, oligomeric proanthocyanidins, osteopathic manipulation, picrorhiza, quercetin, reishi, relaxation therapy, selenium, sublingual immunotherapy, vitamin B_6, vitamin B_{12}, vitamin E, yerba santa, yoga

Definition: Treatment of severe breathing difficulties caused by bronchial inflammation and contraction.

KEY TERMS

acupuncture: a system of integrative medicine that involves pricking the skin or tissues with needles, used to alleviate pain and to treat various physical, mental, and emotional conditions

anti-inflammatory medication: a drug or substance that reduces inflammation (redness, swelling, and pain) in the body by blocking certain substances in the body that cause inflammation

bronchial tubes: tubes that carry air to your lungs; problems with the bronchi include bronchitis, bronchiectasis, and bronchiolitis

bronchodilator: a drug that causes widening of the bronchi, e.g., any of those taken by inhalation for the alleviation of asthma

Buteyko breathing: a form of complementary or alternative physical therapy that proposes the use of breathing exercises primarily as a treatment for asthma and other respiratory conditions

INTRODUCTION

People who have an asthma attack have real trouble taking a breath. Many people with stuffy noses from hay fever or colds say, "I can't breathe," but they retain the option of breathing through the mouth. For asthmatics, the bronchial tubes in their lungs become swollen and clogged. Breathing can become frighteningly difficult.

Asthma involves two conditions: contraction of the small muscles surrounding the bronchial tubes and inflammation of the lining of those tubes. Traditionally, treatment primarily addressed the first aspect of asthma; recently, however, it has become clear that tissue swelling is the underlying cause.

During an asthma attack, obstructed bronchioles limit or halt airflow, resulting in severely restricted breathing. The conventional treatment of asthma is highly effective for most people. Treatments include short- and long-acting bronchodilators, which relax the bronchial muscles, and anti-inflammatory medication, which helps relieve tissue swelling. Bronchodilators alone may be sufficient treatment for mild asthma or asthma that occurs only with exercise. Anti-inflammatory steroids in the cortisone family taken by inhalation are the mainstay of moderate to severe asthma treatment. Although these are much safer than oral steroids, they may still increase the risk of osteoporosis and other problems when taken in high doses or long. Other drugs used to reduce inflammation include montelukast (*Singulair*) and cromolyn (*Intal*). (cromolyn comes from a Mediterranean herb named khella.) The newest drug treatment for asthma, omalizumab (*Xolair*), appears to be safe and effective. Still, it is costly, and for this reason, it is used sparingly.

PRINCIPAL PROPOSED NATURAL TREATMENTS

None of these treatments is effective for severe asthma. One should not stop standard asthma medication except on the advice of a physician.

Tylophora indica. This herb (also called *T. asthmatica*) appears to offer some promise to treat asthma. It has a long history of use in the traditional Ayurvedic medicine of India. However, all studies on this herb were performed in India long ago and failed to reach modern design and reporting standards.

In a double-blind, placebo-controlled study of 195 persons with asthma, the participants given 40 milligrams (mg) of a *Tylophora* alcohol extract daily for six days showed significant improvement compared with placebo. Similar results were seen in two double-blind, placebo-controlled studies involving more than two hundred persons with asthma. However, the design of these studies was a bit convoluted, and various pieces of information are missing from the reports, causing some difficulty in evaluating the validity of these trials.

Another double-blind study that enrolled 135 persons and followed a more straightforward design found no benefit from *Tylophora*. Although *Tylophora* is promising, more extensive and better studies are necessary to discover whether *Tylophora* is genuinely effective.

Boswellia. The herb *Boswellia* has shown promise as a treatment for rheumatoid arthritis. It might work by inhibiting inflammation. Because asthma involves inflammation and is treated by some of the same drugs that treat rheumatoid arthritis, *Boswellia* has been tried for this purpose, too.

One six-week, double-blind, placebo-controlled study of eighty persons with relatively mild asthma found that treatment with Boswellia at a dose of 300 mg three times daily reduced the frequency of asthma attacks and improved objective measurements of breathing capacity. However, further research must follow up this pilot study before Boswellia is a potential asthma treatment.

Coleus forskohlii. Another herb sometimes recommended for asthma also comes from India, *Coleus forskohlii*. While there is some preliminary evidence that it might have value, this evidence is far too weak to be reliable. Furthermore, as sold, the herb is more like a drug than an herb. Natural *C. forskohlii* contains small amounts of a potent chemical called "forskolin." Manufacturers deliberately modify the herb to increase its forskolin content dramatically; therefore, when using such products, one is essentially using an unlicensed drug. Forskolin appears to be safe, but more studies need to be undertaken before it can be recommended for self-treatment.

Ma huang. The Chinese herb *ma huang*, also called "ephedra," is effective for mild asthma because it contains ephedrine. However, it is not recommended because of safety concerns. This Chinese herb is a member of a primitive family of plants that look like thin, branching, connected straws. A related species, *Ephedra nevadensis*, grows wild in the American Southwest and is widely called "Mormon tea." However, only the Asian species of ephedra contains the active compounds ephedrine and pseudoephedrine. Chinese herbalists traditionally used *Ma huang* in the early stages of respiratory infections and the short-term treatment of certain kinds of asthma, eczema, hay fever, narcolepsy, and edema. Japanese chemists isolated ephedrine from *ma huang* around the beginning of the twentieth century. It soon became a primary treatment for asthma in the United States and abroad. Ephedra's other primary ingredient, pseudoephedrine, became the decongestant Sudafed.

Although ephedrine can still be found in a few over-the-counter asthma drugs, physicians seldom prescribe it today. The problem is that ephedrine mimics the effects of adrenaline and causes symptoms such as rapid heartbeat, high blood pressure, agitation, insomnia, nausea, and loss of appetite. The newer asthma drugs are much safer and easier to tolerate. Therefore, presently synthetic drugs are less dangerous than natural ones. *Ma huang* is not recommended for treating asthma.

OTHER PROPOSED NATURAL TREATMENTS

Other herbs and supplements. In a double-blind trial, thirty-two people with steroid-dependent asthma were given either placebo or essential oil of eucalyptus for twelve weeks. The results showed that people using eucalyptus were more able to reduce their steroid dosage than those taking a placebo gradually.

Two double-blind, placebo-controlled studies enrolling more than eighty people with asthma suggest that oligomeric proanthocyanidins from pine bark might reduce symptoms. An extract made from ivy leaf has been advocated for treating childhood asthma. Still, the meaningful supporting evidence is again limited to one placebo-controlled trial.

Another small, double-blind, placebo-controlled study evaluated the effects of four weeks of treatment with a Japanese herbal mixture traditionally called "Saiboku-To." Researchers tested the tendency of the bronchial tubes to contract in response to an asthma-producing substance called "methacholine." The results indicated that the use of Saiboku-To helped prevent such contractions, and it also reduced lung inflammation. Another study reportedly found benefits with a combination named Mai-Men-Dong-Tang.

Many studies have been conducted on the effects of vitamin C in treating asthma. Still, the evidence that it works remains inconsistent and highly incomplete. There is only weak and inconsistent evidence regarding whether two antioxidants in the carotenoid family, lycopene, and beta-carotene, might help prevent exercise-induced asthma. One double-blind comparative study provides weak evidence that the Ayurvedic herbal combination called "Astha" might be helpful for mild asthma.

Vitamin B_6 is often mentioned as a treatment for asthma. Still, the evidence that it works is weak and contradictory at best. A double-blind study of seventy-six children with asthma found significant benefits from vitamin B_6 after the second month of usage. Children in the treated group were able to reduce their doses of bronchodilators and steroids. However, a recent double-blind study of thirty-one adults who also used inhaled or oral steroids did not benefit. Supplementation with vitamin B_{12} is also often said to be effective for asthma. However, the scientific evidence in its favor consists almost entirely of open studies that did not eliminate the placebo effect.

Preliminary evidence hints that the herb butterbur may be helpful for asthma. Another study found potential benefits with the spice *Carum copticum*.

Essential fatty acids, such as gamma-linolenic acid and those found in fish oil and flaxseed oil, may inhibit inflammatory responses such as those in asthma. However, the studies that tried fish oil as a treatment for asthma failed to find significant clinical benefits; one study found that fish oil can worsen aspirin-related asthma. Nonetheless, there is some evidence from one research group that fish oil might be helpful for exercise-induced asthma. There is also some preliminary evidence that women who take fish oil during late pregnancy may reduce the risk of asthma in their children for up to sixteen years after birth.

A study of seventy-two children with moderate, persistent asthma found that combined or single supplementation with omega-3 oils, zinc, or vitamin C improved their symptoms and lung function. Combined supplementation was associated with the most significant improvement. However, these results are dubious because about 20 percent of the children dropped out before the end of the thirty-eight-week study.

A preliminary double-blind, placebo-controlled trial suggests that green-lipped mussel extract might be helpful for allergic asthma. Another study suggests that the natural substance hyaluronic acid might be helpful for asthma when taken by inhalation.

Natural medicine practitioners frequently recommend flavonoid quercetin as a treatment for asthma. However, the only basis for this recommendation consists of a few older, preliminary test-tube studies that suggest it might inhibit the release of inflammatory substances from special cells called "mast cells." The asthma drug Intal (cromolyn) is believed to work in this way. However, there is significant direct evidence from human trials that Intal taken by inhalation works. In contrast, no such evidence exists for quercetin taken in any manner; and it is doubtful that oral intake of quercetin could produce levels in the body similar to the levels used in those test-tube studies.

Alternative medical literature frequently mentions magnesium as a treatment for asthma. However, this idea seems to be based primarily on intravenous magnesium as an emergency treatment for asthma. (Taking something by mouth is very different from having it injected into the veins.) Studies of oral magnesium for asthma have shown more negative than positive results. Still, some evidence exists that intravenous or inhaled magnesium may be beneficial. Also, preliminary evidence, far too weak to be relied upon, has been used to suggest that the supplement coenzyme Q10 (CoQ10) might be helpful for asthma.

Lobelia inflata is sometimes recommended as an herbal treatment for asthma; according to traditional directions, people should take enough of it to induce vomiting. Other natural products commonly recommended for asthma include aloe, brahmi (*Bacopa monniera*), chamomile, damiana, elecampane, garlic, grindelia, horehound, hyssop, licorice, marshmallow, mullein, onion, reishi, and yerba santa, and the supplements adrenal extract and betaine hydrochloride. None of these treatments has any meaningful supporting evidence.

Antioxidants, such as vitamin E, beta-carotene, and selenium, are frequently recommended for asthma because they may protect inflamed lung tissue. Although one study found that asthmatics placed on a low antioxidant diet for ten days experienced worsening symptoms, there is no direct scientific evidence that antioxidant supplementation improves asthma. A rather theoretical study found evidence that the use of vitamin E might decrease the inflammatory response in children with asthma exposed to ozone. However, a more meaningful double-blind, placebo-controlled study found vitamin E (500 mg of natural vitamin E) ineffective for asthma. Similarly, a large (almost two-hundred-participant) study failed to find selenium helpful for asthma.

The herb picrorhiza has been advocated as a treatment for asthma, based primarily on two studies conducted in the 1970s. However, none of these studies reached modern scientific standards. Two subsequent and better-designed studies of picrorhiza failed to find the herb more effective than placebo.

One study failed to find a mixture of probiotics (friendly bacteria) helpful for asthma in children. Another study, though, found that a mixture of probiotic *Bifidobacterium breve* and the prebiotic galacto- and fructooligosaccharides may help reduce wheezing in infants with eczema.

Children with asthma may have reduced growth, possibly from the use of inhaled steroids. One study failed to find protective benefits with a multivitamin that contained vitamin D. The tested supplement did not contain calcium. Other studies have found that combination treatment with calcium and vitamin D may protect bone density in people taking oral corticosteroids (for various reasons, including asthma).

Two preliminary studies reported by one research group have led to publicized concerns that the insomnia supplement melatonin may worsen night-time asthma. However, one double-blind study of melatonin in asthma found evidence of improved sleep without worsening asthma symptoms.

Acupuncture. Although there have been numerous reports on acupuncture treatment for asthma, the results have been contradictory. A team of three researchers analyzed thirteen trials on acupuncture in the treatment of asthma. These studies were scored based on design quality, with a maximum possible score of 100 points. Criteria for assigning points included the size of the study population, randomization procedure, description of treatment, measurement of effects, and follow-up. Eight studies earned more than 50 points, and the highest score was 72 points. However, the overall quality of these studies is mediocre; in any case, the results were contradictory. The conclusion was that "claims that acupuncture is effective in the treatment of asthma are not based on the results of well-performed clinical trials." A more recent review of acupuncture for asthma came to identical conclusions.

Other alternative therapies. Sublingual immunotherapy, a form of "allergy shot" that involves drops or tablets under the tongue rather than injections, works well to treat asthma. Some people with asthma may also have food allergies. One way to discover a food allergy is to eliminate potentially allergenic foods from the diet and then systematically reintroduce them to see if a reaction occurs. Patients should undertake elimination diets only under a doctor's care because of the risk of severe allergic reactions. Other ways to diagnose a food allergy include the skin scratch test and blood tests (such as Radioabsorbent text [RAST] or enzyme-linked immunoabsorbent assay [ELISA]). Persons with a food allergy who eliminate the offending food from the diet might reduce their asthma symptoms.

Hypnosis, massage, yoga, and other forms of relaxation therapy may offer modest benefits for asthma. A unique breathing technique called "Buteyko breathing" may reduce medication use and subjective symptoms. However, it does not appear actually to improve lung function. The same is true of standard aerobic exercise.

In two controlled studies, chiropractic spinal manipulation has failed to prove more effective than fake manipulation for the treatment of asthma. One study of osteopathic manipulation reportedly found benefits, but the study's design was flawed.

People should understand that "natural" does not axiomatically mean safe. Prescription and over-the-counter drugs are subjected to rigorous and thorough safety and efficacy testing before stores can sell them or doctors prescribe them. However, herbal medicines do not go through such exacting testing. Instead, the U.S. government classifies herbs as dietary supplements and not foods or drugs. This classification difference can pose genuine risks to those with allergies or asthma.

Herbs and vitamins need not conform to drug labeling laws. Ingredient labels for supplements are usually incomplete or incorrect. Herbal remedies made from plants can cause allergic reactions in people with allergies to foods or pollens. Chamomile and other herbal teas may promote a calming effect. However, they can cause an allergic reaction for people with a ragweed pollen allergy. Those with ragweed allergies should also avoid Echinacea since these two plants are closely related. Rather than fighting a cold, Echinacea may cause allergies, causing even more misery.

Although these studies hold promise for using alternative formulas in asthma management, the American Academy of Allergies, Asthma, and Immunology strongly warns against using them as a substitute for your asthma medications.

—*EBSCO CAM Review Board*

Further Information

Biltagi, M. A., et al. "Omega-3 Fatty Acids, Vitamin C and Zn Supplementation in Asthmatic Children." *Acta Paediatrica*, vol. 98, 2009, pp. 737-42.

Campos, F. L., et al. "Melatonin Improves Sleep in Asthma." *American Journal of Respiratory Critical Care Medicine*, 170, 2004, pp. 947-51.

Cowie, R. L., et al. "A Randomised Controlled Trial of the Buteyko Technique as an Adjunct to Conventional Management of Asthma." *Respiratory Medicine*, vol. 102, 2008, pp. 726-32.

Giovannini, M., et al. "A Randomized Prospective Double-Blind Controlled Trial on Effects of Long-Term Consumption of Fermented Milk Containing *Lactobacillus casei* in Pre-school Children with Allergic Asthma and/or Rhinitis." *Pediatric Research*, vol. 62, 2007, pp. 215-20.

Gontijo-Amaral, C., et al. "Oral Magnesium Supplementation in Asthmatic Children." *European Journal of Clinical Nutrition*, vol. 61, 2006, pp. 54-60.

Guiney, P. A., et al. "Effects of Osteopathic Manipulative Treatment on Pediatric Patients with Asthma." *Journal of the American Osteopathic Association*, vol. 105, 2005, pp. 7-12.

Gvozdjakova, A., et al. "Coenzyme Q10 Supplementation Reduces Corticosteroids Dosage in Patients with Bronchial Asthma." *Biofactors*, vol. 25, 2006, pp. 235-40.

Huntley, A., A. R. White, and E. Ernst. "Relaxation Therapies for Asthma." *Thorax*, vol. 57, 2002, pp. 127-31.

Mickleborough, T. D., et al. "Protective Effect of Fish Oil Supplementation on Exercise-Induced Bronchoconstriction in Asthma." *Chest*, vol. 129, 2006, pp. 39-49.

Olsen, S. F., et al. "Fish Oil Intake Compared with Olive Oil Intake in Late Pregnancy and Asthma in the Offspring." *American Journal of Clinical Nutrition*, vol. 88, 2008, pp. 167-75.

"Reactions to Complementary and Alternative Medicines." *American Academy of Allergy, Asthma, and Immunology*, www.aaaai.org/Aaaai/media/MediaLibrary/PDF%20Documents/Libraries/EL-Reactions-to-CAM-patient.pdf. Accessed 2 Sept. 2021.

Sabina, A. B., et al. "Yoga Intervention for Adults with Mild-to-Moderate Asthma." *Annals of Allergy, Asthma, and Immunology*, vol. 94, 2005, pp. 543-48.

Schubert, R., et al. "Effect of N-3 Polyunsaturated Fatty Acids in Asthma After Low-Dose Allergen Challenge." *International Archives of Allergy and Immunology*, vol. 148, 2009, pp. 321-29.

Sienra-Monge, J. J., et al. "Antioxidant Supplementation and Nasal Inflammatory Responses Among Young Asthmatics Exposed to High Levels of Ozone." *Clinical and Experimental Immunology* vol. 138, 2004, pp. 317-22.

"Studies on Asthma and Chinese Herbs." *American Academy of Allergy, Asthma, and Immunology*, 28 Sept. 2020, www.aaaai.org/Tools-for-the-Public/Conditions-Library/Asthma/Studies-on-Asthma-and-Chinese-Herbs. Accessed 2 Sept. 2021.

Van der Aa, L. B., et al. "Synbiotics Prevent Asthma-Like Symptoms in Infants with Atopic Dermatitis." *Allergy*, 17 Jun. 2010.

Vempati, R., R. L. Bijlani, and K. K. Deepak. "The Efficacy of a Comprehensive Lifestyle Modification Programme Based on Yoga in the Management of Bronchial Asthma." *BMC Pulmonary Medicine*, vol. 9, 2009, p. 37.

NATURAL TREATMENTS FOR LUPUS

Category: Alternative and Complementary Medicine
Anatomy or system affected: All tissues
Specialties and related fields: Dermatology, gastroenterology, hematology, immunology, internal medicine, neurology, oncology, ophthalmology, otorhinolaryngology, pharmacology, pulmonary medicine
Principal proposed natural treatment: Dehydroepiandrosterone.
Other proposed natural treatments: Beta-carotene, *Cordyceps*, fish oil, flaxseed, food allergen identification and avoidance, magnesium, pantothenic acid, selenium, vitamin B_3, vitamin B_{12}, and vitamin E.
Natural product to avoid: Alfalfa
Definition: Treatment of an autoimmune disease in which antibodies develop to fight foreign substances in the body.

KEY TERMS

autoantibodies: an antibody produced by the immune system against its tissues

dehydroepiandrosterone: also known as androstenolone, is an endogenous steroid hormone precursor and one of the most abundant circulating steroids in humans

INTRODUCTION

Systemic lupus erythematosus (also known as lupus or SLE) is an autoimmune disease that primarily affects young and middle-aged women. Its cause is unknown but involves both genetic inheritance and factors in the environment. Whatever the cause, people with lupus develop antibodies against substances in their bodies, including deoxyribonucleic acid (DNA). These antibodies cause widespread damage and are primarily responsible for the many symptoms of this disease.

Lupus may begin with such symptoms as fatigue, weight loss, fever, malaise, and loss of appetite. Other common early symptoms include muscle pain, joint pain, and a facial rash. As lupus progresses, symptoms may develop in virtually every part of the body. Kidney damage is one of the most devastating effects of lupus. Still, many other serious problems may develop, including seizures, mental impairment, anemia, and inflammation of the heart, blood vessels, eyes, and digestive tract.

Conventional treatment for lupus centers on a variety of anti-inflammatory drugs. In mild cases, taking nonsteroidal anti-inflammatory drugs (NSAIDs) may help; more severe forms of lupus require long-term use of corticosteroid anti-inflammatory drugs such as prednisone. Cytotoxic agents (azathioprine, cyclophosphamide, and chlorambucil) might also be helpful, but they too have many side effects. The side effects of these medications can be pretty serious themselves. Close physician supervision is always required with lupus because of the risk of complications in so many organs.

PRINCIPAL PROPOSED NATURAL TREATMENTS

A meaningful body of evidence indicates that the hormone dehydroepiandrosterone (DHEA) may be helpful for the treatment of lupus when used as part of a comprehensive, physician-directed treatment approach. DHEA is the most abundant steroid hormone found in the bloodstream. The body uses DHEA as the starting material for making the sex hormones testosterone and estrogen. Clinicians have tested DHEA as a treatment for various medical conditions, including osteoporosis, with mixed results. However, it shows its most significant promise in the treatment of lupus.

A twelve-month, double-blind, placebo-controlled trial of 381 women with mild or moderate lupus evaluated the effects of DHEA at a dose of 200 milligrams (mg) daily. Although many participants in both groups improved (the power of placebo is often notable), DHEA was more effective than placebo, reducing many symptoms of the disease.

Similarly, in a double-blind, placebo-controlled study of 120 women with lupus, the use of DHEA at a dose of 200 mg daily significantly decreased symptoms and reduced the frequency of disease flare-ups. A smaller study found equivocal evidence that a lower dose of DHEA (30 mg daily for women older than age forty-five years and 20 mg daily for women aged forty-five years) might also work.

A 2007 review of all published studies concluded that the use of DHEA may meaningfully improve quality of life in the short term for people with lupus, but that it probably does not alter the long-term course of the disease.

OTHER PROPOSED NATURAL TREATMENTS

Flaxseed contains lignans and alpha-linolenic acid, substances with a wide variety of effects in the body. In particular, flaxseed may antagonize the activity of a substance called "platelet-activating factor" (PAF) that plays a role in lupus kidney disease (lupus nephritis). Preliminary evidence suggests that flaxseed might help prevent or treat lupus nephritis.

Fish oil contains omega-3 fatty acids, which have some anti-inflammatory effects. Fish oil has been found helpful in rheumatoid arthritis, a disease related to lupus. The results of two small double-blind studies suggest that fish oil might also be useful for lupus. However, evidence suggests that fish oil is not effective for lupus nephritis.

Other treatments sometimes recommended for lupus include beta-carotene, *Cordyceps*, magnesium, selenium, vitamin B_3, vitamin B_{12}, vitamin E, pantothenic acid, and food allergen identification and avoidance. However, there is no meaningful evidence that these treatments work for lupus. Another study failed to find copper supplements helpful for lupus symptoms.

HERBS AND SUPPLEMENTS TO AVOID
People with lupus should avoid alfalfa entirely. The herb alfalfa contains L-canavanine, which can worsen lupus or bring it out of remission. Also, various herbs and supplements may interact adversely with drugs used to treat lupus.

—*EBSCO CAM Review Board*

Further Information

Chang, D. M., et al. "Dehydroepiandrosterone Treatment of Women with Mild-to-Moderate Systemic Lupus Erythematosus." *Arthritis and Rheumatism*, vol. 46, 2002, pp. 2924-27.

Crosbie, D., et al. "Dehydroepiandrosterone for Systemic Lupus Erythematosus." *Cochrane Database of Systematic Reviews*, vol. 4, no. CD005114, 2007, p. CD005114, www.cochrane.org/CD005114/MUSKEL_dehydroepiandrosterone-dhea-for-lupus-erythematosus , doi:10.1002/14651858.CD005114.pub2.

Duffy, E. M., et al. "The Clinical Effect of Dietary Supplementation with Omega-3 Fish Oils and/or Copper in Systemic Lupus Erythematosus." *Journal of Rheumatology*, vol. 31, 2004, p. 1551.

Nordmark, G., et al. "Effects of Dehydroepiandrosterone Supplement on Health-Related Quality of Life in Glucocorticoid Treated Female Patients with Systemic Lupus Erythematosus." *Autoimmunity*, vol. 38, 2005, pp. 531-40.

Petri, Michelle A., et al. "Effects of Prasterone on Disease Activity and Symptoms in Women with Active Systemic Lupus Erythematosus." *Arthritis and Rheumatism* vol. 50, no. 9, 2004, pp. 2858-68, doi:10.1002/art.20427.

NATURAL TREATMENTS FOR RHEUMATOID ARTHRITIS

Category: Alternative and Complementary Medicine
Anatomy or system affected: Blood, eyes, immune system, joints, lymphatic system, mouth, skin
Specialties and related fields: Dermatology, hematology, immunology, internal medicine, ophthalmology, orthopedics, pathology, pharmacology, pulmonary medicine, rheumatology

Principal proposed natural treatment: Fish oil
Other proposed natural treatments: Acupuncture, balneotherapy (spa therapy), *Boswellia*, bromelain, cat's claw, curcumin (turmeric), deer velvet, devil's claw, folate, food allergen avoidance, gamma-linolenic acid, glucosamine, krill oil, magnet therapy, olive oil, relaxation therapies, rose hips, *Tripterygium wilfordii*, vegan diet, vitamin B_6, vitamin E, zinc
Definition: Treatment of the disease in which the immune system attacks tissues in the body, especially cartilage in the joints.

KEY TERMS

disease-modifying antirheumatic drugs: a category of unrelated drugs that slow the progression of rheumatoid arthritis

tumor necrosis factor (TNF-α)-alpha: a small signaling protein released by the cells of the immune system in response to infection

INTRODUCTION

Rheumatoid arthritis is an autoimmune disease in the general family of lupus. For reasons that are not understood, in rheumatoid arthritis, the immune system goes awry. It begins attacking tissues, especially cartilage in the joints. Various joints become red, hot, and swollen under the onslaught. The pattern of inflammation is usually symmetrical, occurring on both sides of the body. Other symptoms include inflammation of the eyes, nodules (or lumps) under the skin, and a general feeling of malaise.

Rheumatoid arthritis is more common in women than in men and typically begins between thirty-five and sixty. The diagnosis is made by matching the pattern of symptoms with specific characteristic laboratory results.

Medical treatment consists mainly of anti-inflammatory drugs in the ibuprofen family (nonsteroidal anti-inflammatory drugs, or NSAIDs) and drugs that may put rheumatoid arthritis into complete or partial remission (the disease-modifying antirheumatic drugs, or DMARDs).

Anti-inflammatory drugs relieve symptoms of rheumatoid arthritis but do not change the overall progression of the disease. In contrast, DMARDs seem to affect the disease itself. In rheumatoid arthritis, the drugs believed to alter the course of the disease (to slow it down or stop it) include antimalarials (hydroxychloroquine and chloroquine), sulfasalazine, tumor necrosis factor (TNF) inhibitors (etanercept, infliximab, and adalimumab), interleukin-1 receptor antagonists, leflunomide methotrexate, gold compounds, D-penicillamine, and cytotoxic agents (azathioprine, cyclophosphamide, and cyclosporine). These drugs are unrelated to one another but work somewhat similarly in practice.

Most of the drugs in this category can cause severe side effects. Because of this toxicity, physicians adopted a so-called pyramid approach for people with rheumatoid arthritis for years. Physicians started with NSAIDs to help with the pain and inflammation. They progressed to successively more potent and more toxic medications only when the basic treatments failed. Natural treatments such as those described here might also be useful in the early stages.

However, more recent research has found that severe joint damage occurs early in rheumatoid arthritis. This evidence has caused many authorities to suggest early, aggressive treatment with disease-modifying drugs to prevent joint damage. Nonetheless, this approach has not been universally adopted, and some physicians still prescribe NSAIDs for the early stages of rheumatoid arthritis. The treatments described here may be reasonable alternative options.

PRINCIPAL PROPOSED NATURAL TREATMENTS

Rheumatoid arthritis is a complex disease, and no alternative approach solves it easily. Even if one chooses to use alternative methods, all patients should regularly visit a rheumatologist to watch for serious complications. Medical treatment may be able to slow the progression of rheumatoid arthritis. It is not likely that any of the alternative options have the same ability.

Fish oil. Fish oil is the only natural treatment for rheumatoid arthritis with significant documentation. According to the results of about thirteen double-blind, placebo-controlled studies involving more than five hundred participants, supplementation with omega-3 fatty acids can significantly reduce the symptoms of rheumatoid arthritis. Also, at least one small study suggests that omega-3 fatty acids may help persons with rheumatoid arthritis lower their dose of nonsteroidal anti-inflammatory medication (such as ibuprofen).

However, unlike some of the standard treatments, fish oil has not been shown to slow the progression of rheumatoid arthritis. Omega-3 supplementation is more effective when omega-6 intake (particularly arachidonic acid) is kept low, as with a vegetarian diet. The benefits of fish oil may also be enhanced by simultaneous use of olive oil. One poorly designed human study hints that a relative of fish oil, krill oil, might also be helpful. Flaxseed oil has been offered as a more palatable substitute for fish oil, but it does not seem to work.

OTHER PROPOSED TREATMENTS

Boswellia serrata is a shrub-like tree that grows in the dry hills of the Indian subcontinent. It is the source of a resin called "salai guggal," which has been used for thousands of years in Ayurvedic medicine, the traditional medicine of the region. It is very similar to a resin from a related tree, *B. carteri*, also known as frankincense. Both substances have been used historically for arthritis.

Research has identified boswellic acids as the likely active ingredients in *Boswellia*. In animal studies, boswellic acids have shown anti-inflammatory effects. However, their mechanism of action seems to be quite different from that of standard anti-inflammatory medications.

An issue of the journal *Phytomedicine* devoted to *Boswellia* briefly reviewed previously unpublished studies on the herb. A pair of placebo-controlled trials involving eighty-one people with rheumatoid arthritis found significant reductions in swelling and pain for three months. Furthermore, a comparative study of sixty people over six months found the *Boswellia* extract relieved symptoms about oral gold therapy. However, while gold shots can induce remission in rheumatoid arthritis, there is no evidence that *Boswellia* can do the same.

Another double-blind study found no difference between *Boswellia* and placebo. More research is needed to know whether *Boswellia* is an effective treatment for rheumatoid arthritis.

The herb *devil's claw* may be beneficial in rheumatoid arthritis. One double-blind study followed eighty-nine people with rheumatoid arthritis for two months. The group given devil's claw showed a significant decrease in pain intensity and an improvement in mobility. Another double-blind study of fifty people with various types of arthritis showed that ten days of treatment with devil's claw provided significant pain relief.

Other herbs and supplements. Glucosamine is best known as a proposed treatment for osteoarthritis, but it might also be helpful for rheumatoid arthritis. A double-blind, placebo-controlled study of fifty-one people with rheumatoid arthritis found that glucosamine at a dose of 1,500 milligrams (mg) daily significantly improved symptoms. Glucosamine did not, however, alter measures of inflammation as determined through blood tests.

Some evidence, including small double-blind trials, supports the use of the following herbs and supplements for the treatment of rheumatoid arthritis: gamma-linolenic acid (found in evening primrose oil and borage oil), cat's claw (*Uncaria tomentosa*), rosehip powder, and the Chinese herb *Tripterygium wilfordii* (applied topically or taken orally). *T. wilfordii* is believed to be unsafe for pregnant or nursing women and may also present risks in other groups.

Preliminary evidence suggests potential benefits with the following herbs and supplements: methyl sulfonyl methane, yucca, and a mixture of poplar, ash, and goldenrod.

Vitamin E may reduce pain in rheumatoid arthritis, but it does not seem to reduce inflammation. Some evidence suggests that adding vitamin E, or vitamin E plus other antioxidants, to standard rheumatoid arthritis therapy might improve results. However, an extensive randomized trial involving more than 39,000 women found that taking 600 international units of vitamin E every other day did not reduce the risk of rheumatoid arthritis.

Persons taking the drug methotrexate for treatment of rheumatoid arthritis may benefit by taking folate supplements. Folate appears to reduce methotrexate side effects, including mouth sores, nausea, and liver inflammation. In addition, folate supplements may help reverse a more subtle methotrexate side effect: a rise in blood levels of homocysteine. Elevated levels of homocysteine increase the risk of heart disease.

The following treatments are also sometimes proposed as effective for rheumatoid arthritis. Still, there is little to no scientific evidence for or against their use: adrenal extract, beta-carotene, betaine hydrochloride, boron, burdock, cayenne, chamomile, copper, feverfew, folate, ginger, L-histidine, horsetail, magnesium, manganese, molybdenum, panto- thenic acid, D-phenylalanine, perilla frutescens, pregnenolone, proteolytic enzymes, sea cucumber, and vitamin C. Evidence regarding green-lipped mussel for rheumatoid arthritis is more negative than positive.

Zinc supplements have been evaluated as a treatment for rheumatoid arthritis, but overall, the study results have not been encouraging. One study failed to find vitamin B_6 at a dose of 50 mg daily helpful for rheumatoid arthritis, despite a general vitamin B_6 deficiency seen in people with this condition. Other treatments that have generally failed to prove effective in small double-blind trials include selenium, collagen, probiotics, white willow, and an Ayurvedic herbal mixture containing extracts of ashwagandha, *Boswellia*, ginger, and turmeric. Two studies commonly cited evidence that turmeric alone is helpful for rheumatoid arthritis fail to provide any meaningful supporting evidence. A six-month, double-blind, placebo-controlled study of 168 people with rheumatoid arthritis failed to find that elk velvet antler enhanced the effectiveness of conventional treatment for rheumatoid arthritis.

Other alternative therapies. Adopting a vegan (pure vegetarian) diet might help mild rheumatoid arthritis, although the supporting evidence for this claim is weak. Identifying and avoiding food allergens has also been tried. Still, one controlled trial found no clear evidence of benefit with a low-saturated-fat, hypoallergenic diet.

Balneotherapy (hot baths), relaxation therapy, and magnet therapy have shown some promise for rheumatoid arthritis. Two separate groups of researchers conducting detailed reviews of eight randomized, controlled trials found some beneficial effects of acupuncture for rheumatoid arthritis. However, researchers were not convinced that it was more beneficial than sham acupuncture or other standard treatments.

HERBS AND SUPPLEMENTS TO USE WITH CAUTION

Various herbs and supplements may interact adversely with drugs used to treat rheumatoid arthritis, so one should be cautious when considering the use of herbs and supplements.

—*EBSCO CAM Review Board*

Further Information

Allen, M., et al. "A Randomized Clinical Trial of Elk Velvet Antler in Rheumatoid Arthritis." *Biological Research for Nursing*, vol. 9, 2008, pp. 254-61.

Berbert, A. A., et al. "Supplementation of Fish Oil and Olive Oil in Patients with Rheumatoid Arthritis." *Nutrition*, vol. 21, 2005, pp. 131-36.

Biegert, C., et al. "Efficacy and Safety of Willow Bark Extract in the Treatment of Osteoarthritis and Rheumatoid Arthritis." *Journal of Rheumatology*, vol. 31, 2004, pp. 2121-30.

Canter, P. H., et al. "A Systematic Review of Randomised Clinical Trials of *Tripterygium wilfordii* for Rheumatoid Arthritis." *Phytomedicine*, vol. 13, 2006, pp. 371-77.

Deutsch, L. "Evaluation of the Effect of Neptune Krill Oil on Chronic Inflammation and Arthritic Symptoms." *Journal of the American College of Nutrition*, vol. 26, 2007, pp. 39-48.

Galarraga, B., et al. "Cod Liver Oil (N-3 Fatty Acids) as a Nonsteroidal Anti-inflammatory Drug Sparing Agent in Rheumatoid Arthritis." *Rheumatology*, vol. 47, 2008, pp. 665-69.

Karlson, E. W., et al. "Vitamin E in the Primary Prevention of Rheumatoid Arthritis: The Women's Health Study." *Arthritis and Rheumatism*, vol. 59, 2008, pp. 1589-95.

Lee, M. S., B. C. Shin, and E. Ernst. "Acupuncture for Rheumatoid Arthritis." *Rheumatology*, vol. 47, 2008, pp. 1747-53.

Nakamura, H., et al. "Effects of Glucosamine Administration on Patients with Rheumatoid Arthritis." *Rheumatology International*, vol. 27, 2007, pp. 213-18.

Pradhan, E. K., et al. "Effect of Mindfulness-Based Stress Reduction in Rheumatoid Arthritis Patients." *Arthritis and Rheumatism*, vol. 57, 2007, pp. 1134-42.

Verhagen A. P., et al. "Balneotherapy (or Spa Therapy) for Rheumatoid Arthritis." *Cochrane Database of Systematic Reviews*, vol. 4, no. CD000518, 2015, doi:10.1002/14651858.CD000518.pub2. www.cochrane.org/CD000518/MUSKEL_balneotherapy-or-spa-therapy-rheumatoid-arthritis.

Willich, S. N., et al. "Rose Hip Herbal Remedy in Patients with Rheumatoid Arthritis." *Phytomedicine*, vol. 17, 2010, pp. 87-93.

Bibliography

Abbas, Abul K., Andrew H. Lichtman, and Shiv Pillai. *Basic Immunology: Functions and Disorders of the Immune System.* 6th ed., Saunders/Elsevier, 2019.

———. *Cellular and Molecular Immunology.* 10th ed., Elsevier, 2021.

Aberg, Judith A., Jonathan E. Kaplan, and H. Libman. "Primary Care Guidelines for the Management of Persons Infected with Human Immunodeficiency Virus." *Clinical Infectious Diseases,* vol. 49, no. 5, 2009, pp. 651-81.

"About Allergists/Immunologists." www.aaaai.org/About/About-Allergists-Immunologists. Accessed 2 Sept. 2021.

"About Careers in Allergy/Immunology." *American Academy of Allergy, Asthma, and Immunology,* www.aaaai.org/Professional-Education/careers-in-a-i. Accessed 2 Sept. 2021.

"About MS." *National Multiple Sclerosis Society,* 2013.

"About Psoriasis." *National Psoriasis Foundation,* 2013.

"Acute Sinusitis." *Mayo Clinic,* 27 Aug. 2021, www.mayoclinic.org/diseases-conditions/acute-sinusitis/symptoms-causes/syc-20351671. Accessed 27 Aug. 2021.

A.D.A.M. Medical Encyclopedia. "Cushing Syndrome." *MedlinePlus,* 11 Dec. 2011.

———. "Cytomegalovirus Infections." *MedlinePlus,* 2 May 2013.

Adelman, Daniel C., Thomas B. Casale, and Jonathan Corren, editors. *Manual of Allergy and Immunology.* 5th ed., Lippincott Williams & Wilkins, 2012.

"Advice for Travelers." *Medical Letter on Drugs and Therapeutics,* vol. 61, 2019, pp. 153-60.

Aesoph, Lauri M. *How to Eat Away Arthritis.* Prentice, 1996.

Alan, Rick, and Rimas Lukas. "Multiple Sclerosis-Adult." *Health Library,* 30 Sept. 2012.

Alan, Rick, Rebecca Stahl, and Kari Kassir. "Multiple Sclerosis-Child." *Health Library,* 6 Jun. 2012.

Ali, Tauseef. *Crohn's and Colitis for Dummies.* For Dummies, 2013.

Allen, Arthur. *Vaccine: The Controversial Story of Medicine's Greatest Lifesaver.* Norton, 2007.

Allen, Joseph G., and John D. Macomber. *Healthy Buildings: How Indoor Spaces Drive Performance and Productivity.* Harvard UP, 2020.

Allen, M., et al. "A Randomized Clinical Trial of Elk Velvet Antler in Rheumatoid Arthritis." *Biological Research for Nursing,* vol. 9, 2008, pp. 254-61.

Allenspach, Eric, David J. Rawlings, and Andrew M. Scharenberg. "X-Linked Severe Combined Immunodeficiency." *Gene Reviews,* edited by Roberta A. Pagon, et al., U of Washington, Seattle, 1993-2014. *NCBI Bookshelf.* National Center for Biotechnology Information, 24 Jan. 2013. Accessed 20 Aug. 2014.

"Allergic Reactions." *American Academy of Allergy, Asthma, and Immunology,* 20 Sept. 2020, www.aaaai.org/tools-for-the-public/conditions-library/allergies/allergic-reactions. Accessed 2 Sept. 2021.

"Allergic Reactions: Tips to Remember." AAAAI.org. American Academy of Allergy, Asthma & Immunology, 2013. Accessed 28 Jul. 2014.

"Allergy Testing." *American Academy of Allergy, Asthma, and Immunology,* www.aaaai.org/tools-for-the-public/conditions-library/allergies/allergy-testing. Accessed 6 Sept. 2021.

Almansa, C., K. R. Devault, and S. R. Achem. "A Comprehensive Review of Eosinophilic Esophagitis in Adults." *Journal of Clinical Gastroenterology,* vol. 45, no. 8, pp. 658-64, doi:10.1097/MCG.0b013e318211f95b.

Ambardekar, Nayana. "Who Gets Allergies." *WebMD,* 27 Aug. 2021, www.webmd.com/allergies/who-gets-allergies. Accessed 2 Sept. 2021.

American Academy of Allergy, Asthma, and Immunology, Board of Directors. "Position Paper: Idiopathic Environmental Intolerances." *AAAI,* Jan. 1999, www.aaaai.org/Aaaai/media/Media-Library-PDFs/Allergist%20Resources/Statements%20and%20Practice%20Parameters/Idiopathic-environmental-intolerances-1999.pdf. Accessed 6 Sept. 2021.

American Academy of Dermatology. "Vitiligo."

American Academy of Otolaryngology-Head and Neck Surgery. "Antihistamines, Decongestants, and Cold Remedies." *American Academy of Otolaryngology-Head and Neck Surgery,* Dec. 2010.

American College of Physicians. "Position Paper: Clinical Ecology." *Annals of Internal Medicine,* vol. 111, 1989, pp. 168-78.

American College of Rheumatology. *American College of Rheumatology,* 2013.

American Diabetes Association, *American Diabetes Association Complete Guide to Diabetes.* 5th rev. ed., 2011.

———. "Gestational Diabetes." *Diabetes Care,* vol. 26, 2003, pp. S103-5.

———. *Managing Type 2 Diabetes for Dummies*. For Dummies, 2018.

American Medical Association. *American Medical Association Complete Encyclopedia of Medicine*. Random House Reference, 2003.

———. *American Medical Association Family Medical Guide*. 4th ed., John Wiley & Sons, 2004.

An, Zhiqiang, editor. *Therapeutic Monoclonal Antibodies: From Bench to Clinic*. Wiley, 2009.

Anandan, C., U. Nurmatov, and A. Sheikh. "Omega 3 and 6 Oils for Primary Prevention of Allergic Disease." *Allergy*, vol. 64, 2009, pp. 840-48.

Andersohn, Frank, et al. "Systematic Review: Agranulocytosis Induced by Nonchemotherapy Drugs." *Annals of Internal Medicine* vol. 146, no. 9, 2007, pp. 657-65, doi:10.7326/0003-4819-146-9-200705010-00009.

Andrès, Emmanuel, et al. "State of Art of Idiosyncratic Drug-Induced Neutropenia or Agranulocytosis, with a Focus on Biotherapies." *Journal of Clinical Medicine*, vol. 8, no. 9, 2019, p. 1351, doi:10.3390/jcm8091351.

"Another Reason for Iodine Prophylaxis." *The Lancet*, vol. 335, no. 8703, 16 Jun. 1990, pp. 1433-34.

"Antibodies." *Genetics & Inherited Conditions*. Salem Press, 2010.

"Antihistamines: Understanding Your OTC Options." *American Academy of Family Physicians*, Feb. 2012.

"Anti-Inflammatories and Corticosteroids." *American Association for Respiratory Care*, 2013.

"Antiviral Drugs for Influenza for 2020-2021." *Medical Letter on Drugs and Therapeutics*, vol. 62, no. 1610, 2020, pp. 169-73.

Arceci, Robert J., B. Jack Longley, and Peter D. Emanuel. "Atypical Cellular Disorders." *Hematology*, 2002, pp. 297-314.

Arthritis Foundation. *Raising a Child with Arthritis: A Parent's Guide*. National Book Network, 1998.

"Atopic Dermatitis." *MedlinePlus*, 5 Aug. 2021, medlineplus.gov/ency/article/000853.htm. Accessed 24 Aug 2021.

"Autoimmune Conditions." Medline Plus, 31 Mar. 2021, medlineplus.gov/autoimmunediseases.html. Accessed 20 Aug. 2021.

"Autoimmune Polyglandular Syndrome." *Genetics & Inherited Conditions*. Salem Press. 2010.

Azezli, A. D., T. Bayraktaroglu, and Y. Orhan. "The Use of Konjac Glucomannan to Lower Serum Thyroid Hormones in Hyperthyroidism." *Journal of the American College of Nutrition*, vol. 26, 2007, pp. 663-68.

Badar, V. A., et al. "Efficacy of *Tinospora cordifolia* in Allergic Rhinitis." *Journal of Ethnopharmacology*, vol. 96, 2004, pp. 445-49.

Badash, Michelle. "Cushing's Syndrome." *HealthLibrary*, 1 May 2013.

Baden, Lindsey R. et al. "Efficacy and Safety of the mRNA-1273 SARS-CoV-2 Vaccine." *New England Journal of Medicine*, vol. 384, no. 5, 2020, pp. 403-16, doi:10.1056/NEJMoa2035389.

Bain, Barbara J. *Blood Cells: A Practical Guide*. 5th ed., Wiley Blackwell, 2015.

Bair, Brooke, et al. "Cataracts in Atopic Dermatitis: A Case Presentation and Review of the Literature." *Archives of Dermatology*, vol. 147, no. 5, 2011, pp. 585-88.

Bar, Robert S., editor. *Early Diagnosis and Treatment of Endocrine Disorders*. Humana Press, 2003.

Baraniuk, James N., and Dennis Shusterman, editors. *Nonallergic Rhinitis*. Informa Healthcare, 2007.

Barker, Jennifer M. "Polyglandular Deficiency Syndromes." *Merck Manual for Health Care Professionals*. Merck & Co., Jan. 2014. Accessed 22 Jul. 2014.

Barker, Jonathan, et al., editors. *Rook's Textbook of Dermatology*. 9th ed., Wiley-Blackwell, 2016.

Barnes, Penelope D., and Kieren A. Marr. "Aspergillosis: Spectrum of Disease, Diagnosis, and Treatment." *Infectious Disease Clinics of North America*, vol. 20, 2006, pp. 545-61.

Barnes, Peter J. "Theophylline." *American Journal of Respiratory and Critical Care Medicine*, vol. 188, no. 8, 2013, pp. 901-6.

Baron-Faust, Rita, and Jill P. Buyon. *The Autoimmune Connection*. Contemporary Books, 2003.

Barrett S. *MCS: Multiple Chemical Sensitivity*. American Council on Science and Health, 1994.

Barrett, Stephen M., et al. *Consumer Health: A Guide to Intelligent Decisions*. 9th ed., McGraw-Hill, 2013.

Barry, John M. *The Great Influenza: The Story of the Deadliest Pandemic in History*. Viking Penguin, 2005.

Bass, Pat. "Is Theophylline a Good Choice for Treating Your Asthma?" *Verywell Health*, 24 Apr. 2020, www.verywellhealth.com/theophylline-201158.

Bayliss, R. I. S., and W. M. Tunbridge. *Thyroid Disease: The Facts*. 4th ed., Oxford UP, 2008.

Becker, Gretchen. *The First Year-Type 2 Diabetes: An Essential Guide for the Newly Diagnosed*. 3rd ed., Marlowe, 2015.

Beers, Mark H., et al., editors. *The Merck Manual of Diagnosis and Therapy*. 18th ed., Merck Research Laboratories, 2006.

Behrman, Greg. *The Invisible People: How the U.S. Has Slept Through the Global AIDS Pandemic, the Greatest Humanitarian Catastrophe of Our Time*. Free Press, 2004.

Beigel, John, and Mike Bray. "Current and Future Antiviral Therapy of Severe Seasonal and Avian Influenza." *Antiviral Research*, vol. 78, 2008, pp. 91-102.

"Belimumab (Benlysta) for Systemic Lupus Erythematosus." *Medical Letter on Drugs and Therapeutics*, vol. 53, no. 1366, 2011, pp. 45-46.

Bellenir, Karen, editor. *Cancer Sourcebook: Basic Consumer Health Information about Major Forms and Stages of Cancer*. 6th ed., Omnigraphics, 2012.

Bellenir, Karen, and Peter D. Dresser, editors. *Contagious and Noncontagious Infectious Diseases Sourcebook*. Omnigraphics, 1996.

Bennett, John F., Raphael Dolin, and Martin J., editors. *Mandell, Douglas, and Bennett's Principles and Practice of Infectious Diseases*. 9th ed., Churchill Livingstone/Elsevier, 2019.

Benvenga, S., et al. "Usefulness of L-carnitine, a Naturally Occurring Peripheral Antagonist of Thyroid Hormone Action, in Iatrogenic Hyperthyroidism." *Journal of Clinical Endocrinology and Metabolism*, vol. 86, 2001, pp. 3579-94.

Benvenga, S., M. Lakshmanan, and F. Trimarchi. "Carnitine Is a Naturally Occurring Inhibitor of Thyroid Hormone Nuclear Uptake." *Thyroid*, vol. 10, 2000, pp. 1043-50.

Berbert, A. A., et al. "Supplementation of Fish Oil and Olive Oil in Patients with Rheumatoid Arthritis." *Nutrition*, vol. 21, 2005, pp. 131-36.

Bernhard, Jeffrey D., editor. *Itch: Mechanisms and Management of Pruritus*. McGraw-Hill, 1994.

Bernstein, David, and Gilbert Schiff. "Viral Exanthems and Localized Skin Infections." *Infectious Diseases*, edited by Sherwood L. Gorbach, John G. Bartlett, and Neil R. Blacklow, Saunders, 2004.

Besser, G. Michael, and Michael Thorner, editors. *Clinical Endocrinology*. 2nd ed., Gower-Mosby, 1994.

Bhumbra, Nasreen A., and Sophia G. McCullough. "Skin and Subcutaneous Infections." *Update on Infectious Diseases*, edited by Richard I. Haddy and Karen W. Krigger, W. B. Saunders, 2003.

Bibel, Debra Jan, editor. *Milestones in Immunology*. Springer, 1988.

Bick, Roger L. *Disorders of Thrombosis and Hemostasis: Clinical and Laboratory Practice*. 3rd ed., Lippincott Williams & Wilkins, 2002.

Biegert, C., et al. "Efficacy and Safety of Willow Bark Extract in the Treatment of Osteoarthritis and Rheumatoid Arthritis." *Journal of Rheumatology*, vol. 31, 2004, pp. 2121-30.

Biltagi, M. A., et al. "Omega-3 Fatty Acids, Vitamin C and Zn Supplementation in Asthmatic Children." *Acta Paediatrica*, vol. 98, 2009, pp. 737-42.

Black Jacquelyn G., and Laura J. Black. Microbiology. 10th ed., Wiley, 2018.

Blackstone, Margaret. *The First Year-Multiple Sclerosis: An Essential Guide for the Newly Diagnosed*. 2nd ed., Avalon, 2007.

Blaese, Michael R., et al. "T Lymphocyte-Directed Gene Therapy for ADA SCID: Initial Trial Results After Four Years." *Science*, vol. 270, 1995, pp. 475-80.

Board of the International Society of Regulatory Toxicology and Pharmacology. "Report of the ISRTP Board." *Regulatory Toxicology Pharmacology*, vol. 18, 1993, p. 79.

Boldt, Clayton A. "TIL Therapy: 6 Things to Know." *MD Anderson Cancer Center*, 15 Apr. 2021, www.mdanderson.org/cancerwise/what-is-tumor-infiltrating-lymphocyte-til-therapy—6-things-to-know.h00-159460056.html. Accessed 29 Aug. 2021.

Bond, Allison. "A 'Shark Tank'-Funded Test for Food Sensitivity Is Medically Dubious, Experts Say." *STAT*, 23 Jan. 2018, www.statnews.com/2018/01/23/everlywell-food-sensitivity-test/. Accessed 6 Sept. 2021

Bonilla, F. A., et al. "Practice Parameter for the Diagnosis and Management of Primary Immunodeficiency." *Annals of Allergy, Asthma & Immunology*, vol. 94, no. 5 (Suppl 1), May 2005, pp. S1-63.

Bozek, A. "Pharmacological Management of Allergic Rhinitis in the Elderly." *Drugs & Aging*, Jan. 2017.

Boztug, K., et al. "Multiple Independent Second Site Mutations in Two Siblings with Somatic Mosaicism for Wiskott-Aldrich Syndrome." *Clinical Genetics*, vol. 74, 2008, pp. 68-74.

Braga, Pier Carlo, and Luigi Allegra, editors. *Cough*. Raven Press, 1989.

Braverman, Lewis E., editor. *Diseases of the Thyroid*. 2nd ed., Humana Press, 2003.

Braverman, Lewis E., David S. Cooper, and Peter Kopp, editors. *Werner & Ingbar's The Thyroid*. 11th ed., Lippincott Williams & Wilkins, 2020.

Brewer, Earl J., Jr., and Kathy Cochran Angel. *The Arthritis Sourcebook*. 3rd ed., Lowell House, 2000.

Brewer, Earl J., Jr., Edward H. Giannini, and Donald A. Person. *Juvenile Rheumatoid Arthritis*. 2nd ed., W. B. Saunders, 1982.

Brinkhaus, B., et al. "Acupuncture and Chinese Herbal Medicine in the Treatment of Patients with Seasonal Allergic Rhinitis." *Allergy*, vol. 59, 2004, pp. 953-69.

Brodszki, Nicholas, et al. "Novel Genetic Mutations in the First Swedish Patient with Purine Nucleoside Phosphorylase Deficiency and Clinical Outcome After Hematopoietic Stem Cell Transplantation with HLA-Matched Unrelated Donor." *JIMD Reports*, vol. 24, 2015, pp. 83-89, doi:10.1007/8904_2015_444.

Broides, Amon, Wenjian Yang, and Mary Ellen Conley. "Genotype/Phenotype Correlations in X-Linked Agammaglobulinemia." *Clinical Immunology*, vol. 118, 2006, pp. 195-200.

Brook, Itzhak, editor. *Sinusitis: From Microbiology to Management*. Taylor & Francis, 2006.

Brostoff, Jonathan, and Linda Gamlin. *Food Allergies and Food Intolerance: The Complete Guide to Their Identification and Treatment*. Inner Traditions, 2000.

Brown, Elizabeth E., et al. "Virologic, Hematologic, and Immunologic Risk Factors for Classic Kaposi Sarcoma." *Cancer*, vol. 107, no. 9, 2006, pp. 2282-90.

"BTK." *Genetics Home Reference*. U.S. National Library of Medicine, Feb. 2012. Accessed 14 Jul. 2014.Burman, Kenneth D., and Derek LeRoith, editors. *Thyroid Function and Disease*. Saunders/Elsevier, 2007.

Burton, Thomas. "Immunotherapy Treatments for Cancer Gain Momentum." *Wall Street Journal*, 12 Oct. 2017, www.wsj.com/articles/immunotherapy-treatments-for-cancer-gain-momentum-1507825152?mod=searchresults_pos17&page=1.

Busse, William W., and Stephen T. Holgate, editors. *Asthma and Rhinitis*. Wiley-Blackwell, 2000.

Bussel, J. B., et al. "Eltrombopag for the Treatment of Chronic Idiopathic Thrombocytopenic Purpura." *New England Journal of Medicine*, vol. 357, no. 22, 2007, pp. 2237-47.

Busvine, James R. *Disease Transmission by Insects: Its Discovery and Ninety Years of Effort to Prevent It*. Springer, 1993.

Buyukgebiz, Atilla. "Newborn Screening for Congenital Hypothyroidism." *Journal of Clinical Research in Pediatric Endocrinology*, vol. 5, Mar. 2013, pp. 8-12.

Cakir, Mehtap. *Differential Diagnosis of Hyperthyroidism*. Nova Science, 2010.

Camisa, Charles. *Handbook of Psoriasis*. 2nd ed., John Wiley & Sons, 2004.

Campbell, Jacqueline E. *A Patient's Guide to the Treatment of Diabetes Mellitus*. ? Jacqueline Elaine Campbell, 2009.

Campos, F. L., et al. "Melatonin Improves Sleep in Asthma." *American Journal of Respiratory Critical Care Medicine*, 170, 2004, pp. 947-51.

Canalis, Rinaldo, and Paul R. Lambert, editors. *The Ear: Comprehensive Otology*. Lippincott Williams & Wilkins, 2000.

Canter, P. H., et al. "A Systematic Review of Randomised Clinical Trials of *Tripterygium wilfordii* for Rheumatoid Arthritis." *Phytomedicine*, vol. 13, 2006, pp. 371-77.

Cao, Xue-Yi, et al. "Timing of Vulnerability of the Brain to Iodine Deficiency in Endemic Cretinism." *New England Journal of Medicine*, vol. 331, no. 26, 29 Dec. 1994.

Cao, Y., Q Su, B. Zhang, et al. "Efficacy of Stem Cells Therapy for Crohn's Fistula: A Meta-Analysis and Systematic Review." *Stem Cell Research Therapies*, vol. 12, no. 32, 2021, doi.org/10.1186/s13287-020-02095-7.

Carlson, Emily. "Taking the 'Bite' Out of Vector-Borne Diseases." *National Institute of General Medical Sciences*, 15 May 2013.

Carson-DeWitt, Rosalyn. "Allergic Rhinitis." *Health Library*, 31 Oct. 2012.

———. "Myasthenia Gravis (MG)." *Health Library*, 10 Sept. 2012.

———, and Brian Randall. "Common Cold." *Health Library*, 9 Jan. 2013.

Carvalho Ana L., and Hedrich Christian M. "The Molecular Pathophysiology of Psoriatic Arthritis—The Complex Interplay Between Genetic Predisposition, Epigenetics Factors, and the Microbiome." *Frontiers in Molecular Biosciences*, vol. 8, 2021, p. 190, www.frontiersin.org/article/10.3389/fmolb.2021.662047. DOI=10.3389/fmolb.2021.662047.

Centers for Disease Control and Prevention. "Autism and Vaccines." www.cdc.gov/vaccinesafety/concerns/autism.html.

———. "Immunization Schedules: Resources for Parents." www.cdc.gov/vaccines/schedules/parents-adults/resources-parents.html.

———. "Seasonal Flu: What to Do if You Get Sick." www.cdc.gov/flu/whattodo.htm. Discusses influenza diagnosis, symptoms, medical treatment, recovery, and emergency warning signs.

———. "Vaccine Safety: Measles, Mumps, and Rubella (MMR) Vaccine." www.cdc.gov/vaccinesafety.

———. "Vaccines and Immunizations." www.cdc.gov/vaccines/.

Chabner, Bruce A., and Dan L. Longo, editors. *Cancer Chemotherapy and Biotherapy: Principles and Practice*. Lippincott Williams & Wilkins, 2006.

Challem, Jack. *The Inflammation Syndrome: Your Nutritional Plan for Great Health, Weight Loss, and Pain-Free Living*. Rev. ed., Wiley-Blackwell, 2010.

Chames, Patrick, et al. "Therapeutic Antibodies: Successes, Limitations, and Hopes for the Future." *British Journal of Pharmacology*, vol. 157, no. 2, 2009, pp. 220-33.

Chan, Lawrence S., and Vivian Y. Shi. *Atopic Dermatitis: Inside Out or Outside In?* Elsevier, 2022.

Chang, D. M., et al. "Dehydroepiandrosterone Treatment of Women with Mild-to-Moderate Systemic Lupus Erythematosus." *Arthritis and Rheumatism*, vol. 46, 2002, pp. 2924-27.

Chao, Nelson J., and Robert Zeiser. "Pathogenesis of Graft-Versus-Host Disease (GVHD)." *UpToDate*, 8 Apr. 2021, www-uptodate-com.arbor.idm.oclc.org/contents/pathogenesis-of-graft-versus-host-disease-gvhd?search=GvHD&source=search_result&selectedTitle=3~150&usage_type=default&display_rank=3. Accessed 25 Aug. 2021.

Chatenoud, Lucienne. "Emerging Biological and Molecular Therapies in Autoimmune Disease." The Autoimmune Diseases, edited by Noel R. Rose and Ian R. Mackay, pp. 1437-57, 6th ed., Academic Press, 2020.

"Childhood Arthritis." *Centers for Disease Control and Prevention*, 27 Jul. 2020, www.cdc.gov/arthritis/basics/childhood.htm. 31 Aug. 2021.

Chiu, Zelia K., et al. "Patterns of Vitamin D Levels and Exposures in Active and Inactive Noninfectious Uveitis Patients." *Ophthalmology*, vol. 127, no. 2, 2020, pp. 230-37.

"Chronic Hives." Mayo Clinic, 9 Jun. 2020, www.mayoclinic.org/diseases-conditions/chronic-hives/symptoms-causes/syc-20352719. Accessed 27 Aug. 2021.

"Chronic Thyroiditis (Hashimoto's Disease). *Medline Plus*, 5 Aug. 2021, medlineplus.gov/ency/article/000371.htm. Accessed 26 Aug. 2021.

Chung, Kian Fan, John G. Widdicombe, and Homer A. Boushey, editors. *Cough: Causes, Mechanisms, and Therapy*. Blackwell, 2008.

Cichocki, Mark. *Living with HIV: A Patient's Guide*. McFarland, 2009.

Clark, William R. *In Defense of Self: How the Immune System Really Works*. Oxford UP, 2007.

Clerq, Eric De. "Antiviral Drugs in Current Clinical Use." *Journal of Clinical Virology*, vol. 30, 2004, pp. 115-33.

Cockerell, Clay, and Alvin Friedman-Kien. *Color Atlas of AIDS*. W. B. Saunders, 1996.

Coffin, J. M., S. H. Hughes, and H. E. Varmus, editors. *Retroviruses*. Cold Spring Harbor Laboratory Press, 2002. Also available at www.ncbi.nlm.nih.gov/books/nbk19403.

Cohen, Jeffrey I., et al. "The Need and Challenges for Development of an Epstein-Barr Virus Vaccine." *Vaccine*, vol. 31, Apr. 2013, pp. B194-B196.

Cohen, Philip. "Fresh Blow for Gene Treatments as Safety of a Second Virus Is Questioned." *New Scientist*, vol. 178, 2003, p. 17.

Coico, Richard, and Geoffrey Sunshine. "Antibody Structure and Function." *Immunology: A Short Course*. 6th ed., Wiley-Blackwell, 2009, pp. 41-60.

———. *Immunology: A Short Course*. 6th ed., Wiley-Blackwell, 2009

Colaco, Prisca. *Atlas of Growth and Endocrine Disorders in Children*. Jaypee Brothers Medical Publishers Ltd., 2017.

Committee on Environmental Hypersensitivities. *Report of the Ad Hoc Committee on Environmental Hypersensitivities Disorders*. Ministry of Health, 1985.

"Common Cold." *MedlinePlus*, 23 Apr. 2013.

"Common Colds: Protect Yourself and Others." *Centers for Disease Control and Prevention*, 11 Mar. 2013.

Conley, Mary Ellen. "Antibody Deficiencies." *The Metabolic and Molecular Bases of Inherited Disease*, edited by Charles Scriver, et al., 8th ed., McGraw-Hill, 2001.

———, et al. "Primary B Cell Immunodeficiencies: Comparisons and Contrasts." *Annual Review of Immunology*, vol. 27, 2009, pp. 199-227.

———, and Vanessa C. Howard. "X-Linked Agammaglobulinemia." *Gene Reviews*. U of Washington, Seattle, 17 Nov. 2011. Accessed 14 Jul. 2014.

"Contact Dermatitis." *MedlinePlus*, 5 Aug. 2021, medlineplus.gov/ency/article/000869.htm. Accessed 24 Aug. 2021.

Contie, Vicki, Lesley Earl, Belle Waring, and Harrison Wein. "Red, Itchy Skin? Get the Skinny on Dermatitis." *NIH News in Health*. NIH Office of Communications and Public Liaison, Apr. 2012. Accessed 18 Jul. 2014.

Contopoulos-Ioannidis, D. G., I. N. Kouri, and J. P. Ioannidis. "Genetic Predisposition to Asthma and Atopy." *Respiration*, vol. 74, no. 1, 2007, pp. 8-12.

Cooper, Max D., et al. "Immunodeficiency Disorders." *Hematology*, vol. 1, 2003, pp. 314-30. A thorough presentation on the cell biology behind immunodeficiency disorders with a detailed section on SCID.

Cooper, Megan A., Thomas L. Pommering, and Katalin Koranyi. "Primary Immunodeficiencies." *American Family Physician*, vol. 68, 2003, pp. 2001-8, 2011.

Cooper, Necia Grant, editor. *The Human Genome Project: Deciphering the Blueprint of Heredity*. Rev. ed., University Science Books, 1994.

"Copanlisib (Aliqopa) for Relapsed Follicular Lymphoma." *Medical Letter on Drugs and Therapeutics*, vol. 60, no. 1545, 2018, pp. 74-75.

"Coronavirus Disease (COVID-19)." *World Health Organization*, 12 Oct. 2020, www.who.int/news-room/q-a-detail/coronavirus-disease-covid-19. Accessed 10 Sept. 2021.

"Cough." *Mayo Clinic*, 24 May 2013.

Council on Scientific Affairs, American Medical Association. "Clinical Ecology." *JAMA*, vol. 268, 1992, pp. 1634-35.

Cowie, R. L., et al. "A Randomised Controlled Trial of the Buteyko Technique as an Adjunct to Conventional Management of Asthma." *Respiratory Medicine*, vol. 102, 2008, pp. 726-32.

Cox, L. S., et al. "Sublingual Immunotherapy: A Comprehensive Review." *Journal of Allergy and Clinical Immunology*, vol. 117, 2006, pp. 1021-35.

Cram, David L. *Coping with Psoriasis: A Patient's Guide to Treatment.* Addicus Books, 2000.

Crosbie, D., et al. "Dehydroepiandrosterone for Systemic Lupus Erythematosus." *Cochrane Database of Systematic Reviews*, vol. 4, no. CD005114, 2007, p. CD005114, www.cochrane.org/CD005114/MUSKEL_dehydroepiandrosterone-dhea-for-lupus-erythematosus, doi:10.1002/14651858.CD005114.pub2.

Cutler, Ellen W. *Winning the War against Asthma and Allergies.* Delmar, 1998.

Dahl, R., et al. "Sublingual Grass Allergen Tablet Immunotherapy Provides Sustained Clinical Benefit with Progressive Immunologic Changes Over Two Years." *Journal of Allergy and Clinical Immunology*, vol. 121, 2008, pp. 512-18.

Danquah, Michael K., and Mahato, Ram I., editors. Emerging Trends in Cell and Gene Therapy. Humana Press, 2013.

Dartt, Darlene A. *Immunology, Inflammation and Diseases of the Eye.* Academic Press, 2011.

Dawczynski, J., et al. "Selenium and Zinc in Patients with Acute and Chronic Uveitis." *Biological Trace Element Research*, vol. 113, no. 2, 2006, pp. 131-37.

de Leon, L. M., and E. Feller. "Eosinophilic Esophagitis." *The 5-Minute Clinical Consult*, edited by F. J. Domino, pp. 440-41, 21st ed., Wolters Kluwer Health/Lippincott Williams & Wilkins, 2013.

De Vita, Vincent T., Jr., Samuel Hellman, and Steven A. Rosenberg, editors. Principles and Practice of Oncology. 11th ed., Lippincott Williams & Wilkins, 2018.

Deer, Brian. *The Doctor Who Fooled the World.* Johns Hopkins UP, 2020.

DeFranco, Anthony L., Richard M. Locksley, and Miranda Robertson. *Immunity: The Immune Response in Infectious and Inflammatory Disease.* Oxford UP, 2007.

Delgado, Julio, et al. "Chronic Lymphocytic Leukemia: From Molecular Pathogenesis to Novel Therapeutic Strategies." *Haematologica*, vol. 105, no. 9, 2020, pp. 2205-17, doi:10.3324/haematol.2019.236000.

Delves, Peter J., et al. *Roitt's Essential Immunology.* 13th ed., Wiley-Blackwell, 2017.

DeMaeyer, E. M. *The Control of Endemic Goiter.* World Health Organization, 1988.

"Dengue and Severe Dengue." *World Health Organization*, Nov. 2012.

Derebery, M. J., and K. I. Berliner. "Allergy and Its Relation to Meniere's Disease. *Otolaryngologic Clinics of North America*, vol. 43, no. 5, 2010, pp. 1047-58, doi:10.1016/j.otc.2010.05.004.

DeStefano, Frank, Cristofer S. Price, and Eric S. Weintraub. "Increasing Exposure to Antibody-Stimulating Proteins and Polysaccharides in Vaccines Is Not Associated with Risk of Autism." *Journal of Pediatrics*, vol. 163, no. 2, pp. 561-67.

Dettmer, Philipp. Immune: A Journey into the Mysterious System That Keeps You Alive. Random House, 2021.

Deutsch, L. "Evaluation of the Effect of Neptune Krill Oil on Chronic Inflammation and Arthritic Symptoms." *Journal of the American College of Nutrition*, vol. 26, 2007, pp. 39-48.

Di Lorenzo, Giuseppe, et al. "Management of AIDS-Related Kaposi's Sarcoma." *Lancet Oncology*, vol. 8, 2007, pp. 167-76.

"Diabetes." *MedlinePlus*, 2 Aug. 2021, medlineplus.gov/diabetes.html. Accessed 24 Aug. 2021.

"Diabetes in Children and Teens." *MedlinePlus*, 27 May 2021, medlineplus.gov/diabetesinchildrenandteens.html. Accessed 24 Aug. 2021.

Diamos Andrew G., et al. "High Level Production of Monoclonal Antibodies Using an Optimized Plant Expression System." *Frontiers in Bioengineering and Biotechnology*, vol. 7, 2020, p. 472, www.frontiersin.org/article/10.3389/fbioe.2019.00472.

Dikago, Antan Riux. *Commonly Asked Questions About Cushing Syndrome Finally Answered.* Author, 2020.

Dinulos, James G. H. *Habif's Clinical Dermatology: A Color Guide to Diagnosis and Therapy.* 9th ed., Elsevier, 2020.

"Disorders of the Immune System." *American Academy of Allergy, Asthma, and Immunology*, 17 Jan. 2014, www.niaid.nih.gov/research/immune-system-disorders. Accessed 29 Aug. 2021.

"Disorders of Phagocyte Function and Number." *Hematology: Basic Principles and Practice*, edited by Ronald Hoffman, et al., 5th ed., Churchill Livingstone/Elsevier, 2009.

"Do You Know the Hygiene Hot Spots in Your Home?" *BBC News*, 25 Jun. 2019, www.bbc.com/news/health-48746377.

Dollinger, Malin, et al. *Everyone's Guide to Cancer Therapy*. 5th ed., Andrews McMeel, 2008.

Dossenbach, Hans D. *Beware! We Are Poisonous! How Animals Defend Themselves*. Blackbirch Press, 1999.

Douglas, R. M., et al. "Vitamin C for Preventing and Treating the Common Cold." *The Cochrane Database of Systematic Reviews*, vol. 3, no. CD000980, 2007, doi:10.1002/14651858.CD000980.pub3.

Driscoll, John S. *Antiviral Drugs*. John Wiley & Sons, 2006.

Dror, Yigal, et al. "Purine Nucleoside Phosphorylase Deficiency Associated with a Dysplastic Marrow Morphology." *Pediatric Research*, vol. 55, no. 3, 2004, pp. 472-77.

"Drugs for Allergic Rhinitis and Allergic Conjunctivitis." *Medical Letter on Drugs and Therapeutics*, vol. 63, no. 1622, 2021, pp. 57-64.

"Drugs for Inflammatory Bowel Disease." *Medical Letter on Drugs and Therapy*, vol. 60, no. 1550, 2018, pp. 107-14.

"Drugs for Multiple Sclerosis." *Medical Letter on Drugs and Therapeutics*, vol. 63, no. 1620, 2021, pp. 42-48.

"Drugs for Osteoarthritis." *The Medical Letter on Drugs and Therapeutics*, vol. 62, no. 1596, 20 Apr. 2020, pp. 57-62.

"Drugs for Parasitic Infections: Treatment Guidelines from the Medical Letter." *Medical Letter on Drugs and Therapeutics*, vol. 11 (suppl.), no, 143, 2013, pp. e1-e31.

"Drugs for Psoriasis." *Medical Letters on Drugs and Therapeutics*, vol. 61, no. 1574, 2019, pp. 89-96.

"Drugs for Psoriatic Arthritis." *Medical Letters on Drugs and Therapeutics*, vol. 61, no. 1588, 2019, pp. 203-10.

"Drugs for Rheumatoid Arthritis." Medical Letter on Drugs and Therapeutics, vol. 60, no. 1552, 2018, pp. 123-28.

Dübel, Stefan, and Janice M. Reichert, editors. *Handbook of Therapeutic Antibodies*. 3 vols. Wiley-VCH, 2014.

Duffy, E. M., et al. "The Clinical Effect of Dietary Supplementation with Omega-3 Fish Oils and/or Copper in Systemic Lupus Erythematosus." *Journal of Rheumatology*, vol. 31, 2004, p. 1551.

Dugan, Marcia B. *Living with Hearing Loss*. Gallaudet UP, 2003.

Dykewicz, Mark S., et al. "Rhinitis 2020: A Practice Parameter Update." *The Journal of Allergy and Clinical Immunology*, vol. 146, no. 4, 2020, pp. 721-67, doi:10.1016/j.jaci.2020.07.007.

DynaMed. "Eosinophilic Esophagitis in Adults." *EBSCO Information Services*, 13 Jun. 2014, search.ebscohost.com/login.aspx?direct=true&db=dme&AN=435297. Accessed 17 Mar. 2015.

EBSCO Publishing. *Health Library: Flu*. www.ebscohost.com.

———. *Health Library: Measles Vaccine*. www.ebscohost.com.

Eccles, Ronald, and Olaf Weber, editors. *Common Cold: Birkhäuser Advances in Infectious Diseases*. Birkhäuser Basel, 2009.

"Eczema Types: Atopic Dermatitis Overview." www.aad.org/public/diseases/eczema/types/atopic-dermatitis. Accessed 24 Aug. 2021.

Edgar, J. D. "T Cell Immunodeficiency." *Journal of Clinical Pathology*, vol. 61, 2008, pp. 988-93.

Egeler, R. Maarten, and Giulio J. D'Angio, editors. *Langerhans Cell Histiocytosis*. W. B. Saunders, 1998.

Eggert, Julie, editor. *Cancer Basics*. Oncology Nursing Society, 2010.

Eggleston, P. A., & Wood, R. A. "Management of Allergies to Animals." *Allergy and Asthma Proceedings*, vol. 13, no. 6, Nov. 1992, pp. 289-92.

"Elderberry for Influenza." *The Medical Letter on Drugs and Therapeutics*, vol. 61, no. 1566, 2019, p. 32.

"Endocrine Diseases." *MedlinePlus*, 17 Aug. 2021, medlineplus.gov/endocrinediseases.html. Accessed 24 Aug. 2021.

"Endocrine Glands." *MedlinePlus*, 5 Aug. 2021, medlineplus.gov/ency/article/002351.htm. Accessed 24 Aug. 2021.

Engels E. A., et al. "Trends in Cancer Risk Among People with AIDS in the United States 1980-2002." *AIDS*, vol. 20, no. 12, 2006, p. 1645.

Epstein, M. Anthony, and Bert G. Achong, editors. *The Epstein-Barr Virus*. Springer, 1979

Erem, C., et al. "The Effects of Royal Jelly on Autoimmunity in Graves' Disease." *Endocrine*, vol. 30, 2006, pp. 175-83.

Eyre, Harmon J., Dianne Partie Large, and Lois B. Morris. *Informed Decisions: The Complete Book of CancerDiagnosis, Treatment, and Recovery*. 2nd ed., American Cancer Society, 2002.

Ezzell, Carol. "Hope in a Vial: Will There Be an AIDS Vaccine Anytime Soon?" *Scientific American*, vol. 186, June 2002, pp. 38-45.

"Facts about *Stachybotrys chartarum*." *Centers for Disease Control and Prevention*, 16 Dec. 2019, www.cdc.gov/mold/stachy.htm. Accessed 3 Sept. 2021.

FamilyDoctor.org. "Decongestants: OTC Relief for Congestion." *FamilyDoctor.org*, Feb. 2012.

Fan, Hung Y., Ross F. Conner, and Luis P. Villarreal. *AIDS: Science and Society*. 5th ed., Jones and Bartlett, 2007.

———. *The Biology of AIDS*. 4th ed., Jones and Bartlett, 2000.

FARE: Food Allergy Research & Education. n.d., www.foodallergy.org/. Accessed 26 Aug. 2021.

Farmakidis, Constantine, et al. "Treatment of Myasthenia Gravis." *Neurologic Clinics*, vol. 36, no. 2, 2018, pp. 311-37, doi:10.1016/j.ncl.2018.01.011.

Farnan, Rose, and Maithe Enriquez. *What Nurses Know: HIV/AIDS*. Demos Health, 2012.

Feigal, Ellen, et al., editors. *AIDS-Related Cancers and Their Treatment*. Marcel Dekker, 2000.

Ferrari, Mario. *PDxMD Ear, Nose, and Throat Disorders*. PDxMD, 2003.

Ferri, Fred F., editor. *Ferri's Clinical Advisor 2011: Instant Diagnosis and Treatment*. Mosby/Elsevier, 2011.

Fettner, Ann Giudici. *Viruses: Agents of Change*. McGraw-Hill, 1990.

Feuling, M. B., and R. J. Noel. "Medical and Nutrition Management of Eosinophilic Esophagitis in Children." *Nutrition in Clinical Practice*, vol. 25, no. 2, 2010, pp. 166-74, doi:10.1177/0884533610361608.

Finn, O. J. "Immuno-Oncology: Understanding the Function and Dysfunction of the Immune System in Cancer." *Annals of Oncology*, vol. 23(Suppl 8), 2012, pp. iiv6-iiv9, annonc.oxfordjournals.org/content/23/suppl_8/viii6.full.

Firestein, Gary S., Gabriel S. Panayi, and Frank A. Wollheim, editors. *Rheumatoid Arthritis*. 2nd ed., Oxford UP, 2006.

Fischer, A. M., et al. "Naturally Occurring Primary Deficiencies of the Immune System." *Annual Review of Immunology*, vol. 15, 1997, pp. 93-124.

Fischer, David S., et al. The Cancer Chemotherapy Handbook. 6th ed., Mosby, 2003.

Flajnik, Martin F., Nevil J. Singh, and Steven M. Holland. *Paul's Fundamental Immunology*. Lippincott Williams & Wilkins, 2022.

Fleischer, Alan B., Jr. *The Clinical Management of Itching*. Parthenon, 2000.

Flynn, C. A., G. Griffin, and F. Tudiver. "Decongestants and Antihistamines for Acute Otitis Media in Children." *The Cochrane Library*, Issue 4. John Wiley & Sons, 2003.

Flynn, John A., and Lora Brown Wilder, editors. *Recipes for Arthritis Health*. Rebus, 2003.

Foltz-Gray, Dorothy. *The Arthritis Foundation's Guide to Good Living with Rheumatoid Arthritis*. 3rd ed., Arthritis Foundation, 2006.

"Food Allergy." *MedlinePlus*, 5 Aug. 2021, medlineplus.gov/ency/article/000817.htm. Accessed 26 Aug. 2021.

"Food Allergy." *National Institute of Allergy and Infectious Diseases*, 29 Oct. 2019, www.niaid.nih.gov/diseases-conditions/food-allergy. Accessed 26 Aug. 2021.

Food Allergy Research & Education. *Blood Tests*. 2021, www.foodallergy.org/resources/blood-tests. Accessed 6 Sept. 2021.

"Food Protein-Induced Enterocolitis Syndrome (FPIES)." *American Academy of Allergy, Asthma, and Immunology*. 28 Sept. 2020, www.aaaai.org/tools-for-the-public/conditions-library/allergies/food-protein-induced-enterocolitis-syndrome-(fpies. Accessed 26 Aug. 2020.

Ford, Jodi L., and Raymond P. Stowe. "Racial-Ethnic Differences in Epstein-Barr Virus Antibody Titers Among U.S. Children and Adolescents." *Annals of Epidemiology*, vol. 23, no. 5, May 2013, pp. 275-80.

Fortescue R., K. M. Kew, and MShiu Tsun. "Sublingual Immunotherapy for Asthma." *Cochrane Database of Systematic Reviews*, Issue 9, 2020, CD011293, doi:10.1002/14651858.CD011293.pub3.

Foster, Steven, and Roger A. Caras. *A Field Guide to Venomous Animals and Poisonous Plants: North America, North of Mexico*. Houghton Mifflin, 1994.

Fox, Stuart Ira. *Human Physiology*. 16th ed., McGraw-Hill, 2021.

Frank, Steven A. *Immunology and Evolution of Infectious Disease*. Princeton UP, 2002.

Frankel, David H., editor. *Field Guide to Clinical Dermatology*. 2nd ed., Lippincott Williams & Wilkins, 2006.

Freinkel, Ruth K., and David T. Woodley, editors. *Biology of the Skin*. Parthenon, 2001.

Friedman, Ellen M., and James M. Barassi. *My Ear Hurts! A Complete Guide to Understanding and Treating Your Child's Ear Infections*. Diane, 2004.

Friedman-Kien, Alvin, and Clay J. Cockerell. *Color Atlas of AIDS*. 2nd ed., Elsevier Health Sciences, 1996.

Fries, James F. *Arthritis: A Take-Care-of-Yourself Health Guide to Understanding Your Arthritis*. 5th ed., Addison, 1999.

Fry, Lionel. *An Atlas of Atopic Eczema*. Parthenon, 2004.

Gabrilovich, Dmitry, editor. *The Neutrophils: New Outlook for Old Cells*. 3rd ed., Imperial College P, 2013.

Gaby, A. R. "Nutritional Therapies for Ocular Disorders." *Alternative Medicine Review*, vol. 13, 2008, pp. 191-204.

Gaitan, Eduardo, editor. *Environmental Goitrogenesis*. CRC, 1989.

Galanda, Claudia D., editor. *AIDS-Related Opportunistic Infections*. Nova Biomedical Books, 2009.

Galanter, Joshua M., and Homer A. Boushey. "Drugs Used in Asthma." *Basic and Clinical Pharmacology*, edited by Bertram G. Katzung and Anthony J. Trevor, 13th ed., pp. 341-42, McGraw-Hill Education, 2015.

Galarraga, B., et al. "Cod Liver Oil (N-3 Fatty Acids) as a Nonsteroidal Anti-inflammatory Drug Sparing Agent in Rheumatoid Arthritis." *Rheumatology*, vol. 47, 2008, pp. 665-69.

Gallagher, Jason C., and Conan MacDougall. *Antibiotics Simplified*. 4th ed., Jones and Bartlett Learning, 2016.

Gallin, John I., and Ralph Snyderman, editors. *Inflammation: Basic Principles and Clinical Correlates*. 3rd ed., Raven Press, 1999.

Ganem, Don. "KSHV Infection and the Pathogenesis of Kaposi's Sarcoma." *Annual Review of Pathology*, vol. 1, 2006, pp. 273-96.

Gardner, David, and Dolores Shoback. *Greenspan's Basic and Clinical Endocrinology*. 10th ed., McGraw-Hill Educational, 2017.

Gates, Robert H. *Infectious Disease Secrets*. 2nd ed., Hanley, 2003.

"GeneTests." www.ncbi.nlm.nih.gov/sites/GeneTests.

Genetic Alliance, www.geneticalliance.org.

Genetics Home Reference. "HLA-DRB1." *Genetics Home Reference*. U.S. NLM, 28 Jul. 2014. Accessed. 4 Aug. 2014.

Genetics Home Reference. "Purine Nucleoside Phosphorylase Deficiency." *Genetics Home Reference*. U.S. NLM, 18 Aug. 2014. Accessed 20 Aug. 2014.

George, J. N. "Platelets." *The Lancet*, vol. 355, 2000, pp. 1531-39.

———, et al. "Update on Idiopathic Thrombocytopenic Purpura." www.hematology.org/publications/hematologist/2010/4965.aspx.

Gershon, Anne A., Samuel L. Katz, and Peter J. Hotez, editors. *Krugman's Infectious Diseases of Children*. 11th ed., Mosby, 2004.

Gersten, Todd. "Histiocytosis." *MedlinePlus*, 30 Apr. 2012, Histiocytosis Association, www.histio.org.

Gibbs, W. W. "Plantibodies: Human Antibodies Produced by Field Crops Enter Clinical Trials." *Scientific American*, vol. 277, no. 5, 1997, p. 44.

Gibson, Toby, Chenna Ramu, Christina Gemund, and Rein Aasland. "The APECED Polyglandular Autoimmune Syndrome Protein, AIRE-1, Contains the SAND Domain and Is Probably a Transcription Factor." *Trends in Biochemical Sciences*, vol. 23, no. 7, 1988, pp. 242-44.

Gilbert, Hiram F. *Basic Concepts in Biochemistry*. 2nd ed., McGraw-Hill, 2002.

Giovannini, M., et al. "A Randomized Prospective Double-Blind Controlled Trial on Effects of Long-Term Consumption of Fermented Milk Containing *Lactobacillus casei* in Pre-school Children with Allergic Asthma and/or Rhinitis." *Pediatric Research*, vol. 62, 2007, p. 215.

Glatstein, M., et al. "Pharmacologic Treatment of Hyperthyroidism During Lactation." *Canadian Family Physician*, vol. 55, 2009, pp. 797-98.

Glenn, Jim. *Colds and Coughs*. Springhouse, 1986.

Glick, Bernard R., and Jack J. Pasternak, editors. *Molecular Biotechnology: Principles and Applications of Recombinant DNA*. 4th ed., ASM, 2010.

"Global HIV & AIDS Statistics—Fact Sheet." *UNAIDS*, 2021, www.unaids.org/en/resources/fact-sheet. Accessed 5 Sept. 2021

Goering, Richard, et al. *Mims' Medical Microbiology and Immunology*. 6th ed., Elsevier, 2018.

Goldman, John, and Junia Melo. "Chronic Myeloid Leukemia: Advances in Biology and New Approaches to Treatment." *New England Journal of Medicine*, vol. 349, no. 15, 9 Oct. 2003, pp. 1451-64.

Goldsmith, Lowell A., Gerald S. Lazarus, and Michael D. Tharp. *Adult and Pediatric Dermatology: A Color Guide to Diagnosis and Treatment*. F. A. Davis, 1997.

Gomez, Joan. *Thyroid Problems in Women and Children*. Hunter House, 2003.

Gontijo-Amaral, C., et al. "Oral Magnesium Supplementation in Asthmatic Children." *European Journal of Clinical Nutrition*, vol. 61, 2006, pp. 54-60.

Gormley, Myra Vanderpool. *Family Diseases: Are You at Risk?* Genealogical Publishing, 2007.

Górski, Andrzej, Hubert Krotkiewski, and Michal Zimecki, editors. *Inflammation*. Kluwer, 2001.

"Graft-Versus-Host Disease." *Memorial Sloan Kettering Cancer Center*, n.d., www.mskcc.org/cancer-care/types/graft-versus-host-disease-gvhd. Accessed 25 Aug. 2021.

Grammatikos, A. P. "The Genetic and Environmental Basis of Atopic Diseases." *Annals of Medicine*, vol. 40, no. 7, 2008, pp. 482-95.

Greenberg, S. L., "Medical and Noninvasive Therapy for Meniere's Disease." *Otolaryngologic Clinics of North America*, vol. 43, no. 5, 2010, pp. 1081-90, doi:10.1016/j.otc.2010.05.005.

Greenberger, N. J. "Eosinophilic Esophagitis." *Current Diagnosis & Treatment Gastroenterology, Hepatology, & Endoscopy*, edited by N. J. Greenberger, pp. 183-86, 2nd ed., McGraw-Hill Medical, 2012.

Greene, Alan R. *The Parent's Complete Guide to Ear Infections*. Reprint. People's Medical Society, 2004.

Greenspan, Francis S., Dolores M. Shoback, and David G. Gardner, editors. *Greenspan's Basic and Clinical Endocrinology*. 8th ed., McGraw-Hill, 2007.

Greer, John, et al., editors. *Wintrobe's Clinical Hematology*. 13th ed., Wolters Kluwer/Lippincott Williams & Wilkins Health, 2013.

Griffin, James E., and Sergio R. Ojeda, editors. *Textbook of Endocrine Physiology*. 6th ed., Oxford UP, 2012.

Grimm, W., and H. Muller. "A Randomized Controlled Trial of the Effect of Fluid Extract of Echinacea purpurea on the Incidence and Severity of Colds and Respiratory Infections." *American Journal of Medicine*, vol. 106, 1999, pp. 138-43.

Grob, J. J., et al., editors. *Epidemiology, Causes, and Prevention of Skin Diseases*. Blackwell Science, 1997.

Grossman, Leigh B., editor. *Infection Control in the Child Care Center and Preschool*. 8th ed., Silverchair Science, 2012.

"Growth Disorders." *MedlinePlus*, 17 Aug. 2021, medlineplus.gov/growthdisorders.html. Accessed 24 Aug. 2021.

Grunebaum, E., A. Cohen, and C. M. Roifman. "Recent Advances in Understanding and Managing Adenosine Deaminase and Purine Nucleoside Phosphorylase Deficiencies." Current Opinion in Allergy and Clinical Immunology, vol. 13, no. 6, 2013, pp. 630-38. *Medline*. Accessed 20 Aug. 2014.

Guan, W., et al. "Clinical Characteristics of Coronavirus Disease 2019 in China." *New England Journal of Medicine*, 28 Feb. 2020, doi:10.1056/NEJMoa2002032.

Guha, Sushovan, Sunil Krishnan, and Bharat B. Aggarwal. *Inflammation, Lifestyle, and Chronic Disease: The Silent Link*. CRC Press, 2012.

"Guillain-Barré Syndrome Fact Sheet." *National Institute of Neurological Disorders and Stroke*, 16 Mar. 2021, www.ninds.nih.gov/Disorders/Patient-Caregiver-Education/Fact-Sheets/Guillain-Barr%C3%A9-Syndrome-Fact-Sheet. Accessed 25 Aug. 2021.

"Guillain-Barré Syndrome." *MedlinePlus*, 25 Oct. 2019, medlineplus.gov/guillainbarresyndrome.html. Accessed 25 Aug. 2021.

Guiney, P. A., et al. "Effects of Osteopathic Manipulative Treatment on Pediatric Patients with Asthma." *Journal of the American Osteopathic Association*, vol. 105, 2005, pp. 7-12.

Gullatte, M. M. *Clinical Guide to Antineoplastic Therapy: A Chemotherapy Handbook*. Oncology Nursing Society, 2005.

Gvozdjakova, A., et al. "Coenzyme Q10 Supplementation Reduces Corticosteroids Dosage in Patients with Bronchial Asthma." *Biofactors*, vol. 25, 2006, pp. 235-40.

Hackett, Charles J., and Donald A. Harn Jr., editors. *Vaccine Adjuvants: Immunological and Clinical Principles*. Humana, 2006.

Hadley, Andrew G., and Peter Soothill, editors. *Alloimmune Disorders of Pregnancy: Anaemia, Thrombocytopenia, and Neutropenia in the Fetus and Newborn*. Cambridge UP, 2002.

Hadley, Mac E., and Jon E. Levine. *Endocrinology*. 6th ed., Pearson/Prentice Hall, 2007.

Halbreich, Uriel. *Multiple Sclerosis: A Neuropsychiatric Disorder*. American Psychiatric Press, 1993.

Halder, Rebat M., and Jonathan Chappell. "Vitiligo Update." *Seminars in Cutaneous Medicine and Surgery*, vol. 28, no. 2, Jun. 2009, pp. 86-92.

Hall, R., and J. Köbberling, editors. *Thyroid Disorders Associated with Iodine Deficiency and Excess*. Raven Press, 1985.

Hall, Stephen S. *A Commotion in the Blood: Life, Death, and the Immune System*. Henry Holt, 1997.

Halstead, Bruce W., and Paul S. Auerbach. *Dangerous Aquatic Animals of the World: A Color Atlas*. Darwin Press, 1992.

Hamad, Hussein, and Ankit Mangla. "Lymphocytosis." *StatPearls*, StatPearls Publishing, 21 Jul. 2021.

Hamborsky, Jennifer, Andrew Kroger, and Charles Wolfe, editors. *Epidemiology and Prevention of Vaccine-Preventable Diseases*. 13th ed., Public Health Foundation, 2015. Centers for Disease Control and Prevention. Accessed 31 Dec. 2015.

Hamburger, J. I. *Nontoxic Goiter: Concept and Controversy*. Charles C. Thomas, 1973.

Hamid, M. A. "Meniere's Disease." *Practical Neurology*, vol. 9, no. 3, 2009, pp. 157-62, doi:10.1136/jnnp.2009.176602.

Hanas, Ragnar. *Type 1 Diabetes in Children, Adolescents and Young Adults*. Class Health, 2019.

Handwerger, Stuart, editor. *Molecular and Cellular Pediatric Endocrinology*. Humana Press, 1999.

Hanger, Nancy C. *Lupus-The First Year: An Essential Guide for the Newly Diagnosed*. Marlowe, 2003.

Harder, Ben. "Don't Let the Bugs Bite: Can Genetic Engineering Defeat Disease Spread by Insects?" *Science News*, vol. 166, no. 7, 2004, p. 104.

Harlow, Ed, and David Lane, editors. *Using Antibodies: A Laboratory Manual*. Rev. ed., Cold Spring Harbor Laboratory Press, 1999.

Harmel, Anne Peters, and Ruchi Mathur. *Davidson's Diabetes Mellitus: Diagnosis and Treatment*. 5th ed., W. B. Saunders, 2004.

Harvey, Alan L., editor. *Snake Toxins*. Pergamon Press, 1991.

"Hashimoto's Disease." *National Institute of Diabetes and Digestive and Kidney Diseases*, July 2020, www.niddk.nih.gov/health-information/endocrine-diseases/hashimotos-disease. Accessed 26 Aug. 2021

"Hashimoto's Disease." *Office of Women's Health*, 18 Oct. 2018, www.womenshealth.gov/a-z-topics/hashimotos-disease. Accessed 26 Aug. 2021.

Hawker, Jeremy, et al. *Communicable Disease Control Handbook*. 2nd ed., Blackwell, 2006.

Hawkins Robert E. *Cellular Therapy of Cancer: Development of Gene Therapy Based Approaches*. World Scientific, 2013.

Hawley, Louise, Richard J. Ziegler, and Benjamin L. Clarke. *Microbiology and Immunology*. Lippincott Williams & Wilkins, 2013.

Hawley, Robert G., and Donna A. Sobieski. "Of Mice and Men: The Tale of Two Therapies." *Stem Cells*, vol. 20, 2002, pp. 275-78. Discusses the experimental gene therapy trials for both XCID and ADA SCID.

"Hay Fever." *Mayo Clinic*, www.mayoclinic.org/diseases-conditions/hay-fever/symptoms-causes/syc-20373039. Accessed 27 Aug. 2021.

Healthline Editorial Team. "Hives." *Health Library*, 8 Mar. 2019, www.healthline.com/health/hives. Accessed 27 Aug. 2021.

Hellwig, Jennifer. "Eczema." *Health Library*, 11 Mar. 2013.

Henderson, Edward S., T. A. Lister, and M. F. Greaves. *Leukemia*. 7th ed., Saunders, 2002.

Henochowicz, Stuart I. "Allergic Rhinitis." *MedlinePlus*, 17 Jun. 2012.

———. "Vasomotor Rhinitis." *MedlinePlus*, 17 Jun. 2012.

Henry, Helen L., and Anthony W. Norman, editors. *Encyclopedia of Hormones*. 3 vols., Academic Press, 2003.

Hereditary Disease Foundation, www.hdfoundation.org.

Hershman, Jerome M., editor. *Endocrine Pathophysiology: A Patient-Oriented Approach*. 3rd ed., Lea & Febiger, 1988.

Hetzel, Basil S. "Iodine and Neuropsychological Development." *Journal of Nutrition*, vol. 130, no. 2, 1999, pp. 493S-495S.

Hide, Michihiro, et al. "Autoantibodies against the High-Affinity IgE Receptor as a Cause of Histamine Release in Chronic Urticaria." *New England Journal of Medicine*, vol. 328, no. 22, 1993, pp. 1599-1604.

Hirsch, Larissa. "Endocrine System." *KidsHealth*. Oct. 2018, kidshealth.org/en/parents/endocrine.html?ref=search. Accessed 25 Aug. 2021.

"Hives." *MedlinePlus*, 28 Jul. 2021, medlineplus.gov/hives.html. Accessed 27 Aug. 2021.

Hoekelman, Robert A., editor. *Primary Pediatric Care*. 4th ed., Mosby, 2001.

Holland, Kimberly, "What's Hypothyroidism?" *HealthLine*, 19 Dec. 2020, www.healthline.com/health/hypothyroidism/symptoms-treatments-more. Accessed 27 Aug. 2021.

Holland, Steven, et al. "Immunodeficiencies." *Infectious Diseases*, edited by Jon Cohen, William Powderly, and Steven Opal, Mosby/Elsevier, 2010.

Holshue, M. L., et al. "First Case of 2019 Novel Coronavirus in the United States." *New England Journal of Medicine*, vol. 382, 2020, pp. 929-36, doi:10.1056/NEJMoa2001191.

Holt, Elizabeth H., Beatrice Lupsa, Grace S. Lee, Hanan Bassyouni, and Harry Peery. *Goodman's Basic Medical Endocrinology*. 5th ed., Elsevier, 2021.

Hoogenboom, H. R. "Designing and Optimizing Library Selection Strategies for Generating High-Affinity Antibodies." *Trends in Biotechnology*, vol. 15, no. 2, 1997, pp. 62-70.

Hossenbaccus, L., S, Linton, S. Garvey, et al. "Towards Definitive Management of Allergic Rhinitis: Best Use of New and Established Therapies." *Allergy Asthma Clin Immunol*, vol. 16, no. 39, 2020, doi.org/10.1186/s13223-020-00436-y.

"How Is Cough Treated?" *National Heart, Lung, and Blood Institute*, 1 Oct. 2010.

Howard, Vanessa, et al. "The Health Status and Quality of Life of Adults with X-Linked Agammaglobulinemia." *Clinical Immunology*, vol. 118, 2006, pp. 201-8.

Huang, Chaolin, et al. "Clinical Features of Patients Infected with 2019 Novel Coronavirus in Wuhan, China." *The Lancet*, vol. 395, no. 10223, 15 Feb. 2020, pp. 497-506, www.thelancet.com/journals/lancet/article/PIIS0140-6736(20)30183-5/fulltext.

Hunder, Gene G. *Mayo Clinic on Arthritis*. Rev. ed., Mayo Clinic, 2002.

Huntley, A., A. R. White, and E. Ernst. "Relaxation Therapies for Asthma." *Thorax*, vol. 57, 2002, pp. 127-31.

Husebye, E. S., J. Perheentupa, R. Rautemaa, and O. Kämpe. "Clinical Manifestations and Management of Patients with Autoimmune Polyendocrine Syndrome Type I." *Journal of Internal Medicine*, vol. 265, 2009, pp. 514-29.

Husni, Elaine M. "Psoriatic Arthritis." *Cleveland Clinical Center for Continuing Education*, Oct. 2016, www.clevelandclinicmeded.com/medicalpubs/ diseasemanagement/rheumatology/psoriatic-arthritis/. Accessed 5 Sept. 2021.

"Hygiene Etiquette & Practice." *Centers for Disease Control and Prevention*, 27 Jul. 2016, www.cdc.gov/ healthywater/hygiene/etiquette/index.html.

"Hyperthyroidism." *MedlinePlus*, 24 Aug. 2021, medlineplus.gov/hyperthyroidism.html. Accessed 27 Aug. 2021.

"Hypothyroidism." *MedlinePlus*, 17 Aug. 2021, medlineplus.gov/hypothyroidism.html. Accessed 27 Aug. 2021.

Iams, Betty. *From MS to Wellness*. Iams House, 1998.

Icon Health. *Goiter: A Medical Dictionary, Bibliography, and Annotated Research Guide to Internet References*. Author, 2004.

Ikegame, Kazuhiro, et al. "Allogeneic Stem Cell Transplantation for X-linked Agammaglobulinemia Using Reduced Intensity Conditioning as a Model of the Reconstitution of Humoral Immunity." *Journal of Hematology & Oncology*, vol. 9, no. 9. 13 Feb. 2016, doi:10.1186/s13045-016-0240-y.

"Immune System and Disorders." *MedlinePlus*, 18 Aug. 2021, medlineplus.gov/immunesystemanddisorders.html. Accessed 29 Aug. 2021.

Immune Web, www.*immuneweb*.org.

"Impetigo." *Mayo Clinic*, 21 Apr. 2021, www.mayoclinic.org/diseases-conditions/impetigo/ symptoms-causes/syc-20352352. Accessed 29 Aug. 2021.

Imura, Hiroo, editor. *The Pituitary Gland*. 2nd ed., Raven Press, 1994.

"Infectious Diseases: Neutropenia (Agranulocytosis; Granulocytopenia)." *The Merck Manual of Diagnosis and Therapy*, edited by Mark H. Beers, et al., 18th ed., Merck Research Laboratories, 2006.

"Influenza." *The Merck Manual Home Health Handbook*, edited by Robert S. Porter et al., 3rd ed., Merck Research Laboratories, 2009.

"Influenza Vaccines for 2020-2021." *Medical Letter on Drugs and Therapeutics*, vol. 62, no. 1607, 2020, pp. 145-50.

"Iron." *National Institute of Health, Office of Dietary Supplements*. 22 Mar. 2021, ods.od.nih.gov/factsheets/Iron-Consumer/. Accessed 10 Sept. 2021.

Irvine, Alan, Peter Hoeger, and Albert C. Yan. *Harper's Textbook of Pediatric Dermatology*. Wiley-Blackwell, 2011.

Isenberg, D. A., et al. "International Consensus Outcome Measures for Patients with Idiopathic Inflammatory Myopathies: Development and Initial Validation of Myositis Activity and Damage Indices in Patients with Adult-Onset Disease." *Rheumatology*, vol. 43, no. 1, 2004, pp. 49-54.

Isenberg, David A., et al., editors. *Oxford Textbook of Rheumatology*. 3rd ed., New York: Oxford UP, 2004.

Isenstein, Arin, Dean Morrell, and Craig Burkhart. "Vitiligo: Treatment Approach in Children." *Pediatric Annals*, vol. 38, no. 6, Jun. 2009, pp. 339-44.

Ishida, Yoji, and Yoshiaki Tomiyama, editors. *Autoimmune Thrombocytopenia*. Springer, 2017.

Jackson, Alan C. *Viral Infections of the Human Nervous System*. Springer, 2013.

Jackson, Daniel J., and Leonard B. Bacharier. "Inhaled Corticosteroids for the Prevention of Asthma Exacerbations." *Annals of Allergy, Asthma & Immunology*, S1081-1206(21)00572-X, 13 Aug. 2021, doi:10.1016/j.anai.2021.08.014.

Jaffe, Elaine Sarkin. *Hematopathology*. Saunders/Elsevier, 2011.

Jaffe, Glenn, J., et al. "Adalimumab in Patients with Active Noninfectious Uveitis." *The New England Journal of Medicine*, vol. 375, no. 10, 2016, pp. 932-43, doi:10.1056/NEJMoa1509852.

Jain, Shreshta, et al. "Management of COVID-19 in Patients with Seizures: Mechanisms of Action of Potential COVID-19 Drug Treatments and Consideration for Potential Drug-Drug Interactions with Anti-seizure Medications." *Epilepsy Research*, vol. 174, 2021, p. 106675, doi:10.1016/j.eplepsyres.2021.106675.

James, William D., and Dirk M. Elston. *Andrews' Diseases of the Skin: Clinical Dermatology*. Saunders Elsevier, 2011.

Jameson, J. Larry, and Leslie J. DeGroot. *Endocrinology: Adult and Pediatric*. Elsevier Saunders, 2010.

Jameson, J. Larry, and Tinsley Randolph Harrison. *Harrison's Endocrinology*. McGraw-Hill, 2013.

Janeway, Charles A. *Immunobiology: The Immune System in Health and Disease*. 7th ed., Garland Science, 2007.

Jefferis, Roy, Koicho Kato, and William R. Strohl, editors. Structure and Function of Antibodies. Mdpi AG, 2021.

Jerger, James, editor. *Hearing Disorders in Adults: Current Trends*. College-Hill Press, 1984.

Jiang, M. H., L. Zhu, and J. G. Jiang. "Immunoregulatory Actions of Polysaccharides from Chinese Herbal

Medicine." *Expert Opinion on Therapeutic Targets*, vol. 14, 2020, pp. 1367-1402.

Jilani, T. N., C. V. Preuss, and S. Sharma. "Theophylline." StatsPearls Publishing, Jan. 2021 [Updated 2021 May 15], www.ncbi.nlm.nih.gov/books/NBK519024/.

Joneja, Janice M. V., and Leonard Bielory. *Understanding Allergy, Sensitivity, and Immunity*. Rutgers UP, 1990.

Jorde, Lynn B., John C. Carey, and Michael J. Bamshad. *Medical Genetics*. 4th ed., Mosby/Elsevier, 2010.

Jovanovic-Peterson, Lois, Charles M. Peterson, and Morton B. Stori. *A Touch of Diabetes*. 3rd ed., Chronimed, 1998.

Judd, Sandra J. *Childhood Diseases and Disorders Sourcebook: Basic Consumer Health Information About the Physical, Mental, and Developmental Health of Pre-Adolescent Children*. 2nd ed., Omnigraphics, 2009.

———, editor. *Genetic Disorders Sourcebook: Basic Consumer Information About Hereditary Diseases and Disorders*. 4th ed., Omnigraphics, 2010.

Justiz Vaillant, Angel A., and Christopher M. Stang. "Lymphoproliferative Disorders." *StatPearls*, StatPearls Publishing, 30 Dec. 2020.

"Juvenile Idiopathic Arthritis." National Institute of Arthritis and Musculoskeletal and Skin Diseases, Mar. 2021, www.niams.nih.gov/health-topics/juvenile-arthritis. Accessed 31 Aug. 2021

"Juvenile Rheumatoid Arthritis." *Johns Hopkins Medicine*, www.hopkinsmedicine.org/health/conditions-and-diseases/arthritis/juvenile-idiopathic-arthritis. Accessed 31 Aug. 2021.

Kagen, Lawrence J., editor. *The Inflammatory Myopathies*. Humana Press, 2009.

Kahmini, Fatemeh Rezaei, and Shahab Shahgaldi. "Therapeutic Potential of Mesenchymal Stem Cell-Derived Extracellular Vesicles as Novel Cell-Free Therapy for Treatment of Autoimmune Disorders." *Experimental and Molecular Pathology*, vol. 118, 2011, p. 104566, doi:10.1016/j.yexmp.2020.104566.

Kalb, Robert E., and Jeffery M. Weinberg. *Atopic Dermatitis: New Perspectives on Managing a Chronic Inflammatory Disease*. Integritas Communications, 2018.

Kalb, Rosalind, editor. *Multiple Sclerosis: The Questions You Have, the Answers You Need*. 5th ed., Demos Vermande, 2012.

Kaminski, Henry J., editor. *Myasthenia Gravis and Related Disorders*. 2nd ed., Humana Press, 2010.

Kampf, G., et. al. "Persistence of Coronaviruses on Inanimate Surfaces and Their Inactivation with Biocidal Agents." *Journal of Hospital Infection*, doi.org/10.1016/j.jhin.2020.01.022.

Kane, Melissa, and Tatyana Gotovkina. "Common Threads in Persistent Viral Infections." *Journal of Virology*, vol. 84, 2010, pp. 4116-23. Examines how some viruses establish a permanent host relationship and recurrent infection by avoiding immune system actions.

Kappelman, Michael D., et al. "The Prevalence and Geographic Distribution of Crohn's Disease and Ulcerative Colitis in the United States." *Clinical Gastroenterology and Hepatology*, vol. 5, no. 12, 2007, pp. 1424-29.

Karlson, E. W., et al. "Vitamin E in the Primary Prevention of Rheumatoid Arthritis: The Women's Health Study." *Arthritis and Rheumatism*, vol. 59, 2008, pp. 1589-95.

Karpatkin, S. "Autoimmune (Idiopathic) Thrombocytopenic Purpura." *The Lancet*, vol. 349, 1997, pp. 1531-36.

Kasitanon, Nuntana, Laurence S. Magder, and Michelle Petri. "Predictors of Survival in Systemic Lupus Erythematosus." *Medicine*, vol. 85, no. 3, 2006, pp. 147-56.

Kasper, Dennis L., et al., editors. *Harrison's Principles of Internal Medicine*. 20th ed., McGraw-Hill, 2021.

Kau, Andrew, et al. *The Washington Manual Allergy, Asthma, and Immunology Subspecialty Consult*. 3rd ed., Lippincott Williams & Wilkins, 2021.

Kaushansky, Kenneth, Marshall Lichtman, and Josef Prchal. *Williams Hematology*. 10th ed., McGraw-Hill, 2021.

Kavanaugh, Kevin, editor. *New Insights in Medical Mycology*. Springer, 2007.

Keene, Nancy. *Childhood Leukemia: A Guide for Families, Friends and Caregivers*. 4th ed., O'Reilly, 2010.

Kemper, Kathi J. *The Holistic Pediatrician: A Pediatrician's Comprehensive Guide to Safe and Effective Therapies for the Twenty-five Most Common Ailments of Infants, Children, and Adolescents*. Rev. ed., Quill, 2002.

Kennedy, David W., and Marilyn Olsen. *Living with Chronic Sinusitis: A Patient's Guide to Sinusitis, Nasal Allergies, Polyps, and Their Treatment Options*. Hatherleigh Press, 2007.

Kershaw, Michael H., J. A. Westwood, C. Y. Slaney, and P. K. Darcy. "Clinical Application of Genetically Modified T Cells in Cancer Therapy." *Clinical and Translational Immunology*, vol. 3, 2014, p. e16., www.nature.com/cti/journal/v3/n5/full/cti20147a.html

"Key Findings: Congenital Hypothyroidism." *Centers for Disease Control and Prevention*, 7 Sept. 2011.

Khanna, Reena, et al. "Early Combined Immunosuppression for the Management of Crohn's Disease (REACT): A Cluster Randomised Controlled

Trial." *The Lancet*, vol. 386, no. 10006, 2015, pp. 1825-34.

Kierman, John A., and Nagalingam Rajakumar. *Barr's The Human Nervous System: An Anatomical Viewpoint*. 10th ed., Wolters Kluwer/Lippincott Williams & Wilkins, 2013.

Kimball, Chad T. *Childhood Diseases and Disorders Sourcebook: Basic Consumer Health Information about Medical Problems Often Encountered in Pre-adolescent Children*. Omnigraphics, 2003.

———. *Colds, Flu, and Other Common Ailments Sourcebook*. Omnigraphics, 2001.

Kindt, Thomas J., Richard A. Goldsby, and Barbara A. Osborne. *Kuby Immunology*. 6th ed., W. H. Freeman, 2007.

King, Richard A., Jerome I. Rotter, and Arno G. Motulsky, editors. *The Genetic Basis of Common Diseases*. 2nd ed., Oxford UP, 2002.

Kingsmore, S. F., et al. "Identification of Diagnostic Biomarkers for Infection in Premature Neonates." *Molecular & Cellular Proteomics*, vol. 7, no. 10, Oct. 2008, pp. 1863-75.

Klein, Christian. Monoclonal Antibodies. Mdpi AG, 2018.

Kleine, Bernhard, and Winfried G. Rossmanith. *Hormones and the Endocrine System: Textbook of Endocrinology*. Springer, 2016.

Kliegman, Robert M., et al., editors. *Nelson Textbook of Pediatrics*. 21st ed., Elsevier, 2019.

Klinnert, M. D. "Psychological Impact of Eosinophilic Esophagitis on Children and Families." *Immunology & Allergy Clinics of North America*, vol. 29, no. 1, 2009, pp. 99-107, doi:10.1016/j.iac.2008.09.011.

Klippel, John H., Paul A. Dieppe, and Fred F. Ferri. *Primary Care Rheumatology*. W. B. Saunders, 2002.

Kobayashi, M., et al. "Shoyu Polysaccharides from Soy Sauce Improve Quality of Life for Patients with Seasonal Allergic Rhinitis." *International Journal of Molecular Medicine*, vol. 15, 2005, pp. 463-67.

Koch, Christian A., George P. Chrousos. *Endocrine Hypertension: Underlying Mechanisms and Therapy*. Humana Press, 2013.

Komaroff, Anthony, editor. *Harvard Medical School Family Health Guide*. Free Press, 2005.

Kontermann, Roland, and Stefan Dübel, editors. *Antibody Engineering*. 2nd ed., Springer, 2013.

Koopman, William J., and Larry W. Moreland, editors. *Arthritis and Allied Conditions: A Textbook of Rheumatology*. 15th ed., Lippincott Williams & Wilkins, 2005.

Korpás, Juraj, and Z. Tomori. *Cough and Other Respiratory Reflexes*. S. Karger, 1979.

Kovacs, William J.., and Sergio R. Ojeda, editors. *Textbook of Endocrine Physiology*. 6th ed., Oxford UP, 2012.

Koyoma, Shohei, et al. "Innate Immune Response to Viral Infection." *Cytokine*, vol. 43, no. 3, 2008, pp. 336-41.

Krause, Megan L, and Ashima Makol. "Management of Rheumatoid Arthritis during Pregnancy: Challenges and Solutions." *Open Access Rheumatology: Research and Reviews*. vol. 8, 2016, pp. 23-36, doi:10.2147/OARRR.S85340.

Kravets, I. "Hyperthyroidism: Diagnosis and Treatment." *American Family Physician*, vol. 93, 2016, pp. 363-70.

Krohmer, Jon R., editor. *American College of Emergency Physicians First Aid Manual*. 2nd ed., DK, 2004.

Kronenberg, Henry M., et al., editors. *Williams Textbook of Endocrinology*. 14th ed., Saunders/Elsevier, 2019.

Kumar, Vinay, Abul K. Abbas, and Nelson Fausto, editors. *Robbins and Cotran: Pathologic Basis of Disease*. 8th ed., Saunders/Elsevier, 2010.

"Lack of Consensus about Surgery for Ear Infections." *Health News*, vol. 18, no. 3, June/July 2000, p. 11.

Lagerkvist, Ulf. *Pioneers of Microbiology and the Nobel Prize*. World Scientific, 2003.

Lahita, Robert G. *Rheumatoid Arthritis: Everything You Need to Know*. Rev. ed., Avery, 2004.

———, and Robert H. Phillips. *Lupus Q & A: Everything You Need to Know*. Rev. ed., Avery, 2004.

Lal, B., et al. "Efficacy of Curcumin in the Management of Chronic Anterior Uveitis." *Phytotherapy Research*, vol. 13, 1999, pp. 318-322.

Lane, Nancy E., and Daniel J. Wallace. *All About Osteoarthritis: The Definitive Resource for Arthritis Patients and Their Families*. Oxford UP, 2002.

Lane, Thomas, editor. *Chemokines and Viral infection*. Springer, 2006.

Langewitz, W., et al. "Effect of Self-Hypnosis on Hay Fever Symptoms." *Psychotherapy and Psychosomatics*, vol. 74, 2005, pp. 165-72.

Lankarge, Vicki. *What Every Home Owner Needs to Know About Mold (And What to Do About It)*. McGraw-Hill, 2003.

Larsen, Laura, editor. *Childhood Diseases and Disorders Sourcebook*. Omnigraphics, 2012.

Latchford, Teresa. "Cutaneous Effects of Blood and Marrow Transplantation." *Principles of Skin Care and the Oncology Patient*. Oncology Nursing Society, 2010.

Lattime, Edmund C., and Stanton L. Gerson. Gene Therapy of Cancer: Translational Approaches from Preclinical Studies to Clinical Implementation. Academic Press, 2013.

Laws, Edward R., et al. *Pituitary Disorders: Diagnosis and Management*. Wiley, 2013.

Lebovitz, Harold E., editor. *Therapy for Diabetes Mellitus and Related Disorders*. 5th ed., American Diabetes Association, 2009.

Lee, M. S., B. C. Shin, and E. Ernst. "Acupuncture for Rheumatoid Arthritis." *Rheumatology*, vol. 47, 2008, pp. 1747-53.

Levin, Brian J. *EMRA Antibiotic Guide*. 19th ed., Emergency Medicine Residents' Association, 2020.

Levine, Bruce L., Miskin, James, Wonnacott, Keith, and Christopher Keir. "Global Manufacturing of CAR T Cell Therapy." *Molecular Therapy*, vol. 4, 2017, pp. 92-101.

Lewis, Ricki. *Human Genetics: Concepts and Applications*. 10th ed., McGraw-Hill, 2012.

Lexicomp. *The Drug Information Handbook*. 26th ed., Lexi-Comp, 2017.

Lichtenstein, Gary R., et al. "Management of Crohn Disease in Adults." *American Journal of Gastroenterology*, vol. 104, no. 2, pp. 465-83.

Lichtman, Marshall, et al., editors. *Williams Manual of Hematology*. 9th ed., McGraw-Hill, 2016.

Life, Death, and the Immune System. W. H. Freeman, 1994.

Lights, Verneda. "Hyperthyroidism." *HealthLine*, 22 Mar. 2019, www.healthline.com/health/hyperthyroidism. Accessed 27 Aug. 2021.

———. "What You Need to Know About Anemia." *Heathline*, 2 Aug. 2019, www.healthline.com/health/anemia. Accessed 10 Sept. 2021.

Liska, Ken. *Drugs and the Human Body, with Implications for Society*. 8th ed., Pearson/Prentice Hall, 2009.

Litin, Scott C., editor. *Mayo Clinic Family Health Book*. 4th ed., HarperResource, 2009.

———. "Multiple Sclerosis." *Mayo Clinic Family Health Book*. 4th ed., HarperResource, 2009.

Little, Marjorie. *Diabetes*. Chelsea House, 1991.

Liu, Xiu-Fen, et al. "Curcumin, a Potential Therapeutic Candidate for Anterior Segment Eye Diseases: A Review." *Frontiers in Pharmacology*, vol. 8, no. 66, 14 Feb. 2017.

Llop, Stephanie, M., et al. "Association of Low Vitamin D Levels with Noninfectious Uveitis and Scleritis." *Ocular Immunology and Inflammation*, vol. 27, no. 4, 2019, pp. 602-9.

Lodish, Harvey, Arnold Berk, Chris A. Kaiser, Monty Krieger, and Anthony Bretscher. Molecular Cell Biology. 9th ed., W. H. Freeman & Co., 2021.

Lorig, Kate, and James F. Fries, editors. *The Arthritis Helpbook: A Tested Self-Management Program for Coping with Arthritis and Fibromyalgia*. Updated ed., Da Capo, 2007.

Lu, Roujian, et al. "Genomic Characterization and Epidemiology of 2019 Novel Coronavirus: Implications for Virus Origins and Receptor Binding." *The Lancet*, Jan. 2020, doi.org/10.1016/s0140-6736(20)30251-8.

Lüdecke, Dieter K., George P. Chrousos, and George Tolis, editors. *ACTH, Cushing's Syndrome, and Other Hypercortisolemic States*. Raven Press, 1990.

Lumann, Paula, "What Is Contact Dermatitis?" 14 Dec. 2020, www.aad.org/public/diseases/eczema/types/contact-dermatitis/causes. Accessed 24 Aug. 2021.

Lupi, Chiara, et al. "Medicines for Headache Before and During Pregnancy: A Retrospective Cohort Study (ATENA Study)." *Neurological Sciences: Official Journal of the Italian Neurological Society and of the Italian Society of Clinical Neurophysiology*, vol. 42, no. 5, 2021, pp. 1895-1921, doi:10.1007/s10072-020-04702-0.

Lupus Foundation of America, www.lupus.org.

Maberly, Glen F. "Iodine Deficiency Disorders: Contemporary Scientific Issues." *Journal of Nutrition*, vol. 124, no. 8, Aug. 1994, pp. 1473-78S.

MacDonald, Kelli Pa, et al. "Cytokine Mediators of Chronic Graft-Versus-Host Disease." *The Journal of Clinical Investigation*, vol. 127, no. 7, 2017, pp. 2452-63, doi:10.1172/JCI90593.

Mackie, Rona M. *Clinical Dermatology*. 5th ed., Oxford UP, 2003.

Magee, Elaine. *Tell Me What to Eat If I Have Diabetes: Nutrition You Can Live With*. 4th ed., Career Press, 2014.

Magnusson, A. L., et al. "The Effect of Acupuncture on Allergic Rhinitis." *American Journal of Chinese Medicine*, vol. 32, 2004, pp. 105-15.

Mahler, Donald A. *COPD: Answers to Your Most Pressing Questions about Chronic Obstructive Pulmonary Disease*. Johns Hopkins UP, 2022.

Mahy, Brian W. J., and Marc H. V. van Regenmortel, editors. *Desk Encyclopedia of Human and Medical Virology*. Academic Press/Elsevier, 2010.

Majdalawieh, A. F., and R. I. Carr. "In Vitro Investigation of the Potential Immunomodulatory and Anti-Cancer Activities of Black Pepper (Piper nigrum) and Cardamom (Elettaria cardamomum)." *Journal of Medicinal Food*, vol. 13, 2020, pp. 371-81.

Majno, Guido, and Isabelle Joris. "Part III: Immunopathology." *Cells, Tissues, and Disease: Principles of General Pathology*. 2nd ed., Oxford UP, 2004, pp. 523-610.

Mak, Tak W., and Mary E. Saunders. *Primer to the Immune Response*. Academic Press/Elsevier, 2008.

Male, David. *Immunology: An Illustrated Outline*. 6th ed., CRC Press, 2021.

———, et al., editors. *Immunology*. 8th ed., Elsevier/Saunders, 2018.

Malek, N. Z. H., et al. "Association of Transient Hyperthyroidism and Severity of Hyperemesis Gravidarum." *Hormone Molecular Biology and Clinical Investigation*, vol. 3, 2017, doi:10.1515/hmbci-2016-0050.

Man, Yang-gao, et al. "Tumor-Infiltrating Immune Cells Promoting Tumor Invasion and Metastasis: Existing Theories." *Journal of Cancer*, vol. 4, no. 1, 2013, pp. 84-95.

Mancini, Anthony J., and Daniel P. Krowchuk, editors. *Pediatric Dermatology: A Quick Reference*. 4th ed., American Academy of Pediatrics, 2020.

Marcdate, Karen, and Robert M. Kliegman. *Nelson Essentials of Pediatrics*. 8th ed., Elsevier, 2018.

Marieb, Elaine N., and Katja Hoehn. *Human Anatomy and Physiology*. 11th ed., Pearson/Benjamin Cummings, 2018.

Marieb, Elaine N., and Suzanne Keller. *Essentials of Human Anatomy and Physiology*. 12th ed., Pearson/Benjamin Cummings, 2017.

Marks, Julie, "Roseola." *Health Library*, 30 Aug. 2018, www.healthline.com/health/roseola. Accessed 1 Sept. 2021.

Marks, Ronald. *Psoriasis*. 2nd rev. ed., Sheldon Press, 1994.

Marogna, M., et al. "Preventive Effects of Sublingual Immunotherapy in Childhood." *Annals of Allergy, Asthma, and Immunology*, vol. 101, 2008, pp. 206-11.

Marquardt, William C., editor. *Biology of Disease Vectors*. 2nd ed., Academic Press/Elsevier, 2005.

Marshall, Elizabeth L. *The Human Genome Project: Cracking the Code Within Us*. Franklin Watts, 1997.

Martin, Seamus, Dennis R. Burton, Ivan M. Roitt, and Peter J. Delves. *Roitt's Essential Immunology*. 13th ed., Wiley-Blackwell, 2017.

Martini, Frederic. *Fundamentals of Anatomy and Physiology*. 9th ed., Prentice-Hall, 2012.

Masterson, Susan. *You Mean It Isn't in My Head?: What Sjogren's Syndrome Is and What You Can Do About It*. Independently published, 2021.

Matkovic, Z., V. Zivkovic, and M. Korica. "Efficacy and Safety of *Astragalus membranaceus* in the Treatment of Patients with Seasonal Allergic Rhinitis." *Phytotherapy Research*, vol. 24, 2010, pp. 175-81.

Matthews, Bryan. *Multiple Sclerosis: The Facts*. 4th ed., Oxford UP, 2001.

Matthews, Dawn D., editor. *AIDS Sourcebook*. 3rd ed., Omnigraphics, 2003.

May, Jeffrey C., and Connie L. May. *Mold Survival Guide for Your Home and for Your Health*. Johns Hopkins UP, 2004.

Mayforth, Ruth D. *Designing Antibodies*. Academic, 1993.

Mayo Clinic. *Mayo Clinic on Arthritis*. HarperCollins, 2005.

———. "Meniere's Disease." *Mayo Clinic*, 2012, www.mayoclinic.org/diseases-conditions/menieres-disease/basics/definition/con-20028251. Accessed 10 Jul. 2015.

Mayo Foundation for Medical Education and Research. "Common Cold." www.mayoclinic.com/health/common-cold/ds00056.

———. "HIV/AIDS." www.mayoclinic.com/health/hiv-aids/ds00005.

McAlindon, T. E., M. P. LaValley, W. F. Harvey, et al. "Effect of Intra-articular Triamcinolone vs. Saline on Knee Cartilage Volume and Pain in Patients with Knee Osteoarthritis: A Randomized Clinical Trial." *JAMA*, vol. 317, no. 19, 2017, pp. 1967-75, doi:10.1001/jama.2017.5283.

McCaffrey, Thomas. "Functional Endoscopic Sinus Surgery: An Overview." *Mayo Clinic Proceedings*, vol. 68, 1993, pp. 571-77.

McCance, Kathryn L., and Sue E. Huether, editors. *Pathophysiology: The Biologic Basis for Disease in Adults and Children*. 6th ed., Mosby/Elsevier, 2010.

McCormack, Paul L. "Celecoxib: A Review of Its Use for Symptomatic Relief in the Treatment of Osteoarthritis, Rheumatoid Arthritis and Ankylosing Spondylitis." *Drugs*, vol. 71, no. 18, 2011, pp. 2457-89, doi:10.2165/11208240-000000000-00000.

McCoy, Krisha, and Kari Kassir. "Anemia." *Health Library*, 28 Mar. 2013.

McCrae, Keith R., editor. *Thrombocytopenia*. Taylor & Francis, 2006.

McCulloch, David. *The Diabetes Answer Book: Practical Answers to More than Three Hundred Top Questions*. Sourcebooks, 2008.

McCullough, Kenneth, and Raymond Spier. Monoclonal Antibodies in Biotechnology: Theoretical and Practical Aspects. Cambridge UP, 1990.

McDermott, Michael T. *Endocrine Secrets*. 6th ed., Elsevier Saunders, 2013.

McGovern, Dermot, P. B. "Crohn Disease and NOD2/CARD15." *Medscape*, 11 Dec. 2020. emedicine.medscape.com/article/1790325-overview#showall. Accessed 20 Aug. 2021.

McKusick, Victor A., and Paul J. Converse. "*142857 Major Histocompatibility Complex, Class II, DR Beta-1; HLA-DRB1." *OMIM.org*. Johns Hopkins U, 25 Jun. 2014. Accessed 4 Aug. 2014.

McKusick, Victor A., and Cassandra L. Kniffin. "#613179 Purine Nucleoside Phosphorylase Deficiency." *OMIM*. Johns Hopkins U, 8 Jan. 2013. Accessed 20 Aug. 2014.

McPherson, R. "Inflammation and Coronary Artery Disease: Insights from Genetic Studies." *The Canadian Journal of Cardiology*, vol. 28, no. 6, 2012, pp. 662-66.

McQuaid, K. R. "Gastrointestinal Disorders." *2013 Current Medical Diagnosis & Treatment*, edited by M. A. Papadakis, S. J. McPhee, and M. W. Rabow, p. 600, 52nd ed., McGraw-Hill Medica, 2013.

Meadows, Michelle. "Battling Lupus." *FDA Consumer*, vol. 39, no. 4, 2005, pp. 28-34.

"Measles." *Epidemiology and Prevention of Vaccine-Preventable Diseases*, edited by W. Atkinson et al., 11th ed., Public Health Foundation, 2009.

"Measurement of IgE to Ara h 2 & Diagnostics for Peanut Allergy." *American Academy of Allergy, Asthma, and Immunology*, 19 Jan. 2021, www.aaaai.org/Tools-for-the-Public/Latest-Research-Summaries/The-Journal-of-Allergy-and-Clinical-Immunology/2021/ara. Accessed 6 Sept. 2020.

MedlinePlus. "Addison Disease." *MedlinePlus*, 8 Apr. 2013 (reviewed 3 May 2012).

———. "Arthritis." *MedlinePlus*, 24 Apr. 2013.

———. "Chickenpox." www.nlm.nih.gov/medlineplus/ency/article/001592.htm.

———. "Ear Disorders." *MedlinePlus*, 1 Apr. 2013.

———. "Ear Infections." *MedlinePlus*, 1 Apr. 2013.

———. "Immune System and Disorders." *MedlinePlus*. U.S. NLM/NIH, 20 Aug. 2014. Accessed 20 Aug. 2014.

———. "Kawasaki Disease." *MedlinePlus*, 19 May 2013.

———. "Metabolic Disorders." *MedlinePlus*, 21 May 2013.

———. "Myasthenia Gravis." *MedlinePlus*, 19 Apr. 2013.

———. "Rheumatoid Arthritis." *MedlinePlus*, 26 Aug. 2013.

Meggs, William Joel, and Carol Svec. *The Inflammation Cure*. Contemporary Books, 2004.

Melero, I., G. Gaudemack, W. Gerritsen, et al. "Therapeutic Vaccines for Cancer: An Overview of Clinical Trials." *Nature Reviews Clinical Oncology*, vol. 11, 2014, pp. 509-24.

Melina, Vesanto, Jo Stepaniak, and Dina Aronson. *Food Allergy Survival Guide*. Healthy Living, 2004.

Melmed, Shlomo, Ronald Koenig, Clifford Rosen, Richard Auchus, and Allison Goldfine. *Williams Textbook of Endocrinology*. 14th ed., Elsevier, 2019.

Melvin, Jeanne L., and Virginia Wright, editors. *Pediatric Rheumatic Diseases*. Vol. 3. American Occupational Therapy Association, 2000.

Merenstein, Gerald B., David W. Kaplan, and Adam A. Rosenberg. *Handbook of Pediatrics*. 18th ed., Appleton & Lange, 1999.

Merino, Noël. *Vaccines*. Greenhaven, 2015.

Metchnikoff, Elie. *Lectures on the Comparative Pathology of Inflammation*. Translated by F. A. Starling and E. H. Starling. Dover, 1968.

Mickelson, Samuel, and Michael Benninger. "The Nose and Paranasal Sinuses." *Textbook of Primary Care Medicine*, edited by John Noble, 3rd ed., Mosby, 2001.

Mickleborough, T. D., et al. "Protective Effect of Fish Oil Supplementation on Exercise-Induced Bronchoconstriction in Asthma." *Chest*, vol. 129, 2006, pp. 39-49.

"Middle Eastern Respiratory Syndrome (MERS)." *Center for Disease Control and Prevention*, www.cdc.gov/coronavirus/mers/index.html. Accessed 10 Sept. 2021.

Middlemiss, Prisca. *What's That Rash? How to Identify and Treat Childhood Rashes*. Hamlyn, 2002.

Milunsky, Aubrey, and Jeff M. Milunsky, editors. *Genetic Disorders of the Fetus: Diagnosis, Prevention, and Treatment*. 6th ed., Wiley-Blackwell, 2010.

Mincer, D. L., and I. Jialal. *Hashimoto Thyroiditis*. StatPearls Publishing, 10 Aug. 2020, pubmed.ncbi.nlm.nih.gov/29083758/. Accessed 26 Aug. 2021.

Mohamed, Abdalla J., et al. "Bruton's Tyrosine Kinase (Btk): Function, Regulation, and Transformation with Special Emphasis on the pH Domain." *Immunological Reviews*, vol. 228, 2009, pp. 58-73.

Money, Nicholas P. *Carpet Monsters and Killer Spores: A Natural History of Toxic Mold*. Oxford UP, 2004.

Moore, Andrew. "Immunotherapy Can Provide Lasting Relief." *American Academy of Allergy, Asthma, and Immunology*, 28 Sept. 2020, www.aaaai.org/tools-for-the-public/conditions-library/allergies/immunotherapy-can-provide-lasting-relief. Accessed 28 Aug. 2021.

Moore, Kristeen, "Allergic Rhinitis." 7 Mar. 2019, www.healthline.com/health/allergic-rhinitis. Accessed 27 Aug. 2021.

Mounsey, Anne L., Leah G. Matthew, and David C. Slawson. "Herpes Zoster and Postherpetic Neuralgia: Prevention and Management." *American Family Physician*, vol. 72, 2005, pp. 1075-80.

Mueller, Heidi, editor. *Principles and Practice of Dermatology*. Foster Academics, 2016.

"Multiple Sclerosis." *MedlinePlus*, 7 May 2013.

Murphy, Kenneth, Paul Travers, and Mark Walport. *Janeway's Immunobiology*. 7th ed., Garland Science, 2008.

Murray, Patrick R., Ken S. Rosenthal, and Michael A. Pfaller. *Medical Microbiology*. 9th ed., Mosby/Elsevier, 2020.

"The Myth of IgG Food Panel Testing." *American Academy of Allergy, Asthma, and Immunology*, 28 Sept. 2020, www.aaaai.org/tools-for-the-public/conditions-library/allergies/igg-food-test. Accessed 6 Sept. 2021.

Nagami, Pamela. *Bitten: True Medical Stories of Bites and Stings*. St. Martin's Press, 2004.

Nakamura, H., et al. "Effects of Glucosamine Administration on Patients with Rheumatoid Arthritis." *Rheumatology International*, vol. 27, 2007, pp. 213-18.

Nathanson, Neal, et al. *Viral Pathogenesis and Immunity*. 2nd ed., Academic Press/Elsevier, 2007.

National Anemia Action Council, www.anemia.org.

National Center for Immunization and Respiratory Diseases, Division of Bacterial Diseases. "Ear Infections." *Centers for Disease Control and Prevention*, 23 May 2011.

National Center for Immunization and Respiratory Diseases, Division of Viral Diseases. "Cytomegalovirus (CMV) and Congenital CMV Infection." *Centers for Disease Control and Prevention*, 6 Dec. 2010.

National Eczema Society, eczema.org/. Accessed 24 Aug. 2021.

National Endocrine and Metabolic Diseases Information Service. "Cushing's Syndrome." *National Institutes of Health*, 6 Apr. 2012.

National Institute of General Medical Sciences (US). *The Structures of Life*. U.S. Department of Health and Human Services, Public Health Service, National Institutes of Health, National Institute of General Medical Sciences, 2007. NIH publication no. 07-2778.

National Institute of Neurological Disorders and Stroke. "NINDS Myasthenia Gravis Information Page." *NINDS*, 4 Dec. 2012.

National Library of Medicine and National Institutes of Health. "Vitiligo."

National Multiple Sclerosis Society. www.nationalmssociety.org/. Accessed 6 Sept. 2021.

National Newborn Screening and Global Resource Center. "Families: Newborn Screening." NNSGRC: *National Newborn Screening & Global Resource Center*, 22 Apr. 2013.

National Research Council. *Multiple Chemical Sensitivities*. National Academy Press, 1992.

National Vitiligo Foundation. www.facebook.com/MyNVFI/.

Neal, M. J. *Modern Pharmacology at a Glance*. 6th ed., Wiley-Blackwell, 2009.

Nelson, David L., and Michael M. Cox. *Lehninger Principles of Biochemistry*. 7th ed., W.H. Freeman, 2017.

Nelson, Miriam E., et al. *Strong Women and Men Beat Arthritis*. Putnam, 2003.

"Neonatal Hypothyroidism." *Medline Plus*, 28 Jun. 2011.

Nettis, E., et al. "Double-Blind, Placebo-Controlled Study of Sublingual Immunotherapy in Patients with Latex-Induced Urticaria." *British Journal of Dermatology*, vol. 156, 2007, pp. 674-81.

Nevoltris, Damien, and Patrick Chames, editors. *Antibody Engineering: Methods and Protocols*. 3rd ed., Humana Press, 2018.

Newland, A., et al. "An Open-Label, Unit Dose-Finding Study of AMG 531, a Novel Thrombopoiesis-Stimulating Peptibody, in Patients with Immune Thrombocytopenic Purpura." *British Journal of Haematology*, vol. 135, no. 4, 2006, pp. 547-53.

Ng, Wan-Fai, editor. *Sjögren's Syndrome*. Oxford UP, 2016.

Nicholls, John G., et al. *From Neuron to Brain*. 5th ed., Sinauer, 2011.

Noback, Charles R., et al. *The Human Nervous System: Structure and Function*. 6th ed., Humana Press, 2005.

Nordmark, G., et al. "Effects of Dehydroepiandrosterone Supplement on Health-Related Quality of Life in Glucocorticoid Treated Female Patients with Systemic Lupus Erythematosus." *Autoimmunity*, vol. 38, 2005, pp. 531-40.

"NSAIDs: Nonsteroidal Anti-Inflammatory Drugs." *American College of Rheumatology*, Aug. 2012.

Nussbaum, Robert L., et al. *Thompson and Thompson Genetics in Medicine*. 7th ed., Saunders/Elsevier, 2007.

Nyhan, William L., and Georg F. Hoffmann. *Atlas of Inherited Metabolic Diseases*. 4th ed., CRC Press, 2020.

Ober, Carole, and Tsung-Chieh Yao. "The Genetics of Asthma and Allergic Disease: A 21st Century Perspective." *Immunological Reviews*, vol. 242, no. 1, 2011, pp. 10-30.

Odumade, Oludare A., Kristin A. Hogquist, and Henry H. Balfour, Jr. "Progress and Problems in Understanding and Managing Primary Epstein-Barr Virus Infections." *Clinical Microbiology Review*, vol. 24, no. 1, Jan. 2011, pp. 193-209.

O'Hanlon, Leslie Harris. "Tinkering with Genes to Fight Insect-Borne Disease: Researchers Create Genetically Modified Bugs to Fight Malaria, Chagas, and Other Diseases." *The Lancet*, vol. 363, 2004, p. 1288.

Oksenberg, Jorge R., and David Brassat, editors. *Immunogenetics of Autoimmune Disease*. Springer, 2006.

Olsen, S. F., et al. "Fish Oil Intake Compared with Olive Oil Intake in Late Pregnancy and Asthma in the

Offspring." *American Journal of Clinical Nutrition*, vol. 88, 2008, pp. 167-75.

"Oral Iron for Anemia: A Review of the Clinical Effectiveness, Cost-effectiveness and Guidelines Rapid Response Report: Summary with Critical Appraisal Ottawa (ON)." *Canadian Agency for Drugs and Technologies in Health*, 6 Jan. 2006.

Osband, Michael E., and Carl Pochedly, editors. *Histiocytosis-X*. W. B. Saunders, 1987.

"Osilodrostat (*Isturisa*) for Cushing's Disease." *Medical Letter on Drugs and Therapy*, vol. 63, no. 1617, 8 Feb. 2021, pp. 21-23.

Ossipow, Vincent, and Nicolas Fischer. *Monoclonal Antibodies: Methods and Protocols*. 2nd ed., Humana, 2014.

"Overview of the Immune System." *American Academy of Allergy, Asthma, and Immunology*, 30 Dec. 2013, www.niaid.nih.gov/research/immune-system-overview. Accessed 29 Aug. 2021.

"An Overview of Psoriasis and Psoriatic Arthritis." *National Psoriasis Foundation*, Feb. 2011.

Owen, Judith A., Janis Kuby, Jenni Punt, and Sharon A. Stranford. *Immunology*. 7th ed., Macmillan, 2013.

Pachlopnik Schmid, J., T. Güngör, and R. Seger. "Modern Management of Primary T-Cell Immunodeficiencies." *Pediatric Allergy & Immunology*, vol. 25, no. 4, 2014, pp. 300-313.

Paget, Stephen A., Michael D. Lockshin, and Suzanne Loebl. *The Hospital for Special Surgery Rheumatoid Arthritis Handbook*. John Wiley & Sons, 2002.

Pardi, Norbert, Michael J. Hogan, Frederick W. Porter, and Drew Weissman. "mRNA Vaccines—A New Era in Vaccinology." *Nature Reviews Drug Discovery*, vol. 17, 2018, pp. 261-79.

Pardoll, Drew. "T Cells Take Aim at Cancer." *Proceedings of the National Academy of Sciences*, vol. 99, no. 25, 2012, pp. 15840-42, www.pnas.org/content/99/25/15840.full.

Parham, Peter. *The Immune System*. 3rd ed., Garland Science, 2009.

Parker, James N., and Philip M. Parker, editors. *Juvenile Rheumatoid Arthritis: The Official Patient's Sourcebook*. Icon Health, 2002.

———. *Kawasaki Disease: A Bibliography, Medical Dictionary, and Annotated Research Guide to Internet References*. ICON Health, 2004.

———. *Myasthenia Gravis: A Medical Dictionary, Bibliography, and Annotated Research Guide to Internet References*. ICON Health Publications, 2004.

———. *Myositis: A Medical Dictionary, Bibliography, and Annotated Research Guide to Internet References*. ICON Health, 2004.

———. *The Official Patient's Sourcebook on Addison's Disease*. Icon Health, 2002.

———. *The Official Patient's Sourcebook on Atopic Dermatitis*. Icon Health, 2002.

———. *The Official Patient's Sourcebook on Guillain-Barré Syndrome*. Icon Health, 2002.

———. *The Official Patient's Sourcebook on Kaposi's Sarcoma*. Icon Health, 2003.

———. *The Official Patient's Sourcebook on Psoriasis*. Icon Health, 2004.

———. *The Official Patient's Sourcebook on Rheumatoid Arthritis*. Icon Health, 2002.

———. *The Official Patient's Sourcebook on Sjögren's Syndrome*. Icon Health, 2002.

———. *Roseola: A Medical Dictionary, Bibliography, and Annotated Research Guide to Internet References*. Icon Health, 2004.

Patterson, Thomas F. "*Aspergillus* Species." *Mandell, Douglas, and Bennett's Principles and Practice of Infectious Diseases*, edited by Gerald L. Mandell, John F. Bennett, and Raphael Dolin, 7th ed., Churchill Livingstone/Elsevier, 2010.

Paul, Marla. "Food Allergy Is Linked to Skin Exposure and Genetics." *Northwestern Now*, 6 Apr. 2018, news.northwestern.edu/stories/2018/april/food-allergy-is-linked-to-skin-exposure-and-genetics. Accessed 31 Jan. 2019.

Paul, William E., editor. *Immunology: Recognition and Response*. W. H. Freeman, 1991.

PDxMD. *PDxMD Ear, Nose, and Throat Disorders*. Author, 2003.

Peiris, M., et al., editors. *Severe Acute Respiratory Syndrome*. Blackwell, 2005.

Pelengaris, Stella, and Michael Khan, editors. *The Molecular Biology of Cancer*. Blackwell, 2006.

Penack, Olaf, et al. "Prophylaxis and Management of Graft Versus Host Disease After Stem-Cell Transplantation for Haematological Malignancies: Updated Consensus Recommendations of the European Society for Blood and Marrow Transplantation." *The Lancet (Haematology)*, vol. 7, no. 2, 2020, pp. e157-e167, doi:10.1016/S2352-3026(19)30256-X.

Pender, Daniel J. *Practical Otology*. J. B. Lippincott, 1992.

Peter, G., and P. Gardner. "Standards for Immunization Practice for Vaccines in Children and Adults." *Infectious Disease Clinics of North America*, vol. 15, 2001, pp. 9-19.

Peterson, Pärt, and Eystein S. Husebye. "Polyendocrine Syndromes." *The Autoimmune Diseases*, edited by Noel R. Rose and Ian R. Mackay, Elsevier, 2014, pp. 605-18.

Petri, Michelle A., et al. "Effects of Prasterone on Disease Activity and Symptoms in Women with Active Systemic Lupus Erythematosus." *Arthritis and Rheumatism* vol. 50, no. 9, 2004, pp. 2858-68, doi:10.1002/art.20427.

Petris, Gianluca, editor. *Curing Genetic Diseases through Genome Reprogramming*. Academic Press, 2021.

Pfaar, O., and L. Klimek. "Efficacy and Safety of Specific Immunotherapy with a High-Dose Sublingual Grass Pollen Preparation." *Annals of Allergy, Asthma, and Immunology*, vol. 100, 2008, pp. 256-63.

Phillips, Robert H. *Coping with Lupus: A Practical Guide to Alleviating the Challenges of Systemic Lupus Erythematosus*. 3rd ed., Avery, 2001.

"Physicians and Surgeons." *Occupational Outlook Handbook*, Bureau of Labor Statistics, 11 Jun. 2018, www.bls.gov/ooh/healthcare/physicians-and-surgeons.htm. Accessed 25 Oct. 2018.

Pickering, Larry K., et al., editors. *Red Book: 2009 Report of the Committee on Infectious Diseases*. 28th ed., American Academy of Pediatrics, 2009.

Pines, Maya, editor. *Arousing the Fury of the Immune System*. Howard Hughes Medical Institute, 1998.

"Pituitary Tumors." *MedlinePlus*, 17 Aug. 2021, medlineplus.gov/thyroiddiseases.html. Accessed on 24 Aug. 2021.

Playfair, J. H. L., and B. M. Chain. *Immunology at a Glance*. 10th ed., Wiley-Blackwell, 2013.

Plaza, Jose A., and Victor G. Prieto. *Inflammatory Skin Disorders*. Demos Medical Publishing, 2012.

Plotkin, Stanley A., Walter A. Orenstein, and Paul A. Offit, editors. *Vaccines*. 7th ed., Saunders/Elsevier, 2017.

Poehlmann, Katherine M. *Rheumatoid Arthritis: The Infection Connection*. Satori Press, 2002.

Polack, Fernando P., et al. "Safety and Efficacy of the BNT162b2 mRNA Covid-19 Vaccine." *New England Journal of Medicine*, vol. 383, no. 27, 2020, pp. 2603-15, doi.org/10.1056/NEJMoa2034577.

Polman, Chris H., et al. *Multiple Sclerosis: The Guide to Treatment and Management*. 6th ed., Demos Vermande, 2006.

Polovich, M., J. M. White, and L. O. Kelleher. *Chemotherapy and Biotherapy Guidelines*. 2nd ed., Oncology Nursing Society, 2005.

Poppelaars, Felix, Mariana Gaya da Costa, Siawosh K. Eskandari, Jeffery Damman, Marc Seelen. "Donor Genetic Variants in Interleukin-6 and Interleukin-6 Receptor Associate with Biopsy-Proven Rejection Following Kidney Transplantation." *Scientific Reports*, vol. 11, 2021, p. 16483, doi.org/10.1038/s41598-021-95714-z.

Porter, Robert S., et al., editors. *The Merck Manual Home Health Handbook*. 3rd ed., Merck Research Laboratories, 2009.

Powell, Michael, and Oliver Fischer. *101 Diseases You Don't Want to Get*. Thunder's Mouth Press, 2005.

Pradhan, E. K., et al. "Effect of Mindfulness-Based Stress Reduction in Rheumatoid Arthritis Patients." *Arthritis and Rheumatism*, vol. 57, 2007, pp. 1134-42.

Preddy, Victor R., and Ronald R. Watson. *Bioactive Food as Interventions and Related Inflammatory Diseases*. Elsevier/Academic Press, 2013.

Predergast, G. C., and E. M. Jaffee. *Cancer Immunotherapy*. 2nd ed., Academic Press, 2013.

"Prevention of Allergies and Asthma in Children." *The American Academy of Allergy, Asthma, Immunology*, www.aaaai.org/conditions-and-treatments/library/allergy-library/prevention-of-allergies-and-asthma-in-children. Accessed 31 Jan. 2019.

Provan, Drew, and John Gribben, editors. *Molecular Haematology*. 2nd ed., Blackwell, 2005.

"Psoriasis." *MedlinePlus*, 6 May 2013.

Punt, Jenni, et al. editors. *Kuby Immunology*. 8th ed., W. H. Freeman, 2018.

Qontro Medical Guides. *Vasculitis Medical Guide*. Author, 2008.

Rabson, Arthur, et al. *Really Essential Medical Immunology*. 2nd ed., Blackwell Science, 2005.

Radovick, Sally, and Margaret H. MacGillivray. *Pediatric Endocrinology: A Practical Clinical Guide*. Humana Press, 2013.

Rae-Grant, Alexander et al. "Practice Guideline Recommendations Summary: Disease-Modifying Therapies for Adults with Multiple Sclerosis: Report of the Guideline Development, Dissemination, and Implementation Subcommittee of the American Academy of Neurology." *Neurology*, vol. 90, no. 17, 2018, pp. 777-88, doi:10.1212/WNL.0000000000005347.

Rajan, T. V., et al. "Effect of Ingestion of Honey on Symptoms of Rhinoconjunctivitis." *Annals of Allergy, Asthma, and Immunology*, vol. 88, 2002, pp. 198-203.

Rakel, Robert E., and Edward T. Bope, editors. *Conn's Current Therapy*. Saunders, 2007.

Ramos, Alexis et al. "Acupuncture for rheumatoid arthritis." ("Acupuntura para el tratamiento de la artritis reumatoide.") *Medwave*, vol. 18, no. 6, 2018, p. e7284, doi:10.5867/medwave.2018.06.7283.

Rasmussen, S. K., et al. "Recombinant Antibody Mixtures: Optimization of Cell Line Generation and Single-Batch Manufacturing Processes." *BMC Proceedings*, vol. 5 (Suppl. 8), 2011, p. 02.

Rattue, Petra. "*Prochymal*—First Stem Cell Drug Approved." *Medical News Today*, 22 May 2012, www.medicalnewstoday.com/articles/245704#1. Accessed 3 Sept. 2021.

Raz, E. *Immunostimulatory DNA Sequences*. Springer, 2001.

"Reactions to Complementary and Alternative Medicines." *American Academy of Allergy, Asthma, and Immunology*, www.aaaai.org/Aaaai/media/MediaLibrary/PDF%20Documents/Libraries/EL-Reactions-to-CAM-patient.pdf. Accessed 2 Sept. 2021.

Rennert, Nancy J. "Addison's Disease." *MedlinePlus*, 11 Dec. 2011.

Rennie, Ed. *Beginning of the End of My Life*. Xlibris, 2005. Leukemia and Lymphoma Society of America, www.leukemia.org.

"Rheumatoid Arthritis." *Centers for Disease Control and Prevention*, 19 Nov. 2012.

"Rheumatoid Arthritis." *Health Library*, 30 Sept. 2012.

"Rhinovirus Infections." *HealthyChildren.org*. American Academy of Pediatrics, 11 May 2013.

Richardson, Malcolm D., and Elizabeth M. Johnson. *Pocket Guide to Fungal Infection*. 2nd ed., Blackwell, 2006.

Richer, Alice C. *Food Allergies*. Greenwood Press, 2009.

Riedemann, Therese, Alexandre Patchev, Kwangook Cho, and Osborne F. X. Almeida. "Corticosteroids." *Molecular Brain*, vol. 3, 2020, pp. 2-21.

Rietschel, Robert L., and Joseph F. Fowler, editors. *Fisher's Contact Dermatitis*. 6th ed., Marcel Decker, 2008.

Ring, J., U. Krämer, T. Schäfer, and H. Behrendt. "Why Are Allergies Increasing?" *Current Opinion in Immunology*, vol. 13, no. 6, 2001, pp. 701-8.

Ring, J., B. Przybilla, and T. Ruzicka, editors. *Handbook of Atopic Eczema*. 2nd ed., Springer, 2006.

Roberts, J., et al. "A Systematic Review of the Clinical Effectiveness of Acupuncture for Allergic Rhinitis." *BMC Complementary and Alternative Medicine*, vol. 8, 2008.

Robertson, Erle S., editor. *Epstein-Barr Virus*. Caister Academic Press, 2010.

Rodak, Bernadette, editor. *Hematology: Clinical Principles and Applications*. 4th ed., Elsevier Saunders, 2012.

Rodriguez-Perez, N., et al. "Frequency of Acute Systemic Reactions in Patients with Allergic Rhinitis and Asthma Treated with Sublingual Immunotherapy." *Annals of Allergy, Asthma, and Immunology*, vol. 101, 2008, pp. 304-10.

Roizman, Bernard, editor. *Infectious Diseases in an Age of Change: The Impact of Human Ecology and Behavior on Disease Transmission*. National Academy Press, 1995.

Roizman, Bernard, Richard J. Whitley, and Carlos Lopez, editors. *The Human Herpesviruses*. Raven Press, 1993.

Roland, Peter S., Bradley F. Marple, and William L. Meyerhoff, editors. *Hearing Loss*. Thieme, 1997.

Rose, Noel R., and Ian. R. Mackay, editors. *The Autoimmune Diseases*. 6th ed., Academic Press/Elsevier, 2019.

Rosenberg, Steven A., editor. Principles and Practice of the Biologic Therapy of Cancer. 3rd ed., Lippincott Williams & Wilkins, 2000.

Rosenblum, Laurie B. "Vitiligo." *Health Library*, 12 Sept. 2012.

Rosenthal, M. Sara. *The Thyroid Sourcebook*. 5th ed., McGraw-Hill, 2009.

"Roseola." *MedlinePlus*, 5 Aug. 2021, medlineplus.gov/ency/article/000968.htm. Accessed 1 Sept. 2021.

Royal College of Physicians and Royal College of Pathologists. "Good Allergy Practice-Standards of Care for Providers and Purchasers of Allergy Services within the National Health Service." *Clinical and Experimental Allergy*, vol. 25, 1995, pp. 586-95.

Royen, Barend J. van, and Ben A. C. Dijkmans, editors. *Ankylosing Spondylitis: Diagnosis and Management*. Taylor & Francis, 2006.

Rubin, Alan L. *Thyroid for Dummies*. For Dummies, 2006.

Ruggieri, Paul, and Scott Isaacs. *A Simple Guide to Thyroid Disorders: From Diagnosis to Treatment*. Addicus Books, 2003.

Rüker, Florian, and Gordana Wozniak-Knopp, editors. *Introduction to Antibody Engineering*. Springer, 2020.

Russell, Margot. *When the Road Turns: Inspirational Stories About People with MS*. Health Communications, 2001.

Ryan, Kenneth J., and George Ray. *Sherris Medical Microbiology: An Introduction to Infectious Diseases*. 5th ed., McGraw-Hill Medical, 2010.

Saba, Hussain I., and Harold R. Roberts, editor. *Hemostasis and Thrombosis: Practical Guidelines in Clinical Management*. John Wiley & Sons, Ltd., 2014.

Sabil, Fred. *Crohn's Disease and Ulcerative Colitis: Everything You Need to Know*. 3rd ed., Firefly Books, 2011.

Sabina, A. B., et al. "Yoga Intervention for Adults with Mild-to-Moderate Asthma." *Annals of Allergy, Asthma, and Immunology*, vol. 94, 2005, pp. 543-48.

Safer, Diane A. "Kawasaki Disease." *Health Library*, 26 Nov. 2012.

Sajjadi, H., and M. M. Paparella. "Meniere's Disease." *The Lancet*, vol. 372, no. 9636, 2008, pp. 406-14, doi:10.1016/S0140-6736(08)61161-7.

Salter, Robert Bruce. *Textbook of Disorders and Injuries of the Musculoskeletal System*. 3rd ed., Williams & Wilkins, 1999.

Sandborn, William J. "Crohn Disease Evaluation and Treatment: Clinical Decision Tool." *Gastroenterology*, vol. 147, no. 3, 2014, pp. 702-5.

Sande Merle A., et al. *Sande's HIV/AIDS Medicine: Medical Management of AIDS, 2013*. Elsevier Saunders, 2012.

Sanders, Donald B., et al. "International Consensus Guidance for Management of Myasthenia Gravis: Executive Summary." *Neurology*, vol. 87, no. 4, 2016, pp. 419-25, doi:10.1212/WNL.0000000000002790.

Santangelo, C. M., and E. McCloud. "Nutritional Management of Children Who Have Food Allergies and Eosinophilic Esophagitis." *Immunology & Allergy Clinics of North America*, vol. 29, no. 1, 2009, pp. 77-84, doi:10.1016/j.iac.2008.09.009.

Sauer, Aisha V., Immacolata Brigida, Nicola Carriglio, and Alessandro Aiuti. "Autoimmune Dysregulation and Purine Metabolism in Adenosine Deaminase Deficiency." *Frontiers in Immunology*, vol. 3, 2012, p. 265. www.frontiersin.org/article/10.3389/fimmu.2012.00265, doi:10.3389/fimmu.2012.00265.

Scadding, Glenis K., and Wytske J. Hokkens. *Rhinitis*. Health Press, 2007.

Scanlon, Valerie, and Tina Sanders. *Essentials of Anatomy and Physiology*. 6th ed., F. A. Davis, 2011.

Scheld, W. Michael, Richard J. Whitley, and Christina M. Marra, editors. *Infections of the Central Nervous System*. 3rd ed., Lippincott Williams & Wilkins, 2004.

Scherman, Daniel, editor. Advanced Textbook on Gene Transfer, Gene Therapy and Genetic Pharmacology: Principles, Delivery and Pharmacological and Biomedical Applications of Nucleotide-based Therapies. 2nd ed., World Scientific Publishing Europe Ltd., 2019.

Schmitt, Barton D. *Your Child's Health: The Parents' One-Stop Reference Guide to Symptoms, Emergencies, Common Illnesses, Behavior Problems, Healthy Development*. Rev. ed., Bantam Books, 2005.

Schroeder, K., and T. Fahey. "Over-the-Counter Medications for Acute Cough in Children and Adults in Ambulatory Settings." *The Cochrane Library*, Issue 4. John Wiley & Sons, 2003.

Schubert, R., et al. "Effect of N-3 Polyunsaturated Fatty Acids in Asthma After Low-Dose Allergen Challenge." *International Archives of Allergy and Immunology*, vol. 148, 2009, pp. 321-29.

Schulze-Koops H., and A. Skapenko, "Biosimilars in Rheumatology: A Review of the Evidence and Their Place in the Treatment Algorithm." *Rheumatology*, vol. 56, no. suppl 4, 2017, pp. iv-30.

Schwar, Sheri Lyn. *Vasculitis: Sick and Tired of Being Sick and Tired*. iUniverse, 2006.

Schwarz, Klaus, et al. "Human Severe Combined Immune Deficiency and DNA Repair." *Bioessays*, vol. 25, no. 11, 2003, pp. 1061-70.

Scofield, R. Hal, and James Oates. "The Place of William Osler in the Description of Systemic Lupus Erythematosus." *The American Journal of the Medical Sciences*, vol. 338, no. 5, 2009, pp. 409-12, doi:10.1097/MAJ.0b013e3181acbd71.

Scollay, Roland. "Gene Therapy: A Brief Overview of the Past, Present, and Future." *Annals of the New York Academy of Sciences*, vol. 953, 2001, pp. 26-30.

Scott, Andrew M., Jedd D. Wolchok, and Lloyd J. Old. "Antibody Therapy of Cancer." *Nature Reviews Cancer*, vol. 12, 2012, pp. 278-87, www.nature.com/nrc/journal/v12/n4/full/nrc3236.html.

Scriver, Charles R., et al., editors. *The Metabolic and Molecular Bases of Inherited Disease*. 8th ed., McGraw-Hill, 2002.

Segel, George B., and Jill S. Halterman. "Neutropenia in Pediatric Practice." *Pediatrics in Review*, vol. 29, no. 1, 2008, pp. 12-23, doi:10.1542/pir.29-1-12.

Senchina, D. S., et al. "Herbal Supplements and Athlete Immune Function-What's Proven, Disproven, and Unproven?" *Exercise Immunology Review*, vol. 15, 2009, pp. 66-106.

Seppa, N. "Self-Help: Stem Cells Rescue Lupus Patients." *Science News*, vol. 169, no. 5, 4 Feb. 2006, pp. 67-68.

Shahar, E., G. Hassoun, and S. Pollack. "Effect of Vitamin E Supplementation on the Regular Treatment of Seasonal Allergic Rhinitis." *Annals of Allergy, Asthma, and Immunology*, vol. 92, 2004, pp. 654-58.

Shannon, Joyce Brennfleck, editor. *Thyroid Disorders Sourcebook: Basic Consumer Health Information About Disorders of the Thyroid and Parathyroid Glands*. Omnigraphics, 2005.

Shaw, Michael. *Diabetes Mellitus: An Incredibly Easy! Miniguide*. Springhouse Pub. Co., 2000.

———, editor. *Everything You Need to Know About Diseases*. Springhouse Press, 1996.

"Shingrix—An Adjuvanted, Recombinant Herpes Zoster Vaccine." *Medical Letter on Drugs and Therapeutics*, vol. 59, no. 1535, 2017, pp. 195-96.

Shlotzhauer, Tammi L., and James L. McGuire. *Living with Rheumatoid Arthritis*. 2nd ed., Johns Hopkins UP, 2003.

Shoemaker, Ritchie C. *Mold Warriors: Fighting America's Hidden Health Threat*. Gateway Press, 2007.

Shoenfeld, Yehuda, and Nancy Agmon-Levin. *Vaccines and Autoimmunity*. Wiley, 2015.

Shoman, Shmuel, and Stuart M. Levitz. "The Immune Response to Fungal Infections." *British Journal of Haematology,* vol. 129, 2005, pp. 569-82.

Shuman, Jill, and Purvee S. Shah. "Psoriasis." *Health Library,* 25 Feb. 2013.

Sicherer, Scott H. *Understanding and Managing Your Child's Food Allergies.* Johns Hopkins UP, 2006.

Sienra-Monge, J. J., et al. "Antioxidant Supplementation and Nasal Inflammatory Responses Among Young Asthmatics Exposed to High Levels of Ozone." *Clinical and Experimental Immunology* vol. 138, 2004, pp. 317-22.

Silverstein, Alvin, et al. *Bites and Stings.* Scholastic, 2002.

———. *Paul Ehrlich's Receptor Immunology: The Magnificent Obsession.* Academic Press, 2002.

Silverstein, Arthur M. *A History of Immunology.* Academic Press, 1989.

Singh, Jasvinder A., et al. "Special Article: 2018 American College of Rheumatology/National Psoriasis Foundation Guideline for the Treatment of Psoriatic Arthritis." *Arthritis & Rheumatology,* vol. 71, no. 1, 2019, pp. 5-32, doi:10.1002/art.40726.

Singh, Siddharth, and Edward V. Loftus, Jr. "Crohn Disease: REACT to Save the Gut." *The Lancet,* vol. 386, no. 10006, 2015, pp. 1800-1802.

"Sinus Infection (Sinusitis)." *Cleveland Clinic,* 6 Apr. 2020, my.clevelandclinic.org/health/diseases/17701-sinusitis. Accessed 28 Aug. 2021.

"Sjögren Disease." *Oral Health Topics, American Dental Association,* 16 May 2019, www.ada.org/en/member-center/oral-health-topics/sjogren-disease. Accessed 28 Aug. 2021.

Skoner, D. P. "Allergic Rhinitis: Definition, Epidemiology, Pathophysiology, Detection, and Diagnosis." *Journal of Allergy and Clinical Immunology,* vol. 108, no. 1, 2001, pp. S2-S8.

Smith, Mathew D. "Antibody Production in Plants." *Biotechnology Advances,* vol. 14, no. 3, 1996, pp. 267-81.

Spergel, J. M., and M. Shuker. "Nutritional Management of Eosinophilic Esophagitis." *Gastrointestinal Endoscopy Clinics of North America,* vol. 18, no. 1, pp. 179-94, 2008, doi:10.1016/j.giec.2007.09.008.

Sperling, Mark A., editor. *Pediatric Endocrinology.* 3rd ed., Saunders/Elsevier, 2008.

Speroff, Leon, and Marc A. Fritz. *Clinical Gynecologic Endocrinology and Infertility.* 8th ed., Lippincott Williams & Wilkins, 2011.

Spiders and Other Arachnids, spiders.ucr.edu.

Spielman, Andrew, and Michael D'Antonio. *Mosquito: A Natural History of Our Most Persistent and Deadly Foe.* Hyperion, 2001.

Springer, Timothy. *Hybridoma Technology in the Biosciences and Medicine.* Springer, 2013.

Springhouse Corporation. *Everything You Need to Know About Diseases.* Author, 1996.

Steinitz, Michael, editor. *Human Monoclonal Antibodies: Methods and Protocols.* 2nd ed., Humana Press, 2019.

Stern, Peter L., Peter C. L. Beverley, and Miles W. Carroll, editors. Cancer Vaccines and Immunotherapy. Cambridge UP, 2000.

"Steroids." *National Health Service (UK),* 14 Jan. 2020, www.nhs.uk/conditions/steroids/. Accessed 22 Aug. 2021.

Stetson D. B., and R. Medzhitov. "Type I Interferons in Host Defense." *Immunity,* vol. 25, 2006, pp. 373-81.

Sticherling, Michael, and Enno Christophers, editors. *Treatment of Autoimmune Disorders.* Springer, 2003.

Stigbrand, T., et al. "Twenty Years with Monoclonal Antibodies: State of the Art." *Acta Oncologica,* vol. 35, no. 3, 1996, pp. 259-65.

Stine, Gerald J. *AIDS Update 2013.* McGraw-Hill Higher Education, 2013.

"Stinging Insect Allergy." *American Academy of Allergy, Asthma, and Immunology,* 28 Sept. 2020, www.aaaai.org/tools-for-the-public/conditions-library/allergies/stinging-insect-allergy. Accessed 2 Sept. 2021.

Story, Lachel. "Body Defenses." *Pathophysiology: A Practical Approach.* 2nd ed., Jones, 2015, pp. 31-50.

Strauss, James, and Ellen Strauss. *Viruses and Human Disease.* 2nd ed., Academic Press/Elsevier, 2008.

"Studies on Asthma and Chinese Herbs." *American Academy of Allergy, Asthma, and Immunology,* 28 Sept. 2020, www.aaaai.org/Tools-for-the-Public/Conditions-Library/Asthma/Studies-on-Asthma-and-Chinese-Herbs. Accessed 2 Sept. 2021.

Stukus, David. "The Pitfalls of Food Allergy Panel Testing." *YouTube,* American Academy of Allergy, Asthma, and Immunology, 7 Nov 2017, www.youtube.com/watch?v=22I-9JkRyU4.

———. "Pearls and Pitfalls in Diagnosing IgE-Mediated Food Allergy." *Current Allergy and Asthma Reports,* vol. 16, no. 5, 2016, p. 34, doi:10.1007/s11882-016-0611-z.

Subak-Sharpe, Genell J., and Thomas O. Morris, editors. "Drug Therapy." *The Columbia University College of Physicians and Surgeons Complete Home Medical Guide.* 3rd ed., Crown, 1995.

"Sublingual Immunotherapy (SLIT) Allergy Tablets." *American Academy of Allergy, Asthma, and Immunology,* Mar. 2020, www.aaaai.org/Tools-for-the-Public/Drug-Guide/Sublingual-Immunotherapy-(SLIT)-Allergy-Tablets. Accessed 28 Aug. 2021.

Sur, D. K., and M. L. Plesa. "Treatment of Allergic Rhinitis." *American Family Physician*, Dec. 2015.

Sutton, Amy L., editor. *Arthritis Sourcebook: Basic Consumer Health Information About Osteoarthritis, Rheumatoid Arthritis, Other Rheumatic Disorders, Infectious Forms of Arthritis, and Diseases with Symptoms Linked to Arthritis*. 3rd ed., Omnigraphics, 2012.

Swart, Myrna. *There Must Be a Reason: My Daughter's Battle with Wegener's Granulomatosis*. iUniverse, 2008.

Swartz, Morton N., and Mark S. Pasternack. "Cellulitis and Subcutaneous Tissue Infection." *Mandell, Douglas, and Bennett's Principles and Practice of Infectious Diseases*, edited by Gerald L. Mandell, John E. Bennett, and Raphael Dolin, 7th ed., Churchill Livingstone/Elsevier, 2010.

Taneja, A., E. Muco, and A. Chhabra. *Bruton Agammaglobulinemia*. StatPearls Publishing, Jan. 2021 [Updated 29 Jul. 2021], www.ncbi.nlm.nih.gov/books/NBK448170/.

Tarp, S., et al. "Efficacy and Safety of Biological Agents for Systemic Juvenile Idiopathic Arthritis: A Systematic Review and Meta-Analysis of Randomized Trials." *Rheumatology*, vol. 55, no. 4, 2016, p. 669.

Tauber, Alfred I. *Metchnikoff and the Origins of Immunology: From Metaphor to Theory*. Oxford UP, 1991.

Taverner, D., L. Bickford, and M. Draper. "Nasal Decongestants for the Common Cold." *The Cochrane Library*, Issue 4. John Wiley & Sons, 2003.

Taylor, Julie Scott. "Interventions for Impetigo." *American Family Physician*, vol. 70, 9, 1 Nov. 2004.

Taïeb, Alain, and Mauro Picardo. "Clinical Practice: Vitiligo." *New England Journal of Medicine*, vol. 360, no. 2, 8 Jan. 2009, pp. 160-69.

Templeton, Nancy Smyth, editor. Gene and Cell Therapy: Therapeutic Mechanisms and Strategies. 4th ed., CRC Press, 2015.

Territo, Mary. "Neutrophilic Leukocytosis." *Merck Manual*, www.merckmanuals.com/home/blood-disorders/white-blood-cell-disorders/neutrophilic-leukocytosis. Accessed 19 Jan. 2017.

"Theophylline (Oral Route) Side Effects." *Mayo Clinic*, Mayo Foundation for Medical Education and Research, 1 Feb. 2020, www.mayoclinic.org/drugs-supplements/theophylline-oral-route/side-effects/drg-20073599?p=1.

"Theophylline: MedlinePlus Drug Information." *MedlinePlus*, U.S. National Library of Medicine, 15 Nov. 2019, medlineplus.gov/druginfo/meds/a681006.html.

Thevarajan, Irani, et al. "Breadth of Concomitant Immune Responses Prior to Patient Recovery: A Case of Non-Severe COVID-19." *Nature Medicine*, Mar. 2020, doi.org/10.1038/s41591-020-0819-2.

Thomsen, S. F., K. O. Kyvik, and V. Backer. "Etiological Relationships in Atopy: A Review of Twin Studies." *Twin Research and Human Genetics*, vol. 11, no. 2, 2008, pp. 112-20.

"Thyroid Diseases." *MedlinePlus*, 17 Aug. 2021, medlineplus.gov/thyroiddiseases.html. Accessed 24 Aug. 2021.

Torres-Borrego, J., A. B. Molina-Terán, and C. Montes-Mendoza. "Prevalence and Associated Factors of Allergic Rhinitis and Atopic Dermatitis in Children." *Allergologia et Immunopathologia*, vol. 36, no. 2, 2008, pp. 90-100.

Tortora, Gerard J., and Bryan Derrickson. *Principles of Anatomy and Physiology*. 16th ed., John Wiley & Sons, 2020.

Trivedi, Bijal P. *Breath from Salt: A Deadly Genetic Disease, a New Era in Science, and the Patients and Families Who Changed Medicine*. ?BenBella Books, 2020.

Tsai, Sue, and Pere Santamaria. "MHC Class II Polymorphisms, Autoreactive T-Cells, and Autoimmunity." Frontiers in Immunology, vol. 4, no. 321, 2013, pp. 1-7.

Tselis, Alex C., and Hal B. Jenson, editors. *Epstein-Barr Virus*. Taylor & Francis, 2006.

Tu, Anthony T., editor. *Reptile Venoms and Toxins*. Marcel Dekker, 1991.

Turkington, Carol A., and Jeffrey S. Dover. *Skin Deep: An A-Z of Skin Disorders, Treatments, and Health*. 3rd ed., Checkmark, 2007.

———. *The Encyclopedia of Skin and Skin Disorders*. 3rd ed., Facts On File, 2007.

Turkington, Carol A., and Rebecca J. Frey. "Malaria." *The Gale Encyclopedia of Medicine*, edited by Jacqueline L. Longe, 3rd ed., Thomson Gale, 2006.

Turner, R. B., D. K. Riker, and J. D. Gangemi. "Ineffectiveness of Echinacea for Prevention of Experimental Rhinovirus Colds." *Antimicrobial Agents and Chemotherapy*, vol. 44, 2000, pp. 1708-9.

"Types of White Blood Cells." *New Health Advisor*, www.newhealthadvisor.com/Types-of-White-Blood-Cells.html. Accessed 21 Sept. 2017.

Tyring, S. K. "Management of Herpes Zoster and Postherpetic Neuralgia." *Journal of the American Academy of Dermatology*, vol. 57, no. 6, suppl., 2007, pp. S136-S142.

Tyrrell, David, and Michael Fielder. *Cold Wars: The Fight Against the Common Cold*. Oxford UP, 2002.

U.S. Department of Health and Human Services, National Institutes of Health (NIH). National Institute of

Diabetes and Digestive and Kidney Diseases (NIDDK). *Crohn Disease*. NIH Publication No. 14-3410. The National Digestive Diseases Information Clearinghouse (NDDIC), Sept. 2014, www.niddk.nih.gov/health-information/health-topics/digestive-diseases/crohns-disease/Pages/facts.aspx.

U.S. Department of Health and Human Services. "AIDSInfo, 2013." *MedlinePlus*. "HIV/AIDS." *MedlinePlus*, 30 Apr. 2013

Umar, Constantine S., editor. *New Developments in Epstein-Barr Virus Research*. Nova Science, 2006.

"Vaccines." *National Institute of Allergy and Infectious Disease*. National Institutes of Health, 13 Aug. 2020, www.niaid.nih.gov/research/vaccines.

Van de Winkel, J. G., et al. "Immunotherapeutic Potential of Bispecific Antibodies." *Immunology Today*, vol. 18, 1997, pp. 562-74.

Van der Aa, L. B., et al. "Synbiotics Prevent Asthma-Like Symptoms in Infants with Atopic Dermatitis." *Allergy*, 17 Jun. 2010.

Van der Linden, S., and D. van der Heijde. "Ankylosing Spondylitis: Clinical Features." *Rheumatic Disease Clinics of North America*, vol. 24, no. 4, 1998, pp. 663-76.

Van Rooij, J., et al. "Oral Vitamins C and E as Additional Treatment in Patients with Acute Anterior Uveitis." *British Journal of Ophthalmology*, vol. 83, 1999, pp. 1277-82.

Van Schoor, Jacky. "Superficial Skin Infections in the Pharmacy." *SAPA*, vol. 13, no. 1, 2013, pp. 39-40.

"Vasculitis." *MedlinePlus*, 16 May 2013.

"Vasculitis Syndromes of the Central and Peripheral Nervous Systems Fact Sheet." *National Institute of Neurological Disorders and Stroke*, 7 Feb. 2012.

Vempati, R., R. L. Bijlani, and K. K. Deepak. "The Efficacy of a Comprehensive Lifestyle Modification Programme Based on Yoga in the Management of Bronchial Asthma." *BMC Pulmonary Medicine*, vol. 9, 2009, p. 37.

Verhagen A. P., et al. "Balneotherapy (or Spa Therapy) for Rheumatoid Arthritis." *Cochrane Database of Systematic Reviews*, vol. 4, no. CD000518, 2015, doi:10.1002/14651858.CD000518.pub2. www.cochrane.org/CD000518/MUSKEL_balneotherapy-or-spa-therapy-rheumatoid-arthritis.

Vincent, Angela. "Unravelling the Pathogenesis of Myasthenia Gravis." *Nature Reviews Immunology*, vol. 2, Oct. 2002, pp. 797-804.

Vinson, Gavin P., Barbara Whitehouse, and Joy Hinson. *The Adrenal Cortex*. Prentice Hall, 1992.

"Vitiligo." *Mayo Clinic*, 21 Apr. 2011.

"Vitiligo." *MedlinePlus*, 11 Jul. 2012.

"Voclosporin (Lupkynis) for Lupus Nephritis." *Medical Letter on Drugs and Therapeutics*, vol. 63, no. 1631, 2021, pp. 134-36.

Vonau, B., et al. "Does the Extract of the Plant Echinacea purpurea Influence the Clinical Course of Recurrent Genital Herpes?" *International Journal of STD and AIDS*, vol. 12, 2001, pp. 154-58.

Wagman, Richard J., editor. *The New Complete Medical and Health Encyclopedia*. 4 vols. J. G. Ferguson, 2002.

Wagner, Carina, et al. "Systemic corticosteroids for the treatment of COVID-19." *The Cochrane Database of Systematic Reviews*, vol. 8, CD014963, 16 Aug. 2021, doi:10.1002/14651858.CD014963.

Wagner, Edward K., and Martinez J. Hewlett. *Basic Virology*. 3rd ed., Blackwell Science, 2008.

Wales, Jeremy K. H., and Jan Maarten Wit. *Pediatric Endocrinology and Growth*. 2nd ed., W. B. Saunders, 2004.

Walker, P. L., et al. "Purine Nucleoside Phosphorylase Deficiency: A Mutation Update." *Nucleosides, Nucleotides & Nucleic Acids*, vol. 30, no. 12, 2011, pp. 1243-47. *Medline*. Accessed 20 Aug. 2014.

Wallace, Daniel J. *The Lupus Book: A Guide for Patients and Their Families*. 3rd ed., Oxford UP, 2005.

———, et al., editors. *The New Sjogren's Syndrome Handbook*. 3rd ed., Oxford UP, 2005.

Walsh, William. *The Food Allergy Book*. J. Wiley, 2000.

Wang, Henry Y., and Tadayuki Imanaka, editors. *Antibody Expression and Engineering*. American Chemical Society, 1995.

Wang, Manli, et al. "Remdesivir and Chloroquine Effectively Inhibit the Recently Emerged Coronavirus (2019-nCoV) In Vitro." *Cell Research*, vol. 30, 2020, pp. 269-71, doi.org/10.1038/s41422-020-0282-0.

Wang, X. Y., and P. B. Fisher, editors. *Immunotherapy of Cancer*. (Advances in Cancer Research). Vol. 128. Academic Press, 2015.

Wapner, Jessica, and Robert A. Weinberg. *The Philadelphia Chromosome: A Mutant Gene and the Quest to Cure Cancer at the Genetic Level*. Workman, 2013.

Ward, M. M., et al. "2019 Update of the American College of Rheumatology/Spondylitis Association of America/Spondyloarthritis Research and Treatment Network Recommendations for the Treatment of Ankylosing Spondylitis and Nonradiographic Axial Spondyloarthritis." *Arthritis and Rheumatology*, vol. 71, no. 10, 2019, p. 1599.

Wass, John A. H., and Paul M. Stewart, editors. *Oxford Textbook of Endocrinology and Diabetes*. Oxford UP, 2011.

Watson, Stephanie. "Autoimmune Diseases: Types, Symptoms, Causes, and More." Healthline, 26 Mar. 2019, www.healthline.com/health/autoimmune-disorders?print=true. Accessed 20 Aug. 2021.

Weaver, Bethany A. "Herpes Zoster Overview: Natural History and Incidence." *Journal of the American Osteopathic Association*, vol. 109, 2009, pp. S2-S6.

Web MD, "Antihistamines for Allergies." www.webmd.com/allergies/antihistamines-for-allergies. Accessed 20 Sept. 2017.

Weedon, David. *Skin Pathology*. 3rd ed., Churchill Livingstone/Elsevier, 2010.

Weeks, Benjamin S., and Teri Shors. *AIDS: The Biological Basis*. 6th ed., Jones and Bartlett Learning, 2013.

Wei R., et al. "Pediatric Drug Safety Signal Detection of Non-chemotherapy Drug-induced Neutropenia and Agranulocytosis Using Electronic Healthcare Records." *Expert Opinion on Drug Safety*, vol. 18, no. 5, 2019, p. 435.

Weinblatt, Michael E. *The Arthritis Action Program: An Integrated Plan of Traditional and Complementary Therapies*. Fireside, 2001.

Weisman, Michael H., Désirée van der Heijde, and John D. Reveille, editors. *Ankylosing Spondylitis and the Spondyloarthropathies*. Mosby/Elsevier, 2006.

Wells, Ken R. "Endocrine System." *Gale Encyclopedia of Nursing and Allied Health*, edited by Kristine Krapp, Gale Group, 2002.

"West Nile Virus: What You Need to Know." *Centers for Disease Control and Prevention*, 12 Sept. 2012.

Westcott, Patsy. *Eczema: Recipes and Advice to Provide Relief*. Welcome, 2000.

———. *Living with Leukemia*. Raintree-Steck-Vaughn, 1999.

Westly, Erica. "Seeking a Gene Genie." *Nature*, vol. 479, no. 7374, 2011, pp. S10-S11.

Whalen, Karen. *Pharmacology*. (Lippincott Illustrated Reviews Series). 7th ed., Lippincott Williams & Wilkins, 2018.

"What Are Corticosteroids?" *healthychildren.org*, 21 Jan. 2020. www.healthychildren.org/English/health-issues/conditions/allergies-asthma/Pages/Corticosteroids.aspx. Accessed 22 Aug 2021.

"What Is Cancer Immunotherapy?" *Cancer Research Institute*, Oct. 2020, www.cancerresearch.org/immunotherapy/what-is-immunotherapy. Accessed 29 Aug. 2021.

"What Is Cough?" *National Heart, Lung, and Blood Institute*, 1 Oct. 2010.

"What Is Home and Everyday Life Hygiene?" *International Scientific Forum on Home Hygiene*, www.ifh-homehygiene.org/what-home-hygiene.

"What Is an Inflammation?" *PubMed Health*, Jan. 2015.

"What Is Psoriasis?" *National Institute of Arthritis and Musculoskeletal and Skin Diseases*, Sept. 2009.

"What Is Rheumatoid Arthritis?" *National Institute of Arthritis and Musculoskeletal and Skin Diseases*, Dec. 2009.

"What Is Vasculitis?" *National Heart, Lung, and Blood Institute*, 1 Apr. 2011.

"What Is Vasculitis?" *The Johns Hopkins Vasculitis Center*, 2013.

Wheeler, Patricia G. "Newborn Screening Tests." *KidsHealth from Nemours*, Sept. 2012.

"White Blood Cell Disorders." *Dana-Farber/Boston Children's Cancer and Blood Disorders Center*, www.danafarberbostonchildrens.org/conditions/blood-disorders/white-blood-cell-disorders.aspx. Accessed 19 Jan. 2017.

"Why Home Hygiene Is Important." *Healthy House Institute*, 20 Jan. 2012, www.healthyhouseinstitute.com/blog-1156-Why-Home-Hygiene-is-Important.

Wiernik, Peter H., et al. *Neoplastic Diseases of the Blood*. Springer, 2013.

Wilcox, Christie. *Venomous: How Earth's Deadliest Creatures Mastered Biochemistry*. Scientific American/Farrar, Straus and Giroux, 2016.

Williams, J. "Principles of Genetics and Cancer." Seminars in Oncology Nursing, vol. 13, no. 2, 1997, pp. 68-73.

Willich, S. N., et al. "Rose Hip Herbal Remedy in Patients with Rheumatoid Arthritis." *Phytomedicine*, vol. 17, 2010, pp. 87-93.

Wilson, Joanna B., and Gerhard H. W. May, editors. *Epstein-Barr Virus Protocols*. Humana Press, 2001.

Wingerson, Lois. *Mapping Our Genes: The Genome Project and the Future of Medicine*. Plume, 1991.

Woeber, K. A. "Iodine and Thyroid Disease." *Medical Clinics of North America: Thyroid Diseases*, vol. 75, no. 1, Jan. 1991, pp. 169-78.

Wood, Lawrence C., David S. Cooper, and E. Chester Ridgway. *Your Thyroid: A Home Reference*. 4th rev. ed., Ballantine Books, 2005.

Wood, Robert A. *Food Allergies for Dummies*. Wiley, 2007.

Woolf, Alan D., et al., editors. *The Children's Hospital Guide to Your Child's Health and Development*. Perseus, 2002.

Xiumei Hong, et al. "Genome-Wide Association Study Identifies Peanut Allergy-Specific Loci and Evidence of Epigenetic Mediation in US Children." *Nature Communications*, vol 6, no. 1, 2015, doi:10.1038/ncomms7304.

Yadav, U. C. S., et al. "Emerging Role of Antioxidants in the Protection of Uveitis Complications." *Current Medicinal Chemistry*, vol. 18, no. 6, 2011, pp. 931-42.

Yamaguchi, Y., editor. *Immunotherapy of Cancer: An Innovative Treatment Comes of Age*. Springer, 2016.

Yian, Gu, and Nikolas Scarmeas. "Dietary Inflammation Factor Rating System and Risk of Alzheimer Disease in Elder." *Alzheimer Disease and Associated Disorders*, vol. 25, no. 2, 2011, pp. 149-54.

Yin-Murphy, Marguerite, and Jeffrey W. Almond. "Picornaviruses-Classification and Antigenic Types." *Medical Microbiology*, edited by Samuel Baron, U of Texas Medical Branch, 1996.

Yoshimura, M., et al. "An Evaluation of the Clinical Efficacy of Tomato Extract for Perennial Allergic Rhinitis." *Allergology International*, vol. 3, 2007, pp. 225-30.

Yost, Raymond, et al. "A Coreceptor CCR5 Antagonist for Management of HIV Infection." *American Journal of Health-System Pharmacy*, vol. 66, no. 8, Apr. 2009, pp. 715-26.

Young, Stuart H., Bruce S. Dobozin, and Margaret Miner. *Allergies: The Complete Guide to Diagnosis, Treatment, and Daily Management*. Rev. ed., Plume, 1999.

Younis, Ramzi T., editor. *Pediatric Sinusitis and Sinus Surgery*. Taylor & Francis, 2006.

Yung, Raymond L. "What Is a Rheumatologist?" *American College of Rheumatology*, Aug. 2012.

Zack, Eric, "Emerging Therapies for Autoimmune Disorders". Journal of Infusion Nursing, vol. 37, no. 2, 2012, pp. 109-19.

Zappi, Eduardo. *Dermatopathology: Classification of Cutaneous Lesions*. Springer, 2013.

Zen, X. X., et al. "Chinese Herbal Medicines for Hyperthyroidism." *The Cochrane Database of Systematic Reviews*, vol. 2007, no. 2, CD005450, doi:10.1002/14651858.CD005450 pub2.

Zhao, Lijun, and Yu J. Cao. "Engineered T Cell Therapy for Cancer in the Clinic." *Frontiers in Immunology*, vol. 10, 2019, p. 2250, doi.org/10.3389/fimmu.2019.02250.

Zinser, Stephanie. *The Good Gut Guide: Help for IBS, Ulcerative Colitis, Crohn's Disease, Diverticulitis, Food Allergies, and Other Gut Problems*. Thorsons, 2012.

Zlotogora, J., and M. S. Shapiro. "Polyglandular Autoimmune Syndrome Type I among Iranian Jews." *Journal of Medical Genetics*, vol. 29, 1992, pp. 824-26.

Zonali, M. "Taming Lupus." *Scientific American*, vol. 292, no. 3, 2005, pp. 70-77.

Zucker-Franklin, D., et al. *Atlas of Blood Cells: Function and Pathology*. 3rd ed., Lea & Febiger, 2003.

Glossary

abscess: a localized collection of pus (dead cells and a mixture of live and dead bacteria)

acetylcholine: a chemical released by motor neuron terminals that cause muscle contractions and by neurons in the central nervous system that mediate REM sleep, motivation, arousal, attention, learning and memory

acetylcholine receptor: a protein on the surface of muscle cells and some central nervous system neurons; binding of acetylcholine to this receptor on muscle cell surfaces causes muscle cells to contract

acetylcholinesterase: an enzyme that degrades acetylcholine

acquired immune deficiency syndrome (AIDS): a chronic, life-threatening condition caused by the human immunodeficiency virus (HIV) characterized by the functional collapse of the immune system and the overwhelming of the human body by opportunistic infections and tumors.

acupuncture: a system of integrative medicine that involves pricking the skin or tissues with needles, used to alleviate pain and to treat various physical, mental, and emotional conditions

acute disease: a short and sharp disease process

adaptive immunity: acquired immunity to a previous infection or vaccination; involves specialized immune cells and antibodies that destroy foreign cells and remember what those substances look like to prevent future infection

Addison's disease: a condition characterized by insufficiency of the adrenal cortex, causing a drop in glucocorticoid and mineralocorticoid hormones, causing fatigue, low blood pressure, and other symptoms

adjunctive: referring to the treatment of symptoms associated with a condition, not the condition itself

adjuvant: a substance given with a vaccine that enhances the immune response elicited by it

adoptive cell therapy: a type of immunotherapy in which T cells (a type of immune cell) are given to a patient to help the body fight diseases, such as cancer; also called cellular immunotherapy

adrenal cortex: the outer layer of the adrenal glands that synthesize and secrete two main types of steroid hormones, glucocorticoids, and mineralocorticoids

adrenal gland: paired endocrine glands situated immediately above the upper pole of each kidney; they consist of an inner part or medulla that produces epinephrine and norepinephrine, and an outer part or cortex that produces steroid hormones

adrenocorticotropic hormone (ACTH): a peptide hormone secreted by the corticotropes anterior lobe of the pituitary gland that signals to the adrenal cortex to secrete glucocorticoid hormones

agranulocytosis: an extremely low number of granulocytes in the blood

alleles: a distinct form of a gene, inherited from either parent and present in pairs in each person

allergen: an ordinarily harmless substance-such as pet dander, pollen, or food proteins-that can cause an allergic reaction in some patients

allergen immunotherapy: treatment for allergies, also known as allergy shots, in which a small amount of allergen is injected into a patient to develop immunity

Allergic bronchopulmonary aspergillosis: an allergic reaction to the presence of *Aspergillus* components (e.g., spores or hyphae) in the lower respiratory tract

allergic rhinitis: acute or seasonal nasal stuffiness and sneezing that follows the exposure to allergens such as pollen or animal dander; hay fever is one form of allergic rhinitis

allergies: a damaging immune response to a substance, such as pollen, fur, food, or dust, to which it has become hypersensitive

amoeboid movement: a type of cellular movement that features crawling-like movement caused by extensions of the cytoplasmic projections called pseudopodia

anabolic: the metabolic processes by which small molecules are combined to produce larger molecules; used for energy storage or growth of the organism

anaphylaxis: a severe and potentially life-threatening allergic reaction that occurs within seconds or minutes of exposure to an allergen

androgenic hormones: any of several hormones that regulate the expression of male characteristics

anterior chamber: the from part of the eye between the cornea and the iris

anthracyclines: a class of anticancer drugs that are effective against a broad range of different types of cancer and derived from molecules synthesized by members of the bacterial genus *Streptomyces*

antibodies: secreted glycoproteins that bind to foreign substances in our bodies and inactivate them, clump them, mark them for destruction, and facilitate their disposal; also known as immunoglobulins

antigen: a foreign substance that elicits an immune response when inoculated into a living organism

antigen presentation: the process by which antigen-presenting cells introduce protein antigens to lymphocytes in the form of short peptide fragments

antigenic drift: the gradual accumulation of point mutations during the circulation of influenza virus. It results from the high error rates associated with RNA-dependent RNA polymerase during virus replication

antigenic shift: a process by which two or more different strains of a virus combine to form a new strain that has a mixture of the surface antigens of the two or more original strains

antigen-presenting cell: a varied collection of immune cells including dendritic cells, macrophages, and B lymphocytes that process and present antigens for recognition by T lymphocytes.

antigens: foreign substances in the body that elicit an immune response

antihistamine: medications that nullify the effects of histamine, including itching

anti-inflammatory drugs: drugs to counter the effects of inflammation locally or throughout the body; these drugs can be applied locally or introduced by electric currents (in a process called iontophoresis), by injections into the joint or into the muscles, or by mouth; the three classes of these drugs are steroidal, immunosuppressant, and nonsteroidal

antinuclear antibody (ANA): an unusual antibody that is directed against structures within the nucleus of cells

antiretroviral therapy (ART): combinations of drugs that inhibit replication of the human immunodeficiency virus (HIV) and the infection from transitioning to full-blown acquired immune deficiency syndrome (AIDS)

antisera: a complex mixture of heterogeneous antibodies that react with various parts of an antigen; each type of antibody protein in the mixture is made by a different type (clone) of plasma cell

apoptosis: cell death that is programmed as a natural consequence of growth and development through normal cellular pathways or signals from neighboring cells

areflexia: loss of reflex

arrhythmias: problems with the rhythm of the heart, such as irregular heartbeat

arthritis: a painful condition that involves inflammation of one or more joints.

articular: of or relating to a joint or joints

asbestos: a natural material once widely used as insulation that can cause asbestosis and mesothelioma

Aspergillus: a genus of fungus commonly found indoors and outdoors and a wide range of climates

atopy: a condition that underlies allergic diseases, characterized by high levels of immunoglobulin E (IgE), that is highly influenced by genetics

attenuated: weakened or partial organisms

autoantibodies: antibodies that attack the body's cells and tissues

autoimmune disorders: conditions in which the body attacks its cells and tissues

autoimmune regulator (AIRE) gene: a transcription factor expressed in thymus gland cells that causes them to express an array of self-antigens; plays a critical role in self-tolerance

autoimmune: a term describing a disease in which the body produces antibodies against its cells

autoimmunity: a condition in which the immune system fails to recognize its tissues as "self" and mounts an immune response against its cells

autosomal recessive disease: a disease that is expressed when two copies of a defective gene are inherited, one from each parent; present on non-sex-determining chromosomes

autosomal recessive inheritance: a genetic trait or condition that occurs when someone inherits one copy of a mutated, or changed, gene from each parent

B cells: also known as B lymphocytes; the antibody-producing cells of the immune system

B memory cells: descendants of activated B cells that are long-lived and that synthesize large amounts of antibodies in response to subsequent exposure to the antigen, thus playing an important role in secondary immunity

basophil: a type of white blood cell that contains mediators associated with allergic reactions; represents 1 percent or less of total white cells

benign: in reference to a neoplasm, having a non-malignant character

beta-cells: the insulin-producing cells located at the core of the islets of Langerhans in the pancreas; the alpha, or glucagon-producing, cells form an outer coat

biphasic reaction: delayed allergic reaction to an allergen, between one to four hours after the initial reaction

bites: when an animal uses its teeth to inflict an injury

blast cell: an immature dividing cell

blood group antigen: glycolipid surface markers on the outer surface of red blood cell membranes that determine an individual's blood group; two main groups of blood surface antigens are called ABO (blood type A, B, AB, and O) and Rh (Rh-positive or Rh-negative)

blood group system: a classification of individuals into groups based on the presence or absence of blood group antigens found on the surfaces of red blood cells

blood typing: identification of surface blood group antigens of an individual for classification into specific blood groups

blood vessels: tubular structures that carry blood throughout the body, into tissues and organs, consisting of veins, arteries, or capillaries.

blood: the fluid that circulates through the cardiovascular system; composed of a fluid and a cellular fraction that consists of erythrocytes, leukocytes, and thrombocytes

B-lymphocytes: see B-cells

bone marrow: the tissue within bones that produces blood cells; in children, all bones have active marrow, but in adults, blood cell production occurs only in the trunk

bone marrow transplant: a procedure whereby a recipient receives multipotent hematopoietic stem cells derived from the bone marrow of a donor

bronchial tubes: tubes that carry air to your lungs; problems with the bronchi include bronchitis, bronchiectasis, and bronchiolitis

bronchodilation: relaxation of the smooth muscle surrounding the airways, increasing the diameter of the airways, and facilitating the passage of gases to and from the lungs

bronchodilator: a drug that causes widening of the bronchi, e.g., any of those taken by inhalation for the alleviation of asthma

bursitis: inflammation of the sac of lubricating fluid located between joints.

Buteyko breathing: a form of complementary or alternative physical therapy that proposes the use of breathing exercises primarily as a treatment for asthma and other respiratory conditions

cancer: any malignant cellular tumor

capillary exudate: a group of substances secreted by the capillaries as part of the inflammatory process

cartilage: material covering the ends of bones; it does not have a blood supply or nerve supply but may swell or break down

catabolic: the metabolic processes by which food and stored products are broken down to release energy for use by the cell

cellular response: does not involve antibodies; utilizes the activation of phagocytes, antigen-sensitized cytotoxic T cells and the release of cytokines in response to an antigen

chemotaxis: movement of white blood cells toward a gradient of increasing or decreasing concentration of a particular substance

chemotherapy: the use of drugs to kill rapidly growing cancer cells; this treatment will also kill some normal cells, producing undesirable side effects

chickenpox: an infectious disease caused by herpes zoster virus that produces a mild fever and a rash of itchy inflamed blisters

choroid body: a structure within the eye that connects the iris to the choroid and consists of the ciliary muscles, radial ciliary processes to which the lens is attached by ligaments, and the ciliary ring that merges with the choroid

chromosomes: rod-shaped structures in each cell that contain genes, the chemical elements that determine traits

chronic atrophic gastritis: an autoimmune disease characterized by chronic inflammation of the stomach lining, leading to loss of stomach tissue and its replacement by intestinal-type epithelium, pyloric-type glands, and scar tissue

chronic disease: a lingering illness

ciliary muscles: muscles that attach to the lens from the choroid body and alter the curvature of the lens to accommodate differing focal distances

clinical ecologist: proponents of the claim that exposure to low levels of certain chemicals harm susceptible people

common variable immunodeficiency: an immune system disorder caused by abnormally low blood levels of antibodies

complement: a complex of more than thirty proteins in the blood that coordinate to attack invading cells and destroy them

conductive loss: a hearing loss caused by an outer-ear or middle-ear problem which results in reduced transmission of sound

congenital: something that is present at birth

conidiophore: an asexual spore-bearing hypha in fungi

conidium: spores

conjugate: the attachment of molecules that tend to elicit weak immune responses, such as carbohydrates, to large molecules that enhance the immunogenicity of the attached molecules.

connective tissue: the substance holding the body and organs together

constant region: The highly conserved C-terminal portion of the antibody

contraindication: a condition that makes a particular treatment not advisable; contraindications may be absolute (should never be used) or relative (should be used only with caution when the benefits outweigh the potential problems)

cornea: the transparent part of the eye that covers the iris and transmits light to the eye's interior

corticosteroids: a group of synthetic, or natural steroid hormones produced by the adrenal cortex, that regulate metabolic functions, salt balances, and treat inflammation

corticotropin-releasing hormone (CRH): a peptide hormone secreted by the paraventricular nuclei of the hypothalamus that stimulates corticotropes in the anterior lobe of the pituitary to secrete ACTH

cortisol: the main glucocorticoid hormone made by the adrenal cortex, also known as hydrocortisone; that has many physiological actions

coryza: runny nose caused by hay fever or infections

COVID-19: coronavirus disease discovered in 2019 caused by SARS-CoV-2

cretinism: congenital hypothyroidism

cross-linking: a chemical reaction triggered by the binding of glucose to tissue proteins that results in the attachment of one protein to another and the loss of elasticity in aging tissues

crusting: the appearance of slightly elevated skin lesions made up of dried serum, blood, or pus; they can be brown, red, black, tan, or yellowish

CSF protein: a protein in the cerebrospinal fluid which is usually very low

Cushing's syndrome: a disorder characterized by hyperadrenalism caused by an excess secretion or exogenous administration of cortisol

cyclic adenosine monophosphate (cAMP): a small molecule made inside cells in response to specific stimuli that elicits changes in cell behavior and function

cyclic AMP: a chemical that acts as a second messenger to bring about a response by the cell to the presence of some hormones at their receptors

cytokines: soluble intercellular molecules produced by cells such as lymphocytes that regulate the immune response

cytopenia: a condition in which the production of one or more types of blood cells either stops or is significantly reduced

cytotoxic: having a damaging effect on cells

cytotoxic T-cells: a type of lymphocyte that kills foreign cells, cancer cells, and virally-infected cells

decongestants: drugs that are taken to reduce swelling of the nasal passages and decrease the production of mucus, the fluids commonly found in the sinuses during allergic reactions and colds

dehydroepiandrosterone: also known as androstenolone, is an endogenous steroid hormone precursor and one of the most abundant circulating steroids in humans

demyelination: a loss of the myelin coating of nerves

deoxyribonucleic acid (DNA): the chemical molecule that transmits hereditary information from generation to generation

dermatologist: a physician who treats the skin and its structures, functions, and diseases

dermatology: the study of the skin, its chemistry, physiology, histopathology, cutaneous lesions, and the relationships of these lesions to systemic disease

dermatomyositis: inflammation of the skin and underlying muscle tissue due to collagen destruction, leading to discoloration, and swelling, typically results from an autoimmune condition or associated with cancer.

dermis: the layer of skin directly beneath the epidermis, consisting of dense connective tissue and numerous blood vessels

determinant: a region on the surface of an antigen capable of creating an immune response or of combining with an antibody produced by an immune response

deviated septum: a condition that causes a shift of the bones and cartilage from the middle of the nose to either side, making one side of the nasal passages much smaller than the other

diaphragm: a muscular partition separating the thorax from the abdomen; plays a major role in breathing as its contraction increases the volume of the thorax and so inflates the lungs

discoid rash: raised red patches

disease-modifying antirheumatic drugs: a category of unrelated drugs that slow the progression of rheumatoid arthritis

disseminated sclerosis: another name for multiple sclerosis (MS)

dominant gene: a gene that can express its effect when an individual has only one copy of it

downstream: describes the left-to-right direction of DNA whose nucleotides are arranged in sequence with the 5' carbon on the left and the 3' on the right; the direction of RNA transcription of a genetic message with the beginning of a gene on the left and the end on the right

drug synergy: a process by which drugs taken in combination with each other interact and can have a greater effect than the drugs taken separately

drying agent: astringents or water-based products that remove excess oil from the skin and tighten pores

dust: airborne pollutants that can include dead skin, hair, ash, pollen, fibers, and minerals from outdoor soils that can lead to allergies, respiratory diseases, and asthma.

dust mites: microscopic bugs that live in household dust; the primary cause of allergies related to house dust

dyshidrotic eczema: a type of dermatitis in which blisters form on the hands and feet

dysphagia: difficulty or discomfort when swallowing

electrocardiogram: a test that measures the electrical activity of the heart

electromyogram: a technique that measures the electrical activity produced by skeletal muscles

emollient: preparations that smooth and soften the skin

endemic: occurring naturally in a geographic area or population group

endocrine pancreas: specialized secretory tissue dispersed within the pancreas called islets of Langerhans, which are responsible for the secretion of glucagon and insulin

endocrine: the secretion of hormones directly into the bloodstream, rather than by way of a duct

endothelial cell: cells that line blood and lymph vessels

endothelium: a thin, cellular membrane that lines the insides of the heart and blood vessels

Enterovirus: a genus of viruses similar to rhinoviruses

enthesitis: inflammation of the insertion sites of tendons and ligaments to the bone surface

enzymes: substances, usually proteins or RNA molecules, that act as catalysts to acceleration the rate of specific biochemical reactions

eosinophil: a type of white blood cell responsible for combating multicellular parasites and plays a significant role in allergies

epidemic: any disease, injury, or health-related event occurring suddenly in numbers more than normal

epidermis: the outermost part of the skin, composed of four or five different layers called strata

epinephrine: a hormone that acts as a vasoconstrictor and cardiac stimulant

Epi-Pen: a device that administers a prescribed dose of injectable epinephrine

erythematosus: characterized by redness of the skin

erythrocyte sedimentation rate: a laboratory test that measures the rate at which red blood cells in anticoagulated whole blood descend in a standardized tube over one hour. It is a non-specific measure of inflammation

erythrocytes: red blood cells of the circulatory system that contain hemoglobin and are responsible for delivering oxygen to the tissues

erythropoietin: the hormone protein that is produced in the kidneys and acts on the bone marrow helping in red blood cell synthesis

esophagus: the tube that leads from the pharynx to the stomach

essential: referring to an amino acid, lipid, or vitamin that is necessary for proper cell functioning, but which the human body is ordinarily unable to produce on its own; must be supplied through the diet

evidence-based medicine: a method of basing clinical medical practice decisions on systematic reviews of published medical studies

excipient: an inactive substance that serves as the vehicle or medium for a drug, vaccine, or other material

Fc-fusion proteins: specific proteins of interest fused to the Fc region of the antibody at its C-terminal end

feedback: the mechanism whereby a hormone inhibits its production; often involves the inhibition of the hypothalamus and tropic hormones

fissure: a break in the surface tissue of the anal canal or the wall of the gastrointestinal tract

fistula: an abnormal connection between two hollow structures or between a tubular organ and the skin surface

food allergy action plan: a care plan outlining life-saving strategies when experiencing a food allergy reaction

food allergy: an abnormal response to a food triggered by the body's immune system

frequency: the number of vibrations per second of a source of sound, measured in hertz; correlates with perceived pitch

fungal spores: a microscopic body, usually the product of sexual or asexual reproduction, that is specially adapted for dispersal, survival, extended periods of dormancy.

gamma-globulin: antibodies:

gastroesophageal reflux disease: a chronic disease that results from stomach acid or bile flowing into the esophagus, irritating, and damaging it

gene: the hereditary unit, composed of DNA, that resides on chromosomes

gene deletions: the loss of all or part of a gene, possibly resulting in a change in RNA and protein made from that gene; found in cancer and in other genetic diseases and abnormalities

glottis: the part of the larynx consisting of the vocal cords and the opening between them; affects voice modulation through expansion or contraction

glucocorticoid: a steroid hormone such as cortisol from the adrenal cortex that has many physiological actions, including the regulation of glucose metabolism

glucosuria: a condition in which the concentration of blood glucose exceeds the ability of the kidney to reabsorb it; as a result, glucose spills into the urine, taking with it body water and electrolytes

goiter: abnormal enlargement of the thyroid gland

goitrogenic: referring to a factor (typically food or chemicals) that produces goiter

graft-versus-host disease: a condition that occurs when transplanted organs or cells are recognized by the host's immune system as invaders, resulting in the donor cells being attacked by the host's immune system

granulocytes: Granulocytes are a type of white blood cell with granules that contain enzymes released during infection or other immune responses such as allergy. The different types of granulocytes include neutrophils, eosinophils, and basophils.

granulocytopenia: a reduced absolute number of all circulating cells of the granulocyte series, including neutrophils, eosinophils, and basophils

Graves' disease: an autoimmune disease of the thyroid that causes overproduction of thyroid hormone

haplotype: a group of genes within an organism inherited together from a single parent.

Hashimoto's thyroiditis: an autoimmune disease resulting in chronic inflammation of the thyroid; the most common cause of hypothyroidism in the United States

heavy chain: the larger polypeptide chain of an antibody

helper T cells: a type of immune cell that stimulates killer T cells, macrophages, and B cells to make immune responses

hemagglutinin: a surface glycoprotein of the influenza virus that causes red blood cells to clump together.

hematopoiesis: the process of red blood cell production by bone marrow

hematopoietic cells: immature cells that can develop into all types of blood cells, including white blood cells, red blood cells, and platelets

hemoglobin: the pigmented protein that imparts red color to the blood and carries oxygen from the lungs to the rest of the body

hemolytic anemia: anemia attributable to increased destruction of red blood cells

hemoptysis: the expectoration of blood, alone or mixed with mucus, from the lower respiratory tract

hepatitis: inflammation of the liver; usually caused by viral infections, toxic substances, or immunological disturbances

hepatosplenomegaly: enlargement of the liver and spleen such that they may be felt below the rib margins

herbs: any plant with leaves, seeds, or flowers used for flavoring, food, medicine, or perfume

herpes zoster: chickenpox

heterophil antibodies: antibodies that are detected using antigens other than the antigens that induced them

highly active antiretroviral treatment (HAART): a treatment with two or more drugs that stops HIV replication in infected persons

histamine: an amino acid-derived bioactive amine released from mast cells when the body encounters an allergen that causes smooth muscle constriction and blood vessel leakiness

histiocyte: large white blood cells resident in tissues, including Langerhans cells, monocytes/macrophages, and dermal/interstitial dendritic cells

histocompatibility leukocyte antigens: cell surface molecules expressed by antigen-presenting cells that present antigenic peptides to T lymphocytes; also known as major histocompatibility complex (MHC) proteins

hormone: a substance made by the body that travels through the bloodstream to reach its target organ and have its effect.

human herpesvirus 6 (HHV-6): human herpesvirus 6 (HHV-6) is a set of two closely related herpes viruses known as HHV-6A and HHV-6B. HHV-6B infects nearly 100% of human beings, typically before the age of three, and often results in fever, diarrhea, and sometimes with roseola.

human herpesvirus 8 (HHV-8): a small herpes virus common to human populations that plays a role in the development of Kaposi sarcoma

human immunodeficiency virus: a type of lentivirus that infects humans and causes acquired immunodeficiency syndrome (AIDS), a condition resulting in progressive failure of the immune system

human leukocyte antigen (HLA): highly polymorphic cell surface proteins that antigen-presenting cells use to present antigen to lymphocytes (class II HLAs) or are found on the surfaces of every nucleated cell in the body (class I HLAs) and act as identification tags by which the immune system distinguishes between self and non-self; also known as major histocompatibility complex (MHC proteins)

humoral response: targets pathogens circulating in bodily fluids, or "humors"; involves the transformation of B lymphocytes into plasma cells that produce and secrete antibodies to a specific antigen

hyperglycemia: excessive levels of glucose in the circulating blood

hyper-IgM syndrome: a group of rare primary immunodeficiency disorders characterized by an inability of B lymphocytes to mature and make secondary, high-affinity antibodies

hyperlipidemia: an excess of lipids (for example, cholesterol and triglycerides) in the blood

hypersecretion: the excess production and secretion of a hormone or other chemical

hypersensitivity: reactions in which the immune system response is exaggerated

hyperthyroidism: a condition characterized by overactivity of the thyroid gland

hyphae: thin tubes in fungi that secure food and grow, expanding mold size

hypoparathyreosis: a state resulting from a malfunction of the parathyroid glands

hypothalamohypophysial: relating to the hypothalamus and the hypophysis (pituitary gland)

hypothalamus: the region of the brain called the diencephalon, forming the floor of the third ventricle, including neighboring associated nuclei

hypothyroidism: a condition characterized by underactivity of the thyroid gland

iatrogenic: a condition caused by healthcare-based interventions

IgE: an antibody subtype made by the immune system in response to allergens or worm infections

immune modulator: a substance that stimulates or suppresses the immune system and may help the body fight cancer, infection, or other diseases

immune system: a complex network of cells and proteins that defends the body against infection

immunity: the ability of an immune system to recognize, neutralize, and destroy an infecting organism, protecting the individual from infection

immunodeficiency: a condition, inherited or induced, in which the immune system fails to function normally, increasing the risk of life-threatening infections and cancers

immunoglobulin antibody: a protein activated during allergic reactions by the immune system

immunoglobulin E (IgE): see IgE

immunoglobulin G: the most common type of antibody in the body, made by B lymphocytes in response to a repeated bacterial, fungal, or viral infection

immunoglobulin replacement: intravenous or subcutaneous treatment to increase antibodies with immunoglobulins, a blood product derived from blood donors

immunomodulators: a substance that affects the functioning of the immune system

immunosuppression: the partial or complete suppression of someone's immune response to help the survival of an organ after a transplant operation

immunotherapy: therapy using antibodies or other immune system components or using antigens designed to stimulate an immune response to a tumor

immunotolerance: an active state of unresponsiveness to specific antigens

immunotoxic: an event or substance that harms the immune system and kills, or injures immune cells

inflammation: the body's response to injury that may include redness, pain, swelling, and warmth in the affected area.

influenza: a highly contagious viral infection of the respiratory passages that causes fever, runny nose, and severe achiness

inheritance: the passing down of traits from generation to generation

innate immunity: nonspecific immunity in the sense that prior contact with an infectious agent is not required for proper innate immune response

inoculation: the introduction of a substance or group of substances into a living organism

insulin: a hormone that is essential in regulating blood glucose, as well as in assimilating carbohydrates for growth and energy

insulin-dependent diabetes mellitus (IDDM): type 1 diabetes, a state of absolute insulin deficiency in which the body does not produce sufficient insulin to move glucose into the cells

insulin resistance: a lack of insulin action; a reduction in the effectiveness of insulin to lower blood glucose concentrations; characteristic of type 2 diabetes

insulitis: the selective destruction of the insulin-producing beta cells in type 1 diabetes

intensity of sound: the physical phenomenon that correlates approximately with perceived loudness; measured in decibels

interferons: a family of proteins; some of which induce an antiviral state within a cell, while others serve to regulate aspects of the immune response

interleukins: a type of small glycoproteins, secreted by leukocytes that regulate immune response

intralesional chemotherapy: treatment of small, localized tumors in the skin with focused radiation, the injection of anticancer directly into the tumor, or the application of antitumor gels of the tumor

iris: a flat, colored, ring-shaped membrane behind the cornea of the eye that has an adjustable circular opening or pupil in its center

islets of Langerhans: clusters of cells scattered throughout the pancreas; they produce three hormones involved in sugar metabolism: insulin, glucagon, and somatostatin

isotypes: the different classes of antibodies

isotype switching: when activated B cells, by their interaction with T-helper cells change the type of antibody they are secreting to some other antibody subtype

jaundice: yellow staining of the skin, eyes, and other tissues and excretions with excess bile pigments in the blood

joint: the conjunction of two or more bones

Kaposi's sarcoma: a form of blood vessel tumor that produces pink to purple splotches or plaques on the skin in about 25 percent of persons with AIDS and may also affect internal organs; caused by sexual transmission of human herpesvirus 8 (HHV8)

ketoacidosis: high levels of ketones in the blood that result from a lack of circulating insulin

killer T cells: a type of immune cell that can kill certain cells, including foreign cells, cancer cells, and cells infected with a virus; can be separated from other blood cells, grown in a laboratory, and given to patients

Koplik spots: small, white spots on the inside of the cheeks early in the course of measles

Langerhans cell histiocytosis: a disorder characterized by a buildup of excess immune system cells called Langerhans cells that damage tissues or cause lesions in multiple locations in the body

larynx: the hollow muscular organ forming an air passage to the lungs and holding the vocal cords

latency: following an acute infection by a virus, a period of dormancy from which the virus may be reactivated during times of stress or immunocompromise

lentivirus: a classification of retroviruses characterized by a very long incubation period (ten to twenty years) before symptoms of a disease appear

lesion: any pathologic change in tissue

leukemia: a malignant, progressive disease caused by bone marrow production of abnormal, immature white blood cells that inhibit the production of normal blood cells, leading to anemia and other symptoms.

leukocytes: colorless, nucleated, amoeboid cells that circulate throughout the blood and body fluids and destroy or isolate foreign substances and infectious agents, including lymphocytes, granulocytes, monocytes, and macrophages

light chain: the smaller polypeptide chain of an antibody

lipid nanoparticles: a shell of cholesterol and other fat-soluble molecules that house an internal mRNA core, and fuse with host cells to deliver the mRNA payload

long COVID: Those who had COVID-19 recovered from it but continue to feel symptoms long after the days or weeks that represent a typical course of the disease.

lower esophageal sphincter: a bundle of muscles at the bottom of the esophagus, where it meets the stomach that closes to prevent acid and stomach contents from refluxing into the esophagus

L-thyroxine (T4): a less potent thyroid hormone than the T3 form that cells convert to T3

L-triiodothyronine (T3): the most potent of the thyroid hormones

lymph glands: a small bean-shaped structure that filters substances that travel through the lymphatic fluid; lymph glands contain lymphocytes (white blood cells) that help the body fight infection and disease

lymphocytes: small white blood cells that have a single, round nucleus and inhabit the lymphatic system and bloodstream

lymphoma: cancer of the lymphatic system

lymphopoiesis: the process of B lymphocyte development

macrocytic anemia: anemia with red blood cells of increased size

macrophage: a type of white blood cell that surrounds and kills microorganisms, removes dead cells, and regulates the action of other immune cells

major histocompatibility complex (MHC proteins): cell surface proteins that come in two types, class I and II that help antigen-presenting cells present antigen to lymphocytes (class II) and mark every nucleated cell in the body (class I); also called human leukocyte antigens (HLAs)

malar rash: a redness or rash on the face covering the cheeks and the bridge of the nose; also called butterfly rash

malignant: in reference to a neoplasm, having the property of uncontrollable growth and dissemination, recurrence after removal, or both

manifestation: an outward or visible expression

mast cells: cells found in numbers in connective tissue and filled with basophil granules that release histamine and other substances during inflammatory and allergic reactions

Medical College Admission Test (MCAT): a standardized examination for prospective medical students in the United States, Australia, Canada, and Caribbean Islands designed to assess problem solving, critical thinking, written analysis and knowledge of scientific concepts and principles

melanin: the substance in the skin responsible for color (pigment); melanin causes tanning from sun exposure

MERS: Middle East Respiratory Syndrome caused by the beta-coronavirus MERS-CoV

metabolism: the process of extracting energy that can be used to power the cells of the body; includes both anabolic and catabolic processes

metacarpophalangeal: referring to the joints of the fingers closest to the body or knuckles

metastasis: the shifting of a disease, or its local manifestations, from one portion of the body to another; in cancer, the appearance of neoplasms in parts of the body remote from the primary tumor

methicillin-resistant *Staphylococcus aureus*: a strain of the common skin microorganism S. aureus that has acquired new genes that render it resistant to standard antibiotics and more virulent

methotrexate: a powerful drug originally developed to treat cancer that treats patients with severe cases of psoriasis

microcephaly: a congenital condition involving an abnormally small head associated with an incompletely developed brain

microcytic anemia: anemia with red blood cells of decreased size

mineralocorticoid: an adrenal cortex hormone that regulates the retention of minerals such as potassium and sodium

mold: one of a large group of fungi that can proliferate on food or in moist areas; can cause an allergic reaction

monoclonal antibodies: antibodies made by a single B-lymphocyte clone that are homogeneous and recognize only one antigen

monocytes: large, phagocytic white blood cell with a simple oval nucleus and clear, grayish cytoplasm that regulates and participated in the immune response

motor weakness: muscle weakness resulting from the failure of motor nerves

mucosae: the innermost, mucus-secreting layer that lines the gastrointestinal tract

mucous membranes: the inner lining of the mouth and nasal passages, as well as any membrane or lining containing mucus-secreting glands

multigenic: referring to a trait or characteristic that requires the product of more than one gene to be expressed

mycelium: mold colonies consisting of numerous meshed hyphae

mycologists: scientists who study the biological field specializing in fungi and similar spore producers that do not undergo photosynthesis

mycotoxins: poisons released by fungi

myelin: a fatty substance wrapping nerves as a sheath that accelerates electric impulse propagation

N95 respirators: a respiratory protective device designed to achieve a very close facial fit and very efficient filtration of airborne particles

nasal polyps: noncancerous growths inside the nose; usually associated with allergies or asthma, which can block the sinus drainage tract

nasopharyngeal: referring to the nose and pharynx (the upper part of the throat that leads from the mouth to the esophagus)

natural killer cells: a type of white blood cell with enzymes that can kill tumor cells or cells infected with a virus

nerve conduction velocity: the speed at which a nerve impulse travels along a nerve

neuraminidase: an enzyme on the surface of influenza viruses that catalyzes the breakdown of complex sugars that contain neuraminic acid.

neurogenic atrophy: shrinkage of muscle caused by a loss of nervous stimulation

neuropathy: a condition in which nerves are diseased, are inflamed, or show abnormal degeneration

neutropenia: an abnormally low number of neutrophils in the blood

neutrophils: the most abundant white blood cell in the bloodstream, filled with microscopic granules, that gobble up and digest invading microorganisms and debris

nonallergic rhinitis: acute nasal stuffiness produced because of the common cold or flu

non-Hodgkin lymphoma: cancer that starts in the lymphocytes and is most commonly appears in adults

non-insulin-dependent diabetes mellitus (NIDDM): type 2 diabetes, which is the state of a relative insulin deficiency; although insulin is released, its target cells do not adequately respond to it by taking up blood glucose

normocytic anemia: anemia with red blood cells of normal size

nummular eczema: a kind of dermatitis in which itchy, coin-shaped spots or patches appear on the skin

onchonylysis: pitting and destruction of the fingernails or toenails

oncogenes: genes found in every cell that can cause cancer if activated or mutated

oncoviruses: viruses causing the growth of cancerous cells

opportunistic infection: an infection caused by any type of pathogen in individuals who have an impaired immune system

orbit: the bones and other tissues that surround the eye, commonly known as the eye socket

orthobiosis: sound and correct living that leads to longevity and well-being

orthomyxovirus: a family of negative-sense RNA viruses that infect animal species

otitis: any inflammation of the outer or middle ear

pancreas: a large gland near the stomach that has both exocrine and endocrine functions and which produces insulin

paraneoplastic syndrome: a cluster of rare disorders triggered by an abnormal immune system response induced by a tumor

parasite: an organism that obtains food and shelter from another organism or host

parathyroid gland: one of four small endocrine glands situated underneath the thyroid gland, whose main product is parathyroid hormone, which regulates serum calcium levels

patch test: skin test used to diagnose allergies in which a substance is placed in a small metal disk and applied to the skin for a few days

pathogen: a disease-producing microorganism such as bacteria, viruses, algae, and fungi

phagocyte: any cell capable of surrounding, ingesting, and digesting microbes or cell debris; in a certain sense, phagocytes function as scavengers

phagocytosis: a form of ingestion of bacteria or other foreign material by white blood cells

Philadelphia chromosome: a translocation, or swap of parts, between nonhomologous chromosomes 9 and 22 that generates a fusion between the ABL and BCR genes. The resultant BCR-ABL gene product is an unregulated protein kinase that drives cells to divide uncontrollably.

phosphodiesterase: an enzyme that degrades second messenger molecules like cAMP

photosensitivity: sensitivity to light or sunlight

physical modalities: the physical means of addressing a disease, which include heat, cold, electricity, exercises, braces, assistive devices, and biofeedback

picornavirus: the family of viruses that includes the

pituitary gland: a tiny gland at the base of the brain that, with the hypothalamus, regulates most of the endocrine systems

plasma: the protein-containing fluid portion of the blood in which blood cells are suspended

plasma cells: descendants of activated B cells that synthesize and secrete a single antibody type in large quantities and play an important role in primary immunity

plasmacytoma: a plasma cell tumor that can be grown continuously in a culture

platelet: cells in the blood that initiate the clotting cascade

pneumocystis pneumonia: a form of pneumonia caused by the fungus *Pneumocystis carinii* and commonly seen in persons with AIDS

pneumonia: an infection of the lower respiratory system that includes the bronchial tubes and alveoli of the lung

pollen: a fine powder produced by certain plants; one of the most common cause of allergies

polymorphic: genes that exist in multiple forms or alleles within a population; genes that show extensive variability within a population

polymorphonuclear leukocytes: Polymorphonuclear leukocyte, or PMN, is another term for neutrophil, based on the irregularly-shaped multi-lobed nuclei characteristic of this cell type.

polymyositis: a muscle disease characterized by chronic muscle inflammation and muscle weakness

polyneuropathy: neuropathy found in many areas

postherpetic neuralgia: lasting pain after resolution of shingles in the same patches of the skin that formerly suffered from shingles

postnasal drip: the discharge of nasal mucus into the back of the throat

prenatal/neonatal screening: a tool whereby small volume fluid samples (prenatal) or blood samples (neonatal) are drawn and studied to determine the genetic traits carried by the child; neonatal screening is often mandated by law and used to find metabolic diseases as early in life as possible

preventative vaccine: a vaccine to create immunity by introducing a weakened or killed form of a bacteria or virus, which the immune system uses to create antibodies

primary progressive MS: the most aggressive form of MS, characterized by the absence of remissions and continual decline

protease inhibitors: any of several drugs that inhibit the HIV protease, an enzyme encoded by the HIV genome that cleaves proteins into smaller polypeptide changes, and prevents the assembly of HIV virions

proximal interphalangeal: referring to the middle joints of the fingers

pruritic: itchy

psoralens: chemicals found in plants that make the skin more sensitive to light

psoriatic arthritis: a subtype of psoriasis characterized by the extension of the inflammation that involves the skin to the joints and nails

purines: nitrogen-containing, heterocyclic aromatic organic compounds with two rings fused that form one of the two main bases in DNA and RNA

PUVA: a treatment for psoriasis that exposes the patient to ultraviolet A (UVA) light after receiving one of the psoralens

radon: a colorless, odorless, radioactive element produced by the decay of radium that occurs in minute amounts in soil, rocks, and the air near the ground; can seep into a building though floors, causing health concerns including lung cancer

RAST: the most accurate blood test available to diagnose allergies

Raynaud's phenomenon: discoloration and pain in the fingertips induced by cold

receptor: a membrane-bound protein that normally mediates interactions between the cell in which it is bound and specific, external signals, such as hormones

recombinase: the RAG-1 and RAG-2 protein complex that cuts and paste gene segments from the antibody gene cluster together to form unique antibodies that bind a wide range of antigens

rehabilitation: a physician-led program to evaluate, treat, and educate patients and their families about the sequelae of birth defects, trauma, disease, and degenerative conditions, with the goals of alleviating pain, preventing complications, correcting deformities, improving function, and reintegrating individuals into the family and society

relapsing-remitting MS: the most common form of MS, characterized by unpredictable attacks (relapses) followed by periods free of symptoms (remission)

remyelination: the repair of myelin

replication: the viral insertion of genetic information into host cell nuclei to create additional similar viruses

reservoir: the host species in which a parasite is maintained in each area and from which it may infect other species, initiating an epidemic

respiratory tract: the passage formed by the mouth, nose, throat, and lungs, through which air passes during breathing

retrovirus: a virus with ribonucleic acid (RNA) as its genetic material that produces a deoxyribonucleic acid (DNA) copy of the RNA to be integrated into a chromosome of the host cell, from which it will make new infectious copies of the RNA during the viral life cycle

reverse transcriptase: a polynucleotide polymerase that utilizes an RNA template to synthesize a DNA copy of it

Reye syndrome: a rare but serious condition characterized by the swelling in the liver and brain, caused when children or adolescents take aspirin or other non-steroidal anti-inflammatory drugs while infected by viruses

rheumatoid factor: an antibody found in the blood that identifies an inflammatory process

rheumatoid nodule: a small hard growth under the skin of the hands and elbows that may be present in those with rheumatoid arthritis

rhinovirus: a group of picornaviruses that cause some forms of the common cold

salicylates: a group of drugs (including aspirin) derived from salicylic acid, used to relieve pain, reduce inflammation, and lower fever.

salvage pathway: enzyme-catalyzed reactions that form a biosynthetic pathway for purines and pyrimidines that use preformed purine or pyrimidine bases or nucleosides to form nucleotides.

SARS: a severe acute respiratory syndrome caused by the beta coronavirus SARS-CoV

scaling: a buildup of hard, horny skin cells

sclerosis: a process of hardening of tissues

seborrheic eczema: A skin condition that causes scaly patches and red skin, mainly on the scalp

second messenger: a small molecule made by cells after they are stimulated by hormones, physical stimuli, cytokines, or other types of cell signals

secondary infection: a bacterial, viral, or other infection that results from or follows another disease

secondary progressive MS: a form that occurs in patients who initially had relapsing-remitting MS and transition to a more aggressive MS

selection: the process by which developing immune system cells are either allowed to continue to maturation or destroyed before they can enter the circulation

sensorineural loss: a hearing loss caused by a problem in the inner ear; this impairment is caused by a hair cell or nerve problem and is usually not amenable to surgical correction

seroconversion: the detection of anti-HIV antibodies in the blood of an HIV-infected person, who is then said to be HIV-positive

serositis: inflammation of the lining of the lung or heart

serotype: a group of viruses that can be characterized by common cell surface antigens

serum: the clear, yellowish fluid obtained from blood after it has been allowed to clot thrombocytes: platelets; small, irregularly shaped cells in the blood that participate in blood clotting

severe combined immune deficiency: a group of rare disorders caused by mutations in various genes involved in the development and function of infection-fighting immune cells that cripples the immune system, increasing the risk of grave infections and tumors

sicca syndrome: a condition characterized by dryness of the mouth and eyes

sick building syndrome: a condition in which people in a building suffer from symptoms of illness or develop chronic disease from living or working in a building

sinus infection: inflammation or swelling of the tissue lining the sinuses resulting in nasal congestion, drainage, facial pain/pressure, and decreased sense of smell

Sjögren's syndrome: dry eyes and mouth-related to rheumatoid arthritis

spleen: an abdominal organ that forms part of the immune system and produces and removes blood cells

spondyloarthropathies: a family of long-term (chronic) diseases of joints that occur in children and adults

sputum: a mixture of saliva and mucus coughed up from the respiratory tract, typically because of infection

stem cell transplant: a procedure in which a patient receives healthy blood-forming cells (stem cells) from a donor to replace their stem cells that have been destroyed by disease, chemicals, or radiation

steroids: a class of hormones produced by the adrenal glands; can also be made synthetically.

stings: a small sharp-pointed organ at the end of the abdomen of some arthropods, including bees, wasps, ants, and scorpions, that can inflict a painful or dangerous wound by injecting poison.

stratum corneum: the outermost layer of the epidermis; its cells are generally dead, hard, and removed by regular bathing

subacute sclerosing panencephalitis: a very rare, but fatal central nervous system disease caused by measles virus infection

sublingual: placing something under the tongue

supplements: a manufactured of natural product that augments one's diet or medicines by taking a pill, capsule, tablet, powder, or liquid

suppressor T cells: a lymphocyte that can suppress antibody production by other lymphoid cells; blocks the actions of other lymphocytes to keep the immune response from becoming overactive

symmetric: occurring on both sides of the body at the same time

syndrome: a collection of symptoms associated with a particular disease state; an individual patient may show some, but not necessarily all, of these symptoms

synovial membrane: a sac in a joint space filled with synovial fluid that reduces friction during movement of the joint

synovium: the cellular lining of a joint, having a blood supply and a nerve supply; the synovium secretes fluid for lubrication and protects against injury and injurious agents

systemic lupus erythematosus (SLE): commonly called lupus; a chronic inflammatory disease characterized by an arthritic condition and a rash

systemic: relating to the body as a whole, not limited to a particular part

T cells: one of the two subclasses of lymphocytes, distinguished by the exacting developmental program they undergo within the thymus gland before their release into the bloodstream, where they actively participate in cellular immunity and regulation of the immune response

T lymphocyte: see T-cells

T4 cells: also called CD4 cells or T-helper cells; a specific type of white blood cell (lymphocyte) which regulates the entire immune system and is the preferred target for HIV infection, resulting in immunodeficiency

tachycardia: an excessively high heart rate, usually over 100 beats per minute for an adult

target cell or organ: a cell or organ possessing the specific hormone receptors needed to respond to a given hormone

targeted antibodies: a form of cancer immunotherapy treatment that can disrupt cancer cell activity and alert the immune system to target and eliminate cancer cells

T-cell receptor: a T lymphocyte-specific cell surface protein that recognizes and binds specific antigens

T-cytotoxic cell: a subtype of T lymphocyte that has the CD8 cell surface glycoprotein, and attacks and destroys tumor cells and viral-infected cells

tendinitis: inflammation of a tendon, a tough band of tissue that connects muscle to bone.

T-helper cell: a subtype of T lymphocyte that secretes signaling molecules called lymphokines that induce the maturation and activation of B lymphocytes, macrophages, and T-cytotoxic cells

therapeutic vaccine: a vaccine administered after a disease or infection has already occurred; works by activating the immune system of a patient to fight an infection

thrombocytopenia: a deficiency of platelets

thymus: a lymphoid organ that lies just over the upper part of the heart and produces mature T cells for the immune system

thyroid eye disease: an autoimmune disorder characterized by ocular inflammation and protrusion

thyroid gland: a small, butterfly-shaped gland in the front of the neck that controls how your body uses energy

thyroiditis: inflammation of the thyroid gland

thyroid-stimulating hormone: a peptide hormone secreted by the anterior lobe of the pituitary gland that stimulates the thyroid to produce thyroid hormone

thyroxine: the primary hormone released by the thyroid gland

tinnitus: ringing or buzzing in the ears

titer: antibody or viral particle concentration

tolerance: the ability of the immune system to remain unresponsive to self-antigens

topical: referring to treatments applied directly to the skin or mucous membranes that affect primarily the area in which they are applied

trachea: the airway that leads from the larynx to the bronchi; also called the windpipe

transposon: a sequence of nucleotides flanked by inverted repeats capable of being removed or inserted within a genome

tropic: hormones that feed a particular physiological state

tropin: hormones that cause a "turning toward" a particular physiological state

tumor necrosis factor-alpha: a small signaling protein released by the cells of the immune system in response to infection

ultraviolet light: invisible light composed of waves that are shorter than the ordinary light waves able to be seen by humans

umbilical cord blood transplant: a procedure in which hematopoietic stem cells collected from the blood left in the umbilical cord after a baby's birth are used to replace someone's damaged bone marrow

upper respiratory tract: the nose, sinuses, throat, ears, Eustachian tubes, and trachea

uric acid: an insoluble molecule that is a breakdown product of purine metabolism

urticaria: a rash consisting of round, red welts on the skin that itch and are often swollen, caused by an allergic reaction, usually to specific foods.

variable region: the N-terminal portion of the antibody, which possesses antigen-binding sites and has variable amino acid sequences

varicella-zoster virus: the virus that causes chickenpox or herpes zoster and shingles

vector: an organism that transmits a disease from one host to another

venom: a poisonous substance secreted by animals such as snakes, spiders, and scorpions that is injected into prey or aggressors by biting or stinging.

vesicopustules: a blister filled with pus

vestibular system: a sensory system that contributes to balance and spatial orientation to coordinate movement with balance.

viral load: a measurement of the amount of HIV present in the blood; often used to monitor the effectiveness of anti-HIV therapy

viral tropism: the tendency of or efficiency with which a specific virus productively infects a particular cell type or tissue.

virion: a viral particle that contains genetic information inside a protective structure

wheal: a flat, firm, and raised area of the skin

white blood cells: White blood cells function in the immune system and are made in the bone marrow. There are many types of white blood cells, including granulocytes, monocytes, and lymphocytes.

xerophthalmia: dry eyes

xerostomia: dry mouth

X-linked gene: a gene located on the X chromosome

ORGANIZATIONS

Academy of Nutrition & Diabetes
120 South Riverside Plaza
Chicago, IL 60606-6995
312-899-0040
www.eatright.org

American Academy of Dermatology
PO Box 1968
Des Plaines, IL 60017
847-240-1280
www.aad.org

American Association of Neuromuscular & Electrodiagnostic Medicine
2621 Superior Dr. NW
Rochester, MN 55901
507-288-0100
www.aanem.org

American Autoimmune Related Diseases Association, Inc.
22100 Gratiot Ave.
Eastpointe, MI 48201
586-776-3900
www.aarda.org

American Celiac Society
266 Midway Dr.
New Orleans, LA 70123
504-305-2968
www.americanceliacsociety.org

American Chronic Pain Association
PO Box 850
Rocklin, CA 95677
www.theacpa.org

American Diabetes Association
2451 Crystal Dr.
Arlington, VA 22202
888-342-2383
www.niddk.nih.gov

American Fibromyalgia Syndrome Association
PO Box 32698
Tucson, AZ 85751
520-733-1570
www.afsafund.org

American Heart Association
7272 Greenville Ave.
Dallas, TX 75231
800-242-8721
www.heart.org

American Juvenile Arthritis Organization
Arthritis Foundation
1355 Peachtree St. NE
Atlanta, GA 30309
800-283-7800
www.arthritis.org

American Lyme Disease Foundation
175 Church St.
New Haven, CT 06510
www.aldf.com

American Skin Association
335 Madison Ave.
New York, NY 10017
212-889-4858
www.americanskin.org

American Thyroid Association
2000 Duke St.
Alexandria, VA 22314
800-849-7643
www.thyroid.org

Arthritis Foundation
1355 Peachtree St. NE
Suite 600
Atlanta, GA 30309
www.arthritis.org

Arthritis Society
393 University Ave.
Toronto, Ontario M5G-1E6
416-979-7228
www.arthritis.ca

Canadian Addison Society
2 Palace Arch Dr.
Etobicoke, Ontario, ON M9A 2S1
888-550-5582
www.addisonsociety.ca

Canadian Celiac Association
1450 Meyerside Dr.
Suite 503
Mississauga, ON L5T 2N5
905-507-6208
www.celiac.ca

Centers for Disease Control and Prevention
1600 Clifton Rd.
Atlanta, GA 30333
404-639-3311
www.cdc.gov

Christopher & Dana Reeve Foundation
636 Morris Tpke
Short Hills, NJ 07078
800-539-7309
www.christopherreeve.org

Crohn's & Colitis Foundation
733 Third Ave.
Suite 510
New York, NY 10017
800-932-2423
www.crohnscolitisfoundation.org

Dermatology Foundation
1560 Sherman Ave.
Evanston, IL 60201-4808
847-328-2256
www.dermatologyfoundation.org

Diabetes Education and Research Center
PO Box 897
Philadelphia, PA 19105
215-829-3426
diabeteseducationandresearchcenter.org

Digestive Disease National Coalition
507 Capitol Court NE
Suite 200
Washington, DC 20002
202-544-7497
www.ddnc.org

Endocrine Society
2055 L Street NW
Washington, DC 20036
202-971-3636
www.endocrine.org

Endometriosis Association
8585 N 76th Pl
Milwaukee, WI 53223
414-355-2200
www.endometrisisassn.org

Eunice Kennedy Shriver National Institute of Child Health and Human Development
PO Box 3006
Rockville, MD 20847
800-370-2943
www.nichd.nih.gov

GBS/CIDP Foundation International
375 East Elm St.
Conshohocken, PA 19482
610-667-0131
www.gbs-cipd.org

Genetic Alliance
4301 Connecticut Ave.
Washington, DC 20008
202-966-5557
www.geneticalliance.org

Genetic and Rare Disease Information Center
National Institutes of Health
PO Box 8126
Gaithersburg, MD 20898-8126
888-205-2311
rarediseases.info.nih.gov

Global Lyme Alliance
1290 E. Main St.
Stamford, CT 06902
202-969-1333
globallymealliance.org

Gluten Intolerance Group
31214 124th Ave. SE
Auburn, WA 98092
253-833-6655
gluten.org

Heart and Stroke Foundation of Canada
110-1525 Carling Ave.
Ottawa, Ontario K1Z-8R9
888-473-4636
www.heartandstroke.ca

Hormone Health Network
800-467-6663
www.hormone.org

HypoPARAthyroidism Association
695 Montecito Ct.
Lemoore, CA 93245
599-817-7171
www.hypopara.org

Inflammatory Bowel Disease Program
Digestive Health Center
Winfield, IL 30190
630-933-1600
www.nm.org

International Foundation for Functional Gastrointestinal Disorders
3015 Dunes West Blvd.
Mount Pleasant, SC 29466
414-964-1799
www.iffgd.org

International Scleroderma Network
7455 France Ave.
Edina, MN 55435-4702
952-831-3091
www.intsocderm.org

Juvenile Diabetes Research Foundation
200 Vesey St.
New York, NY 10281
800-533-2873
www.jdrf.org

Lupus Foundation of America
2121 K Street NW
Suite 200
Washington, DC 20037
800-558-0121
www.lupus.org

Lupus Research Alliance
275 Madison Ave.
10th Floor
New York, NY 10016
212-218-2840
800-867-1743
www.lupusresearch.org

Lyme Disease Association, Inc.
PO Box 1438
Jackson, NJ 08527
888-366-6611
www.lymediseaseassociation.org

March of Dimes Foundation
1550 Crystal Dr.
Suite 1300
Arlington, VA 22202
914-997-4488
www.marchofdimes.org

Multiple Sclerosis Association of America
375 Kings Highway North
Cherry Hill, NJ 08034
800-532-7667
mymsaa.org

Multiple Sclerosis Foundation
6520 N. Andrews Ave.
Fort Lauderdale, FL 33309-2132
954-776-6805
www.msfocus.org

Muscular Dystrophy Association
161 N. Clark
Suite 3550
Chicago, IL 60601
800-572-1717
www.mda.org

Myasthenia Gravis Foundation of America, Inc.
355 Lexington Ave.
15th floor
New York, NY 10017
800-541-5454
www.myasthenia.org

Myasthenia Gravis Society of Canada
247 Harold Ave.
Stouffville, Ontario L4A-1C2
905-642-2545
www.mgcanada.org

Myositis Association of America
2000 Duke St.
Alexandria, VA 22314
800-821-7356
www.myositis.org

National Capital Lyme Disease Association
PO Box 211
McLean, VA 22106-8211
703-8833
www.natcaplyme.org

National Celiac Association
20 Pickering St.
Needham, MA 02492
617-262-5422
nationalceliac.org

National Center for Complementary and Integrative Health
9000 Rockville Pike
Bethesda, MD 20892
nccih.nih.gov

National Digestive Diseases Information Clearinghouse
National Institutes of Health
2 Information Way
Bethesda, MD 20892-2560
800-860-8747
www.niddk.nih.gov

National Eczema Association
505 San Marin Dr.
Novato, CA 94945
415-499-3474
www.national.eczema.org

National Eye Institute
National Institutes of Health
31 Center Dr.
Rm. 6A32 MSC 2510
Bethesda, MD 20892-2510
301-496-5248
nei.nih.gov

National Fibromyalgia Association
3857 Birch St.
Newport Beach, CA 92660
www.fmaware.org

National Health Information Center
Office of Disease Prevention & Health Promotion
1101 Wootton Pkwy.
Rockville, MD 20852
www.health.gov/nhic

National Heart, Lung, and Blood Institute
National Institutes of Health
31 Center Dr.
Bethesda, MD 20892
877-645-2448
www.nhlbi.nih.gov

National Institute of Allergy and Infectious Diseases
National Institutes of Health
5601 Fishers Lane
MSC 9806
Bethesda, MD 20892-9806
301-496-5717
866-284-4107
www.niaid.nih.gov

National Institute of Arthritis and Musculoskeletal and Skin Diseases
National Institutes of Health
1 AMS Circle
Bethesda, MD 20892-3675
301-495-4484
www.niams.nih.gov

National Institute of Diabetes and Digestive and Kidney Diseases
National Institutes of Health
31 Center Dr.
Bethesda, MD 20892-2560
888-828-0904
www.endocrine.niddk.nih.gov

National Institute of Environmental Health Sciences
National Institutes of Health
PO Box 12233
Mail Drop K3-16
Research Triangle Park, NC 27709
919-541-3345
niehs.nih.gov

National Institute of Neurological Disorders and Stroke
National Institutes of Health
PO Box 5801
Bethesda, MD 20824
800-352-9424
www.ninds.nih.gov

National Library of Medicine
National Institutes of Health
8600 Rockville Pike
Bethesda, MD 20894
301-594-5983
www.nim.nih.gov

National Multiple Sclerosis Society
733 Third Ave.
New York, NY 10017
800-344-4867
www.nationalmssociety.org

National Organization for Rare Disorders
55 Kenosia Ave.
Danbury, CT 06810
203-744-0100
orphan@rarediseases.org

Office on Women's Health
US Department of Health and Human Services
200 Independence Ave. SW
Washington, DC 20201
800-994-9662
www.womenshealth.gov

Pediatric Endocrine Society
6728 Old McLean Vg. Dr.
McLean, VA 22101
703-556-9222
www.pedsendo.org

PRO-kIIDS
773 Third Ave.
New York, NY 10017
646-943-7454
www.crohnscolitisfoundation.org

Scleroderma Foundation
300 Rosewood Dr.
Suite 105
Danvers, MA 01923
978-463-5843
800-722-4673
www.scleroderma.org

Scleroderma Research Foundation
220 Montgomery St.
Suite 484
San Francisco, CA 94104
415-834-9444
800-441-2873
www.srfcure.org

Sjögren's Syndrome Foundation
10701 Parkridge Blvd
Reston, VA 20191
301-530-4420
www.Sjögrens.org

Thyroid Foundation of Canada
PO Box 298
Bath, Ontario K0H-1G0
800-267-8822
www.thyroid.ca

United Ostomy Associations of America, Inc.
PO Box 525
Kennebunk, ME 04043-0525
800-826-0826
www.ostomy.org

US Food and Drug Administration
10903 New Hampshire Ave.
Silver Spring, MD 20993
888-463-6332
www.fda.gov

Vasculitis Foundation
PO Box 28660
Kansas City, MO 64188
816-436-9474
www.vasculitisfoundation.org

Vasculitis Foundation Canada
877-572-9474
vasculitis.ca

Subject Index

acquired immunodeficiency syndrome (AIDS), 173-179
acupuncture, 383, 384, 448, 460, 461, 463, 464, 465, 468, 469, 472, 475
acute inflammation, 65, 66, 71, 76
adaptive immune response, 44, 61, 100, 112, 217, 225, 334
adaptive immunity, 42, 43
Addison's disease, 221-223
adoptive cell therapy (ACT), 81, 440, 441
adrenal gland, 12, 13, 14, 15, 139, 221, 222, 225, 232, 233, 241, 242, 244, 291, 409, 433, 434, 435, 436
adrenocorticotropic hormone (ACTH), 11, 16, 222, 241, 242, 434
agammaglobulinemia, 91-93
agranulocytosis, 200, 210
allergen, 23, 93, 94, 95, 96, 118, 119, 120, 121, 123, 124, 125, 126, 128, 131, 133, 134, 136, 137, 139, 140, 141, 148, 150, 151, 152, 153, 154, 155, 156, 157, 158, 160, 161, 255, 372, 388, 389, 390, 415, 447, 448, 449, 461, 462, 465, 470, 471, 472, 475
allergic bronchopulmonary aspergillosis, 117-118
allergic rash, 124, 386
allergic reactions, 23, 30, 94, 96, 98, 113, 117, 118, 120, 121, 124, 131, 149, 150, 151, 153, 154, 155, 160, 161, 162, 251, 299, 319, 334, 360, 370, 388, 403, 410, 414, 415, 432, 435, 448, 450, 463, 469
allergic response, 95, 119, 121, 130, 131, 160, 161, 386, 388, 390, 449, 461
allergy symptoms, 96, 125, 152, 154, 156, 157, 414, 416, 449, 462, 463
American College of Medical Genetics, 208
aminoguanidine, 252, 253
amoeboid movement, 67
ampicillin, 355, 375
anaphylaxis, 63, 93, 96, 118, 120, 125, 126, 131, 151, 152, 153, 156, 157, 158, 386, 447
androstenolone, 470
anthracyclines, 186, 189, 191, 195, 196
antibacterial agents, 146
antibiotics, 26, 50, 54, 63, 69, 83, 102, 133, 134, 136, 137, 145, 146, 174, 176, 200, 211, 213, 220, 239, 255, 331, 340, 343, 354, 355, 356, 362, 364, 365, 369, 372, 374, 375, 376, 377, 385, 387, 391, 392, 399, 400, 401, 404, 405, 452, 456
antibodies, 3-5, 97-103
antibody-mediated immune response, 100

anticholinesterase drugs, 59
antigenic drift, 356, 357
antigenic shift, 356, 357
antigens, 3, 4, 5, 6, 7, 9, 25, 27, 30, 33, 34, 35, 37, 39, 40, 42, 43, 44, 45, 46, 47, 48, 50, 52, 53, 55, 56, 57, 58, 60, 61, 63, 74, 78, 79, 80, 83, 85, 86, 87, 97, 98, 99, 100, 101, 102, 110, 111, 112, 113, 118, 120, 122, 126, 131, 160, 213, 224, 226, 227, 231, 237, 256, 261, 295, 313, 332, 335, 337, 345, 348, 349, 350, 351, 356, 392, 393, 426, 427, 430, 432, 442, 444, 446, 447, 462
antihistamines, 414-418
anti-inflammatory drugs, 409-414
antineutrophil cytoplasmic antibody (ANCA), 320
antinuclear antibody (ANA), 305, 320
antithymocyte globulin (ATG), 41, 258
antiviral drugs, 418-426
apoptosis, 33, 47, 48, 109, 110, 111, 112, 228, 229
appendectomies, 238
areflexia, 259, 260
arrhythmias, 152, 177, 280, 414, 452
asthma, 464-470
atherosclerosis, 247, 309, 405
atrophic rhinitis, 388, 391
autism, 54, 86, 87
autoantibody, 56, 57, 223
autoimmune diseases, 4, 9, 34, 56, 57, 58, 59, 60, 61, 66, 112, 113, 123, 212, 213, 219, 225, 226, 227, 230, 231, 233, 238, 281, 285, 286, 316, 322, 397, 459
autoimmune disorders, 223-231
autoimmune polyglandular syndrome (APS), 231-233
autoimmune theory, 74
autoimmunity, 37, 56, 64, 109, 112, 218, 219, 224, 225, 227, 230, 276, 320
autosomal recessive disease, 103, 105, 107
azathioprine, 59, 60, 139, 228, 233, 239, 240, 283, 284, 286, 297, 298, 299, 307, 308, 309, 315, 317, 320, 397, 471, 473

basophil, 25, 38, 65, 70, 118, 119, 120, 121, 125, 126, 156, 160, 200, 328, 334, 388, 461
biological therapies, 426-433
bites and stings, 129-132
black mold spores, 166
blood donors, 91
blood group system, 332, 335
B lymphocytes, 5-10

bone deterioration, 75
bone marrow biopsy, 194, 328, 330
bronchial tubes, 125, 132, 133, 341, 415, 465, 467
bronchodilation, 450, 452
Burnet, Frank Macfarlane, 60, 109
bursitis, 409, 435
Buteyko breathing, 465, 469

cardiology, 189, 285, 302, 304, 318, 327
cellular immunity, 27, 30, 56, 58, 62, 67, 69, 224
Centers for Disease Control and Prevention (CDC), 166, 168, 175, 248, 346, 357, 370, 373, 424
cerebrospinal fluid filtration, 263
chemotaxis, 64, 65, 66, 124
chemotherapy, 10, 47, 51, 71, 117, 168, 174, 176, 184, 186, 187, 189, 191, 193, 194, 195, 196, 197, 198, 199, 200, 201, 202, 211, 216, 220, 243, 258, 266, 267, 323, 351, 397, 404, 427, 430, 432, 435, 440, 443
chickenpox, 85, 100, 164, 167, 168, 169, 346, 370, 386, 396, 398
chimeric antigen receptor (CAR), 81, 198, 441
chromosomes, 91, 103, 104, 106, 110, 177, 191, 218
chronic inflammation, 65, 66, 231, 296, 299, 310, 329
chronic otitis, 144, 146, 373, 376
clinical trials, 4, 34, 55, 81, 139, 140, 141, 176, 181, 196, 240, 250, 274, 279, 282, 304, 323, 324, 384, 432, 437, 443, 469
clonal selection theory, 109
Common Cold Research Unit (CCRU), 393
complete blood count (CBC), 92, 203, 213, 239, 271, 314, 320, 340
computed tomography (CT), 19, 21, 272, 400
congenital hypothyroidism (CH), 234-236
congenital immune deficiencies, 26
conidiophore, 165
conjugated vaccines, 51, 52
contact dermatitis, 63, 121, 125, 135, 136, 137, 139, 140, 152, 156, 163, 164, 255, 403
coronaviruses, 338-341
corticosteroids, 433-438
corticotropin-releasing hormone (CRH), 16, 241, 242, 434
COVID-19, 341-345
Crohn's disease (CD), 236-241
Cushing, Harvey, 19, 244
Cushing's syndrome, 241-244
cyclic adenosine monophosphate (cAMP), 139, 450, 451
cyclophosphamide, 187, 195, 196, 197, 228, 258, 307, 308, 317, 320, 397, 471, 473
cyclosporine, 59, 139, 197, 258, 262, 263, 293, 297, 298, 299, 301, 308, 315, 317, 397, 473

cystic fibrosis, 105, 107, 117, 399
cytokines, 3, 8, 44, 47, 48, 80, 100, 109, 110, 113, 121, 126, 139, 140, 185, 192, 230, 273, 274, 290, 294, 334, 427, 431, 432, 441, 442, 443, 444, 450
cytomegalovirus (CMV), 345-348
cytoxin, 307

decongestants, 438-440
dehydroepiandrosterone, 16, 437, 470, 471
dendritic cells, 27, 78, 79, 80, 81, 111, 266, 415, 427
deoxyribonucleic acid (DNA), 8, 36, 52, 59, 82, 95, 102, 103, 109, 110, 173, 180, 195, 206, 212, 215, 220, 225, 228, 250, 263, 280, 297, 329, 349, 419, 422, 423, 431, 443, 470
depigmentation therapy, 323
dermatitis, 134-141
dermatology, 31, 45, 62, 93, 118, 134, 148, 155, 162, 163, 167, 173, 183, 187, 200, 211, 254, 256, 267, 285, 287, 304, 318, 321, 338, 354, 368, 385, 396, 402, 409, 418, 422, 440, 455, 458, 461, 464, 470, 472
dermatomyositis, 225, 285, 286, 301, 378
Dexcom System, 22, 229
diabetes mellitus, 245-254
diaphragm, 39, 132, 133
DiGeorge syndrome, 62, 218, 220
disease-modifying antirheumatic drugs (DMARDs), 228, 274, 288, 297, 472, 473
DNA vaccines, 52, 53, 55, 85
Duchenne muscular dystrophy (DMD), 106, 108
dyshidrotic eczema, 254, 255
dysphagia, 148, 149

ear infection, 141-148
eardrum, 142, 143, 144, 145, 146, 373, 376
eating disorders, 152
eczema, 254-255
electrocardiogram (ECG or EKG), 189, 190
electromyogram (EMG), 259, 262, 285, 286
ellipsoidal joints, 73
endocrine disorders, 10-14
endocrinology, 15-22
endothelium, 188, 319
enzyme adenosine deaminase (ADA), 29, 215
eosinophil, 25, 27, 38, 70, 117, 148-150, 153, 154, 200, 266, 319, 334, 447, 448, 461
eosinophilic esophagitis (EoE), 148-150
epinephrine (adrenalin), 15, 125, 132, 151, 153, 154, 156, 157, 158, 159, 162, 242, 384, 438
epinephrine autoinjector, 125, 158, 159
Epstein-Barr virus, 348-352

erythrocyte sedimentation rate (ESR), 239, 285, 286, 296, 303, 320
erythrocytes, 37, 191, 192, 194, 196, 327, 332, 333, 335
erythromycin, 355, 437, 452
Escherichia coli, 102
euthyroid goiter, 353

fibrositis, 380
food allergies, 151-155
Food Allergy Research and Testing, 158
Food and Drug Administration (FDA), 4, 9, 22, 34, 53, 81, 113, 124, 139, 177, 181, 198, 229, 240, 244, 249, 251, 269, 279, 291, 298, 307, 312, 315, 359, 384, 387, 390, 398, 401, 420, 427, 443
food protein-induced allergic proctocolitis (FPIAP), 153
food protein-induced enterocolitis syndrome (FPIES), 153
formaldehyde, 83, 85, 456

gamma-globulin, 41, 189, 190
gastroesophageal reflux disease (GERD), 148
gene deletions, 91, 92
gene therapies, 431
genetic diseases, 103-109
genetic tests, 107
glucosuria, 245, 246
goiter, 352-354
Graft-versus-host disease (GVHD), 255-259
granulocytes, 27, 37, 38, 65, 70, 71, 191, 192, 193, 197, 200, 210, 333, 334
granulocytopenia, 200, 210
Graves' disease, 12, 17, 18, 224, 225, 228, 229, 233, 263, 267, 268, 270, 310, 312, 353, 459
Guillain-Barré syndrome (GBS), 259-264
Guillemin, Roger C. L., 14

haplotype, 95, 109, 111, 112, 224, 226
Hashimoto's thyroiditis, 264-266
hay fever (allergic rhinitis), 159-162
hematopoiesis, 191, 192, 193, 199, 327, 338
hematopoietic cells, 91
hemoglobin, 60, 61, 105, 192, 250, 327, 328, 329, 330, 331, 332, 333, 336, 337, 429
hemolytic anemia, 58, 213, 225, 327, 328, 329, 330, 331, 346
hemophilia, 106, 108, 174, 178, 181, 184, 336, 378
hemoptysis, 132, 134
hepatitis B, 9, 30, 48, 52, 55, 84, 85, 227, 228, 319, 422, 423, 425, 441, 443
hepatosplenomegaly, 345, 346
herd immunity, 50, 83

highly active antiretroviral therapy (HAART), 173, 177, 180, 182, 186, 189, 268, 419, 422, 424
histamine, 64, 65, 74, 96, 118, 120, 123, 124, 125, 126, 136, 151, 152, 153, 156, 157, 160, 161, 162, 163, 201, 388, 389, 390, 414, 415, 416, 451, 461, 462
histiocytosis, 266-267
History of Immunology, 69
hives (urticaria), 162-163
home hygiene, 22
human immune system, 34, 36, 37, 42, 47, 48, 63, 224, 230, 237
human immunodeficiency virus (HIV), 179-183
human leukocyte antigen (HLA), 5, 79, 93, 95, 224, 225, 232, 256, 295
hybridomas, 31-36
hydration, 138, 153, 164, 246, 247, 251, 289, 395
hyperglycemia, 207, 245, 246, 435, 452
hyperlipidemia, 105, 246, 305, 307
hypersensitivity, 62, 63, 64, 118, 119, 122, 123, 125, 126, 127, 128, 228, 229, 230, 299, 319, 334, 403, 455, 456
hyperthyroidism, 267-271
hypogammaglobulinemia, 91, 92
hypophysis, 10, 11, 15, 311
hypothyroidism, 12, 13, 18, 19, 21, 22, 219, 234-236, 264, 265, 268, 269, 310, 311, 312, 329, 388

idiopathic environmental intolerance (IEI), 455-458
idiopathic thrombocytopenic purpura (ITP), 271-273
immune response, 37-42
immunization, 49-55
immunodeficiency, 62, 63, 91, 92, 109, 112, 128
immunogenetics, 109-114
immunogens, 49, 82, 261
immunoglobulin antibody, 151
immunoglobulin E (IgE), 63, 93, 94, 134, 135, 138, 151, 156, 160, 218, 389, 415, 447, 448, 461
immunology, 56-62
immunomodulators, 239, 255, 314, 315, 419, 443, 458, 461
immunopathology, 62-64
immunosuppression, 37, 60, 93, 184, 186, 187, 209, 228, 240, 256, 347, 398
immunotherapy, 440-447
impetigo, 354-356
inactivated vaccines, 51, 52, 85
inactivated whole-agent vaccines, 51 52
inflammation, 64-67
inflammatory bowel diseases (IBDs), 313, 411
influenza (or flu), 356-361
insect-borne diseases, 361-367

insulin, 12, 13, 14, 15, 17, 20, 21, 57, 112, 207, 209, 210, 226, 229, 230, 233, 245, 246, 247, 248, 249, 251, 252, 253, 269, 312, 434
interferons (IFNs), 26, 48, 113, 277, 279, 425, 427, 431, 444
International Prognostic Index, 187
intravenous drug use, 178, 181, 184, 189
itching, 163-165

Jenner, Edward, 30, 50, 432
juvenile idiopathic arthritis, 273-275

Kaposi's sarcoma, 175-178, 184-186, 187-189
karyotype analysis, 106
Kawasaki disease, 189-191
ketoacidosis, 46, 245, 251, 374
ketonemia, 246
Köhler, Georges, 31, 32
Koplik spots, 368

lactose intolerance, 152, 156
langerhans cell histiocytosis (LCH), 266
larynx, 11, 133, 147, 310, 371, 372, 375
lentivirus, 167, 173, 180, 198, 419, 422
leprosy, 29, 66, 140, 294, 405
leukemia, 191-199
leukocytes, 6, 37, 38, 39, 40, 43, 64, 65, 66, 68, 70, 71, 78, 124, 191, 192, 193, 194, 196, 200, 239, 273, 319, 332, 333, 334, 337, 392
leukopenia, 200-202
Lewis, Thomas, 162
lifelong immunity, 51, 84
live attenuated vaccines, 51, 82, 84
lower esophageal sphincter (LES), 148, 149
lymph glands, 213, 362, 363, 394
lymph node, 5, 8, 35, 39, 40, 63, 75, 78, 99, 135, 175, 186, 187, 188, 189, 190, 191, 193, 194, 196, 203, 224, 266, 321, 334, 336, 371, 372, 395, 415, 427, 442
lymphocytes, B and T, 5-10, 78-82
lymphocytosis, 202-203
lymphomas, 9, 30, 164, 185, 186, 203, 212, 291, 299, 336, 338, 351, 427, 443
lymphopenia, 212, 280
lymphopoiesis, 5, 7, 99

macrocytic anemia, 327, 329
maculopapular diseases, 404
magnetic resonance imaging (MRI), 19, 21, 277, 286, 290, 379

malaria, 50, 76, 130, 201, 229, 297, 307, 309, 343, 362, 365, 366, 367, 473
malnutrition, 63, 152, 217, 238, 240, 336
mast cells, 65, 66, 98, 118, 119, 120, 121, 123, 125, 126, 136, 151, 156, 157, 160, 161, 162, 388, 389, 390, 415, 451, 461, 462, 463, 467
measles, 368-370
Medical College Admission Test (MCAT), 128, 129
medical technology, 19, 106
melanin, 322, 402, 403, 404
melanocytes, 11, 322, 324, 402, 403, 404, 405, 406
melanocyte-stimulating hormone (MSH), 11, 16, 403
Ménière's disease, 204-205
messenger ribonucleic acid (mRNA), 49, 53, 82, 85, 110, 315, 343
metabolic disorders, 205-210
metastasis, 82, 186, 402
Metchnikoff, Élie, 30, 50, 67
methotrexate (MTX), 59, 60, 139, 195, 229, 239, 240, 274, 286, 287, 288, 293, 297, 298, 299, 308, 317, 320, 329, 473, 474
methylprednisolone, 139, 222, 228, 258, 262, 279, 291, 298, 307, 320, 384, 411, 435, 436
microcephaly, 219, 346
microcytic anemia, 327, 328
Milstein, Cesar, 31, 32
MMR (measles, mumps, rubella) vaccine, 54
monoclonal antibodies, 31-36
monocytes, 26, 27, 38, 39, 43, 65, 70, 192, 266, 333, 334, 427
multiple sclerosis (MS), 276-282
myasthenia gravis, 282-285
mycelium, 165
mycologists, 165
mycoses, 45
mycotoxins, 165, 166
myositis, 285-287

nasal obstruction, 371, 372, 374, 376
nasal symptoms, 388, 389, 390
nasopharyngeal disorders, 371-377
National Childhood Vaccine Injury Act, 54
National Institute of Neurological and Communicative Disorders and Stroke, 260
National Institutes of Health, 169, 281, 382
neutropenia, 210-211
neutrophils, 70-72
The New York Times, 178

nonsteroidal anti-inflammatory drugs (NSAIDs), 76, 96, 201, 274, 290, 293, 297, 300, 302, 303, 304, 307, 313, 356, 384, 409, 410, 471, 472
normocytic anemia, 327, 329
nucleoside reverse transcriptase inhibitors, 176, 421, 423
nummular eczema, 254, 255

oncoviruses, 348
ophthalmology, 31, 45, 93, 127, 167, 173, 183, 212, 231, 267, 273, 285, 287, 302, 316, 318, 338, 368, 396, 409, 418, 422, 458, 461, 464, 470, 472
opioids, 384, 418
oral antihistamines, 139, 390
orthobiosis, 67, 69
orthomyxovirus, 356
osteoarthritis, 377-385

paraneoplastic syndrome, 283
patch test, 93, 96, 128, 140, 148
pathogen, 4, 23, 24, 37, 40, 41, 43, 46, 47, 48, 50, 51, 52, 53, 55, 65, 72, 82, 83, 84, 85, 86, 98, 103, 123, 173, 183, 215, 220, 232, 256, 342, 349, 355, 361, 362, 363, 366, 367, 372, 374, 376, 395, 403, 419
penicillin, 41, 58, 120, 123, 125, 165, 200, 305, 355, 375, 376
phagocytes, 25, 26, 27, 28, 43, 46, 47, 100, 125, 151, 334
phagocytosis, 4, 27, 37, 39, 67, 68, 70, 71, 210, 259, 378
phenylketonuria (PKU), 206, 404
phospholipids, 379
photosensitivity, 60, 305, 306
phototherapy, 139, 255, 292, 410
pineal gland tumors, 13
pituitary gland, 10, 11, 15, 16, 20, 221, 222, 223, 226, 241, 242, 244, 266, 267, 268, 311, 353, 434, 435
plant biotechnology, 102
plasma cells, 4, 5, 8, 9, 31, 32, 35, 44, 47, 98, 101, 110, 259
plasmacytoma, 31, 32, 35
pneumonia, 52, 75, 92, 113, 149, 173, 174, 175, 176, 177, 178, 213, 338, 339, 340, 341, 342, 343, 346, 358, 363, 370, 376, 392, 419
polio vaccine, 28, 51, 53, 84, 85, 93
polymorphisms, 95
polymyositis, 225, 285, 286, 301
postherpetic neuralgia (PHN), 396, 397
Prausnitz-Giles, Carl, 155
prenatal testing, 107
preventative vaccine, 81, 155, 441
protease inhibitors, 173, 174, 177, 180, 182, 419, 421, 422, 423, 425, 426

psoriasis, 287-295
psoriatic arthritis (PsA), 287-295
purine nucleoside phosphorylase (PNP), 211-214
pustular diseases, 404

radiation therapy, 19, 186, 189, 197, 200, 201, 258, 397, 404
radioallergosorbent test (RAST), 123, 126, 151, 153
rashes, 385-387
Raynaud's phenomenon, 305, 306
recombinant vector vaccines, 53, 82, 86
registered dietician (RD), 150
respiratory tract, 117, 123, 132, 133, 149, 167, 168, 229, 230, 299, 343, 370, 410, 415, 438, 456, 462
retrovirus, 102, 173, 179, 180, 419, 421, 422
reverse transcriptase-polymerase chain reaction (RT-PCR), 393
Reye's syndrome, 356, 359, 370, 411
rheumatoid arthritis (RA), 296-300, 472-475
rheumatology, 72-78
rhinitis, 388-391
rhinovirus, 391-393
ribonucleic acid (RNA), 102, 109, 168, 173, 180, 208, 212, 215, 228, 281, 297, 338, 339, 342, 356, 359, 419, 422, 423
roseola, 393-396

salicylates, 76, 309, 314, 409, 414
salicylic acid, 292, 307, 409, 411
Schally, Andrew V., 14
scleroderma, 4, 224, 225, 228, 286, 301, 405
seborrheic eczema, 254, 255
serositis, 305, 306, 307
severe combined immunodeficiency syndrome (SCID), 214-217
sexual dimorphism, 277
sexual transmission, 173, 181, 346
shingles, 396-398
Sicca syndrome, 300
sinus infection, 128, 402, 416, 438
sinusitis, 399-402
Sjögren's syndrome, 300-302
skin biopsy, 106, 188
skin cancer, 30, 292, 323, 405, 406, 441, 444
skin disorders, 402-406
smallpox, 28, 30, 31, 41, 50, 51, 53, 55, 87, 135, 136, 154, 155
social distancing, 344
spondylitis, 302-304
spondyloarthropathies, 302

sporadic goiter, 352, 353
sputum, 117, 133, 134
Staphylococcus aureus (or streptococcus), 26, 135, 354, 355, 376, 404
sublingual immunotherapy (SLIT), 447-450
subunit vaccines, 51, 52, 82, 85
sulfasalazine, 76, 201, 239, 293, 297, 299, 315, 329, 415, 473
surgical interventions, 299
synovial joints, 73
systemic lupus erythematosus (SLE), 304-310

T lymphocytes, 78-82
T-cell immunodeficiency syndrome, 217-220
T-cell receptors (TCR), 79, 80, 111, 112
tendinitis, 409
theophylline, 450-453
therapeutic vaccine, 430, 441
thrombocytopenia, 58, 196, 213, 219, 228, 271, 346
thymocytes, 112
thymus, 5, 11, 28, 29, 37, 39, 40, 57, 59, 62, 64, 78, 79, 80, 99, 111, 112, 121, 191, 203, 213, 215, 217, 218, 220, 224, 231, 256, 283, 284, 285, 313
thyroid autoimmune diseases, 233
thyroid gland, 4, 11, 15, 16, 18, 225, 228, 229, 234, 235, 264, 267, 268, 269, 270, 310, 311, 312, 352, 353, 354
thyroiditis, 56, 57, 213, 224, 225, 228, 229, 233, 264-266, 267, 268, 269, 310, 311, 459
thyroid-stimulating hormone (TSH), 11, 228, 267, 268, 311, 352, 353, 354
thyrotropin-releasing hormone (TRH), 16
thyroxine, 11, 12, 13, 16, 264, 265, 310, 311, 312, 352, 353, 354
tinnitus, 145, 146, 204, 411
tissue injury, 74
toxic goiter, 352, 353, 354

toxoids, 51, 52, 85
trachea, 15, 133, 175, 310, 371, 372, 375, 415, 438
tuberculosis, 29, 51, 66, 75, 117, 134, 176, 203, 221, 229, 240, 298, 405, 430, 437, 452

ulcerative colitis (UC), 313-316
ultraviolet (UV) light, 255, 291, 323
urticaria, 124, 156, 162
uveitis, 316-318

vaccination, 5, 9, 28, 30, 31, 41, 42, 49, 50, 51, 54, 55, 64, 82, 83, 84, 85, 87, 155, 168, 183, 220, 229, 260, 262, 271, 277, 344, 360, 368, 370, 377
varicella-zoster virus (VZV), 168, 396, 397, 420
variolation, 30, 50, 53
vasculitis, 318-321
venom, 28, 63, 120, 121, 125, 129, 130, 131, 336
vesiculobullous diseases, 404
viral antigens, 47, 48, 55, 58
viral infections, 47-49, 167-169
viral nerve deafness, 145
vitiligo, 321-324
vocal cords, 133, 262, 371, 372

whooping cough, 28, 52, 87, 203
World Health Organization (WHO), 169, 179, 253, 362

X chromosomes, 91, 104, 218
xerophthalmia, 300
xerostomia, 300, 301
X-linked disorder, 105, 106, 108, 218
X-linked gene, 103, 105, 215, 218

Y chromosome, 91, 104, 105

Zika virus, 53, 86